Barkley's Curriculum Review for Family Nurse Practitioners

Thomas W. Barkley, Jr., PhD, ACNP-BC, ANP, FAANP
President, Barkley & Associates
Los Angeles, California
and
Professor
Director of Nurse Practitioner Programs
California State University, Los Angeles
School of Nursing

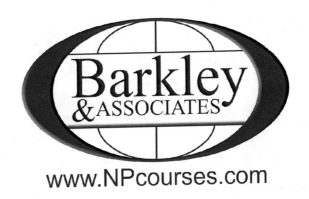

www.NPcourses.com

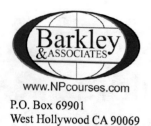

www.NPcourses.com

P.O. Box 69901
West Hollywood CA 90069

BARKLEY'S CURRICULUM REVIEW FOR FAMILY NURSE PRACTITIONERS
NATIONAL CERTIFICATION
ISBN 978-0-9864021-2-8
Copyright ©2015 by Barkley & Associates

Notice

International Standard Book Number: 978-0-9864021-2-8
Printed in the United States of America

Managing Editor: Taylor Spining
Staff Coordinator: Christopher Cudé
Cover Design: Andres Morgan
Contributing Writers: Andrey Gordienko, Roberto A. Rael, Justin R. Searles, Kaitlyn C. Sullivan

Preface

Barkley's Curriculum Review for Family Nurse Practitioners is a long-overdue resource in advanced practice nurse practitioner education. The text is written at a level appropriate for family nurse practitioner (FNP) students, faculty, and practicing nurse practitioners.

For students and faculty, the text can be strategically utilized in several ways to enhance nurse practitioner curricula. First, the text can be used as an excellent culminating work to review key subject areas of the entire FNP curriculum prior to national certification.

For most faculty who adopt a modular approach to systems and special topics learning, the book can be extremely valuable throughout the FNP student's entire course of studies. Assigning chapter by chapter, in conjunction with course topical outlines, serves to reinforce classroom lectures and other learning activities as either pre- or post-class assignments.

For the certified FNP, a comprehensive review of the FNP curriculum is always rewarding to assist in revisiting those "not-so-commonly seen" patient diagnoses in individual practice. Whether being used by student, faculty, or certified nurse practitioner, *Barkley's Curriculum Review for Family Nurse Practitioners* is an outstanding asset.

In light of the varied needs of the readers, the text is designed for both practicality and flexibility. *Barkley's Curriculum Review for Family Nurse Practitioners* is essentially two books in one, comprising a Practice Question/Rationale Section and a comprehensive Discussion Section. Extensive question rationales feature not only why the correct answer is correct, but also why all other answer choices are either incorrect or not the best answer. After the Practice Question Section in each chapter, an extensive Discussion Section includes the following: Overview (incidence/predisposing factors), Presentation (signs and symptoms), Workup (laboratory/diagnostic tests), and Treatment (management options) for all common diagnoses presented in the chapter. Further, the book is supplemented with relevant figures, tables, and diagrams in color.

Unique to other nurse practitioner review texts, two chapters are especially noteworthy: Special Considerations in Gerontology, along with Evidence-based Practice and Health Care Policy/Issues. With today's increasing need to particularly focus on the care of older adults, in addition to the need to make clinical decisions based on the latest research, *Barkley's Curriculum Review for Family Nurse Practitioners* is especially distinct.

As editor, I sincerely thank the Distinguished Reviewers of this text who represent some of the most exceptional nurse practitioner experts in the country. In addition, I am extremely grateful to the talented staff of Barkley & Associates, Inc. who tirelessly produced this work with never-ending enthusiasm. I trust that you will find *Barkley's Curriculum Review for Family Nurse Practitioners* to be an invaluable educational tool.

Thomas W. Barkley, Jr., PhD, ACNP-BC, ANP, FAANP
Editor

Acknowledgments

We gratefully acknowledge the combined efforts of the staff of Barkley & Associates whose knowledge and dedication provided the foundation for this review guide. We would additionally like to thank the outstanding contributors and reviewers of this text. Without the expertise of these scholars, this work would not have been possible.

We also thank the following people:

Pediatric Content Experts: Sharyn Flavin, Molly K. Rothmeyer, Joetta D. Wallace, Stacey A. Warner
Managing Editor: Taylor Spining
Staff Coordinator: Christopher Cudé
Cover Design: Andres Morgan
Contributing Writers: Andrey Gordienko, Roberto A. Rael, Justin R. Searles, Kaitlyn C. Sullivan

whose combined efforts have produced what we believe is a state-of-the-art,
evidence-based, excellent resource for the profession.

Reviewers

Adult-Gerontology Primary Care

Molly Bradshaw, RN, MSN, FNP-BC, WHNP-BC
Family Nurse Practitioner Track
Rutgers School of Nursing
Newark, NJ

Latina M. Brooks, PhD, CNP
Associate Professor and Director, DNP Program
Ashland University, Dwight Schar College of Nursing
and Health Sciences
Mansfield, OH

Sharon K. Byrne, DrNP, APN, NPC, AOCNP, CNE
Assistant Professor
The College of New Jersey
Ewing, NJ

Angela L. Caires, MSN, RN, CRNP, FNP-BC
Clinical Assistant Professor
University of Alabama in Huntsville, College of
Nursing
Huntsville, AL

Sandy Carollo, PhD, MSN, FNP-BC
Associate Professor
Washington State University
Pullman, WA

Connie S. Cole, DNP, RN-BC, NP-C
Clinical Assistant Professor of Nursing
Indiana University-Purdue University Fort Wayne
Fort Wayne, IN

Mary DiGiulio, DNP, ANP-BC
Director of AGPCNP Program
Rutgers University, School of Nursing
New Brunswick, NJ

Sherry L. Donaworth, DNP, ACNP-BC, FNP-BC
Assistant Professor of Clinical Nursing
University of Cincinnati, College of Nursing
Cincinnati, OH

Cheryl S. Emich, MSN, ANP-BC
Clinical Assistant Professor
University of Alabama in Huntsville, College of
Nursing
Huntsville, AL

Karen D French, FNP-C, MSN
Assistant Professor
Azusa Pacific University
Azusa, CA

Melanie Gilmore, PhD, FNP-BC
Associate Professor, Department of Advanced
Practice College of Nursing
The University of Southern Mississippi
Hattiesburg, MS

Patricia Griffith, MSN, CRNP, ACNP-BC
Clinical Coordinator and Associate Course Director
Senior Lecturer
Adult Gerontology Acute Care Nurse Practitioner
Program
University of Pennsylvania, School of Nursing
Philadelphia, PA

Anna S. Hamrick, DNP, FNP-C, ACHPN
Assistant Professor of Nursing, Director of FNP
Program
Gardner-Webb University
Boiling Springs, NC

Addie P. Herrod, DNP, FNP-BC, NE
Assistant Professor of Nursing
Delta State University, Robert E. Smith School of
Nursing
Cleveland, MS

Monica M. Jones, DNP, FNP-BC
Assistant Professor of Nursing
Delta State University, Robert E. Smith School of
Nursing
Cleveland, MS

Debora Corison Kilborn, RN, MSN, FNP-BC
Department of Nursing
Holy Names University
Oakland, CA

Kimberly J Langer, MSN, APRN, ACNP-BC
Associate Professor
Winona State University
Winona, MN

Shirley Levenson, PhD, APRN, FNP-BC
Professor, Nurse Practitioner Program Director
Texas State University
San Marcos, TX

Kathleen Marollo, MS, ANP-BC, FNP-BC
Clinical Instructor
State University of New York, Polytechnic Institute
Utica, NY

Mary Anne McCoy, PhD, ACNS-BC, ACNP-BC
Assistant Professor
Wayne State University, College of Nursing
Detroit, MI

Helen Miley, RN, PhD, AG-ACNP, CCRN
Clinical Assistant Professor, Director Acute Program
Division of Advanced Nursing Practice
Rutgers University
Newark, NJ

S. Lori Neal, RN, MSN, ACNP-BC, FNP-BC
Trauma Nurse Practioner
Erlanger Health Systems
Chattanooga, TN

Marilyn Perkowski, RN, Med, MSN
Instructor
University of Akron, School of Nursing
Akron, OH

Lisa R. Roberts, Dr.Ph, MSN, FNP-BC, RN
FNP and AGNP Program Director
Loma Linda University
Loma Linda, CA

Jennifer Ruel, DNP, FNP-BC, ENP-BC
Associate Clinical Professor
University of Detroit Mercy
Detroit, MI

Debra Lee Servello, DNP, MSN, ACNP, RN
Assistant Professor, Acute Care Nurse Practitioner
Coordinator
Rhode Island College
Providence, RI

Patricia Sweeney, PhD, CRNP, FNP-BC
Assistant Professor of Nursing
Wilkes University
Wilkes-Barre, PA

Bernard P. Tadda, DNP, FNP-BC
Clinical Instructor
University of Illinois at Chicago (UIC), College of
Nursing
Chicago, IL

Frankie Wallis, DNP, RN
Associate Professor
Samford University, Ida V. Moffett School of Nursing
Birmingham, AL

Sandra Kay Sexton Welling, PhD, RN, CCM
Davenport University
Grand Rapids, MI

Mary Ellen Wilkosz, RN, FNP-BC, BSN, MSN, PhD
Director FNP Program
Sonoma State University
Rohnert Park, CA

Yakima (Kim) Young-Shields, Ed.D.(c), APRN, ANP-BC
Assistant Teaching Professor, Adult-Geriatric Nurse
Practitioner Coordinator
University of Missouri-St. Louis
St. Louis, MO

Primary Care Pediatrics

Sharyn Flavin, APRN, DNP, AGNP, CPNP
Long Beach Memorial & Miller Children's Hospital
Long Beach, CA

Donna Susan Freeborn, PhD, FNP
Assistant Professor, Coordinator FNP Program
Brigham Young University
Provo, UT

Jane T. Garvin, PhD, RN, FNP-BC
Assistant Professor of Nursing
Georgia Regents University
Augusta, GA

Gay L. Goss, PhD, APRN-BC
Professor
Cal State University Dominguez Hills
Carson, CA

Paula Gray, FNP/DNP, CRNP, NP-C
Clinical Assistant Professor of Nursing, Director
Family (Individual Across the Lifespan) CRNP
Program
Widener University, School of Nursing
Chester, PA

Yvonne L. Joy, MBA, MSN, APRN
Assistant Professor of Nursing
University of Saint Joseph
West Hartford, CT

Vanessa M. Kalis, DNP, PNP-AC, ACNP-BC, CNS, RN
Assistant Professor, Director Acute Care DNP
Programs: Pediatric and Adult-Gerontologic
Brandman University
Irvine, CA

Pamela L. King, PhD, FNP, PNP, FAANP
MSN Program Director
Spalding University, School of Nursing
Louisville, KY

Deborah Lee-Ekblad, MSN, FNP, ACNP-BC
Clinical Instructor, Acute Care Nurse Practitioner
Program
University of Michigan, School of Nursing
Ann Arbor, MI

Denise M. Linton, DNS, FNP-BC
Assistant Professor and Nurse Practitioner
Coordinator
University of Louisiana at Lafayette, College of
Nursing and Allied Health Professions
Lafayette, LA

Ildiko E. Monahan, MS, ANP-C, FNP
Instructor
SUNY Institute of Technology, College of Health
Sciences and Management
Utica, NY

Martha J. Morrow, PhD, FNP-BC, CNE
Associate Professor Graduate Nursing Program
Shenandoah University, Eleanor Wade Custer
School of Nursing
Winchester, VA

Mary B. Neiheisel, BSN, MSN, EdD, FNP-BC, CNS-BC, FAANP, FNAP
Professor
University of Louisiana at Lafayette
Lafayette, LA

Michelle Pardee, DNP, FNP-BC
Clinical Assistant Professor
University of Michigan, School of Nursing
Ann Arbor, MI

Gloria M. Rose, PhD, NP-C, FNP-BC
Assistant Professor, Coordinator of FNP Program
Prairie View A&M University
Prairie View, TX

Molly K. Rothmeyer, DNP, APRN, FNP-BC, CPNP-AC
Assistant Professor
University of Alaska
Anchorage, AK

Sharon L. Stager, DNP, FNP-BC
Assistant Professor of Nursing
Salve Regina University
Newport, RI

Twila Sterling-Guillory, RN, FNP-BC, PhD
Associate Professor
McNeese State University
Lake Charles, LA

Joetta D. Wallace, RN, MSN, NP-C
Program Coordinator
Pediatric Palliative Care Service
Miller Children's and Women's Hospital
Long Beach, CA

Frankie Wallis, DNP, RN
Associate Professor
Samford University, Ida V. Moffett School of Nursing
Birmingham, AL

Stacey A. Warner, RN, MSN, CPNP
Assistant Professor
California State University, Los Angeles
Los Angeles, CA

Ann Weltin, DNP, FNP-BC, CNM
Assistant Professor of Nursing, DNP Program
Coordinator
Clarke University
Dubuque, IA

Johnnie Sue Wijewardane, PhD, APRN, FNP-BC
Associate Professor
Mississippi University for Women
Columbus, MS

Mary Ellen Wilkosz, RN, FNP-BC, BSN, MSN, PhD
Director FNP Program
Sonoma State University
Rohnert Park, CA

Alyssa N. Wislander, MS, BSN, APN, RN, ACNP, CPNP
University of Illinois at Chicago, Quad Cities
Regional Campus
Moline, IL

Carmen Wycoff, DNP, MBA, ARNP, CPNP
Pediatric Nurse Practitioner, Assistant Professor of
Nursing
Clarke University
Dubuque, IA

Table of Contents

Adult-Gerontology Primary Care

Primary Care Pediatrics

SECTION ONE
Adult Curriculum Review

Chapter 1

Contraceptive Options

1. A patient using the calendar method for contraception has determined that her shortest cycle lasts 28 days, her longest cycle lasts 32 days, and that her cycle starts on day 5 of the month. During which range of days of the month should she abstain from intercourse to best avoid pregnancy?

   a. Day 14 to day 27

   b. Day 21 to day 27

   c. Day 15 to day 28

   d. Day 19 to day 28

2. Which of these statements is true regarding the use of condoms?

   a. There is a higher reported failure rate of female condoms than male condoms.

   b. Natural skin condoms give the most protection against sexually transmitted diseases.

   c. The failure rate of condoms is the lowest of all barrier contraceptives.

   d. Leaving empty space at the end of the condom increases the risk of breakage.

3. A patient with an intrauterine device learns that she is pregnant. If the device is not removed, which of these complications is most likely to occur?

   a. Placenta previa

   b. Ectopic pregnancy

   c. Spontaneous abortion

   d. Abruptio placentae

4. An 18-year-old patient comes to your office to inquire about spermicides, and asks about the failure rate of spermicides when used alone. As a nurse practitioner, you tell her the typical first-year failure rate is:

   a. Approximately 11%

   b. Approximately 16%

   c. Approximately 21%

   d. Approximately 32%

5. Which of the following is the least likely undesirable effect to expect in a female patient using spermicides?

   a. Incomplete dissolution of suppositories

   b. Increased risk for candidiasis

   c. Vaginal skin irritation

   d. Unpleasant taste

6. Which of these patients would most likely need to have her diaphragm refitted, given that all of these patients already have a diaphragm and want to continue to use one?

   a. A patient who experiences an allergic reaction

   b. A patient who has gained approximately 25 lb

   c. A patient who has lost approximately 8 lb

   d. A patient who has contracted herpes

7. Patients are at increased risk for what fungal infection when using the sponge?

    a. Toxic shock syndrome

    b. Candidiasis

    c. Skin irritation

    d. Urinary tract infections

8. Which of the following types of contraceptives may be used to prevent the recurrence of Asherman's syndrome?

    a. Injected contraception

    b. Cervical caps

    c. Disposable barriers

    d. Intrauterine devices

9. A patient starting the contraceptive patch places her first patch on the first Sunday of the month. Assuming she maintains the recommended schedule, she would replace this patch with a new one on each of the following Sundays except:

    a. Second Sunday

    b. Third Sunday

    c. Fourth Sunday

    d. Fifth Sunday

10. What effect does Depo-Provera have specifically on the endometrium?

    a. Creates a thin, atrophic lining

    b. Thickens the cervical mucus

    c. Promotes local foreign body inflammatory responses

    d. Causes lysis of implanted blastocysts

11. Depo-Provera and NuvaRing share all of the following mechanisms of action except:

    a. Release of synthetic estrogen and progestin

    b. Thickening of cervical mucus

    c. Suppression of follicle-stimulating hormone

    d. Suppression of luteinizing hormone

12. For which of the following types of condoms is use of oil-based lubricants most strongly discouraged?

    a. Synthetic condoms

    b. Polyurethane condoms

    c. Natural membrane condoms

    d. Latex condoms

13. Although progestin-only contraceptive pills are not as effective in suppressing unscheduled bleeding, these are a more viable option for patients with certain conditions that are exacerbated by estrogen. Which of these conditions does not usually warrant the need for progestin-only pills?

    a. Migraine headaches

    b. Hypertension

    c. Endometriosis

    d. Obesity

14. Which of these most strongly reflects the theory behind natural family planning?

    a. Pregnancy is less likely when the cervical mucus is thin.

    b. Pregnancy is less likely when the female's temperature drops and rises prior to ovulation.

    c. Pregnancy is less likely when there are "strawberry patches" on the cervix.

    d. Pregnancy is less likely when the female is lactating.

15. All of the following are definitive reasons to re-examine and possibly replace a diaphragm as a contraceptive method except:

    a. Use of oil-based lubricants

    b. Wear and tear

    c. Being diagnosed with vulvovaginitis

    d. Gaining weight exceeding 20 lb

16. Which of the following contraceptives has two products commonly named ParaGard and Mirena?

    a. Diaphragm

    b. Disposable barriers

    c. The patch

    d) Intrauterine device

17. Which of the following is not a typical advantage of contraceptive rings?

    a. Alleviation of depression symptoms

    b. Lighter menstrual periods

    c. Fewer mood swings than oral contraceptives

    d. Decreased menstrual cramps

18. Undesirable side effects of oral contraceptives such as depression, fatigue, and decreased libido usually primarily result from:

    a. Excessive estrogen

    b. Estrogen deficiency

    c. Excessive progesterone

    d. Progesterone deficiency

19. In which of the following patients would the NuvaRing be contraindicated?

    a. A 32-year-old female who has just undergone a first trimester abortion

    b. A 33-year-old female who gave birth 8 weeks ago and is not breastfeeding

    c. A 34-year-old female who uses tampons

    d. A 36-year-old female who smokes

20. What is the typical initial dosage of ethinyl estradiol for combined oral contraceptives?

    a. Dose of 35 mcg or less

    b. Dose of 40 mcg or less

    c. Dose of 45 mcg or less

    d. Dose of 50 mcg or less

21. Which of these methods of natural family planning uses both the basal body temperature graph and cervical mucus test?

    a. Lactational amenorrhea method

    b. Symptothermal method

    c. Calendar method

    d. Billings test

22. If the sponge is left in place for too long, a patient is typically at serious risk for which of the following conditions?

    a. Toxic shock syndrome

    b. Trichomoniasis

    c. Anemia

    d. Amenorrhea

23. High amounts of estrogen may cause several adverse effects associated with oral contraceptive use. Which of the following adverse effects is not typically caused by high amounts of estrogen?

    a. Nausea

    b. Acne

    c. Edema

    d. Breast tenderness

24. Which of the following choices is not a standard advantage of using a diaphragm or cervical cap?

    a. It is relatively safe and easy to use.

    b. It provides immediate protection.

    c. When used with spermicidal gel, it may protect against sexually transmitted diseases.

    d. It remains in place during intercourse.

25. Which of the following contraceptive methods should not typically be suggested to a woman who weighs more than 90 kg?

    a. Depo-Provera

    b. Implanon

    c. The patch

    d. Mirena

26. A patient arrives for a regular injection of Depo-Provera. However, in consulting your records, you find that it has been 14 weeks since the patient received her last injection. When you ask when her cycle begins, she says, "I don't know." After administering the injection, you should caution her to use backup contraception for how long?

    a. During the first 2 days after injection

    b. During the first 5 days after injection

    c. During the first week after injection

    d. During the first 2 weeks after injection

27. Which of the following contraceptives almost always contains the chemicals nonoxynol-9 and octoxynol?

    a. The sponge

    b. Condoms

    c. Diaphragms

    d. Spermicides

28. Ashley, a 22-year-old female, is discussing various forms of contraception with you. She says she has heard some great things about intrauterine devices (IUDs) but would like to be informed about the disadvantages of such devices. Which of the following disadvantages is most commonly associated with IUDs?

    a. Increased risk of pelvic inflammatory disease after insertion

    b. Annual need for maintenance and reinsertion

    c. Increased risk of Asherman's syndrome

    d. High levels of adverse estrogenic effects

29. When using intrauterine devices, which of the following mechanisms of action is typically caused by local foreign body inflammatory responses?

    a. Lysis of the blastocyst

    b. Thickening of cervical mucus

    c. Atrophy of the endometrial lining

    d. Inhibition of sperm binding to egg

30. A patient taking oral contraceptives may be at increased risk for which of the following conditions as the patient's age, dose, and length of therapy increase?

    a. Hypertension

    b. Type 2 diabetes

    c. Abnormal menstrual bleeding

    d. Hypercholesterolemia

31. Jennifer, an 18-year-old female, arrives at your clinic seeking emergency contraception. She claims that she was engaging in intercourse with her boyfriend last night and the condom broke during the act. You believe that levonorgestrel would best address her concerns. Which of the following statements would be most accurate?

    a. "You will likely need a prescription to get the drug."

    b. "This pill works by terminating an implanted fertilized egg."

    c. "You may experience menstrual irregularities during your next cycle."

    d. "The drug should work up to 4 days after intercourse."

32. Nancy, a 24-year-old female, was engaging in intercourse with her boyfriend 3 days ago when the condom broke. She seeks emergency contraception; however, in the past, she has experienced severe nausea and vomiting after using levonorgestrel products. Which of the following products would be best suited for Nancy at this time?

    a. ParaGard

    b. Implanon

    c. Mirena

    d. The patch

33. How should a spermicide be applied in conjunction with use of a diaphragm for maximum efficacy?

    a. The spermicide should be applied to the vagina immediately following intercourse while leaving the diaphragm in place.

    b. The spermicide should be placed around the outside of the diaphragm, which is then removed immediately after intercourse.

    c. The spermicide should be placed inside the diaphragm, which is then removed at least 6 hours after intercourse.

    d. The diaphragm should be removed immediately following intercourse so that spermicide can be applied.

34. A patient who has recently started on the patch mentions that she is also pursuing an herbal regimen for various health issues. Which of the following herbs would be most likely to affect her treatment with the patch?

    a. St. John's Wort

    b. Ginger

    c. Echinacea

    d. Ginseng

35. A patient is using the NuvaRing as a contraceptive and asks you how long she is allowed to have the ring in her vagina at one time. As a nurse practitioner, you would know that this contraceptive could typically be left in place for how many days?

    a. As long as 11 days

    b. As long as 16 days

    c. As long as 21 days

    d. As long as 26 days

36. As a practitioner, you know that the approximate theoretical and actual failure rates for oral contraceptives are:

    a. Perfect use: 0.1%, typical use: 10%–15%

    b. Perfect use: 5%, typical use: 10%

    c. Perfect use: 1%–3%, typical use: 1.5%–3%

    d. Perfect use: 0.1%, typical use: 3%–5%

37. Implanon usually offers continuous birth control for how long?

    a. Three years

    b. Four years

    c. Five years

    d. Six years

38. A patient arrives at your clinic to discuss long-term options for contraception. In evaluating her circumstances, you decide that Implanon might work best for her. You might tell her all of the following regarding the implant except:

    a. "Odds are you will be able to maintain a regular cycle."

    b. "I would hold off on agreeing to Implanon before I tell you everything about it."

    c. "This drug will be more expensive than the pill – at least, at first."

    d. "The implant may be visible, so take that into consideration."

39. A 19-year-old patient is using a cervical cap as a contraceptive. She asks you how long must the cervical cap be left in the vagina following intercourse. You should tell her which of the following?

    a. Two hours at most

    b. Three hours at most

    c. At least 4 hours

    d. At least 6 hours

40. Sharon, a 24-year-old female, calls the clinic inquiring about her NuvaRing. She says that her ring, which had been in place for 2 weeks, fell out about 4 hours prior. She is worried that this will throw off her contraceptive schedule. What instructions would be most effective in helping Sharon continue on her contraceptive schedule?

    a. Rinse the ring with cool water, reinsert, and use a spermicide or barrier for 1 week.

    b. Reinsert the ring immediately.

    c. Discard the ring and insert a new ring immediately.

    d. Wait until the current 21 day period is over and start a new ring.

RATIONALES

1. c

A patient using the calendar method whose cycle begins on day 5 of the month, whose shortest cycle lasts 28 days and whose longest cycle lasts 32 days, should avoid intercourse between days 15 and 28 of the month to best avoid pregnancy. When using the calendar method, the patient should subtract 18 days from her shortest cycle and 11 days from her longest cycle. Both those totals should be added to the day of the month her cycle begins, counting that day as part of the totals, thus determining the window of fertility.

2. a

The failure rate of the female condom is substantially higher than the failure rate of male condoms. Latex condoms provide the greatest degree of protection from sexually transmitted diseases (STDs), whereas natural skin condoms do not protect against STDs. Condoms do not have the lowest failure rates of the barrier contraceptives, which include spermicides and the sponge. The sponge has the lowest possible failure rate of these, whereas spermicides used alone have a higher failure rate than male condoms. Leaving a ½-inch of space at the end of the condom decreases the risk of breakage.

3. c

In the event of pregnancy, spontaneous abortion occurs in up to 50% of all users of intrauterine devices (IUDs) if the device is left in the uterus. Ectopic pregnancies, on the other hand, occur in 5% of all pregnancies in IUD users. Pregnant patients with IUDs are at increased risk for abruptio placentae compared to other pregnant patients, but this outcome does not occur in 50% of all such patients. Placenta previa is not associated with use of an IUD.

4. c

The typical first-year failure rate of spermicides is approximately 21%. When combined with other barrier contraceptives such as condoms or diaphragms, the failure rate is reduced to approximately 5%. Male condoms have an estimated failure rate of 11%. The cervical cap has an estimated 16% failure rate in patients who have not given birth, and an estimated 32% failure rate in patients who have.

5. b

Although spermicides may increase a patient's risk of developing candidiasis, this risk is not significant compared to the risk of other undesirable effects. Instead, spermicides significantly increase a female patient's risk for urinary tract infections. Vaginal or penile skin irritation, incomplete dissolution of suppositories, and unpleasant taste are other common undesirable effects of spermicides.

6. b

Although guidelines may vary, it is often considered necessary to refit a diaphragm if the patient using it gains or loses weight in excess of 20 lb. Whether or not a patient contracts a sexually transmitted infection would not directly affect whether the patient needs to have her diaphragm refitted. Although an allergic reaction may result from exposure to latex or spermicides, such reactions may require a change of formulation or removal of the diaphragm, not a refitting.

7. b

The risk of candidiasis is increased when the sponge is used as a contraceptive. Toxic shock syndrome may ensue from leaving the sponge in for too long, but this condition is bacterial, not fungal, in nature. Although the sponge may produce vaginal irritations and urinary tract infections, these reactions are not typically fungal in nature.

8. d

An intrauterine device can be used to prevent the recurrence of Asherman's syndrome because of the ability to be placed in the uterine cavity to create a barrier between the walls of the uterus. Implantation after the initial removal of scar tissue in the uterus may help with healing and facilitate separation of the tissues. Injected contraceptive methods are not a form of physical barriers and would not help prevent Asherman's syndrome. Cervical caps and disposable barriers are placed over the cervix to prevent sperm from entering the uterus, but there is no evidence of their effectiveness in preventing recurrences of Asherman's syndrome.

9. c

Proper use of the patch requires changing the patch out once each week on the same day of the week it was first applied; on the fourth "change day," however, the patch is removed and not replaced until 1 week later. The patch would be replaced on the second and third change day, and the fifth change day would mark a new administration of the patch and the start of a new cycle.

10. a

Depo-Provera alters the endometrium by creating a thin, atrophic lining. Depo-Provera also thickens the cervical mucus, but this mechanism of action does not directly alter the endometrium; rather, it interferes with sperm transport and penetration. Intrauterine devices, not Depo-Provera, prevent implantation either by causing lysis of the blastocyst before it implants or by promoting local foreign body inflammatory responses.

11. a

Although NuvaRing acts by releasing synthetic estrogen and progestin, Depo-Provera is a progestin-only formulation. Both methods of contraception act to prevent fertilization via suppression of follicle-stimulating hormone and luteinizing hormone, as well as promote thickening in the cervical mucus.

12. d

Oil-based lubricants, such as baby oil, lotions, and petroleum jelly, should not be used with latex condoms, as these can increase the risk of condom breakage. The other types of condoms, such as synthetic, natural membrane, and polyurethane, do not significantly weaken when exposed to oil-based lubricants as compared to latex.

13. c

A combination of estrogen and progestin contraceptives actually decreases the pain resulting from endometriosis; therefore, the use of estrogen is often recommended for endometriosis. Patients who have migraine headaches, hypertension, or obesity would most likely benefit from progestin.

14. d

The lactational amenorrhea method of natural family planning holds that pregnancy is less likely when the female is not menstruating and fully breast feeeding her infant. The cervical mucus method indicates that pregnancy is more likely when there is a lot of clear, stretchy mucus; fertility is low when there is a scant amount of thick, white mucus. The basal body temperature method of contraception instructs couples seeking to prevent pregnancy to obstain from sexual intercourse during the expected rises and drops in basal body temperature. Lastly, "strawberry patches" on the cervix usually indicate thrichomoniasis and are not used in natural family planning.

15. c

Although use of a diaphragm may increase the risk of contracting vulvovaginitis, contraction of the disease is not an absolute reason to re-examine or replace the device. Diaphragms should regularly be checked for tears and holes resulting from repeated use. Furthermore, latex diaphragms should be examined and possibly replaced following use of oil-based lubricants, as such lubricants may weaken the latex. Finally, although precise figures vary, diaphragms should also be examined for refitting if a patient gains or loses weight in excess of 20 lb.

16. d

ParaGard (copper-releasing) and Mirena (progestin-releasing) are two brands of intrauterine devices. Diaphragms, disposable barriers, and the patch do not have two products with these names.

17. a

Although the NuvaRing may provide fewer mood swings than oral contraceptives, it may worsen, not alleviate, symptoms of depression and should be used with caution in patients with pre-existing cases of the condition. The NuvaRing may also lead to lighter menstrual periods and decreased menstrual cramps.

18. c

Excessive progesterone may produce depression, fatigue, and decreased libido through its androgenic properties. Undesirable effects that are related to estrogen use include nausea, hypertension, and increased propensity to develop deep vein thromboses. Some adverse effects, such as breast tenderness, headaches, and hypertension, may be caused by a combination of both hormones.

19. d

NuvaRing is contraindicated in smokers 35 years of age and older, as these patients are at an increased risk for arterial or venous thrombotic diseases that may be exacerbated by the content of the NuvaRing. Females may start the NuvaRing within the first 5 days after a first trimester miscarriage or abortion, or after 4 weeks postpartum if not breastfeeding. Studies show that tampons do not affect the placement or hormonal agents of the NuvaRing.

20. a

The typical initial dose of ethinyl estradiol (estrogen) in a combined oral contraceptive is 35 mcg. Products containing less than 50 mcg of estrogen are considered "low-dose" and are considered less likely to cause significant adverse events. Higher doses do not typically invoke a higher efficacy rate in most women, but may cause more adverse effects associated with hormonal contraceptives; as such, initial doses greater than 35 mcg are not typically prescribed.

21. b

The symptothermal method of natural family planning uses both the basal body temperature graph and cervical mucus test as mechanisms. These two mechanisms are not typically used in either the calendar method, which records serial cycles, or the lactational amenorrhea method, in which patients rely on breastfeeding for natural family planning. Lastly, the Billings test is another name for the cervical mucus test.

22. a

A patient is at serious risk for toxic shock syndrome if the sponge is left in place for too long. Using the sponge may also increase risk for candidiasis. Intrauterine devices, not the sponge, may increase the risk of anemia due to increased menstrual bleeding, whereas Depo-Provera can increase the risk of amenorrhea.

23. b

The development of or worsening of facial acne is typically a result of excess androgens, not a higher dose of estrogen. Although earlier progestins commonly promoted androgenic activity, some modern progestins have antiadrenergic activity. These progestins are often used alongside estrogen to combat severe acne and other adverse androgenic effects. High amounts of estrogen may cause nausea, edema, and breast tenderness.

24. d

Remaining in place during intercourse is not a standard advantage of using either a diaphragm or a cervical cap, as both can be disturbed during the act; rather, it is an advantage of using the sponge contraceptive. The advantages of being relatively safe and easy to use, providing immediate protection, and guarding against sexually transmitted infections (STIs) when used with spermicidal gel are advantages from using the diaphragm. Likewise, the cervical cap is relatively safe, easy to use, and provides immediate protection. Although the cervical cap's activity against STIs is limited, it may provide some protection from gonorrhea and chlamydia.

25. c

The patch is often less effective than other contraceptive methods in women weighing more than 90 kg, which is possibly related to pharmacokinetic differences associated with increased adipose tissue. Obesity is also a predisposing factor for the development of venous thromboembolism and may therefore increase the risk for this adverse effect of hormonal contraception. Intrauterine devices, implanted contraceptives, and injected contraceptives do not routinely demonstrate significantly reduced efficacy in obese women. As such, Depo-Provera, Implanon, and Mirena are contraceptive options better suited for women who are obese.

26. d

For full efficacy, the Depo-Provera shot must be administered every 12–13 weeks; should the patient miss this window, she is encouraged to use backup contraception for 2 weeks after the shot is administered. For patients who receive the Depo-Provera shot within the first 7 days of the menstrual cycle, or within the first 5 days following abortion or miscarriage, the drug should typically provide immediate protection from pregnancy. For all others, backup contraception is recommended for 1 week following administration.

27. d

Spermicides may contain the chemicals nonoxynol-9 and octoxynol for the purpose of destroying sperm cells. The sponge typically contains nonoxynol-9, but does not typically contain octoxynol. Some condoms come with spermicides, but most do not, and the diaphragm regularly requires outside administration of spermicides to be fully effective.

28. a

Patients who use intrauterine devices (IUDs) commonly have a risk of pelvic inflammatory disease for some time after insertion because of the effect of the IUD on the microbiologic environment of the vagina. Although some reports link IUDs with the development of the intrauterine adhesions characteristic of Asherman's syndrome, such devices are more commonly used to prevent the formation of such adhesions. Annual maintenance or reinsertion is not a common concern, as some IUDs can remain in the uterus for up to 10 years without need for adjustment. Lastly, hormonal IUDs typically release levonorgestrel, a progestin-like compound, instead of estrogen, meaning estrogenic side effects are not a common concern.

29. a

Intrauterine devices (IUDs) typically cause lysis of the blastocyst due to local foreign body inflammatory responses. Progestin-producing IUDs typically induce thickening of cervical mucus, formation of an atrophic endometrial layer, and inhibition of sperm binding to egg; however, these mechanisms more commonly occur as a result of progestins, not as a direct inflammatory response.

30. a

The risk of hypertension in patients taking oral contraceptives often increases with age, dose, and length of therapy. Concomitant use of oral contraceptives in patients with type 2 diabetes and hypercholesterolemia has not been significantly shown to increase the exacerbation of these conditions. Although abnormal menstrual bleeding is also a potential adverse effect of oral contraceptives, this effect does not increase specifically because of age or course of treatment.

31. c

Oral levonorgestrel as an emergency contraceptive, or "Plan B," may result in changes to the patient's menstrual flow and the development of other irregularities, such as spotting, during the next cycle. Patients of child-bearing age can purchase it over-the-counter. Levonorgestrel does not terminate an implanted fertilized egg; rather, it works by preventing release of eggs from the ovary, preventing fertilization of the egg by sperm, and by altering the uterine lining to prevent implantation. Levonorgestrel is often effective for up to 72 hours following conception, not 96 hours.

32. a

Copper-releasing intrauterine devices (IUDs), such as ParaGard, may be used as an alternative form of emergency contraception within 5–6 days of intercourse. Mirena, a progestin-releasing IUD, is not useful for emergency contraception and would not be recommended for a patient with levonorgestrel hypersensitivity. Implanon, an etonogestrel-containing implant, and the patch that releases ethinyl estradiol and norelgestromin, are similarly ineffective as emergency contraceptives.

33. c

Spermicide should be placed inside, rather than outside, of the diaphragm before it is inserted into the vagina preceding intercourse; once intercourse is complete, the diaphragm should remain inside the vagina for at least 6 hours. Spermicide can be applied inside the vagina without removing the diaphragm, but this is only recommended for repeated intercourse, not first encounters.

34. a

St. John's Wort may diminish the therapeutic effect of estrogens while decreasing the serum concentration of CYP3A4 substrates, thus creating the risk of contraceptive failure in treatment with the patch. Ginseng, ginger, and echinacea do not typically have any significant interaction with the patch.

35. c

The NuvaRing must be taken out after 21 days to allow the menstrual cycle to continue. Proper usage of the NuvaRing is to keep it in the vagina for 21 days, then remove it for a 1 week break. The ring is kept in for 21 days so that it may continually release hormonal contraceptives in low doses; to remove it before that time could significantly lower the efficacy of the drugs, and keeping the ring in longer than 21 days could throw off the timeline of administration for the next cycle. If the ring is removed, accidentally or otherwise, within those 21 days, it may be reinserted within 3 hours of removal without losing efficacy; if too much time has elapsed, however, the patient should either adopt barrier methods to compensate for reduced efficacy or acquire a new NuvaRing and continue the cycle.

36. d

Oral contraceptives (OCs) are one of the most reliable forms of birth control, with a theoretical failure rate of approximately 0.1%; however, due to the need to take OCs at the same time every day and the associated risk of nonadherence, the actual failure rate ranges from approximately 3% to 5%.

37. a

By suppressing ovulation, altering the viscosity of cervical mucus, and preventing embryo implantation in the endometrium through controlled release of etonogestrel, Implanon usually offers up to 3 years of continuous birth control. After the 3 years have elapsed, the device loses its effectiveness and may not successfully prevent pregnancy.

38. a

As the Implanon implant may lead to irregular or absent periods, a regular menstrual cycle cannot be guaranteed for somebody taking the drug. Informed consent from the patient is required before Implanon can be implanted; as such, the nurse practitioner should inform the patient about all aspects of the implant, which include potentially higher initial expenses than other contraceptive methods and the possibility that the implant will be slightly visible under the skin for a short period following implantation.

39. d

The general recommendation is that a cervical cap be left in the vagina for at least 6 hours post intercourse. Studies have not shown the cervical cap to be as effective if removed before this recommended time.

40. a

If the NuvaRing is displaced for more than 3 hours within the first 2 weeks of using it, the best course of action would be to rinse the ring with cool water, reinsert it as soon as possible, and use a spermicide or barrier form of contraceptive in conjunction with the ring for the next 7 days. If the ring is displaced for less than 3 hours, the ring should be re-inserted as soon as possible, as contraceptive effectiveness would not necessarily be decreased; however, the ring should still be rinsed with cool water before re-insertion to minimize the risk of infection. If the ring is displaced for more than 3 hours during the third week of use, the ring should be discarded and a new ring should be inserted immediately. Waiting until the 3 week period is over is not necessary under the circumstances presented.

DISCUSSION

Oral Contraceptives

Overview

Oral contraceptives (OCs) (i.e., "the pill") are daily tablets that interfere with fertilization and implantation.

There are two general categories of OCs based on formulation and dosage. Combination pills (e.g., Ortho-Cyclen, Ortho Tri-Cyclen, Ortho Tri-Cyclen Lo) contain a synthetic estrogen and a progestin. Combination pills suppress ovulation and alter the cervical mucus and uterine lining to prevent fertilization. The other type of OC is a progestin-only formulation (i.e., minipills) that contains a lower dose of progestin than the dose in a combination pill. The minipill is not as effective as the combination pill because it does not always suppress ovulation; the minipill prevents fertilization by altering the cervical mucus and cervical lining.

Ethinyl estradiol is the most common synthetic estrogen in combination pills, followed by mestranol The combination pill and the minipill mainly use norgestimate for progestin; other types of progestin used in OCs include norethindrone, norethindrone acetate, ethanedial diacetate, norethynodrel, norgestrel, levonorgestrel, desogestrel, and gestodene.

The mechanism of action in OCs relies on estrogenic effects and progestational effects. Estrogen causes progesterone levels to drop and inhibits ovulation via suppression of follicle-stimulating hormone (FSH), luteinizing hormone (LH), or both. Estrogen also inhibits implantation via alteration of the endometrium, acceleration of ovum transport, and promotion of luteolysis.[1] Progestin promotes the secretion of thick cervical mucus to interfere with sperm transport, and inhibits the process of capacitation. Other progestational effects include the suppression of the endometrium, and hypothalamic-pituitary-ovarian disturbances that inhibit ovulation.[2]

Advantages

The use of OCs allows women to control their own fertility. Preparations offer excellent reversibility, are easy to use, and are considered safe for most women. The biggest advantage of using OCs is the excellent protection they provide against unwanted pregnancies; OCs have a first-year failure rate of approximately 3% in women older than 22 years of age, and a failure rate of approximately 4.7% in women younger than age 22. The use of OCs can provide other benefits, such as fuller sexual satisfaction, and may help regulate abnormal menstrual cycles and reduce menstrual blood flow. Additional advantages of OCs include decreased menstrual cramps and pain, and improvement in facial acne.

In addition to providing some therapeutic benefits, OCs have been proven to protect against ovarian and endometrial cancers, ectopic pregnancy, pelvic inflammatory disease (PID), functional ovarian cysts, endometriosis, and uterine fibroids.[3]

Disadvantages

One of the disadvantages of using OCs is that they offer no protection against HIV or other STDs. Pills must be taken every day to ensure full efficacy, and the cost of OCs can be a burdensome expense for some women.

The use of OCs increases the risk of developing some forms of cancer, such as liver tumors and breast cancer, as well as rare and potentially dangerous circulatory complications. Possible side effects include mood changes, nausea, headaches, and breakthrough bleeding.[4]

Side Effects

Because OCs affect hormone function, the use of OCs can produce side effects associated with excessive levels of estrogen, progestin, or androgen. Conversely, OCs can lead to a deficiency in estrogen or progesterone.

Women with an estrogen deficiency could present with complaints of no withdrawal bleeding, decreased duration in menstrual bleeding, continuous spotting and/or bleeding, breakthrough bleeding on day of cycle (DOC) anywhere between days 1 and 9, and atrophic vaginitis.

Excessive progesterone could lead to breast tenderness, transient hypertension, depression, fatigue, decreased libido, decreased duration in menstrual bleeding, and increased appetite. A deficiency in progesterone could lead to breakthrough bleeding on DOC 10–21 and delayed menses.

Signs and symptoms of excessive androgenic side effects include hirsutism, acne, oily skin, edema, and an increased libido.

Women with a combination of excess estrogen and deficient progesterone could present with dysmenorrhea or menorrhagia, nausea, vomiting, headache, irritability, bloating with or without edema, and syncope.[4]

Long-term complications associated with OCs include chloasma, cerebrovascular accident (CVA), deep venous thrombosis, thromboembolic disease, pulmonary emboli, telangiectasias, hepatic adenoma, adenocarcinoma, and cervical changes.

Contraindications

Contraindications for OCs include a history of thromboembolic disorders, CVA, and coronary artery disease. OCs should not be prescribed to patients with known or suspected breast cancer, or other cancers. Other contraindications include known or suspected estrogen-dependent neoplasia,

pregnancy, benign or malignant liver tumor or impaired liver function, previous cholelithiasis during pregnancy, and undiagnosed abnormal uterine bleeding.[4]

Management Guidelines

The three primary management or prescriptive guidelines for OCs are general considerations, patient education, and adverse effects.

General considerations call for OC regimens to begin with low-dose combined or multiphasic pills (35 mcg or less). Progestin-only pills should be considered for women with a history of migraine headaches, who are breast-feeding, or who have some contraindication to combination pills.[5] Additionally, the risk of hypertension increases with age, dose, and length of therapy. OCs are also known to have drug-to-drug interactions. For example, interactions with certain antibiotics and anticonvulsants can reduce the effectiveness of OCs. Alternatively, OCs can reduce the effectiveness of warfarin, insulin, and certain oral hypoglycemics.[6]

Patients should be educated about the use of OCs and their adverse effects. Breakthrough bleeding and spotting are common with abnormal menstrual bleeding and would require a higher dose, if necessary.[7] Some OCs are used to manage amenorrhea, which is caused by low amounts of progesterone. Immediately discontinue OCs if the patient is pregnant to avoid birth defects caused by excessive estrogen levels.

Contraceptive Ring

Overview

The contraceptive ring is a flexible, prescriptive contraceptive that is approximately 2 inches in diameter. The most popular known brand is the NuvaRing. Contraceptive rings are highly effective at preventing pregnancy; the typical failure rate is less than 1%–2%, and the reported manufacturer effectiveness is 92%–99.7%.[8]

The four mechanisms of action for the contraceptive ring are: the ring releases synthetic estrogen and progestin, which provides protection from pregnancy for up to 1 month. Second, vaginal contact activates the release of hormones in a sudden burst, with concentration gradually decreasing over the course of use. Third, the ring suppresses ovulation and thickens the cervical mucus to help with preventing fertilization. Lastly, the ring may alter the endometrium to affect implantation.[9]

Advantages

The contraceptive ring is convenient to use and provides advantages over other forms to prevent pregnancy. The contraceptive ring is reversible and discreet, and generally cannot be felt by the user or the partner. Use of the contraceptive ring has a once per month insertion, which allows for uninterrupted sexual activity. Another advantage of the contraceptive ring is that it is associated with causing fewer mood swings than those associated with OCs.

Therapeutic benefits of the contraceptive ring aside from birth control include the possibility of shorter, lighter, and more regular menstrual periods. In some patients, the contraceptive ring has also been associated with decreased menstrual cramps, and an improvement in facial acne, among other benefits.[10]

Disadvantages

Side effects of the contraceptive ring are similar to those associated with some OCs (e.g., breast tenderness, headaches, weight gain, nausea, mood changes, breakthrough bleeding), but these side effects occur at a lower incidence. The contraceptive ring is known to increase the risk of vaginal discharge, irritation, or infection in some patients. Some methods of contraception, such as diaphragms, cervical caps, and shields, cannot be used simultaneously with the ring. Use of the contraceptive ring is also known to worsen depression in some patients with a history of the disorder. Lastly, the contraceptive ring offers no protection against HIV/AIDS, STDs, or other sexually transmitted infections (STIs).[10]

Contraindications

Uncontrolled hypertension and smoking are two main contraindications for using the contraceptive ring; smoking more than 15 cigarettes a day is a contraindication even in patients with controlled hypertension. A history of blood clots or any cardioembolic disorder (e.g., myocardial infarction, CVA) should be considered as strong contraindications, and the risk of side effects increases in women older than 35 years of age.[4]

Management Guidelines

The contraceptive ring is vaginally inserted once a month; the ring is then left in place for 21 days—no more, no less. The patient should remove the ring after 3 weeks to allow menstruation to occur. A new ring is then inserted for continuous pregnancy protection, but must be inserted on the same day of the week as it was inserted in the last cycle or else pregnancy may occur. If the ring falls out, it must be reinserted within 3 hours; a backup method of contraception must be used if the ring was left out for more than 3 hours. Unopened packages of the ring must be protected from direct sunlight or very high temperatures.[11]

The Patch

Overview

Transdermal contraceptive patches releases synthetic estrogen and progestin. The mechanism of

action for the patch is to prevent ovulation and works similarly to combination OCs.[12] The patch has a typical failure rate of less than 1%–2%.

Advantages

The patch also does not interfere with sexual activity. The patch is applied only once per week and can be worn for 3 weeks. It is also easily reversible.[12]

Disadvantages

The patch may cause mild to moderate site reactions and offers no protection from HIV/AIDS and other STDs or STIs. Effectiveness is reduced in women who weigh more than 90 kg, and is not as effective with concurrent use of certain antibiotics, antifungals, and other medications. The patch also increases the risk for serious cardioembolic events (e.g., myocardial infarction, CVA, pulmonary embolus).[12] The risk for estrogenic side effects is also increased because 60% more estrogen is released in the patch than in OCs.

Contraindications

The patch should be discontinued or not used in patients who are taking certain antibiotics, antifungals, or other medications. Also, women older than 35 years of age should not use the patch. Other contraindications include smoking, high blood pressure, and a history of blood clots or any cardioembolic disorder, among others.[13]

Management Guidelines

This contraceptive method may be applied to the arm, buttocks, torso (but not breast), or abdomen on either the first day of the patient's menstrual cycle (i.e., day 1) or on the first Sunday following the first day, whichever is preferred. The date of application is known from that point on as patch change day. The patch is removed 7 days later, and another patch is applied to an approved body location. The process is repeated again on the next patch change day. The patch is removed without being replaced on the following patch change day. After waiting for 7 days, a new patch is applied on the next patch change day. If the patch stays off for more than 24 hours, restarting a new 4-week cycle is often necessary in addition to using a backup method of contraception.[13]

Injection Contraception

Overview

Injection contraception (Depo-Provera) is a long-acting progestin administered intramuscularly. This method of birth control also provides more control of hormone levels throughout the menstrual cycle. Injection contraception is highly effective, as it has a typical first-year failure rate that is less than 1%.

The mechanism of action involves a suppression

of FSH and LH, thus blocking the LH surge and inhibiting ovulation and altering the endometrium by creating a thin, atrophic lining.[14] Progestin thickens cervical mucus, which interferes with sperm transport and penetration.

Advantages

Injection contraception is highly effective, long-acting, and convenient. Prolonged amenorrhea is seen in some patients, as well as concomitant effects such as a general decrease in anemia, cramps, and ovulatory pain. This form of contraception is often useful in reducing pain associated with endometriosis and generally does not cause estrogen-related side effects. Injected contraceptives are known to reduce the risk of PID and other endometrial and ovarian cancers.[15]

Disadvantages

Injection contraception can cause menstrual irregularities, usually amenorrhea, and can delay fertility for up to 1 year. The injection must be performed every 3 months, which can make this method of birth control inconvenient for some patients.[15]

Side Effects

Potential side effects of Depo-Provera include variable and individualized menstrual irregularities, adverse effects associated with progestin, decreases in high-density lipoprotein cholesterol, and possible diminishment of bone density after long-term use. In some patients, an anaphylactic reaction can occur immediately after the injection; however, allergic reactions are rare.[16]

Contraindications

There are two common types of contraindications for the use of Depo-Provera: relative contraindications and absolute contraindications. Relative contraindications involve planning pregnancy within a year of receiving the injection and inability to cope with menstrual irregularities. Absolute contraindications include pre-existing allergies to Depo-Provera, unexplained abnormal uterine bleeding, and pregnancy.[13]

Management Guidelines

Women should be screened regularly to identify risk factors that would contraindicate use of injection contraception. For instance, a pregnancy test should be performed if menstruation has not occurred more than 2 weeks after the 3-month contraceptive period of effect has ended.

The patient receiving the injection should be warned to avoid massaging the site of injection. The injection must be repeated every 3 months. There is a 2-week grace period; any longer, and the patient would have to take a pregnancy test before further administration.[14] For sexually active patients, a backup method of contraception should be implemented during the first 2 weeks after the injection unless the contraceptive was administered by DOC 5.

Implant Contraception

Overview

Implant contraception (e.g., Nexplanon) is a thin, flexible rod that contains etonogestrel. The rod is implanted in the upper arm and diffuses progestin to prevent pregnancy. The typical failure rate of Nexplanon is 0.01%, and the mechanism of action is the same as other progestins.[9]

Advantages

The advantages of using implant contraception include continuous protection for 3 years with no estrogen-related side effects. Implant contraceptives produce fewer serious system complications than most other birth control methods. Additionally, scanty or absent menses may occur with decreased anemia. Use of a contraceptive implant could provide some beneficial effects, such as a general reduction in menstrual cramps, ovulatory pain, and risk of endometrial cancer.[4]

Disadvantages

Some of the side effects associated with implant contraception include irregular menstrual periods, prolonged menses, spotting between periods, and absent periods. Cosmetically, the implant may be slightly visible when initially administered. Implant contraception is more expensive than other methods of contraception.[13]

Management Guidelines

Implant contraception requires informed consent, with the patient receiving a full briefing on the benefits, risks, effectiveness, and processes associated with the implant.[15]

Intrauterine Device

Overview

The intrauterine device (IUD) is an artificial T-shaped device with either a metal wrapping or chemically-impregnated surface that is inserted into the uterus to prevent pregnancy.[17] The first-year failure rate for this type of contraception is between 1% and 3%.

There are two common types of IUDs: the copper-releasing device, known as ParaGard, and the progestin-releasing device, known as Mirena. ParaGard is a plastic device wrapped with fine copper wire that can remain in the uterus for up to 10 years. Mirena (also known as a levonorgestrel-releasing intrauterine system) is a plastic device that can remain in the uterus for up to 5 years.[17]

The mechanism of action for IUDs involves the immobilization of sperm; IUDs interference with sperm migration from the vagina to the fallopian tubes. IUDs also accelerate the transport of the ovum through the fallopian tube and inhibits fertilization. Lastly, IUDs often cause lysis of the blastocyst and/or prevent implantation due to local foreign body inflammatory responses.[18]

Advantages

Mirena has been shown to decrease menstrual loss and dysmenorrhea. This type of IUD can also potentially prevent the severity of Asherman's syndrome, which is the formation of scar tissue in the uterine cavity.

Disadvantages

Side effects of IUDs include pain and cramping—up to 40% of all removals of the device are related to pain. An increase in menstrual bleeding that leads to anemia may occur with the use of an IUD. With pregnancy, spontaneous abortions occur in up to 50% of all cases if the IUD is left in the uterus, and ectopic pregnancies occur in up to 5% of all users.[17]

Side Effects

Possible side effects of IUDs include spotting, bleeding, hemorrhage, anemia, cramping, and pain. These side effects may also include expulsion of the IUD, with an expulsion rate of up to 10% in the first year. A lost IUD string complicates removal of the device, and pregnancy can still occur while using the IUD. IUDs increase the risk of developing PID, which is often highest in the first 6 weeks after insertion.[13]

Contraindications

The IUD comes with both absolute and strong relative contraindications. Absolute contraindications include active, recent, or recurrent pelvic infection (e.g., gonorrhea, chlamydia). Pregnancy is also an absolute contraindication for the IUD. Strong relative contraindications for IUDs include undiagnosed, irregular, or abnormal uterine bleeding, as well as risk for PID.[13]

Management Guidelines

The management guidelines for IUDs should include patient education. Patients should be informed on how the IUD works, with instructions that focus on how to check the string, monitor bleeding, and control pain. IUDs can be inserted anytime during a woman's menstrual cycle. It should be noted, however, that the risk of expulsion is greater during menses. For women who have recently given birth, the device may be inserted 4–8 weeks postpartum. Patients should also be taught to recognize danger signs associated with IUDs, such as late menses, abdominal pain or dyspareunia, fever, and chills.[13]

Diaphragm/Cervical Cap

Overview

A diaphragm or cervical cap is a flexible, dome-shaped cup constructed of latex rubber. Its purpose is to prevent pregnancy by blocking the transport of sperm through the cervical os. The typical first-year failure rate for this contraceptive method is approximately 18%. The mechanism of action works to make a barrier against sperm transport. When used with spermicidal cream or gel, the cell membrane of the sperm is often destroyed as well.[19]

Advantages

Diaphragms and cervical caps are barrier methods of contraception that provide immediate protection against pregnancy and minimal protection against STDs when used with spermicidal gels.[19] Both are safe and easy to use, and neither option interrupts sexual activity because both forms of birth control are inserted into the vagina prior to sexual intercourse.

Disadvantages/Side Effects

Diaphragms and cervical caps can cause skin irritations in patients who have an allergic reaction to latex or spermicides, and overall increase the risk of urinary tract infections and vulvovaginitis.[19]

Contraindications

The diaphragm or cervical cap should not be used if the patient exhibits an allergy to rubber, latex, or spermicide, or is unable to insert the device.[19]

Management Guidelines

General considerations for the use of a diaphragm or cervical cap include periodically checking for holes and tears. If the patient gains or loses more than 20 lb. while using the diaphragm, the diaphragm should be refitted. The use of oil-based lubricants should be avoided because these may destroy the latex of the diaphragm or cervical cap.

The cervical cap must remain in the vagina for at least 6 hours following intercourse. If the patient attempts repeated intercourse, she must again instill spermicide into the vagina without removing the diaphragm.[19]

Spermicides

Overview

Spermicides are preparations that primarily use nonoxynol-9 as the main ingredient to destroy sperm cells.[20] Spermicides have a typical first-year failure rate of 21% when used alone.

Advantages

Spermicides are available for over-the-counter purchase and help to provide immediate protection against pregnancy and transmission of STDs.

Spermicides are relatively safe, and can be used with barrier methods of birth control to improve effectiveness.[20]

Disadvantages

Temporary vaginal or penile skin irritation is a common side effect. Spermicides that are available in suppository form may not dissolve completely. Lastly, spermicides have an unpleasant taste.[20]

Contraindications

The only contraindication for the use of spermicides is an allergy.[20]

Condoms

Overview

Condoms have sheath-like coverings that are inserted over the penis or into the vagina to act as an obstructive barrier for sperm. Most condoms are made of latex and are available with or without a spermicide. The failure rate is 12% for male condoms and 21% for female condoms.[21]

Advantages

Condoms are safe and easily available as an over-the-counter birth control option. Condoms provide immediate protection against pregnancy and help to protect against the transmission of most STDs.[21]

Disadvantages

Condoms may interfere with sensation, and it's possible for some condoms to break upon use. Foreplay and sexual activity are often interrupted when putting on the condom.[21] Natural skin condoms provide minimal protection against STDs.

Contraindications

Allergies to rubber or spermicide are the major contraindications to condom use.[21]

Management Guidelines

Latex condoms provide a greater degree of protection against STDs than natural or lamb skin condoms. Patient education is also very important. Patients who use condoms should be informed of the following: to avoid the use of oil-based lubricants, that sensation is increased with lubricant use, that condom breakage risk is reduced by leaving 1/2 inch of empty space at the end of the condom, and that spermicide use often increases effectiveness.[21]

The Sponge

Overview

The contraceptive sponge is a disposable, round barrier of soft polyurethane that fits over the cervix, similar to a diaphragm, and contains spermicides.

A common brand name for the sponge is Today. The typical failure rate of the sponge is 10%, but effectiveness is raised if used in conjunction with a condom.

Advantages

One of the main advantages of the sponge is not feeling its presence during intercourse. It can be inserted up to 6 hours before intercourse, which avoids interrupting foreplay or sexual activity and provides some protection against gonorrhea and chlamydia.[22]

Disadvantages

Common disadvantages of this contraceptive method include increased risk for candidiasis and slight risk for toxic shock syndrome from leaving the sponge in place too long. The sponge also does not protect against most STDs.[22,23]

Contraindications

The sponge is contraindicated in patients who are allergic to spermicides.[22]

Management Guidelines

The management guidelines when using the sponge includes instructing the patient on how to insert the sponge into the vagina while using a cord loop attachment. Patients should understand that the sponge is inserted up to 6 hours before intercourse, and that the sponge should be left in place for at least 6 hours after intercourse. The sponge provides protection for up to 12 hours. Lastly, patients should know not to leave the sponge in the vagina for more than 30 hours.[22]

Emergency Contraception

Overview

Mechanisms of emergency contraception commonly work to prevent either fertilization or the implantation of a fertilized egg in the uterus. Preparations do not cause abortion.

Two common types of emergency contraception are levonorgestrel (Plan B One Step, Ella), which is also known as "the morning after pill," and the copper-releasing IUD.

Emergency contraception pills are commonly sold over-the-counter to women 17 years of age and over. Females younger than 17 years of age need a prescription. Plan B should be taken within 72 hours of unprotected intercourse for greatest efficacy. One should stress that Plan B is not the "abortion pill" (i.e., mifepristone). The typical effectiveness of Plan B is 85%.

The copper-releasing IUD is an alternative form of emergency contraception that must be inserted within 5–6 days of intercourse.[24] The typical effectiveness of the copper-releasing IUD is 99%.

Side Effects

Possible side effects of using Plan B and intrauterine devices include nausea and vomiting, fatigue, headaches, dizziness, diarrhea, breast tenderness, and fluid retention. The timing or flow of the patient's menstrual period could also change, and duration of the menstrual cycle could also increase.[24]

Sterilization

Overview

Sterilization is a method of birth control that involves a variety of medical techniques that intentionally interrupt a person's ability to reproduce. Sterilization can be achieved through surgical and non-surgical means.

Surgical procedures of sterilization are an effective method of birth control and are intended to be permanent. In females, tubal ligation (i.e., "having one's tubes tied") involves closure of the fallopian tubes to prevent fertilization. In males, vasoligation (i.e., vasectomy) is the process in which the vas deferens is cut and closed to prevent the passage of oocytes and sperm in semen.

The failure rate for surgical sterilization is low: For females, the failure rate is often less than 1%; for males, the failure rate is 1:600.[13]

Advantages

The main advantage of using the sterilization method is that it is a permanent form of contraception for both males and females with a low failure rate.[13]

Disadvantages

Indecision regarding future childbearing should be carefully considered because sterilization is meant to be permanent. Procedures to reverse surgical sterilization are both are costly and complicated.[13]

Sterilization does not provide protection from STDs. Safe sexual practices with a condom should be used to prevent unwanted infections.

Natural Family Planning

Overview

Natural family planning involves planned abstinence from sexual intercourse while the female is most fertile. When used alone, the typical first-year failure rate is 20%.

The mechanisms that comprise natural family planning include the calendar method, which consists of recording serial cycles and identifying the longest and shortest cycles. Abstinence occurs during the fertile phase of a woman's menstrual cycle, which is determined by subtracting 18 days from the shortest cycle, which is the earliest day of fertility, and 11 days from the longest cycle, which is the latest day of fertility.

The basal body temperature (BBT) graph is another method of natural family planning contraception. This method involves a daily record of BBT prior to rising in the morning over a 3- to 4-month period. The temperature commonly drops 12–24 hours prior to ovulation, and increases after ovulation due to production of progesterone. It is strongly recommended that patients avoid intercourse from between 2 and 3 days prior to the expected drop and approximately three days following the rise.

The cervical mucus test (Billings ovulation method) involves documenting changes in cervical mucus (i.e., spinnbarkeit) over a 3- to 4-month period. The patient must also notice when mucus changes from sparse and thick amounts to thin with increasing spinnbarkeit. The patient must abstain from intercourse from the time of mucus change until approximately four days thereafter, when mucus will resume its standard thickness.

The symptothermal method is a method that uses both the basal body temperature and cervical mucus techniques.

The lactational amenorrhea method (i.e., prolonged breast-feeding) is when the patient plans via breastfeeding for natural family planning because breastfeeding often delays ovulation and menstruation for approximately six months.[20]

Disadvantages

There are a few disadvantages to using the natural family planning method for contraception. Unintended pregnancy is a possibility, and this contraceptive method offers no protection against HIV/AIDS or STDs/STIs. Sexual activity could also be limited to 25% of the month if this method is rigidly followed.[20]

Management Guidelines

When using the natural family planning method, the patient must be properly educated in the mechanisms of action and logistics for this contraceptive method to work.[20]

References

1. Zieman M. Overview of contraception. In: Basow DS, ed. *UpToDate*. Waltham, MA: UpToDate; 2015. http://www.uptodate.com/contents/overview-of-contraception. Last updated February 24, 2015. Accessed March 11, 2015.

2. Stone RH, Rafie S, El-Ibiary SY, Karaoui LR, Shealy KM, Vernon VP. Oral contraceptive pills and possible adverse effects. *J Symptoms Signs*. 2014; 3(4): 282–291.

3. Armstrong C. ACOG guidelines on noncontraceptive uses of hormonal contraceptives. *Am Fam Physician*. 2010; 82(3); 288–295. http://www.aafp.org/afp/2010/0801/p288.html

4. United States Department of Health and Human Services, Centers for Disease Control and Prevention. Contraception. http://www.cdc.gov/ reproductivehealth/UnintendedPregnancy/ Contraception.htm. Reviewed February 24, 2015. Updated February 24, 2015. Accessed March 11, 2015.

5. Kaunitz AM. Progestin-only pills (POPs) for contraception. In: Basow DS, ed. *UpToDate*. Waltham, MA: UpToDate; 2015. http://www.uptodate.com/contents/progestin-only-pills-pops-for-contraception. Last updated August 29, 2014. Accessed March 11, 2015.

6. Martin KA. Douglas PS. Risks and side effects associated with estrogen-progestin contraceptives. In: Basow DS, ed. *UpToDate*. Waltham, MA: UpToDate; 2015. http://www.uptodate.com/contents/risks-and-side-effects-associated-with-estrogen-progestin-contraceptives?source=search_result&search=Risks+and+side+effects+associated+with+estrogen-progestin+contraceptives&selectedTitle=1~150. Last updated November 11, 2014. Accessed March 11, 2015.

7. Edelman A, Kaneshiro B. Management of unscheduled bleeding in women using contraception. In: Basow DS, ed. *UpToDate*. Waltham, MA: UpToDate; 2015. http://www.uptodate.com/contents/management-of-unscheduled-bleeding-in-women-using-contraception. Last updated May 20, 2014. Accessed March 11, 2015.

8. Carroll JL. *Discovery Series Introduction to Human Sexuality*. Belmont, CA: Wadsworth, Cengage Learning; 2013.

9. Darney PD. Etonogestrel contraceptive implant. In: Basow DS, ed. *UpToDate*. Waltham, MA: UpToDate; 2015. http://www.uptodate.com/contents/etonogestrel-contraceptive-implant. Last updated April 29, 2014. Accessed March 11, 2015.

10. Kerns J., Darney PD. Contraceptive vaginal ring. In: Basow DS, ed. *UpToDate*. Waltham, MA: UpToDate; 2015. http://www.uptodate.com/contents/contraceptive-vaginal-ring. Last updated December 5, 2014. Accessed March 11, 2015.

11. Patient information: NuvaRing. Merck. http://www.merck.com/product/usa/pi_circulars/n/nuvaring/nuvaring_ppi.pdf. Revised October 2014. Accessed March 11, 2015.

13. Burkman RT. Transdermal contraceptive patch. In: Basow DS, ed. *UpToDate*. Waltham, MA: UpToDate; 2015. http://www.uptodate.com/contents/transdermal-contraceptive-patch. Last updated March 18, 2014. Accessed March 11, 2015.

14. Centers for Disease Control and Prevention. U.S. selected practice recommendations for contraceptive use, 2013. *MMWR Morb Mortal Wkly Rep*. 2013; 62(RR05): 1–46. http://www.cdc.gov/mmwr/preview/mmwrhtml/rr6205a1.htm

15. Kaunitz AM. Depot medroxyprogesterone acetate for contraception. In: Basow DS, ed. *UpToDate*. Waltham, MA: UpToDate; 2015. http://www.uptodate.com/contents/depot-medroxyprogesterone-acetate-for-contraception. Last updated March 6, 2014. Accessed March 11, 2015.

16. Barkley TW Jr. Contraceptive options. In: Barkley TW Jr., ed. *Adult-Gerontology Primary Care Nurse Practitioner Certification Review/Clinical Update*. West Hollywood, CA: Barkley & Associates; 2014: 5–17.

17. Depo-Provera. Pfizer. http://labeling.pfizer.com/ShowLabeling.aspx?id=522. Revised January 2015. Accessed March 11, 2015.

18. Milton SH, Karjane NW. Intrauterine device insertion. In: Chelmow D, ed. Medscape. http://emedicine.medscape.com/article/1998022-overview. Updated April 9, 2013. Accessed March 11, 2015.

19. Searle ES. The intrauterine device and the intrauterine system. *Best Pract Res Clin Obstet Gynaecol*. 2014; 28(6): 807–824. doi: 10.1016/j.bpobgyn.2014.05.004

20. Barrier contraceptives. In: Porter RS, Kaplan JL, eds. The Merck Manual Online. http://www.merckmanuals.com/professional/gynecology_and_obstetrics/family_planning/barrier_contraceptives.html. Last full review June 2013. Content last modified August 2013. Accessed March 11, 2015.

21. Samra-Latif OM, Wood E. Contraception. In: Lucidi RS, ed. Medscape. http://emedicine.medscape.com/article/258507-overview. Updated May 2, 2014. Accessed March 11, 2015.

22. Condoms – male. A.D.A.M. Medical Encyclopedia. http://www.nlm.nih.gov/medlineplus/ency/article/004001.htm. Updated February 4, 2014. Accessed March 11, 2015.

23. Mayo Clinic Staff. Contraceptive sponge. Mayo Clinic. http://www.mayoclinic.org/tests-procedures/contraceptive-sponge/basics/definition/prc-20014127. Updated January 8, 2013. Accessed March 11, 2015.

24. French, LM. Yeast infections. HealthyWomen. http://www.healthywomen.org/condition/yeast-infections. Updated September 14, 2011. Accessed March 11, 2015.

25. Emergency contraception. A.D.A.M. Medical Encyclopedia. http://www.nlm.nih.gov/medlineplus/ency/article/007014.htm. Updated March 11, 2014. Accessed March 11, 2015.

Chapter 2
Obstetrics and Pregnancy Pearls

QUESTIONS

1. Which of the following best depicts Hegar's sign?

   a. Cervical cyanosis

   b. Softening of the cervicouterine junction

   c. Amenorrhea

   d. Softening of the cervix

2. During a prenatal exam, your patient says: "I've been getting some really bad headaches lately. They start at the base of my skull, and then spread through my head." She is 36 weeks pregnant, and her history shows that she has been seen for high blood pressure on previous visits. You note that she's gained 5 lb since her last visit the week prior, and that she has edema of the hands and feet. These findings most likely indicate what condition?

   a. Hemolysis, elevated liver enzymes and low platelets syndrome

   b. Eclampsia

   c. Pregnancy-induced hypertension

   d. Preeclampsia

3. A patient in her 28th week of pregnancy arrives to your clinic with concerns of vaginal bleeding. Upon questioning, she tells you that the bleeding is not accompanied with any pain and that the bleeding occurred after vaginal intercourse. Based on these signs, you should screen the patient for which of the following conditions?

   a. Placenta previa

   b. Premature labor

   c. Spontaneous abortion

   d. Abruptio placentae

4. How often should prenatal checks be traditionally scheduled for a patient who is 30 weeks pregnant?

   a. Every week

   b. Every 2 weeks

   c. Every 3 weeks

   d. Every 4 weeks

5. Approximately 95% of ectopic pregnancies occur in which location?

   a. Cervix

   b. The cornua of the uterus

   c. Ovaries

   d. Fallopian tubes

6. Which of the following is more likely to cause a pregnancy loss in the second trimester?

   a. A patient with uterus didelphys

   b. Implantation of the fertilized egg in the fallopian tubes

   c. The fetus is missing a second X chromosome

   d. The placenta is located in the lower uterine segment

7. At which point during pregnancy should women expect to see the most significant abdominal growth?

   a. 20 weeks

   b. 24 weeks

   c. 28 weeks

   d. 32 weeks

8. In following your patient who is 32 weeks pregnant who is admitted to the hospital for convulsions, you note that her medical record shows that she has preeclampsia. Which of the following drugs is most likely to be ordered in the plan of care to stabilize the patient at this time?

   a. B-methasone

   b. Diazepam

   c. Magnesium sulfate

   d. Phenytoin

9. All of the following factors are associated with an increased incidence of placenta previa except:

   a. Chronic hypertension

   b. Previous uterine surgery

   c. Multiparity

   d. Malpresentation

10. Which of the following conditions is least associated with causing spontaneous abortions in the second trimester of pregnancy?

    a. Chromosomal abnormalities

    b. Cervical incompetence

    c. Infection

    d. Uterine abnormalities

11. You are examining a patient whose complaints include pelvic cramps and heavy vaginal bleeding that she says is "dark." She says she thought she was pregnant because she missed her period the month prior, and that this is the first time she has seen any bleeding in 8 weeks. When asked if she has any other pain, she says "Come to think of it, my shoulder's been hurting since the cramps began." The exam indicates an adnexal mass. Considering that the patient is likely pregnant, these findings most indicate which of these?

    a. Spontaneous abortion

    b. Preeclampsia

    c. Ectopic pregnancy

    d. Eclampsia

12. The results of a prenatal exam for a patient who is 16 weeks pregnant show normal findings. The nurse practitioner should schedule the patient's next prenatal visit _____ from today.

    a. One week

    b. Two weeks

    c. Three weeks

    d. One month

13. Considering that age is a risk factor for some pregnancy-related complications, a 16-year-old and a 45-year-old who are pregnant are both at risk of developing which complication due to their ages?

    a. Ectopic pregnancy

    b. Spontaneous abortion

    c. Premature labor

    d. Placentia previa

14. Which of the following typically occurs in the first trimester but may also return in the third trimester?

    a. Abdominal growth

    b. Back pain

    c. Urinary frequency

    d. Breast tenderness

15. In cases of abruptio placentae, separation of the placenta from the uterine wall usually occurs at which point in pregnancy?

    a. First trimester

    b. First or second trimester

    c. Second or third trimester

    d. Third trimester

16. When are Leopold maneuvers first able to be performed?

    a. 15 weeks

    b. 20 weeks

    c. 25 weeks

    d. 34 weeks

17. A patient in the third trimester of pregnancy presents with a swollen face and complaints of nausea and headaches that she says originate at the back of her head. You note that the patient's skin is slightly yellow, which is most likely a sign of what pregnancy-related complication?

    a. Preeclampsia

    b. Eclampsia

    c. Hemolysis, elevated liver enzymes and low platelets syndrome

    d. Pregnancy-induced hypertension

18. Which of the following tests is most useful in providing a specific diagnosis of ectopic pregnancy and ruling out other conditions?

    a. Clinical examination

    b. Serum quantitative human chorionic gonadotropin

    c. Ultrasound

    d. Biophysical profile

19. A patient in the early second trimester of pregnancy is experiencing seizures. She says that she experiences a severe, unrelenting headache and blurred vision prior to each episode. The blood pressure readings indicate that her BP is consistently elevated above 160/100 mmHg. Based on these findings, for what condition should she be treated?

    a. Pregnancy-induced hypertension

    b. Preeclampsia

    c. Hemolysis, elevated liver enzymes, and low platelets syndrome

    d. Eclampsia

20. Both cocaine use and poor nutrition are known risk factors for which pregnancy-related complication?

    a. Placentia previa

    b. Preeclampsia

    c. Hemolysis, elevated liver enzymes and low platelets syndrome

    d. Premature labor

21. Sandra, a patient who is 34 weeks pregnant, arrives at your clinic with complaints of bleeding. She does not report any pain. Given your concern regarding possible placenta previa, which of the following should not be performed at this time?

    a. Biophysical profile

    b. Vaginal rest

    c. Bimanual exam

    d. Hospitalization

22. An ultrasound examination for fetal survey is typically performed at:

    a. Weeks 10–12

    b. Weeks 18–20

    c. Weeks 20–22

    d. Weeks 22–24

23. Which of the following is <u>not</u> typically performed either during the first trimester of pregnancy or upon a new visit?

   a. Quantitative human chorionic gonadotropin blood titer

   b. Sexually transmitted disease screening

   c. Hepatitis B surface antigen screening

   d. Dating ultrasound

24. All of the following factors are known to contribute to pregnancy-induced hypertension <u>except</u>:

   a. Diabetes

   b. Multiparity

   c. Maternal age

   d. Uterine tumor

25. Which of the following poses the greatest risk of ectopic pregnancy among the general population?

   a. History of infertility

   b. Previous ectopic pregnancy

   c. Use of an intrauterine device

   d. Tubal surgery

26. Which major pregnancy-related complication is known to occur in no more than 2% of the general population?

   a. Spontaneous abortion

   b. Pregnancy-induced hypertension

   c. Ectopic pregnancy

   d. Abruptio placentae

27. What two drugs are typically prescribed to induce an elective abortion within the first 49 days of pregnancy?

   a. Mifepristone and B-methasone

   b. B-methasone and magnesium sulfate

   c. Prostaglandin and mifepristone

   d. Prostaglandin and B-methasone

28. Fetal monitoring commonly involves the conjunction of a non-stress test, biophysical profile, and which other diagnostic procedure?

   a. Blood pressure surveillance

   b. Complete blood count

   c. Liver function test

   d. Kick count

29. Syncopal episodes are most likely to occur in which trimester?

   a. First trimester

   b. Second trimester

   c. Third trimester

   d. Postpartum

30. Which of the following statements is <u>not</u> true regarding abruptio placenta?

   a. An abruption is most likely to occur in the second or third trimester.

   b. The recurrence rate increases after it occurs more than once.

   c. It is most often precipitated by a previous uterine surgery.

   d. Cocaine, alcohol, and cigarette use contribute to the incidence of abruptio placentae.

31. The first day of your pregnant patient's last normal menstrual period was on March 24. Using Naegele's rule, you estimate the date of confinement to occur on:

   a. December 18

   b. December 24

   c. December 31

   d. January 1

32. Vacuum curettage and dilation may usually be used to perform an induced or selective abortion until what week of pregnancy?

   a. Up to 12 weeks

   b. Up to 14 weeks

   c. Up to 20 weeks

   d. Up to 22 weeks

33. When should fetal heart tones be able to be first detected?

   a. Between 8 and 10 weeks of pregnancy

   b. Between 10 and 12 weeks of pregnancy

   c. Between 12 and 14 weeks of pregnancy

   d. Between 14 and 16 weeks of pregnancy

34. As a nurse practitioner, you know that an intrauterine pregnancy typically presents with the following specific indications in the first trimester except:

   a. Amenorrhea

   b. Change in skin pigmentation

   c. Urinary frequency

   d. Breast tenderness

35. Which of the following is least useful as an initial test for providing a diagnosis of suspected placenta previa?

   a. Complete blood count

   b. Ultrasound

   c. Rh blood test

   d. Electronic fetal monitoring

36. All of the following situations constitute a high risk situation in pregnancy except:

   a. Multiple gestations

   b. Thrombocytopenia

   c. Premature rupture of membranes

   d. Rh desensitization

37. Which of the following tests would usually be performed during a prenatal exam for a patient who is 28 weeks pregnant?

   a. Human chorionic gonadotropin test

   b. Ultrasound

   c. Glucose tolerance test

   d. Triple/quad screening

38. Which of the following methods would be most appropriate to use for an induced or elective abortion on a patient who is 22 weeks pregnant?

   a. Vacuum dilation and curettage

   b. Administration of mifepristone and prostaglandin

   c. Tocolytic therapy and steroid injections

   d. Dilation and evacuation procedure

39. A patient who is 32 weeks pregnant is hospitalized for severe preeclampsia. Based on your knowledge of this condition, you know that she should be initiated on which type of therapy to stabilize her condition?

   a. B-methasone

   b. Magnesium sulfate

   c. Lumirubin

   d. Calcium gluconate

40. Softening of the cervix and the vagina indicates which sign?

   a. Chadwick's sign

   b. Goodell's sign

   c. Braxton-Hicks sign

   d. Hegar's sign

RATIONALES

1. b

Hegar's sign is softening of the cervicouterine junction, which usually occurs around the fourth to sixth week of pregnancy. Cervical cyanosis (i.e., Chadwick's sign) may onset by the sixth week of pregnancy, but may also appear after 8 weeks. Amenorrhea is often an initial sign of pregnancy and would occur prior to Hegar's sign. Softening of the cervix (i.e., Goodell's sign) usually occurs by the eighth week of pregnancy.

2. d

The patient's findings indicate preeclampsia.
Although the patient has a history of high blood pressure and may have been seen previously for pregnancy-induced hypertension (PIH), the patient's symptoms of occipital headaches, sudden weight gain, and generalized edema on the hands and feet would indicate that the patient's condition has progressed from PIH to preeclampsia. Furthermore, the absence of seizures or abdominal pain suggests that the patient's condition has not yet progressed to eclampsia. And although edema with secondary weight gain may present in hemolysis, elevated liver enzymes, and low platelets syndrome, occipital headaches are not associated with this syndrome.

3. a

Pregnant patients who present with bleeding that is unaccompanied by pain and seen after vaginal intercourse should be screened for placenta previa. Painless bleeding after vaginal intercourse usually accompanies this condition in the late second trimester to the early third trimester. Both abruptio placentae and spontaneous abortion are least likely to be responsible for the patient's condition because both generally present with bleeding that may be heavy and accompanied by pain. Premature labor may be indicated by vaginal spotting or discharge, but uterine cramping and contractions are absent.

4. b

Prenatal checks should be traditionally scheduled for every 2 weeks for patients who are 28 to 36 weeks pregnant. However, some obstetricians may schedule prenatal visits every 3 weeks, but such is based on the obstetrician's discretion. Prenatal visits should be every 4 weeks up to 28 weeks, and then weekly after 36 weeks.

5. d

Approximately 95% of all ectopic pregnancies occur in the fallopian tubes. An ectopic pregnancy, which is any pregnancy that occurs outside of the uterine cavity, may occur in the cervix, one of the ovaries, or even the cornua of the uterus, but these are rarely seen.

6. a

Uterine abnormalities, such as uterus didelphys, are more likely to cause a pregnancy loss in the second trimester. Chromosomal abnormalities (e.g., Turner syndrome) account for the majority of pregnancy losses in the first trimester. Pregnancy loss due to ectopic pregnancy is more likely to occur in the first trimester, as it is usually detected by the eighth week. Placenta previa is less likely to result in pregnancy loss in the second trimester; however, signs of a complication often occur in the late second to early third trimester, and pregnancy loss can often be avoided if the patient is immediately treated.

7. c

Pregnant patients should expect to see significant abdominal growth by the 28th week of pregnancy, although abdominal growth may be seen prior to this time. Significant abdominal growth is least likely to be expected at week 20 or 24 because the fetus is not yet fully developed, although fetal movement should be expected. Significant abdominal growth should already have occurred by week 32.

8. c

Magnesium sulfate ($MgSO_4$) is usually administered intravenously to break seizures and to stabilize the patient due to preeclampsia or eclampsia. Diazepam and phenytoin are least likely to see initial use, but these drugs may be used as a second-line treatment for patients who either cannot take or are unresponsive to $MgSO_4$. B-methasone may see initial use to promote fetal lung maturity if the patient is less than 34 weeks pregnant, but would not be used to break seizures or stabilize the patient.

9. a

Chronic hypertension is a known risk factor for abruptio placentae, not placenta previa. Known risk factors of placenta previa incidence include multiparity, malpresentation, and previous uterine surgery.

10. a

Although chromosomal abnormalities are the cause of the majority of pregnancy losses in the first trimester, they are least associated with spontaneous abortions occurring in the second trimester. The majority of pregnancy losses in the second trimester are attributed to cervical incompetence, infection, and uterine abnormalities.

11. c

Heavy vaginal bleeding accompanied by pelvic and shoulder pain and findings of an adnexal mass most likely indicate an ectopic pregnancy. Furthermore, shoulder pain may indicate bleeding into the abdomen underneath the diaphragm. A spontaneous abortion may present similarly to ectopic pregnancy, such as with heavy vaginal bleeding and pain, but an adnexal mass is indicative of ectopic pregnancy. Preeclampsia and eclampsia are characterized by hypertension and are characterized by hypertension, but neither condition would directly cause vaginal bleeding.

12. d

Under normal circumstances, a patient in her 16th week of pregnancy should be seen for a prenatal visit every 4 weeks. Prenatal visits should be scheduled for every 2 weeks from 28–36 weeks of pregnancy, but some obstetricians may allow a visit every 3 weeks during this window. Once the patient reaches the 36th week, the patient should be seen weekly until delivery.

13. c

Adolescent females and those who are advanced in maternal age are both at a higher risk of experiencing premature labor due to their ages. Age is not considered a risk factor of ectopic pregnancy, but the incidence of ectopic pregnancy is highest among women with a history of infertility. Spontaneous abortions are associated with risk factors that include chromosomal abnormalities and cervical incompetence. Although advanced maternal age also increases the risk of spontaneous abortion, there is no known correlation between spontaneous abortions and adolescent pregnancy. Lastly, the risk of placenta previa is high with adolescent pregnancies, but not necessarily with pregnancy in older females.

14. c

Of the choices, urinary frequency typically occurs in the first trimester but may also return in the third trimester as the uterus expands and applies more pressure to the bladder. Abdominal growth and back pain are both normally expected in the third trimester. Breast tenderness is an early sign of pregnancy and would be seen early in the first trimester.

15. c

In cases of abruptio placentae, separation of the placenta from the uterine wall usually occurs in the second or third trimester and rarely in the first trimester.

16. b

Leopold maneuvers are first able to be performed at 20 weeks of pregnancy. Prior to 20 weeks, the fetal outline may not be palpable, thus making the maneuver not as effective at 15 weeks. The maneuver may be performed at 25 weeks, but are generally more effective at 34 weeks due to mobility of the fetus.

17. c

Jaundice is most likely indicative of hemolysis, elevated liver enzymes, and low platelets (HELLP) syndrome, which also may present with nausea. Findings of preeclampsia include occipital headaches and mild facial edema, which may suggest preeclampsia as a pre- or co-existing condition. Pregnancy-induced hypertension may occasionally present with nausea and vomiting as well, but does not typically present with jaundice. Eclampsia also does not present with nausea or jaundice and is additionally characterized by experiencing a seizure.

18. c

An ultrasound is most useful in providing a specific diagnosis of ectopic pregnancy in addition to ruling out other conditions that present with similar findings, such as spontaneous abortion. A clinical examination may show findings of tender adnexa with possible palpable mass, but this finding may not be noted during a clinical examination and would not provide a specific diagnosis if unable to be detected. Although a serum quantitative human chorionic gonadotropin test would be administered to test for pregnancy, it is less specific in providing a diagnosis of ectopic pregnancy. A biophysical profile combines an ultrasound and a non-stress test; however, a non-stress test would not be included in the diagnostic process for ectopic pregnancy.

19. d

Seizures precluded by severe headaches and blurred vision in pregnant patients are most likely indicative of eclampsia. Findings of pregnancy-induced hypertension (PIH) and preeclampsia are both preexisting conditions that may present with eclampsia; however, seizures are more specific to eclampsia. The patient does not display symptoms of hemolysis, elevated liver enzymes, and low platelets syndrome, which would include jaundice, nausea, and fatigue.

20. d

Cocaine use and poor nutrition increase the risk of premature labor. Risk factors for placenta previa include previous caesarean birth and uterine surgery, multiparity, malpresentation, and history of previous previa. Neither cocaine use nor poor nutrition are risk factors associated with either preeclampsia or hemolysis, elevated liver enzymes, and low platelets syndrome.

21. c

In cases of suspected placenta previa, which is suggested by painless bleeding, a bimanual exam should not be performed because it may increase the risk of bleeding. Patients who present with indications of placenta previa are usually hospitalized and a biophysical profile is performed to assess the patient. Vaginal rest is generally advised to prevent further complications.

22. b

An ultrasound examination for fetal survey is typically performed between 18 and 20 weeks of pregnancy. The fetal survey will evaluate fetal structures, assess fetal measurements, and access the amniotic fluid volume. An ultrasound may be performed prior to 12 weeks to confirm a due date, but is not typically required as part of a prenatal check at this time. Patients who are between 20 and 24 weeks pregnant may undergo a diagnostic ultrasound if complications such as ectopic pregnancy or placenta previa occur, but are not required during a prenatal exam.

23. a

Although a quantitative human chorionic gonadotropin blood titer is performed in the first trimester, it is not usually performed upon a new visit. Screening for sexually transmitted diseases, screening for the hepatitis B surface antigen, and the dating ultrasound all should occur within the first trimester or upon a new visit.

24. d

Uterine tumor is not a contributing factor for pregnancy-induced hypertension (PIH); however, such tumors are known to lead to abruptio placentae. Predisposing factors known to contribute to PIH include diabetes and maternal age.

25. a

Among the general population, a history of infertility is considered to pose the highest risk for ectopic pregnancy. Among women with medical histories involving the oviducts, the rate of occurrence for ectopic pregnancy is approximately 30% in those with previous tubal surgery; 15% in those with a previous ectopic pregnancy; and 9% in women who have used intrauterine contraceptive devices.

26. c

The incidence of ectopic pregnancy among the general population is no more than 2%. Approximately 15% of pregnancies will experience a spontaneous abortion, usually due to a chromosomal abnormality. Pregnancy-induced hypertension is seen in approximately 12% of all pregnancies. And the occurrence rate of abruptio placentae ranges from 5%–17% in women who have already experienced one occurrence.

27. c

Prostaglandin and mifepristone are typically prescribed to induce an elective abortion within the first 49 days of pregnancy. B-methasone may be used to promote fetal lung maturity if the fetus is less than 34 weeks gestation, and magnesium sulfate is used to stabilize patients with preeclampsia or eclampsia.

28. d

Fetal monitoring includes a non-stress test, biophysical profile, and kick counts to determine fetal activity at home. Blood pressure surveillance, complete blood counts, and liver function tests are not typically seen as derivatives of fetal monitoring.

29. b

Syncopal episodes are most likely to occur in the second trimester due to a decrease in blood pressure and vascular resistance. Syncopal episodes less commonly occur during in the first and third trimesters, as well as postpartum.

30. c

Because abruptio placentae has an unknown etiology, previous uterine surgery is not known to precipitate the condition but, rather, is associated with increased incidence of placenta previa. Cocaine, alcohol, and tobacco use are considered risk factors of abruptio placentae. An abruption is more likely to occur in the second or third trimester, and the recurrence rate of abruptio placentae increases after more than one incidence.

31. c

According to Naegele's rule, if the first day of the patient's last menstrual period is on March 24, the estimated date of confinement is December 31. Naegele's rule, which provides a rough estimate of a patient's date of confinement, is determined by subtracting 3 months from the first day of the patient's last menstrual period, then adding 7 days to the resulting date. All of the other answer choices do not reflect a correct calculation of Naegele's rule.

32. a

Vacuum curettage and dilation can be used until the patient is 12 weeks pregnant. Vacuum dilation and evacuation may be performed after 16 weeks gestation, and medical induction after 16 weeks is typically used for induced abortion.

33. b

Fetal heart tones are initially able to be assessed by 10–12 weeks of pregnancy. Although the fetus has a heartbeat as early as 8–10 weeks of pregnancy, the heart tones are more usually able to be heard at 10–12 weeks. Fetal heart tones would also be heard between 12–14 weeks of pregnancy and 14–16 weeks of pregnancy.

34. b

Change in skin pigmentation typically occurs in the second trimester, not the first trimester. Amenorrhea, urinary frequency, and breast tenderness are presenting indications of intrauterine pregnancy in the first trimester, but are non-specific. Patients presenting with these signs should be administered a pregnancy test to rule out other conditions.

35. c

An Rh blood test is least likely to provide evidence of placenta previa. The initial diagnostics for placenta previa would include an ultrasound for localization of placental implantation, a complete blood count, and electronic fetal monitoring.

36. d

Rh sensitization, rather than Rh desensitization, constitutes a high-risk pregnancy because it could potentially lead to incompatible blood between the mother and the fetus. High-risk pregnancies include multiple gestations, thrombocytopenia, and a premature rupture of membranes, among others.

37. c

A glucose tolerance test (GTT) is usually performed during a prenatal exam at 28 weeks as part of a routine check-up. However, a GTT or other glucose check may be performed at 20 weeks for patients with a family history of diabetes or who weigh more than 200 lb. A human chorionic gonadotropin test is performed very early in the first trimester to detect pregnancy. An ultrasound for fetal survey is typically performed at 18–20 weeks. A triple/quad screening test is performed at 16–20 weeks for women with a family history of chromosomal abnormalities or those who are advanced in maternal age.

38. d

At 22 weeks of pregnancy, dilation and evacuation is the most appropriate procedure for an induced or elective abortion. Dilation and evacuation may be performed at 13–14 to 20–22 weeks. Vacuum dilation and curettage is the appropriate procedure prior to 12 weeks of pregnancy. Mifepristone and prostaglandin may be administered to induce abortion only within the first 49 days. Lastly, tocolytic therapy and steroid injections are used to treat premature labor, not to induce abortion.

39. b

Hospitalized patients with severe preeclampsia are typically initiated on magnesium sulfate therapy for stabilization. At 32 weeks, the patient would receive weekly steroid injections of B-methasone to ensure fetal lung maturity, but not to be stabilized. Lumirubin is indicated for neonatal jaundice, not fetal lung maturity. Calcium gluconate, on the other hand, is used to counteract magnesium toxicity in preeclampsia and eclampsia.

40. b

Softening of the cervix and the vagina confirms Goodell's sign, which is a positive indication of pregnancy that usually appears by the eighth week of gestation. Chadwick's sign is confirmed by a finding of vaginal and cervical cyanosis resulting from increased blood flow. Braxton-Hicks contractions are "practice" contractions that may begin during the first trimester, but are not noticeable until the second or third trimester. Hegar's sign is the softening of cervicouterine junction and may indicate pregnancy, but is not always a reliable indicator.

DISCUSSION

General Overview

While the family nurse practitioner (FNP) is knowledgeable in the management of the obstetric patient, adult-gerontology primary care nurse practitioners (AGPCNPs) must also have general knowledge of the basic pearls of pregnancy. It is reasonable that both FNPs and AGPCNPs be able to order initial laboratory and diagnostic tests for the newly diagnosed pregnant patient. With regard to scope of practice, AGPCNPs would then appropriately refer the patient to an obstetrics expert. Further, all nurse practitioners should be able to provide basic information and answer simple patient questions about the course of pregnancy, as well as identify potential life-threatening emergencies such as ectopic pregnancy, placenta previa, and placenta abruptio.

Intrauterine Pregnancy

Overview

Intrauterine pregnancy refers to the normal phenomenon that occurs when a fetus grows and develops within the mother's uterus. Pregnancy starts at the last menstrual period and lasts about 40 weeks. Many females suspect pregnancy following the absence of a menstrual period. The gestational age, and subsequently the delivery date, is estimated based on when the last known menstrual period began and the findings on an ultrasound. If delivery occurs within a 2-week window before or after the estimated date, the delivery is considered "full term," as opposed to premature or late.[1]

Presentation

Breast enlargement and tenderness is often the first indication of a pregnancy. Amenorrhea serves as another common early indicator; however, this sign may be difficult to determine because many females have cycle variation, indicated by variation of more than 5 days in the length of each cycle period. Other signs and symptoms generally experienced by women in the first trimester include nausea, urinary frequency, fatigue, and lower abdominal cramping. The second trimester is characterized by the emergence of presentations such as increased pigmentation of the skin, back pain, syncopal episodes, constipation, food cravings, and abdominal bloating.[2] Abdominal growth, bloating, and back discomfort typically continue into the third trimester.[3] The third trimester might also see the return of urinary frequency and the presence of round ligament pain, carpal tunnel syndrome, and vaginal discharge.[4] Two other symptoms germane to the third trimester are the occurrence of Braxton-Hicks contractions and a shortness of breath due to placental pressure on the diaphragm.[4]

Many of the physical findings associated with pregnancy are directly correlated to the symptoms presented and experienced by the pregnant woman. Although a confirmation of pregnancy requires methods such as an ultrasonography, the positive, probable, and presumptive signs indicate that pregnancy is likely the diagnosis. Presumptive signs are the subjective signs indicated by the woman whereas probable signs are those observed by the examiner.[5]

After 4 weeks of gestation, the uterus should expand in size at a rate of approximately 1 centimeter (cm) per week. By around 6 weeks, the cervix begins to soften; this is Goodell's sign. Hegar's sign, the softening of the lower uterine segment, also occurs around this time.[2] After 12 weeks of gestation, the uterus becomes large enough to extend over the symphysis pubis, giving the woman a pregnant appearance.[2] Breast enlargement can result in breast tenderness as well as simultaneous visible changes, such as increased pigmentation in the areola and increased visibility of the venous pattern under the skin of the breasts. Striae gravidarum, which often present in the second trimester, will also appear on the breasts, as well as on the hips and abdomen. At around 8–12 weeks of gestation, the mucus membranes of the vulva, vagina, and cervix become more congested. The increased blood flow that brings about the congestion yields a bluish discoloration of the cervix; this is Chadwick's sign. By 10–12 weeks of gestation, fetal heart activity can be detected using a Doppler device.[6] Fetal movement is traditionally felt by 18–20 weeks of gestation. After the palpable uterine fundus has presented at about 20 weeks, it is possible to employ Leopold maneuvers.[3] Most of these findings will continue into the third trimester; some of the findings will cease completely, and some will temporarily cease and reappear again later.

In the last few weeks of pregnancy, women often experience an increase in Braxton-Hicks contractions, or false labor, as the body prepares for delivery. The fetus will likewise engage at about 36 weeks by dropping into the pelvic area in preparation for delivery; this is called lightening. An increase in vaginal discharge is an additional sign of approaching labor. A mucus plug accumulates in the cervix over the course of the pregnancy. When the cervix begins to dilate closer to delivery, the plug is pushed into the vagina, and may pass by approximately one week prior to labor. This passage is called the bloody show, due to the streaks of old, brown-tinted blood often present in the mucus.[7]

Workup

A pregnancy is made by the detection of human chorionic gonadotropin (hCG) in either urine or serum and by ultrasound. A qualitative hCG test will determine whether hCG is present, whereas a quantitative hCG test will determine the amount of the hormone present. The urine test used by patients at home is qualitative, whereas serum tests can be either qualitative or quantitative. After the pregnancy diagnosis, the mother will then begin a routine of obstetric visits and testing over the course of her pregnancy term. These visits aim to ensure optimal health for the fetus and for the mother, as well as supply the mother with the resources and information necessary to make informed decisions regarding her pregnancy.

For a nulliparous woman, the recommended frequency of obstetric visits in the first 28 weeks of gestation is one visit every 4 weeks. From weeks 28 to 36, the recommended frequency is one visit every 2 weeks. Nulliparous women should make weekly obstetric visits from 36 weeks of gestation up until delivery. Prior delivery history is a key consideration for multiparous women with regard to the schedule for obstetric visits.[8]

First Trimester Tests

A variety of baseline studies are conducted at the first obstetric visit after pregnancy is confirmed. A dating ultrasound is performed on the first obstetric visit. This test works to confirm the status of the intrauterine pregnancy and is more accurate than providing a diagnosis based on the woman's last menstrual period. A standard urinalysis, urine culture, and urine screening with dipstick are likewise ordered. Blood and Rhesus (Rh) typing and antibody screening is performed to detect antibodies that can cause hemolytic disease in the infant. A complete blood count (CBC) is ordered as well to assess for anemia or thalassemia.

Pregnant women with an incomplete history of infection or vaccination should be tested for rubella, varicella, and hepatitis B.[9,10] Screening should also be performed for various sexually transmitted infections (STI) and diseases, such as syphilis and HIV, as many women may be asymptomatic, increasing the risk of transmission from mother to fetus.[11]

Papanicolaou smears and cervical cultures are ordered to detect pre-cancerous or cancerous cells.[9] Specialty screening is recommended to detect chromosomal abnormalities such as Trisomy 21 or Trisomy 18. Chorionic villus sampling may be ordered in the first trimester. The test is generally ordered if other screening tests have suggested an anomaly, if there is an increased maternal age, or if there is a history of pregnancy complications.[12]

Second Trimester Tests

Ultrasonography, amniocentesis, quad screening, and a glucose tolerance test are tests regularly ordered during the second trimester.

Although ultrasounds performed within the first trimester may be able to detect early fetal anomalies, the second trimester ultrasound, also known as the anatomy ultrasound, would more accurately determine these malformations. The optimal time to perform the second trimester ultrasound is between 18 and 20 weeks of gestation.[8]

Amniocentesis, when necessary, is generally performed within the second trimester, preferably at 15–17 weeks. Amniotic fluid is analyzed for genetic disorders, fetal lung maturity, blood or platelet type, and neural tube defects.[13]

One of the two multiple marker tests is ordered during the second trimester, preferably between gestation weeks 16 and 20.[3] The quad screen and the triple screen both work to provide information that informs risk and aids in assessing the fetus's chance of having genetic disorders such as spina bifida, anencephaly, and Down syndrome; the quad screen, however, provides more accuracy in the screening for Down syndrome due to supplemental evaluation of inhibin-A.[14] If these tests indicate a condition, other tests should be ordered.

A glucose tolerance test may be ordered at 20 weeks of gestation if there is a family history of diabetes or if the patient's weight exceeds 200 lb.[3] Otherwise, the recommended period for a glucose tolerance test is in the third trimester from 24 to 28 weeks gestation for multiparous women.[8,15]

Third Trimester Tests

After an Rh-negative test in the first trimester, the woman is tested for antibodies that may attack Rh-positive blood; the presence of antibodies indicates the woman is sensitized to Rh-positive blood. If the father is Rh-positive, then the fetus is Rh-positive. A woman who is sensitized to Rh-positive blood and is carrying an Rh-positive fetus requires additional monitoring. If the woman is Rh-negative and is not yet determined to be Rh-sensitized, the repeat test is ordered at 28 weeks gestation; if the woman is still not sensitized, she should be given an anti-D immune globulin injection (RhoGAM), which reduces the risk of becoming Rh-sensitized before delivery.[16]

Hemoglobin and hematocrit levels should be reevaluated in the third trimester as well. Lastly, in some cases, a biophysical profile is ordered after 32 weeks to evaluate fetal well-being.[17] The test is recommended for women who are overdue or when there is a suspicion of decreased fetal heart activity.[18]

Treatment

During the first obstetric visit, an estimated due date can be determined using Naegele's rule. The due date is calculated by adding a year to the date when the last normal menstrual period began, then subtracting 3 months and subsequently adding 7 days. Also during the first visit, a thorough history and physical exam should be taken. The history should include social, medical, obstetrical, and family histories; it should also detail diet, work, and living environment.[9] The history should be reviewed on every return visit. The physical exam should include height, weight, vital signs, and pelvic exam. The physical exam should also be repeated on every return visit, with focus on the changing fundal height, as well as fetal activity, heart tones, and position.[19] The aforementioned laboratory tests are administered throughout the course of the pregnancy, but a urinalysis should be performed at every obstetric visit to monitor protein, glucose, and ketones.[3]

The importance of adhering to the scheduling of visits is highlighted in the presence of a high-risk situation in the pregnancy. Consistent monitoring allows for early detection and prevention of high-risk situations. Upon detection of circumstances that may be threatening to the mother or fetus, an obstetrical consultation should be arranged accordingly for additional testing, treatment, abortion of pregnancy, or early delivery as needed. The patient's history of previous pregnancy losses, preterm labor and delivery, or family histories of genetic anomalies should allow practitioners to be attentive to the possibility of these situations recurring. Blood laboratory tests help to identify high-risk situations such as Rh sensitization, HIV, hemoglobinopathies, or thrombocytopenia. Other laboratory results can indicate high-risk situations or situations that may necessitate further consultation and referral (e.g., multiple gestation pregnancy, uterine bleeding, polyhydramnios or oligohydramnios, intrauterine growth retardation, pre-eclampsia, or pregnancy-induced hypertension). Abnormal multiple marker tests can indicate gestational diabetes. Conditions late in the pregnancy may also call for close monitoring or referral, such as preterm labor leading to premature rupture of membranes or the fetus not dropping after 34 weeks.[3]

Ectopic Pregnancy

Overview

An ectopic pregnancy is a pregnancy in which the fertilized egg implants outside the uterus. About 95% of all ectopic pregnancies occur in the fallopian tube; however, it is possible for implantation to occur in the ovaries, cervix, or abdominal cavity.[20] The incidence of ectopic pregnancy within the general population is less than 2%; women with medical histories involving the oviducts and with histories of infertility are at higher risk for the condition than the general population.[3,21]

Presentation

Signs and symptoms generally appear 6–8 weeks after the last menstrual period. As with intrauterine pregnancy, amenorrhea is common in the early stages of the condition. For many patients, the first sign of ectopic pregnancy is abnormal uterine bleeding; this bleeding usually presents as spotting, and is often dark brown to tarry in color. This discharge is often accompanied by pain and discomfort in the shoulder and abdomen.[22] Heavy uterine bleeding is not likely, although when it happens, it is indicative of a possible tubal rupture, which can result in shock and intra-abdominal hemorrhaging.[23] Acute manifestations of pelvic pain, unilateral lower quadrant pain, and lower back pain are other indicative symptoms of ectopic pregnancy.

Physical examination may reveal adnexal and/or cervical motion tenderness, as well as an adnexal mass. When Hegar's sign begins to present at about eight weeks, as indicated by the softening of the cervicouterine junction, concurrent presentation of uterine enlargement suggests ectopic pregnancy.[3] Vaginal bleeding can also present along with pelvic pain. Signs and symptoms of peritonitis, such as abdominal tenderness, bloating, nausea, vomiting, and diarrhea, indicate that rupture may have occurred.[24]

Workup

The best way to diagnose an ectopic pregnancy, especially early on, is through the utilization of both a quantitative analysis of hCG serum and a transvaginal ultrasound.[22] A deviation from the standard escalation of hCG serum levels in pregnant women usually indicates an ectopic pregnancy.[25] A CBC and screening for blood type and Rh should also be ordered. For women who are Rh-negative, antenatal RhoGAM should be ordered because of the increased risk of fetomaternal hemorrhaging in ectopic pregnancy.

Treatment

Ectopic pregnancy requires aggressive treatment, as the potential for morbidity and mortality are high. Patients should be evaluated by an obstetrician-gynecologist (OB/GYN) and assessed for the need for medical or surgical intervention.

Abortion

Overview

Abortion is defined as the termination of pregnancy at any time prior to age of viability, either through spontaneous expulsion or medical or surgical removal. Some abortions, however, may occur spontaneously but initially go undetected and unexpelled.[24] Approximately 15% of all pregnancies are spontaneously aborted, with 80% of those abortions occurring in the first 12 weeks of gestation.[26,27] The majority of first trimester spontaneous abortions are related to chromosomal abnormalities that are not compatible with life and are not necessarily indicative of complications in future pregnancies. Loss after 24 weeks of gestation generally results from cervical incompetence, infection, or uterine abnormalities.

Elective abortions account for approximately half of all abortions per every 100 live births among unmarried women.[3]

Presentation

Although it does not necessarily indicate spontaneous abortion or any other detrimental condition, vaginal bleeding while a patient is pregnant is a hallmark sign of spontaneous abortion and necessitates further evaluation. If heavy bleeding occurs as a result of hemorrhage, the patient's vital signs will be marked by hemodynamic changes suggesting shock.[3] Other symptoms of the condition include pelvic or lower back pain and severe cramping. In cases of spontaneous abortion, severe cramping often heralds or accompanies membrane rupture and passing of fetal tissue.[28]

Workup

A pelvic ultrasound is the most useful diagnostic utilized in evaluating women who present with indications of spontaneous abortion.[29] In cases where the ultrasound findings are nondiagnostic, evaluation of hCG is helpful in determining whether or not all placental tissue has been passed.[28] A CBC may be ordered to assess levels of hemoglobin and hematocrit.[30] Additionally, if a patient has a history of bleeding or recurrent loss, a coagulation profile should be ordered.[31] Blood type and Rh screening is also ordered. If the patient is Rh-negative and has miscarried before, RhoGAM will be administered.[30]

Treatment

For patients who are not experiencing complications, it is possible to allow the spontaneous abortion process to progress on its own. Because this can take 3–4 weeks, the patient should be monitored for signs and symptoms of infection. The use of medication is an option for patients undergoing an elective abortion. In the first trimester, within 49 days from the first day of the last known menstrual period, a mix of the medications mifepristone and misoprostol serves as the preferred option; if the procedure is being performed in the second trimester, misoprostol alone is the standard regimen.[32] Another option is dilation and curettage surgery, which is the preferred and safest treatment for patients experiencing infection or heavy bleeding.[28] This method, however, is only an option up to 12 weeks of gestation. In patients between 13 and 22 weeks of gestation seeking abortion, a dilation and evacuation procedure should be ordered.

Complications of Pregnancy

Significant complications of pregnancy include hypertensive disorders such as pregnancy-induced hypertension, preeclampsia, eclampsia, and hemolysis, elevated liver enzymes, and low platelets (HELLP) syndrome. Placenta previa, abruptio placentae, and premature labor are also considered significant complications. All of these require the intervention of an OB/GYN specialist. Pregnancy-induced hypertension may require nothing more than a consultation with a specialist, but the other complications will require a referral.

Pregnancy-Induced Hypertension

Overview

Pregnancy-induced hypertension, also known as gestational hypertension, is denoted by a systolic blood pressure exceeding 140 mmHg or a diastolic blood pressure exceeding 90 mmHg after the 20th week of pregnancy. Although the condition resembles preeclampsia in many regards, pregnancy-induced hypertension is distinguished by a lack of elevated protein in the patient's urine.[33,34] Pregnancy-induced hypertension can also be indicated by a rise in systole of over 30 mmHg or a rise in diastole of over 15 mmHg above an established baseline on two different occasions, at least 4 hours apart.[35] This condition manifests in approximately 12% of all pregnancies.[3] Conditions such as renal or cardiovascular disease, diabetes, lupus, and autoimmune disorders are predisposing factors for pregnancy-induced hypertension. Other predisposing factors include multiple gestation, first pregnancy, pregnancy in adolescence or past 40 years of age, and a personal or family history of either pregnancy-induced hypertension or preeclampsia.[3,34]

Presentation

An initial indication of pregnancy-induced hypertension usually includes increased blood pressure, edema, and weight gain. The woman may also experience changes in vision, oliguria, nausea, vomiting, and abdominal pain. Although such findings suggest pregnancy-induced hypertension, some women with the condition have few or no symptoms.[36]

Workup

An OB/GYN specialist should usually be consulted in cases of pregnancy-induced hypertension. Pregnancy-induced hypertension warrants regular blood pressure monitoring due to the increased demand on the cardiovascular system.[37] A 24-hour urinalysis evaluation for protein and creatinine is additionally necessary and may aid in detecting preeclampsia.[34,38] A CBC and liver function testing should be ordered as well. Non-stress tests are performed at 32–34 weeks, or as needed. A biophysical profile should be ordered as needed to evaluate and detect fetal growth complications.

Treatment

Pregnancy-induced hypertension is generally managed with therapeutic lifestyle changes and bed rest. Resting in the left, lateral recumbent position allows for improved blood flow by non-compression of the vena cava. Patients are instructed to perform daily "kick counts" and report to the NP if the number of kicks has decreased. A non-stress test, along with an ultrasound, should be performed to eradicate the possibility of placental insufficiency and assure that fetal activity is present.[35]

Preeclampsia

Overview

Preeclampsia is the presence of hypertension and proteinuria in a woman after her 20th week of pregnancy when the patient was normotensive before pregnancy.[39] The condition develops from pregnancy-induced hypertension and is distinguishable primarily by the elevated levels of protein in the urine. Preeclampsia and other hypertensive disorders during pregnancy affect about 5%–8% of all births in the United States.[40]

Presentation

In addition to the presence of hypertension and proteinuria, preeclampsia is often accompanied by findings of generalized edema. Preeclampsia is also suggested by sudden weight gain, qualified by a gain of more than 2 lb per week or more than 6 lb per month.[3,41] Other findings of preeclampsia may include severe headaches, upper abdominal and epigastric pain, nausea, and vomiting.[39]

As pregnancy-induced hypertension is a predisposing factor for preeclampsia, a systolic blood pressure higher than 140 mmHg or a diastolic blood pressure higher than 90 mmHg are required findings for the condition. Preeclampsia is also diagnostically supported by proteinuria of at least 1+, with higher ratings indicating a worsening condition.[38] The diagnostic edema ratings are similar to those of proteinuria, with a 1+ indicating nondependent edema. Despite the presence of sudden weight gain, a lack in fundal height is a standard finding with preeclampsia. Although reflexes are generally within normal limits, findings of hyperreflexia indicate a worsening condition, as do visual disturbances.[3]

Workup

All baseline pregnancy tests should be ordered as usual in cases of preeclampsia to assess for hemolysis, elevated liver enzymes, and low platelets (HELLP) syndrome.[42] Once the patient has been referred to an OB/GYN specialist, testing will include coagulation studies, blood pressure monitoring, urinalysis, non-stress tests, and biophysical profile, among others.[3]

Treatment

In severe cases, hospitalization with referral is necessary, and therapy with magnesium sulfate is often necessary for prevention of eclampsia. Delivery is the best treatment for preeclampsia. Therefore, in cases where preeclampsia manifests before 34 weeks of gestation, weekly injections of the beta-methasone steroid may be given to accelerate fetal lung maturity.[43,44] Bedrest, left lateral positioning, and daily kick counts are critical. Once fetal maturity is assured, delivery will likely be recommended.[45]

Eclampsia

Overview

Eclampsia is the combination of pregnancy-induced hypertension, preeclampsia, and the onset of a seizure.[3] Eclampsia develops in 2%–3% of all women diagnosed with preeclampsia and manifests in 1.6–10 cases per 10,000 deliveries in developed countries. The incidence of eclampsia is higher and more variable in developing countries.[46]

Presentation

Eclampsia echoes many of the signs and symptoms of pregnancy-induced hypertension and preeclampsia. Elevated blood pressure is a key sign of all these conditions. However, distinguishing features of eclampsia include a systolic reading greater than 160 mmHg and a diastolic reading greater than 100 mmHg. Other findings include severe headaches, epigastric or right upper quadrant pain, oliguria, and visual disturbances.[3,46] Tonic-clonic seizures likewise serve to distinguish eclampsia from preeclampsia and other conditions of pregnancy.[3] During and after the seizures, it is common for the fetus to experience bradycardia for a few minutes, indicating fetal distress in utero.[46]

Workup

The diagnostic testing profile for eclampsia is very similar to that for pregnancy-induced hypertension and preeclampsia. Upon referral, a variety of blood and urine studies will be conducted.[47]

Treatment

Patients with eclampsia are referred to an OB/GYN specialist and usually hospitalized for management of their condition. In treating the condition, magnesium sulfate therapy may be used to decrease the amount of recurring convulsions associated with eclampsia.[46] Once maternal and fetal stability is determined, delivery follows treatment.

Hemolysis Elevated Liver Enzymes and Low Platelets (HELLP) Syndrome

Overview

Hemolysis elevated liver enzymes and low platelets (HELLP) syndrome is closely related to preeclampsia. HELLP syndrome occurs in approximately 0.1%–0.8% of all pregnancies, and 10%–20% of all cases of the condition are accompanied by severe preeclampsia or severe eclampsia.[48] A personal or family history of preeclampsia or HELLP syndrome serves as a major risk factor for the condition.[49,50,51,52]

Presentation

The hallmark findings for HELLP syndrome are mid-epigastric and right upper quadrant pain.[53] Nausea, vomiting, and malaise are also common findings, potentially resulting in misdiagnosis and consequent maternal death. Severe cases of the syndrome can produce symptoms associated with preeclampsia and eclampsia, such as headaches and visual disturbances. However, these manifestations, as well as findings such as jaundice, ascites, and extreme fatigue, are not standard presentations of the condition.[54] Hepatomegaly may be discovered upon percussion.[55]

Workup

A standard diagnostic panel for HELLP syndrome includes a CBC, a peripheral blood smear, and tests for serum levels of aspartate aminotransferase (AST), alanine transaminase (ALT), and bilirubin, all of which serve to isolate the diagnostic criteria for the condition.[48]

Patients with suspected HELLP syndrome should be referred to an OB/GYN specialist. Under the specialist's care, a variety of other tests and diagnostics will be ordered, such as a 24-hour urinalysis, liver function tests, platelet counts, and frequent blood pressure monitoring.[3]

Treatment

Symptomatic care and delivery as soon as reasonable are the cornerstones of treatment for HELLP syndrome.[56]

Placenta Previa

Overview

Placenta previa is a condition in which the placenta of the fetus partially, marginally, or wholly covers the mother's cervix, which deters passage from the uterus to the vagina. This condition stems from cases where the conceptus implants itself on the lower part of the uterus; when the placenta grows around the fetus, it can potentially cover the cervix.[57] A higher risk of placenta previa is associated with women who are multiparous or have had previous cases of cesarean delivery, uterine surgery, abortion, or placenta previa. Placenta previa is also known to increase the incidence of fetal malpresentation.[58] Multiple gestation, cocaine use, smoking, increased maternal age, and non-white ethnicity are all additional risk factors for placenta previa.[59]

Presentation

The chief sign of placenta previa is painless vaginal bleeding that occurs after 20 weeks of gestation. This bleeding often occurs following intercourse but may also present without any clear precipitating factor and is not characteristically accompanied by uterine tenderness.[3] Premature contractions have been reported in cases of placenta previa, but are not standard symptoms of the condition. There is typically little to no fetal compromise, unless bleeding is severe or other sources of fetal distress are present.

Workup

In cases of placenta previa, an ultrasound is generally the first diagnostic ordered. Once placenta previa or other abnormalities have been detected through a transabdominal ultrasound, a transvaginal ultrasound is often concluded to more precisely locate the placenta.[60] Electronic fetal heart monitoring is ordered to detect fetal distress. A CBC is ordered as a baseline.[3]

A speculum examination is performed to determine the extent of the patient's bleeding.[3] If little to no bleeding occurs and no other complications are present, bed rest at home is an. In any other case, the patient is required to be hospitalized for close monitoring.[57] A fetal non-stress test and a biophysical profile are ordered and subsequently performed weekly until delivery.[3]

Treatment

Patients with placenta previa should be referred to an OB/GYN specialist. In cases where placenta previa is diagnosed early in the pregnancy and the placenta is near the cervix, rather than overlapping or covering it, it is possible for the condition to resolve on its own. The likelihood of vaginal delivery is high in this circumstance. However, when the placenta is covering the cervix and the condition does not resolve on its own, cesarean delivery is required at fetal maturity. In cases where the patient is experiencing heavy vaginal bleeding, cesarean delivery before fetal maturity may be necessary, as well as use of corticosteroid therapy to speed fetal lung development before delivery. After diagnosis of placenta previa, it is strongly encouraged and very important for the patient to have vaginal rest.[57]

Abruptio Placentae

Overview

Abruptio placentae, also known as placental abruption, is the partial or total detachment of the placenta from the uterine wall. Abruption occurs during the second and third trimester, and results in hemorrhage that threatens the life of both the fetus and the mother. In cases where hemorrhage is uncontrolled, disseminated intravascular coagulation can occur. There is no direct known etiology of abruptio placentae. This condition can manifest from abdominal trauma that produces a rupture in maternal vessels. Rapid loss of amniotic fluid may also lead to abruptio placentae. Factors that put women at a higher risk of abruptio placentae include cocaine and alcohol use, increased maternal age, asthma, preeclampsia, and eclampsia. Women who smoke are 2 ½ times more likely to experience abruption than non-smokers, and hypertensive women are 5 times more likely to experience abruption than normotensive women.[61,62,63] A history of placental abruption also puts women at a higher risk for a recurrence. Women who experienced a previous abruption are 5%–17% more likely to have another; women who experienced two previous abruptions are 25% more likely to have another.[3]

Presentation

The indicative findings of abruptio placentae are severe abdominal pain, contractions, and vaginal bleeding.[61] However, it is important to note that the amount of vaginal bleeding does not correlate specifically with the severity of the abruption; in cases of concealed abruption, the placenta traps the blood from exiting through the cervix and vagina, yielding less visible vaginal bleeding.[23] A tender or rigid uterus is a stronger indicator for a concealed abruption.[3,64] If the abruption is not concealed, bleeding may be heavy, which can result in shock and, consequently, death for both the mother and the fetus.[65] Shock-like symptoms are common, and can indicate abruption in non-concealed cases when vaginal bleeding is minimal.[64] Back pain accompanied by uterine tenderness can also present in cases of abruptio placentae.[61] Fetal distress occurs in about half of all abruption cases. The abruption can lead to a deprivation of oxygen and nutrients for the fetus, stillbirth, or preterm delivery. Surviving infants have approximately a 40%–50% chance of complications.[23,65]

Workup

An ultrasound is generally the first step of the diagnostic process for abruptio placentae.[3] Severe separation and hemorrhaging are often indicated by a coagulation panel. If fibrinogen levels are decreased, it is likely the patient is at substantial risk for postpartum hemorrhaging. Other hemodynamic changes will be monitored with other parts of the coagulation profile as well. Severe abruption can lead to disseminated intravascular coagulation and, consequently, fetal death.[61]

Electronic fetal monitoring likewise assists in the evaluation of abruptio placentae. Maternal hypotensive and fetal heart abnormalities are suggestive of severe separation, which can lead to fetal death and maternal mortality.

Treatment

Patients with abruptio placentae should be referred to an OB/GYN specialist immediately. Hospitalization and continuous monitoring are necessary for any case of abruptio placentae. Similar to other pregnancy complications, the best treatment of abruptio placentae is delivery. Severe abruption calls for delivery as soon as possible, as this condition can rapidly progress and threaten both the fetus and the mother.[66] In non-severe abruptions at or later than 36 weeks of gestation, vaginal delivery is considered acceptable. In non-severe cases earlier than 36 weeks of gestation, the patient may be treated as an outpatient with frequent monitoring. In severe cases, the patient should be hospitalized immediately. Severe cases in which hemorrhaging or fetal distress is present often call for cesarean delivery upon stability of the mother.[3,66]

Premature Labor

Overview

Premature labor, or preterm labor, is indicated by the presence of contractions and true labor after 20 weeks of pregnancy and more than 3 weeks before the estimated due date.[67] Premature labor is the leading cause of neonatal mortality in the United States.[68] The exact etiology of premature labor is not known, although there are many factors that put a woman at higher risk for premature labor.

A history of premature labor is a risk factor for subsequent premature labor; the chances increase considerably when the birth occurs before 34 weeks of pregnancy.[69] Multiple gestation is another strong risk factor for premature labor; multiple gestation pregnancies account for approximately 2%–3% of all births, as well as approximately 23% and 17% of all births under 32 and 37 weeks of pregnancy, respectively. Genitourinary findings such as bacteriuria, bacterial vaginosis, *Chlamydia trachomatis*, *Neisseria gonorrhoeae*, syphilis, and *Trichomonas vaginalis* have an association with premature labor.[70] Studies have shown that both underweight and obese mothers are at higher risk than the rest of the population for premature labor and birth.[71,72] Poor weight gain, poor nutrition, and low income are other risk factors. Similar to the mother's weight, extremes in maternal age are associated with higher premature labor.[68]

Substance abuse and smoking also contribute to

higher rates of premature labor. Increased frequency of cigarette smoking correlates with an increased risk of premature birth.[73] Although various substances may increase the risk of premature birth, cocaine is seen more often in toxicology reports in women who have experienced premature labor. Congenital or acquired uterine malformations and cervical trauma are additional risk factors for premature labor.[3,70]

Presentation

The main findings of preterm labor are constant or rhythmic uterine cramping, lower back pain when the patient had not previously experienced back pain, increased occurrence of contractions, pelvic pressure, cervical effacement and dilatation, and vaginal spotting or change in vaginal discharge.[74] These findings are non-specific and may persist for hours before any type of cervical change occurs.

Workup

The patient should be referred to an OB/GYN specialist. If the patient is not experiencing placenta previa or if a rupture of membranes has not occurred, a pelvic exam should be conducted to determine whether cervical changes have occurred. The patient's contractions will also be monitored, and an ultrasound will be conducted.[75,76]

Treatment

Hospitalization is generally required if the contractions do not cease before cervical changes occur.[3] Weekly checks are conducted to monitor cervical changes and other signs of preterm labor. If the patient is less than 34 weeks pregnant, betamethasone steroid injections are considered in order to expedite fetal lung maturity until 34 weeks. Tocolytic therapy may be administered with steroids to stop premature labor.[77] Bedrest and abstinence are recommended for managing the condition at home.

The NP's recognition and control of risk factors early in the pregnancy is crucial to prevention of preterm labor. Even after measures are taken early in the pregnancy to eliminate these risk factors, they should be reassessed every trimester. The patient should also be well-educated about the warning signs of preterm labor to ensure early identification of such signs for optimal management.[3]

References

1. Brown HL. Physical changes during pregnancy. In: Porter RS, Kaplan JL, eds. The Merck Manual Online. http://www.merckmanuals.com/home/womens_health_issues/normal_pregnancy/physical_changes_during_pregnancy.html. Revised April 2014. Accessed March 12, 2015.

2. Bastian LA, Brown HL. Clinical manifestations and diagnosis of early pregnancy. In: Basow DS, ed. UpToDate. Waltham, MA: UpToDate; 2015. http://www.uptodate.com/contents/clinical-manifestations-and-diagnosis-of-early-pregnancy. Accessed March 12, 2015.

3. Barkley TW Jr. Obstetrics and pregnancy pearls. In Adult-Gerontology Primary Care Nurse Practitioner: Certification Review/Clinical Update Continuing Education Course. West Hollywood, CA: Barkley & Associates; 2015: 18–26.

4. Mayo Clinic Staff. Pregnancy week by week. Mayo Clinic. http://www.mayoclinic.com/health/pregnancy/PR00009. Reviewed May 5, 2014. Accessed March 12, 2015.

5. Antipuesto DJ. Signs of pregnancy. Nursingcrib. http://nursingcrib.com/nursing-notes-reviewer/maternal-child-health/signs-of-pregnancy. Published January 10, 2011. Accessed March 12, 2015.

6. Jarvis C. Physical Examination and Health Assessment. 6th ed. Philadelphia, PA: W. B. Saunders; 2011.

7. How to tell when labor begins. American College of Obstetricians and Gynecologists web site. http://www.acog.org/Patients/FAQs/How-to-Tell-When-Labor-Begins. Published May 2011. Accessed March 12, 2015.

8. Lockwood C J, Magriples U. Prenatal care (second and third trimesters). In: Basow DS, ed. UpToDate. Waltham, MA: UpToDate; 2015. http://www.uptodate.com/contents/prenatal-care-second-and-third-trimesters. Accessed March 12, 2015.

9. Lockwood CJ, Magriples U. Initial prenatal assessment and first trimester prenatal care. In: Basow DS, ed. UpToDate. Waltham, MA: UpToDate; 2015. http://www.uptodate.com/contents/initial-prenatal-assessment-and-first-trimester-prenatal-care. Accessed March 12, 2015.

10. Pregnancy and HBV: FAQ. Hepatitis B Foundation web site. http://www.hepb.org/patients/pregnant_women.htm. Last updated October 17, 2012. Accessed March 12, 2015.

11. Norwitz ER. Syphilis in pregnancy. In: Basow DS, ed. UpToDate. Waltham, MA: UpToDate; 2015. http://www.uptodate.com/contents/syphilis-in-pregnancy. Accessed March 12, 2015.

12. Mayo Clinic Staff. Chorionic villus sampling. Mayo Clinic. http://www.mayoclinic.com/health/chorionic-villus-sampling/MY00154/DSECTION=why-its-done. Reviewed October 10, 2012. Accessed March 12, 2015.

13. Ghidini A. Diagnostic amniocentesis. In: Basow DS, ed. UpToDate. Waltham, MA: UpToDate; 2015. http://www.uptodate.com/contents/diagnostic-amniocentesis. Accessed March 12, 2015.

14. Healthwise, Inc. Triple or quad screening for birth defects. WebMd. http://www.webmd.com/a-to-z-guides/triple-or-quad-screening-for-birth-defects-topic-overview. Last updated April 4, 2012. Accessed March 12, 2015.

15. Coustan DR, Jovanovic L. Diabetes mellitus in pregnancy: Screening and diagnosis. In: Basow DS, ed. *UpToDate*. Waltham, MA: UpToDate; 2015. http://www.uptodate.com/contents/screening-and-diagnosis-of-diabetes-mellitus-during-pregnancy. Accessed March 12, 2015.

16. Healthwise, Inc. Exams and tests. WebMD. http://www.webmd.com/baby/guide/rh-sensitization-during-pregnancy-exams-and-tests. Last updated September 24, 2013. Accessed March 12, 2015.

17. Biophysical profile. American Pregnancy Association web site. http://americanpregnancy.org/prenatal-testing/biophysical-profile. Last updated August 2013. Accessed March 12, 2015.

18. Mayo Clinic Staff. Biophysical profile. Mayo Clinic. http://www.mayoclinic.com/health/biophysical-profile/MY01919/DSECTION=why-its-done. Reviewed March 5, 2015. Accessed March 12, 2015.

19. Group Health Cooperative. Prenatal care: Screening and testing guideline. GroupHealth. http://www.ghc.org/all-sites/guidelines/prenatal.pdf. Published October 2013. Accessed March 12, 2015.

20. Mayo Clinic Staff. Ectopic pregnancy. Mayo Clinic. http://www.mayoclinic.com/health/ectopic-pregnancy/DS00622. Reviewed January 20, 2015. Accessed March 12, 2015.

21. Capmas P, Bouyer J, Fernandez H. Treatment of ectopic pregnancies in 2014: New answers to some old questions. *Fertil Steril*. 2014; 101(3): 615–620. doi: 10.1016/j.fertnstert.2014.01.029

22. Tulandi, T. Ectopic pregnancy: Clinical manifestations and diagnosis. In: Basow DS, ed. *UpToDate*. Waltham, MA: UpToDate; 2015. http://www.uptodate.com/contents/clinical-manifestations-diagnosis-and-management-of-ectopic-pregnancy. Accessed March 12,2015.

23. Mayo Clinic Staff. Placental abruption. Mayo Clinic. http://www.mayoclinic.com/health/placental-abruption/DS00623. Reviewed December 13, 2014. Accessed March 12, 2015.

24. Dulay AT. Ectopic pregnancy. In: Porter RS, Kaplan JL, eds *Merck Manual Online*. http://www.merckmanuals.com/professional/gynecology_and_obstetrics/abnormalities_of_pregnancy/ectopic_pregnancy.html. Last reviewed January 2014. Accessed March 12, 2015.

25. Sepilian VP, Wood E. Ectopic pregnancy. In: Rivlin ME, ed. Medscape. Retrieved from http://emedicine.medscape.com/article/2041923-workup#aw2aab6b5b2

26. Tulandi T, Al-Fozan HM. Spontaneous abortion: Risk factors, etiology, clinical manifestations, and diagnostic evaluation. In: Basow DS, ed. *UpToDate*. Waltham, MA: UpToDate; 2015. http://www.uptodate.com/contents/spontaneous-abortion-risk-factors-etiology-clinical-manifestations-and-diagnostic-evaluation. Accessed March 12, 2015.

27. Dulay AT. Spontaneous abortion (miscarriage). In: Porter RS, Kaplan JL. The Merck Manual Online. https://www.merckmanuals.com/professional/gynecology-and-obstetrics/abnormalities-of-pregnancy/spontaneous-abortion. Last reviewed January 2014. Accessed March 12, 2015.

28. Mayo Clinic Staff. Miscarriage. Mayo Clinic. http://www.mayoclinic.com/health/pregnancy-loss-miscarriage/DS01105. Reviewed July 9, 2013. Accessed March 12, 2015.

29. Raptis CA, Mellnick VM, Raptis DA, et al. Imaging of trauma in the pregnant patient. *Radiographics*. 2014; 34(3): 748–763. doi: 10.1148/rg.343135090

30. Todd N. Understanding miscarriage—diagnosis & treatment. http://www.webmd.com/baby/understanding-miscarriage-treatment. Last reviewed March 11, 2014. Accessed March 12, 2015.

31. Bick, RL. Miscarriages caused by blood coagulation protein or platelet deficits workup. In: Besa EC, ed. Medscape. http://emedicine.medscape.com/article/210857-workup. Updated November 13, 2014. Accessed March 12, 2015.

32. Clark W, Shannon C, Winikoff B. Misoprostol as a single agent for medical termination of pregnancy. In: Basow DS, ed. *UpToDate*. Waltham, MA: UpToDate; 2015. http://www.uptodate.com/contents/misoprostol-as-a-single-agent-for-medical-termination-of-pregnancy. Accessed March 12, 2015.

33. Scantlebury DW, Schwartz GL, Acquah LA, White WM, Moser M, Garovic VD. The treatment of hypertension during pregnancy: When should blood pressure medications be started? *Curr Cardiol Rep*. 2013; 15(11): 412. doi: 10.1007/s11886-013-0412-0

34. Rosser ML, Katz NT. Preeclampsia: An obstetrician's perspective. *Adv Chronic Kidney Dis*. 2013; 20(3): 287–296. doi: 10.1053/j.ackd.2013.02.005

35. Magloire L, Funai, EF. Gestational hypertension. In: Basow DS, ed. *UpToDate*. Waltham, MA: UpToDate; 2015. http://www.uptodate.com/contents/gestational-hypertension. Accessed March 12, 2015.

36. Trevino H. Gestational hypertension. University of Rochester Medical Center Health Encyclopedia. http://www.urmc.rochester.edu/Encyclopedia/Content.aspx?ContentTypeID=90&ContentID=P02484. Last updated March 12, 2015. Accessed March 12, 2015.

37. Palmer, CM. Coexisting disease and other issues. In: Palmer CM, D'Angelo R, Paech MJ, eds. *Obstetric Anesthesia*. New York, NY: Oxford University Press; 2011: 314–341.

38. Turner JA. Diagnosis and management of pre-eclampsia: An update. *Int J Womens Health.* 2010; 2: 327–337. doi:10.2147/IJWH.S8550

39. August P, Sibai BM. Preeclampsia: Clinical features and diagnosis. In: Basow DS, ed. *UpToDate.* Waltham, MA: UpToDate; 2015. http://www.uptodate.com/contents/preeclampsia-clinical-features-and-diagnosis. Accessed March 12, 2015.

40. FAQs. Preeclampsia Foundation web site. http://www.preeclampsia.org/health-information/faqs. Last updated December 20, 2013. Accessed March 12, 2015.

41. Healthwise, Inc. Preeclampsia – symptoms. WebMD web site. http://www.webmd.com/baby/tc/preeclampsia-and-high-blood-pressure-during-pregnancy-symptoms. Last updated June 4, 2014. Accessed March 12, 2015.

42. HELLP syndrome. American Pregnancy Association web site. http://americanpregnancy.org/pregnancy-complications/hellp-syndrome. Last updated March 2009. Accessed March 12, 2015.

43. ACOG Committee on Obstetric Practice. ACOG Committee Opinion No. 475: Antenatal corticosteroid therapy for fetal maturation. *Obstet Gynecol.* 2011; 117(2): 422–424.

44. Ornoy A, Weber-Schöndorfer C. Hormones. In: Schaefer C, Peters P, Miller RK, eds. *Drugs During Pregnancy and Lactation: Treatment Options and Risk Assessment.* 3rd ed. Waltham, MA: Academic Press; 2015: 414–451.

45. Norwitz ER, Repke JT. Preeclampsia: Management and prognosis. In: Basow DS, ed. *UpToDate.* Waltham, MA: UpToDate; 2015. http://www.uptodate.com/contents/preeclampsia-management-and-prognosis. Accessed March 12, 2015.

46. Norwitz ER. Eclampsia. In: Basow DS, ed. *UpToDate.* Waltham, MA: UpToDate; 2015. http://www.uptodate.com/contents/eclampsia. Accessed March 12, 2015.

47. Ross MG. In: Ramus RM, ed. Medscape. http://emedicine.medscape.com/article/253960-overview#a30. Updated September 22, 2014. Accessed March 12, 2015.

48. Sibai BM. HELLP syndrome. In Basow DS, ed. *UpToDate.* Waltham, MA: UpToDate; 2015. http://www.uptodate.com/contents/hellp-syndrome. Accessed March 12, 2015.

49. Giannubilo SR, Landi B, Ciavattini A. Preeclampsia: What could happen in a subsequent pregnancy? *Obstet Gynecol Surv.* 2014; 69(12): 747–762.

50. Abildgaard U, Heimdal K. Pathogenesis of the syndrome of hemolysis, liver enzymes, and low platelet count (HELLP): A review. *Eur J Obstet Gynecol Reprod Biol.* 2013; 166(2): 117–123. doi: 10.1016/j.ejogrb.2012.09.026

51. Aydin S, Ersan F, Ark C, Aydin CA. Partial HELLP syndrome: Maternal, perinatal, subsequent pregnancy and long-term maternal outcomes. *J Obstet Gynaecol Res.* 2014; 40(4): 932–940.

52. Takahashi K, Ohkuchi A, Kobayashi M, Matsubara S, Suzuki M. Recurrence risk of hypertensive disease in pregnancy. *Med J Obstet Gynecol.* 2014; 2(2): 1023.

53. Gyamlani G, Geraci SA. Kidney disease in pregnancy. *South Med J.* 2013; 106(9): 519–525. doi: 10.1097/SMJ.0b013e3182a5f137

54. Edlow JA, Caplan LR, O'Brien K, Tibbles CD. Diagnosis of acute neurological emergencies in pregnant and post-partum women. *Lancet Neurol.* 2013; 12(2): 175–185. doi: 10.1016/S1474-4422(12)70306-X\

55. HELLP Syndrome. A.D.A.M. Medical Encyclopedia. http://www.nlm.nih.gov/medlineplus/ency/article/000890.htm. Updated November 8, 2012. Accessed March 12, 2015.

56. Khan H, Meirowitz NB. HELLP syndrome treatment & management. In: Ramus RM, ed. Medscape. http://emedicine.medscape.com/article/1394126-treatment#showall. Updated July 22, 2013. Accessed March 12, 2015.

57. Mayo Clinic Staff. Placenta previa. Mayo Clinic. http://www.mayoclinic.com/health/placenta-previa/DS00588. Reviewed May 9, 2014. Accessed March 13, 2015.

58. Rosenberg T, Pariente G, Sergienko R, Wiznitzer A, Sheiner E. Critical analysis of risk factors and outcome of placenta previa. *Arch Gynecol Obstet.* 2011; 284(1): 47–51. doi:10.1007/s00404-010-1598-7

59. Rosenberg T, Pariente G, Sergienko R, Wiznitzer A, Sheiner E. Critical analysis of risk factors and outcome of placenta previa. *Arch Gynecol Obstet.* 2011; 284(1): 47–51. doi: 10.1007/s00404-010-1598-7.

60. Lockwood CJ, Russo-Stieglitz K. Management of placenta previa. In: Basow DS, ed. *UpToDate.* Waltham, MA: UpToDate; 2015. http://www.uptodate.com/contents/management-of-placenta-previa. Accessed March 13, 2015.

61. Ananth CV, Kinzler WL. Placental abruption: Clinical features and diagnosis. In: Basow DS, ed. *UpToDate.* Waltham, MA: UpToDate; 2015. http://www.uptodate.com/contents/placental-abruption-clinical-features-and-diagnosis. Accessed March 13, 2015.

62. Mukherjee S, Bawa AK, Sharma S, Nandanwar YS, Gadam M. Retrospective study of risk factors and maternal and fetal outcome in patients with abruptio placentae. *J Nat Sc Biol Med.* 2014; 5(2): 425–428. doi: 10.4103/0976-9668.136217

63. Mbah AK, Alio AP, Fombo DW, Bruder K, Dagne G, Salihu HM. Association between cocaine abuse in pregnancy and placenta-associated syndromes using propensity score matching approach. *Early Hum Dev.* 2014; 88(6): 333–337. doi:10.1016/j.earlhumdev.2011.09.005

64. Healthwise Staff. Placenta abruptio. University of Michigan Health System. http://www.uofmhealth.org/health-library/hw180726#hw180728. Last updated June 4, 2014. Accessed March 13, 2015.

65. Placenta abruptio. A.D.A.M. Medical Encyclopedia. http://www.nlm.nih.gov/medlineplus/ency/article/000901.htm. Updated November 8, 2012. Accessed March 13, 2015.

66. Oyelese Y, Ananth CV. Placental abruption: Management. In: Basow DS, ed. *UpToDate.* Waltham, MA: UpToDate; 2015. http://www.uptodate.com/contents/placental-abruption-management. Accessed March 13, 2015.

67. Preterm labor. March of Dimes web site. http://www.marchofdimes.org/pregnancy/preterm-labor-and-premature-birth.aspx. Last reviewed October 2014. Accessed March 13, 2015.

68. Ross MG. Preterm labor. In: Smith CD, ed. Medscape. http://emedicine.medscape.com/article/260998-overview#aw2aab6b4. Updated September 29, 2014. Accessed March 13, 2015.

69. Clark EAS, Esplin S, Torres L, et al. Prevention of recurrent preterm birth: Role of the neonatal follow-up program. *Matern Child Health J.* 2014; 18(4): 858–863. doi: 10.1007/s10995-013-1311-0

70. Robinson JN, Norwitz ER. Risk factors for preterm labor and delivery. In: Basow DS, ed. *UpToDate.* Waltham, MA: UpToDate; 2015. http://www.uptodate.com/contents/risk-factors-for-preterm-labor-and-delivery. Accessed March 13, 2015.

71. Han Z, Mulla S, Beyene J, Liao G, McDonald SD. Maternal underweight and the risk of preterm birth and low birth weight: A systematic review and meta-analyses. *Int J Epidemiol.* 2011; 40(1): 65–101. doi:10.1093/ije/dyq195

72. McDonald SD, Han Z, Mulla S, Beyene J. (2010). Overweight and obesity in mothers and risk of preterm birth and low birth weight infants: Systematic review and meta-analyses. *BMJ.* 2010; 341: c3428. doi:10.1136/bmj.c3428

73. Hodyl NA, Stark MJ, Scheil W, Grzeskowiak LE, Clifton VL. Perinatal outcomes following maternal asthma and cigarette smoking during pregnancy. *Eur Respir J.* 2014; 43(3): 704–716. doi: 10.1183/09031936.00054913

74. Lockwood CJ. Overview of preterm labor and birth. In: Basow DS, ed. *UpToDate.* Waltham, MA: UpToDate; 2015. http://www.uptodate.com/contents/overview-of-preterm-labor-and-birth. Accessed March 13, 2015.

75. American College of Obstetricians and Gynecologists. FAQ—Preterm (premature) labor and birth. American College of Obstetricians and Gynecologists web site. http://www.acog.org/~/media/For%20Patients/faq087.pdf. Published July 2014. Accessed March 13, 2015.

76. Mayo Clinic Staff. Fetal fibronectin test. Mayo Clinic. http://www.mayoclinic.com/health/fetal-fibronectin/MY00128. Reviewed May 10, 2013. Accessed March 13, 2015.

77. Mayo Clinic Staff. Preterm labor. Mayo Clinic. http://www.mayoclinic.com/health/preterm-labor/DS01197/DSECTION=treatments-and-drugs. Reviewed December 4, 2014. Accessed March 13, 2015.

Chapter 3
Eye, Ear, Nose, and Throat Disorders

QUESTIONS

1. A patient states that she is unable to hear well with her left ear. The Weber test shows lateralization to the right ear. The Rinne test shows AC>BC with a ratio of 2:1 in both ears, left AC 4 sec. and BC 2 sec., right AC 20 sec. and BC 10 sec. What would be the best interpretation of these results?

   a. The test results are reflective of normal hearing.

   b. Conduction of sound through bones is impaired.

   c. The patient may have sensorineural hearing loss.

   d. Further testing should be done.

2. Of the following, which condition is most likely to develop as a result of pressure on the cornea in cases of chalazia?

   a. Glaucoma

   b. Astigmatism

   c. Arcus senilis

   d. Presbyopia

3. Which of the following pathogens is least likely to cause acute sinusitis in the adult-gerontology patient?

   a. *Streptococcus pneumoniae*

   b. *Haemophilus influenzae*

   c. *Staphylococcus aureus*

   d. *Moraxella catarrhalis*

4. The American Academy of Ophthalmology recommends that all patients receive a complete screening for glaucoma by at least what age?

   a. By age 25

   b. By age 30

   c. By age 35

   d. By age 40

5. Shawn, a 23-year-old male, has been experiencing nasal mucosal discharge, headache, cough, and malaise for approximately 5 days. You suspect that he has a cold. Which of the following findings would best suggest an alternative diagnosis?

   a. He has a sore throat.

   b. His nasal passages are occasionally blocked.

   c. He continuously sneezes.

   d. He has occasional muscle aches.

6. What are hyperopia and myopia also known as, respectively?

   a. Astigmatism and farsightedness

   b. Farsightedness and nearsightedness

   c. Astigmatism and nearsightedness

   d. Nearsightedness and farsightedness

7. Your patient lives in Palm Desert and presents to your practice with this finding. He describes it as painless, though sometimes it "feels like there's something sticking to my eye." What is the diagnosis?

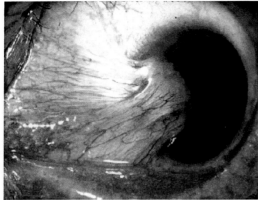

Figure 3.1.

   a. Conjunctivitis

   b. Hordeolum

   c. Pterygium

   d. Cataracts

8. Which of the following findings is present in 90% of all cases of cholesteatoma?

   a. Painful otorrhea

   b. Ear canal filled with cerumen

   c. Tympanic membrane perforation

   d. Localized furuncles

9. When performing an eye exam, if you have difficulty visualizing the macula, what instruction should you give the patient?

   a. "Look into the light."

   b. "Look slightly upward."

   c. "Look at an object on the distant wall."

   d. "Look downward."

10. Which of the following does not accurately describe the usual mucosal findings of a patient with a typical case of sinusitis?

    a. Dry

    b. Reddened

    c. Foul-smelling

    d. Discolored

11. A patient presents with hearing loss and painless otorrhea. Upon physical exam, you note the canal is filled with mucopus and granulation tissue. Tympanic perforation and ossicular damage are also noted. As a nurse practitioner, how would you best treat this patient's condition?

    a. Prescribe antibiotics and recommend hydration

    b. Refer the patient for surgery

    c. Refer the patient for a general neurological exam

    d. Prescribe prednisone

12. A patient presents with complaints of a burning sensation in the left eye. A physical examination reveals redness and watery, nonpurulent discharge. The patient presents with no other physical symptoms or sensations. Based on the patient's signs and symptoms, which type of conjunctivitis is the most likely diagnosis?

    a. Bacterial conjunctivitis

    b. Gonococcal conjunctivitis

    c. Allergic conjunctivitis

    d. Viral conjunctivitis

13. A male patient in his early 20s who was diagnosed with a stye in his left eye has been applying a warm compress to the affected area for more than a week as part of a home remedy. Despite this treatment, the patient's stye is still present. What further treatment would be best to recommend at this time?

    a. Refer the patient for surgical removal.

    b. Prescribe erythromycin topical ointment.

    c. Recommend the patient scrub and rinse his lashes and lid margins.

    d. Begin a course of systemic antibiotics.

14. You are treating a 52-year-old female diagnosed with chronic glaucoma. The patient is most likely to state which of the following?

    a. "My eye hurts really bad."

    b. "My vision has become blurry."

    c. "It's harder to see objects that are on the side of me."

    d. "I've started seeing spots."

15. After observing a red reflex, a fundoscopic exam should proceed from the optic disc and end at which part of the eye?

    a. Macula

    b. Veins

    c. Fovea centralis

    d. Arteries

16. Which of the following findings typically distinguishes a viral form of pharyngitis from a bacterial form of the condition?

    a. Fever

    b. Erythematous pharynx

    c. Painful throat

    d. Rhinorrhea

17. A 48-year-old male presents with difficulty maintaining a clear visual focus at a near distance. He notes that he has never experienced vision-related conditions until recently. You would know that which of these is the most likely diagnosis?

    a. Hyperopia

    b. Myopia

    c. Presbyopia

    d. Arcus senilis

18. For a patient diagnosed with bacterial acute otitis media, which of these medications is usually recommended for first-line treatment?

    a. Amoxicillin

    b. Miconazole

    c. Ceftriaxone

    d. Clotrimazole

19. Of the following, which treatment is best employed to treat severely enlarged tonsils in cases of mononucleosis?

    a. Antibiotics

    b. Hydration

    c. Referral for surgery

    d. Prednisone taper

20. Which of the following medications would be the best first-line treatment for a patient with gonococcal pharyngitis?

    a. Levofloxacin

    b. Penicillin V

    c. Prednisone taper

    d. Ceftriaxone

21. A patient presents with the following abscess and reports that it appeared suddenly, presenting with pain in the surrounding area. Of the following, which condition is the patient most likely experiencing?

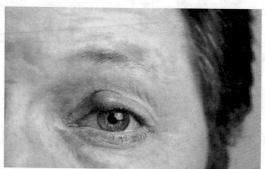

Figure 3.2.

    a. Conjunctivitis

    b. Hordeolum

    c. Chalazion

    d. Blepharitis

22. Neuraminidase inhibitors can shorten the duration of symptoms of influenza by approximately how many days?

    a. Two days

    b. Four days

    c. Six days

    d. Eight days

23. A patient's vision is recorded as 20/40 using the Snellen eye chart. What does this mean?

    a. The patient can read at 40 feet what a person with normal vision can read at 20 feet.

    b. The patient can read the chart from 20 feet in the left eye and 40 feet in the right eye.

    c. The patient can read at 20 feet what a person with normal vision can read at 40 feet.

    d. The patient can read the entire chart at 40 feet, indicating what a person with normal vision can do.

24. Chlamydial conjunctivitis would most likely be treated with all of the following <u>except</u>:

    a. Erythromycin

    b. Doxycycline

    c. Ceftriaxone

    d. Clarithromycin

25. Which of the following is the most frequent site of nose bleeds?

    a. Anterior septum

    b. Superior septum

    c. Posterior septum

    d. Inferior septum

26. Of the following causes of conductive hearing loss, which is the most common?

    a. Perforated tympanic membrane

    b. Hematoma

    c. Foreign body

    d. Otosclerosis

27. A 62-year-old male patient presents with cloudy vision in a single eye. In addition, he complains of glare coming off of bright lights and difficulty with night vision. Which of the following is the most likely diagnosis?

    a. Chalazion

    b. Cataracts

    c. Conjunctivitis

    d. Glaucoma

28. A patient presents with a white, pimple-like, small lesion protruding on his eyelid. It is tender, firm, and discrete. Which of the following should you most likely chart?

    a. Dacryocystitis

    b. Hordeolum

    c. Blepharitis

    d. Ectropion

29. A healthy, fit, 41-year-old male says that he has been experiencing several problems that manifested about two days ago after his head was slammed onto the mat while wrestling at a mixed martial arts school. His initial complaints were dizziness and ringing in the ears. Since then, he has been experiencing short periods of dizziness and disorientation, ringing in the ears, and blurred vision. An ear exam shows no signs of inflammation or exudate. The patient may require a further diagnostic assessment for all of the following conditions <u>except</u>:

    a. Retinal detachment

    b. Vertigo

    c. Otitis externa

    d. Hearing loss

30. Nonviral otitis media is most commonly caused by what pathogenic bacteria?

    a. *Staphylococcus aureus*

    b. *Streptococcus pneumoniae*

    c. *Haemophilus influenzae*

    d. *Moraxella catarrhalis*

31. Your patient complains that his eyes "just aren't the same color anymore." What is the most likely diagnosis, given this picture?

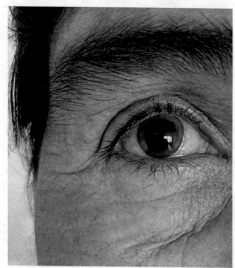

Figure 3.3.

   a. Fovea centralis

   b. Pterygium

   c. Arcus senilis

   d. Presbyopia

32. During an eye exam, a patient's optic cup-to-disc ratio indicates that the size of the optic cup is larger than one half of the diameter of the optic disc. Which optic disease does this finding most strongly indicate?

   a. Cataract

   b. Retinal detachment

   c. Glaucoma

   d. Conjunctivitis

33. An elderly male presents with symptoms that include a burning sensation in the eye and red, scaly flakes around the eyelids, which are covered with thick crusts. Based on the patient's presentation, which of the following medications should be prescribed to treat the patient's condition?

   a. Levofloxacin or ofloxacin

   b. Ofloxacin or erythromycin

   c. Bacitracin or erythromycin

   d. Ciprofloxacin or bacitracin

34. A patient comes to your practice with symptoms of fever, rhinorrhea, and pain in the throat. Suspecting strep pharyngitis, you assess the patient under the guidelines of the Centor criteria. Under these standards, which of these findings would not be confirmatory for strep pharyngitis?

   a. Pharyngo-tonsillar exudate

   b. Presence of persistent cough

   c. Fever of 100.6 °F

   d. Anterior cervical adenopathy

35. Joe, a 54-year-old male, comes to your practice with complaints of frequent drainage in his ear and decreased hearing. Upon looking at his medical history, you notice that he has been experiencing these symptoms on and off for about two years. You examine his ear with an otoscope, and discover that his tympanic membrane is perforated. In addition, his ear canal is filled with mucopus and peeling layers of scaly epithelium. Which of the following conditions does the patient most likely have?

   a. Otitis externa

   b. Furunculosis

   c. Acute otitis media

   d. Cholesteatoma

36. Cataracts are most commonly associated with which condition?

   a. Diabetes

   b. Hypertension

   c. Hypercholesterolemia

   d. Retinal artery occlusion

37. You are treating Peter, a 47-year-old male, who exhibits symptoms of sensorineural hearing loss. In order to determine the cause of his condition, you obtain the patient's history. You know that the following factors may usually contribute to this type of hearing loss except:

   a. Close range to an explosion

   b. Acoustic neuroma

   c. Perforated tympanic membrane

   d. Long-term exposure to loud music

38. If a patient with a sore throat has been advised to avoid contact sports, his condition most likely stems from which of the following viruses?

    a. Respiratory syncytial virus

    b. Adenovirus

    c. Epstein-Barr virus

    d. Rhinovirus

39. During an eye exam, a 65-year-old man complains of blurred vision and flashes of light in his periphery, which began to manifest within the past day. A look over his medical history reveals the patient was diagnosed with type 2 diabetes mellitus at age 55. Given these findings, which of these is the most likely eye condition, and how would the nurse practitioner best manage this condition?

    a. Retinal detachment and should be referred to a surgeon

    b. Glaucoma and should be treated with miotic agents

    c. Cataract and should be referred to the ophthalmologist for glasses or surgery

    d. Subconjunctival hemorrhage and should be treated with an ice compress

40. All of the following treatment options are commonly used to manage vertigo except:

    a. Meclizine

    b. Diazepam

    c. Prednisone

    d. Scopolamine transdermal patch

RATIONALES

1. c

When a patient has sensorineural hearing loss, the Weber test usually causes the sound to lateralize to the unaffected ear, whereas the Rinne test would typically show air conduction (AC) as greater than bone conduction (BC). Normal hearing usually results in equal sound lateralization with the Weber test and AC that is twice as long as BC with the Rinne test. Using the Weber test on a patient with conductive loss would typically result in sound lateralization to the poorer ear, whereas the BC for such a patient would typically be equal to or greater than AC with the Rinne test.

2. b

In cases of chalazia, pressure on the cornea may lead to astigmatism. In contrast, glaucoma usually develops as a consequence of increased intraocular pressure as opposed to corneal pressure. Arcus senilis often develops as a result of lipid deposits, not corneal pressure. Presbyopia usually occurs as a result of aging and results in difficulty maintaining a clear focus of close objects.

3. c

Staphylococcus aureus is not one of the common causes of acute sinusitis; rather, it is more likely to cause chronic sinusitis. *Streptococcus pneumoniae, Haemophilus influenzae,* and *Moraxella catarrhalis* are all more common causes of acute sinusitis than *S. aureus.*

4. d

The American Academy of Ophthalmology recommends a complete screening for glaucoma every 4 years starting at the age of 40. Before that age, patients are expected to receive a screening for visual acuity every 3 years, but not a complete exam.

5. d

The common cold and influenza share similar signs and symptoms that include mucosal discharge, headache, cough, and malaise; however, patients diagnosed with influenza are more likely to experience muscle soreness and body aches, which typically present lightly, if at all, in patients with the common cold. A sore throat, blocked nasal passages, and sneezing would all help to confirm the initial diagnosis of the common cold.

6. b

Hyperopia is known as farsightedness, or difficulty seeing close objects, whereas myopia is known as nearsightedness, or difficulty seeing distant objects. Astigmatism refers to shaping of the cornea or lens that alters the orientation of the light rays.

7. c

Pterygium is typically characterized by raised, wedge-shaped growths of thin, noncancerous tissue over the conjunctiva. Although conjunctivitis also affects the conjunctiva, it is usually characterized by inflammation, infection, and an itching sensation, rather than a growth of noncancerous tissue. Hordeola do not typically affect the conjunctiva, but instead manifest as localized, tender masses that develop in the eyelid. Lastly, cataracts involve clouding and opacification of the normally clear lens of the eye and have little direct effect on the conjunctiva.

8. c

Approximately 90% of cholesteatoma patients present with tympanic membrane perforation. Otorrhea is often noted with cholesteatoma, but it is typically painless. The ear canal of a patient with cholesteatoma is usually obstructed by layers of scaly or keratinized epithelium, not cerumen. Lastly, cholesteatoma does not usually cause localized furuncles.

9. a

A patient should look directly into the light of the ophthalmoscope if the nurse practitioner has difficulty visualizing the macula. Asking a patient to look downward, slightly upward, or at an object on the distant wall will not typically help to visualize the macula.

10. a

A dry nasal mucosa does not typically present in patients with sinusitis. Sinusitis is more often indicated by a nasal mucosa that is reddened, foul-smelling, or discolored.

11. b

Cholesteatoma is a type of chronic otitis media characterized by painless otorrhea, mucopus and granulation tissue in the ear canal, tympanic membrane perforation, and ossicular damage; the best form of management for a patient who presents with these symptoms is usually referral to a surgeon for excision. Although hearing loss (due to ossicular damage) may be an indication for a general neurological exam, this exam is not the first-line protocol when symptoms such as tympanic membrane perforation are experienced by the patient. Although antibiotics and corticosteroids such as prednisone may be recommended for serous otitis media, a condition that often contributes to cholesteatoma, drug therapy is not a mainstay of cholesteatoma treatment.

12. d

A patient experiencing a burning sensation in the eye, as well as redness and watery discharge, is most likely experiencing viral conjunctivitis. Although other forms of conjunctivitis also involve redness and a burning sensation in the eye, these forms typically present with a different quality and quantity of discharge. Bacterial and gonococcal forms of conjunctivitis are both characterized by purulent discharge, with gonococcal conjunctivitis often exhibiting a particularly copious discharge. Allergic conjunctivitis, on the other hand, more commonly presents with string-like discharge and an itching sensation, whereas viral conjunctivitis often presents with watery discharge and no itch.

13. b

Since the warm compress has proven ineffective in treating the patient's hordeolum, the best course of treatment for the patient would be an antibiotic ointment, such as erythromycin. Systemic antibiotics are usually reserved for cases where the patient's hordeolum displays signs of preseptal cellulitis. A referral for surgical removal would not be advised at this time, as the patient should continue conventional treatment first. Scrubbing and rinsing the lashes and lid margins is not typically recommended for treatment of hordeolum, but is often recommended in cases of blepharitis.

14. c

Although chronic glaucoma is usually asymptomatic, patients may complain of a reduction in peripheral vision due to angle closure. Extreme pain, blurred vision, and dilated pupils are all symptoms more commonly found in acute glaucoma than chronic glaucoma.

15. c

A standard fundoscopic exam should proceed from the optic disc and end at the fovea centralis of each eye. Although a patient's veins, macula, and arteries would all be observed in a fundoscopic exam, none of these would traditionally serve as the end point of the exam.

16. d

Of the choices, rhinorrhea is often the most distinguishing sign of viral pharyngitis, as it does not typically produce in cases of bacterial pharyngitis. A painful throat, fever, and an erythematous pharynx can often be found in both forms of the disease and would not serve to distinguish bacterial pharyngitis from viral pharyngitis.

17. c

The patient's difficulty maintaining a clear visual focus at a near distance most likely indicates that he should be evaluated for presbyopia, which most commonly presents after the age of 40. Hyperopia, which is also known as farsightedness, also involves difficulty focusing on nearby objects; however, it is more often a defect of vision present at birth rather than a condition that develops with age. Myopia, also known as nearsightedness, causes difficulty in focusing on far objects, not near ones. Lastly, arcus senilis usually has no effect on vision; rather, the condition presents with a gray or white arc in the periphery of the cornea.

18. a

A patient diagnosed with a bacterial case of acute otitis media (OM) would most likely be treated with amoxicillin. Ceftriaxone may be used to treat OM but is not usually recommended for first-line treatment, due to the rise of multi-drug resistant *Streptococcus pneumoniae*. Clotrimazole and miconazole are antifungal medications and would not be indicated for a bacterial infection.

19. d

Severely enlarged tonsils resulting from mononucleosis would typically be treated with a prednisone taper. Antibiotics see use in cases of bacterial infections that produce enlarged tonsils, such as tonsillitis; however, mononucleosis is a viral infection and would not usually require antibiotics. Although hydration may form a part of supportive care in cases of mononucleosis, it does not usually provide effective treatment for severely enlarged tonsils. Lastly, referral for surgery is not likely to be recommended in cases of enlarged tonsils.

20. d

Gonococcal pharyngitis should typically be treated with ceftriaxone, as it treats the infection itself instead of just maintaining the symptoms produced by the infection. Levofloxacin does not typically see use in the treatment of bacterial pharyngitis and is more often used to treat pneumonia and sinusitis. Although penicillin V is also used to treat pharyngitis, it is typically prescribed only for streptococcal infections. Finally, prednisone tapers may be used to reduce inflammation but would not serve much use in treating the underlying infection.

21. b

A patient presenting with a painful abscess on the upper or lower eyelid is most likely experiencing a hordeolum. Conjunctivitis would more commonly present with inflammation and swelling, rather than a single abscess. Chalazion may present as an abscess but does not typically present with pain. Blepharitis usually produces greasy flakes on the eyelid margins, which are not depicted in the figure.

22. a

Findings show that neuraminidase inhibitors, such as oseltamivir, can shorten the duration of symptoms of influenza by approximately 2 days. Current research does not support the contention that neuraminidase inhibitors shorten influenza symptoms by any duration of time longer than 2 days.

23. c

The term 20/40 means that the patient can see at 20 feet what a normal person with perfect vision can see at 40 feet. The term does not pertain to the difference in vision between the left and right eye.

24. c

Gonococcal, rather than chlamydial, conjunctivitis would typically be treated with an intramuscular dosing of ceftriaxone. Chlamydial conjunctivitis is usually treated with erythromycin, doxycycline, or clarithromycin. Other oral medications that often see use in cases of chlamydial conjunctivitis include azithromycin and tetracycline.

25. a

The most frequent site of nose bleeds is the anterior septum. Nose bleeds that present in the posterior septum are typically less common and more complicated than nosebleeds in the anterior septum. The superior septum and inferior septum do not exist.

26. c

Foreign bodies in the ear canal, along with cerumen build-up, are the most common and most treatable causes of conductive hearing loss. Hematoma, tympanic membrane perforation, and otosclerosis are also likely causes of conductive hearing loss, but are not as common as foreign bodies.

27. b

A patient experiencing cloudy vision in a single eye, glare from bright lights, and difficulty with vision at night is most likely to be diagnosed with cataracts. Although chalazia may present with changes to vision, it usually presents with other distinctive symptoms such as swelling on the eyelid, eyelid tenderness, and increased tearing, which are not part of the patient's presentation. Conjunctivitis is often characterized by blurred vision and sensation of a foreign body in the eye, but does not typically present with glare from bright lights or difficulty with vision at night. Lastly, glaucoma is typically either asymptomatic, if chronic, or presents with pain, if acute.

28. b

White, pimple-like lesions on the eyelid that are tender and discrete are characteristic of hordeolum. Although dacryocystitis may present with a palpable mass, it most commonly results in pain, tenderness, and edema of the lacrimal sac. Blepharitis affects the eyelids, but usually produces red, scaly flakes rather than white lesions. Lastly, ectropion occurs when the eyelid margin turns outwards, which usually causes irritated, red, or watery eyes.

29. c

A patient who experienced head trauma would not typically receive further diagnostic assessment for otitis externa (OE); although OE may be caused by ear trauma, it typically does not present with alterations in vision. Further, pain, itching, and erythema are more prominent symptoms in patients with OE; dizziness, tinnitus, and vision problems are more likely to be attributed to the other listed conditions. Retinal detachment, vertigo, and hearing loss can be caused by head trauma. Retinal detachment could potentially be indicated by blurred vision, hearing loss could cause tinnitus, and vertigo could explain the dizziness and disorientation.

30. b

Streptococcus pneumoniae is the most common bacterial cause of otitis media and is responsible for approximately 40%–50% of all cases. *Staphylococcus aureus* may produce bacterial otitis media, but is not one of the three most common pathogens. Although *Haemophilus influenzae* and *Moraxella catarrhalis* are both known to cause serous otitis media, these pathogenic bacteria are not as prevalent as *S. pneumoniae* in cases of serous otitis media. *H. influenzae* is responsible for 20%–30% of all cases, whereas *M. catarrhalis* is responsible for 10%–15% of all cases.

31. c

Arcus senilis typically presents with a gray or white arc in the periphery of the cornea, which may eventually form a circle. Pterygium, on the other hand, is characterized by a raised, wedge-shaped growth of thin, noncancerous tissue over the conjunctiva. Presbyopia is usually caused by decreasing flexibility of the crystalline lens and weakening of the ciliary muscles that control lens focusing; however, it does not typically present with an arc. Lastly, fovea centralis does not refer to a condition of visual acuity, but a 2.5 mm-diameter reflective area in the center of the macular region of the eye.

32. c

If the size of a patient's optic cup is larger than one half of the optic disc during an eye exam, glaucoma should be considered. The pathology of cataracts typically consists of clouding and opacification of the eye lens, which is normally clear. Retinal detachment is more commonly detected through pupil reaction and an external examination for signs of trauma, particularly in the vitreous. Lastly, conjunctivitis typically manifests as inflammation with possible infection of the conjunctiva.

33. c

Based on the patient's symptoms, blepharitis is the most likely condition, which is typically treated with bacitracin or erythromycin. Levofloxacin, ofloxacin, and ciprofloxacin are antibiotics more commonly used to treat bacterial conjunctivitis, and have not been shown to be more effective than bacitracin or erythromycin in treating blepharitis.

34. b

The lack of cough, rather than the presence of a persistent cough, is considered an indicator for strep pharyngitis under the Centor criteria. However, as the Centor criteria use a points system for positive findings to determine likelihood of strep pharyngitis, the presence of a cough does not rule out the condition. Other positive findings for strep pharyngitis under the Centor criteria include a fever higher than 100.4 °F, pharyngo-tonsillar exudate, and anterior cervical adenopathy.

35. d

Cholesteatoma is the most likely diagnosis in this patient, as it typically presents with otorrhea, hearing loss, layers of scaly epithelium, a mucopus-filled ear canal, and a perforated tympanic membrane. Cholesteatoma is more likely to produce from chronic otitis media and other chronic ear infections than from acute otitis media. Otitis externa is caused by inflammation or infection of the external auditory canal; although the condition may present with hearing loss and discharge, it does not usually present with peeling layers of scaly epithelium. Furunculosis of the ear may likewise present with hearing loss and discharge upon bursting, but does not typically present with perforated membrane or for long-term durations.

36. a

Cataracts may derive from a variety of causes including aging, diabetes, heredity, tobacco use, and alcohol consumption, among others. This phenomenon does not typically occur as a direct result of hypertension, hypercholesterolemia, or retinal artery occlusion.

37. c

A perforated tympanic membrane is considered a conductive cause of hearing loss, not a sensorineural cause of hearing loss. A perforated tympanic membrane involves damage to the middle ear; this type of damage most often results in conductive hearing loss, which occurs when sound is not properly conducted through the outer ear canal to the eardrum and ossicles (tiny bones) of the middle ear. On the other hand, acoustic neuroma and exposure to loud noises, be it short-term or long-term, are considered sensorineural causes of hearing loss; this type of hearing loss is often a result of damage to the cochlea (inner ear), or to the nerve pathways from the inner ear to the brain.

38. c

Patients with mononucleosis, which is an infection caused by the Epstein-Barr virus, are advised to avoid contact sports for up to a month to limit the risk of splenic rupture. The respiratory syncytial virus, which often produces cold-like symptoms in adults and pneumonia in children, does not usually require limiting one's involvement in strenuous activities in order to avoid organ damage. The common cold can be caused by the rhinovirus or the adenovirus; these viruses do not typically increase the risk of splenic rupture.

39. a

The appearance of flashes of light, especially in peripheral vision, and blurred vision are often symptoms of retinal detachment, which may produce as a result of diabetic retinopathy. Glaucoma and cataracts may also be experienced by a patient with advanced diabetes, but both conditions are more likely to present with halos of light rather than flashes of light in the periphery. Finally, subconjunctival hemorrhage does not typically cause changes in vision.

40. c

Prednisone, a corticosteroid, is not regularly used in treating vertigo and is more commonly prescribed to treat inflammatory diseases. Antihistamines, such as meclizine, and benzodiazepines, such as diazepam, may be used to suppress vestibular symptoms of vertigo; given the risks associated with benzodiazepines, however, antihistamines should be used as first-line treatment. Furthermore, scopolamine transdermal patches may be used to prevent nausea and vomiting triggered by the sensation of motion sickness that accompanies vertigo.

DISCUSSION

Assessment of the Eye

Overview

During the fundoscopic exam, the examiner uses his or her right hand for the ophthalmoscope while using his or her right eye to look into the patient's right eye.[1] With the lens wheel set at zero diopters, the examiner begins the procedure at a distance of about 12 inches from the patient and moves in to a distance of 12 inches from the patient's eye.[2] Throughout the procedure, the examiner should function as one with the ophthalmoscope. Upon obtaining a red reflex, the exam should move from the back of the eye to the optic disk. The exam then progresses from the optic disk to the fovea centralis.

Upon inspection, the optic disc should appear to be shaped like a doughnut. The disc should have a white depression in the center of the eye (i.e., the physiologic cup) and an orange or pink area surrounding the cup (i.e., the neuroretinal rim).[3] The physiologic cup should not exceed half the size of the disc diameter; if the physiologic cup exceeds half the size of the disc's diameter, the patient should be considered for a glaucoma screening. The retinal arteries are often thinner and a brighter shade of red than the veins; hence, the arteries-to-veins ratio for visualization is expected to be 2:3 or 3:4.[4]

The macula is an avascular oval-shaped area of the retina that expands temporally from the optic disc, covering an area of approximately two to two-and-a-half disc diameters.[5] The fovea centralis, which is located in the macular region, is a slightly darker reflective area that extends 2.5 mm in diameter. If visualizing the macula during the fundoscopic exam is difficult, the examiner should order the patient to focus his or her gaze directly on the ophthalmoscope's light.

A Snellen eye chart measures visual acuity according to the 20/20 standard—the patient should be able to see at 20 feet what people with normal eyesight can see at 20 feet. Hence, a larger denominator value on the Snellen chart typically indicates visual impairment. Hyperopia (i.e., "farsightedness") and myopia (i.e., "nearsightedness") are common refractive disorders and correctable causes of impaired vision.[6] Presbyopia, on the other hand, is a non-refractive disorder that is common after the age of 40. Due to reduced flexibility in the crystalline lens and weakened ciliary muscles, it is difficult to maintain a distinct focus at a close distance.

Some abnormalities may present with no effect on vision. Arcus senilis, for instance, presents as a cloudy tint to the cornea with a gray or white accumulation that forms an arc or circle around the limbus, stemming from lipid deposits. Similarly, pterygium is a raised growth of noncancerous tissue over the conjunctiva, typically presenting as thin and wedge-shaped.

Hordeolum (Stye)

Overview

A hordeolum is an acute and commonly infectious inflammation of the eyelid that is usually caused by *Staphylococcus aureus*.[7]

Presentation

A hordeolum is characterized by a localized, tender mass developing in the eyelid. This disorder is abrupt in onset and accompanied by pain and erythema of the eyelid.

Workup

A hordeolum may be diagnosed by the clinical presentation, which reveals a focal collection of polymorphonuclear leukocytes and necrotic tissue in a small abscess.[8]

Treatment

A hordeolum is treated with warm compresses, topical bacitracin, or erythromycin ophthalmic ointment during the acute stage. If the hordeolum is not resolved despite continued treatment, the patient should be referred to an ophthalmologist for possible incision.[9]

Chalazion

Overview

A chalazion is a beady, painless nodule on the eyelid stemming from the meibomian gland, typically resulting from infection or from obstruction of the gland's excretory duct.

Presentation

Chalazia usually present on the upper eyelid and are characterized by hard, nontender swelling. Common findings include sensitivity to light, increased tearing, redness, and swelling of adjacent conjunctiva. If very large, chalazia may exert pressure upon the cornea, distorting vision and causing astigmatism.[10]

Workup

Chalazia are normally diagnosed on the basis of appearance. If drainage is present, it should be collected for culture.[11]

Treatment

In most cases, warm compresses are sufficient for the treatment of chalazia. Symptomatic patients can be referred to an ophthalmologist for surgical removal.[12]

Blepharitis

Overview

Blepharitis is an inflammatory condition of the eyelid often caused by staphylococcal infection or obstruction of eyelid glands. A more chronic form of the condition may also present as a result of seborrheic dermatitis of the lid edge.[13]

Presentation

Patients with blepharitis typically present with red, scaly, greasy flakes on the eyelid skin and thickened, crusted lid margins. Other findings may include burning, itching, and tearing.

Workup

Blepharitis does not require laboratory tests or diagnostic procedures, although slit lamp evaluation may be performed when patients are referred to ophthalmology for evaluation.[14]

Treatment

Blepharitis is typically treated with hot, moist compresses to the eyes and baby shampoo scrubs. If there is a bacterial component, erythromycin ointment may be applied at bedtime.[13]

Conjunctivitis

Overview

Conjunctivitis, also known as pink-eye, is the most common eye disorder seen in primary care. Conjunctivitis is usually caused by a virus (e.g., adenovirus), but inflammation can also result from allergies, chemical irritation, bacterial sources (e.g., *Staphylococcus, Streptococcus, Haemophilus influenzae*) and by gonococcal or chlamydial conjunctivitis infection. Less commonly seen viral infections include herpes simplex and zoster.

Presentation

Signs and symptoms of conjunctivitis may include itching, burning, redness, and increased tearing. Patients do not usually complain of pain or loss of vision, although blurred vision is possible in some cases. In addition, patients may present with swelling of eyelids, as well as the sensation of foreign matter on the eye or inside the eyelid. Eyelids may show discharge, which varies depending on the type of conjunctivitis. Bacterial conjunctivitis presents in one eye with purulent discharge, whereas gonococcal and chlamydial conjunctivitis both commonly produce copious amounts of purulent discharge. In contrast, viral conjunctivitis often presents with profuse watery discharge, and allergic conjunctivitis is characterized by stringy discharge and increased tearing.

Workup

Conjunctivitis is diagnosed by exclusion. A patient presenting with a red eye and discharge can often be diagnosed with conjunctivitis if the vision is normal and there is no evidence of keratitis, iritis, or closed angle glaucoma.[15]

Treatment

Specific treatment options depend on the etiology of conjunctivitis. Although bacterial conjunctivitis is often self-limiting, it may be treated with ophthalmic antibiotic drops such as trimethoprim/polymixin (Polytrim), azithromycin, erythromycin (Ilotycin), sulfacetamide sodium (Bleph-10), or tobramycin (Tobrex). Gonococcal conjunctivitis is usually managed with intramuscular ceftriaxone (Rocephin), whereas chlamydial conjunctivitis can be treated with erythromycin or azithromycin ophthalmic ointment, as well as oral antibiotics such as erythromycin (Benzamycin), azithromycin (Zithromax), or doxycycline (Monodox). Allergic conjunctivitis is often treated with oral antihistamines and/or drops including ketotifen (Zaditor, Alaway), ketorolac (Acular), or azelastine (Optivar), whereas viral conjunctivitis calls for symptomatic care with artificial tears, topical antihistamines, or decongestants.[16] Herpetic conjunctivitis should be immediately referred to an ophthalmologist for treatment.

Glaucoma

Overview

Glaucoma is a disease characterized by increased intraocular pressure. The condition causes vision loss and may lead to blindness. Glaucoma is divided into two categories: open-angle glaucoma and closed-angle glaucoma.

Presentation

Open-angle glaucoma is a chronic disease that is often asymptomatic. The condition is characterized by increased intraocular pressure, cupping of the disc, and constriction of visual fields. If untreated, open-angle glaucoma takes approximately 25 years to result in complete blindness.[17] Closed-angle glaucoma is an acute condition that involves extreme pain. In addition, this disorder commonly presents with blurred vision, halos surrounding lights in the field of vision, and dilated or fixed pupils.

Workup

The most reliable screening test for glaucoma is tonometry, which measures intraocular pressure.[18] Tonometry screening is nationally recommended for patients age 40 and older.

Treatment

Open-angle glaucoma is managed with alpha 2-adrenegic agonists (e.g., brimonidine), beta-adrenergic blockers (e.g., timolol), and miotic agents (e.g., pilocarpine). In addition, topical prostaglandins may be prescribed as initial therapy to reduce intraocular pressure.[19] Carbonic anhydrase inhibitors such as dorzolamide and brinzolamide are preferred over systemic acetazolamide (Diamox) and osmotic diuretics (e.g., mannitol). Patients with suspected closed angle glaucoma require immediate referral to the emergency department.[20,21]

Cataracts

Overview

Cataracts are characterized by the manifestation of clouding and opacity in the lens of the eye, which is normally clear. Cataracts are the leading cause of treatable blindness.[22] Senile cataracts are the most common condition requiring surgical intervention in patients over 65 years of age.

Presentation

Cataracts are caused by several factors, including aging, heredity, diabetes, trauma, and ultraviolet sunlight exposure.[23] Toxins, drugs, tobacco, and alcohol consumption may also contribute to the development of this disorder. Cataracts are painless and characterized by clouded, blurred, or dim vision. Other common signs and symptoms include halos surrounding lights in the patient's field of vision, difficulty with vision at night, sensitivity to light and glare, and diplopia in a single eye. The patient may see fading or yellowing of colors and require brighter illumination to carry out normal activities such as reading.

Workup

Cataracts are commonly diagnosed by a non-dilated fundoscopic examination, which would reveal an altered red reflex (e.g., dark spot or generally diminished) and clouding of the lens. With advanced cataracts, the pupil will typically appear white.

Treatment

Cataracts require a referral to an ophthalmologist. As cataracts develop, the patient will require vision correction with corrective lenses. Surgery is necessary when cataracts markedly decrease visual acuity. The surgery may involve cataract extraction and artificial lens implants.[24]

Retinal Detachment

Overview

Retinal detachment is a separation of the light-sensitive membrane from its supporting layers, which are located in the back of the eye.[25]

Presentation

Patients with retinal detachment present with blurred vision, floaters in the eye, flashes of light in their peripheral vision, and discrepancies such as shadows or blindness in a portion of the visual field of one eye.[26]

Workup

Patients presenting with common signs and symptoms of retinal detachment should undergo a test of visual acuity and confrontational evaluation of visual fields. Other screening procedures for retinal detachment include slit-lamp biomicroscopy and a dilated retinal examination.[27]

Treatment

Retinal detachment requires surgical intervention. A minor retinal detachment can be treated with delimiting laser photocoagulation or a cryoretinopexy barrier, whereas advanced retinal detachment may call for a pneumatic retinopexy, temporary peribulbar balloon, scleral buckle placement, or pars plana vitrectomy.[28]

Otitis Externa

Overview

Otitis externa is an inflammation or infection of the external auditory canal.[29] It is commonly differentiated as the following types: acute localized (i.e., furunculosis), acute diffuse bacterial (i.e., swimmer's ear), chronic, fungal, and eczematous. Acute diffuse bacterial otitis externa is most common among swimmers and people living in hot, humid climates.

Presentation

Acute diffuse bacterial otitis externa is caused by a bacterial infection and is characterized by pain with tenderness of the tragus and pinna. Mild cases present with fullness or itchiness. Otorrhea is common, with debris, redness, and edema in the external canal often obscuring the tympanic membrane and causing hearing loss. Preauricular lymphadenopathy and fever may be present, which may indicate local cellulitis.[13]

Acute localized otitis externa is usually caused by *S. aureus* and is characterized by pustules and furuncles manifesting in the ear canal, typically in the outer third of the area. This condition commonly presents with itching, erythema, scaling, crusting, fissuring, severe pain with areas of cellulitis, and possible exudates.

Workup

Otitis externa can usually be diagnosed after completing a patient history and physical examination. Culture screening is recommended for patients with severe otitis externa, immunocompromised patients, and those who do not respond to initial therapy.[30]

Treatment

The initial step in treatment of otitis externa is cleansing and debridement of the ear canal. Additional management options include other topical antibiotic and steroid otic drops (e.g., Cortisporin Otic) or antibiotic drops alone (e.g., Ciloxan or Tobrex), in addition to pain control with oral nonsteroidal anti-inflammatory drugs (NSAIDs) or acetaminophen.[13]

Acute/Serous Otitis Media

Overview

Acute otitis media and serous otitis media are marked by fluid accumulation in the middle ear, presenting alongside signs and symptoms of infection. Chronic otitis media that results in effusion is classified as serous otitis media; this condition typically causes an excess of inflammatory drainage in the middle ear cleft without other signs of inflammation.[31] Otitis media is most commonly caused by an upper respiratory infection, often of viral origin. Bacterial pathogens for the condition include *Streptococcus pneumoniae* (40%–50% of all cases), *H. influenzae* (20%–30% of all cases), and *Moraxella catarrhalis* (10%–15% of all cases).[32]

Presentation

Acute otitis media is most common in infants and children but may occur at any age. Signs and symptoms include otalgia, fever, decreased hearing, and a feeling of pressure in the ear. During the exam, the tympanic membrane may be erythematous with decreased mobility. Rarely, a severe empyema may occur, causing the tympanic membrane to bulge outward to the point of rupture, which often leads to otorrhea and sudden relief of pain. In serous otitis media, the tympanic membrane is typically dull and hypomobile and is characterized by chronic infection. Serous otitis media is often a result of prolonged Eustachian tube dysfunction.[10]

Workup

Erythema of the tympanic membrane is not a sole diagnostic criterion of acute and serous otitis media, as this sign may present from a number of upper respiratory tract infections, crying, or nose-blowing. Examination with a handheld otoscope is the most widely used method of diagnosing otitis media.[33]

Treatment

Most uncomplicated cases of otitis media resolve spontaneously. However, supportive therapy may involve analgesia, irritant avoidance, proper hydration, topical or oral decongestants, and cool mist humidifiers. Antibiotic therapy, such as amoxicillin, should only be used for suspected bacterial cases.[34]

Cholesteatoma

Overview

Cholesteatoma is a type of chronic otitis media characterized by peeling layers of scaly or keratinized epithelium.[35] If untreated, this condition may erode the middle ear, causing facial nerve damage and deafness.

Presentation

The characteristic sign of cholesteatoma is a squamous epithelium-lined sac filled with desquamated keratin. Other signs and symptoms include chronic infection, painless otorrhea, an ear canal filled with keratin debris or granulation tissue,

and hearing loss caused by ossicular damage.[10] Patients with cholesteatoma present with tympanic membrane perforation in 90% of all cases.[32]

Workup

The initial workup for cholesteatoma consists of a careful ear examination. Patients should be referred for a computed tomography (CT) scan to identify areas of erosion and potential fistula formation.[36]

Treatment

Patients are referred to an otolaryngologist for surgery.[10]

Vertigo

Overview

Dizziness is a broad term used to describe faintness, lightheadedness, and other forms of motion intolerance. Vertigo is a subtype of dizziness defined as a sensation of movement, applied by the person experiencing the condition to the environment or to his or her self. Benign paroxysmal positional vertigo (BPPV), characterized by the sensation of motion producing from sudden head movements, is the most common type of vertigo.[37] Common causes of vertigo include brain tumors, medications, otitis media, labyrinthitis, Ménière's disease, acoustic neuroma, migraines, cerebellar hemorrhage, head traumas, and neck injuries.[38]

Presentation

Sensation of disorientation or motion is a hallmark sign of vertigo. In addition, patients experiencing vertigo may present with nausea, vomiting, sweating, abnormal eye movement (nystagmus), hearing loss, tinnitus, weakness, visual disturbances, difficulty walking, decreased level of consciousness, and difficulty speaking.[39]

Workup

The Dix-Hallpike test (also known as the Nylen-Barany maneuver) is a common diagnostic procedure used to identify posterior canal BPPV.[40] Although further testing is not usually necessary, in more complicated cases, a referral may be necessary for a hearing examination, magnetic resonance imaging, and vestibular function testing, among others. A Venereal Disease Research Laboratory test may also be conducted to screen for syphilis. Orthostatic vital sign assessment, blood glucose testing, and electrocardiography may also be helpful in ruling out other causes of dizziness.

Treatment

Treatments vary widely based on the cause of vertigo. First line treatment for BPPV is a reposition maneuver. For symptomatic treatment, antihistamines, such as meclizine hydrochloride

(Antivert) and diphenhydramine (Benadryl), are often the drugs of choice for the management of vertigo.[41] Additional treatment options include a scopolamine transdermal patch, antiemetics, and benzodiazepines such as diazepam (Valium).

Hearing Loss

Overview

Hearing loss is defined as an acquired inability to detect pure tones above 20 decibels. Foreign bodies in the ear canal and cerumen build-up are the two most common reversible causes of hearing loss. Other common conductive causes of hearing loss include hematomas, otitis media, otitis externa, and otosclerosis. Tympanic membrane perforation affects the middle ear and causes varying degrees of hearing loss depending on the extent of the perforation.[42] Damage to hair cells or nerves that sense sound waves is a common sensorineural cause of hearing loss. Other causes of sensorineural hearing loss include acoustic trauma (e.g., exposure to loud sounds), head trauma, Ménière's disease, acoustic neuroma, and barotrauma, which is particularly common in divers.[43] Ototoxic drugs, such as aminoglycosides, diuretics, salicylates, NSAIDs, and antineoplastics, may also be responsible for hearing loss. Lastly, hearing loss due to infections may lead to mumps, measles, herpes zoster, syphilis, and meningitis. Sensorineural hearing loss related to deterioration of the cochlea and loss of hair cells in adults frequently occurs after age 65.

Presentation

The degree of severity and speed of hearing loss indicates the underlying cause. Deviations from normal findings in the Weber and Rinne tests are standard signs of hearing loss. The Weber test is "normal" when sound is heard bilaterally and equally and does not lateralize. Rinne test findings are considered "normal" when air conduction (AC) is greater than bone conduction (BC).

Workup

The initial workup for hearing loss includes a variety of evaluations, such as the whispered voice test, the tone-emitting otoscope, questionnaires, and tuning fork tests.[44] The Weber test is a tuning fork test that can be used as a follow-up to the initial screening. Sound that lateralizes to the affected ear indicates conductive hearing loss in that ear, whereas sound that lateralizes to the unaffected ear indicates sensorineural hearing loss.[45] The Rinne test is another tuning fork test that detects conductive hearing loss versus sensorineural loss.[44] The test results are abnormal when BC exceeds AC. When abnormal, the test indicates conductive hearing loss in the affected ear. Screening with an otoscope, which is used to inspect an ear canal and tympanic membrane, is among the most efficient screening methods for hearing loss.[46] If conductive hearing loss is unexplained, the NP should refer the patient for a CT scan.

Treatment

In cases of conductive hearing loss, management often consists of clearing the ear canal and treating the underlying cause. Sensorineural hearing loss, on the other hand, requires referral to a specialist.

Common Cold

Overview

The "common cold" is a colloquial term for viral rhinosinusitis. This condition is self-limiting and usually lasts 5–10 days. It may be caused by any one of more than 200 viruses that include rhinovirus, coronavirus, respiratory syncytial virus (RSV), and adenovirus, among others.[10]

Presentation

The common cold is characterized by watery rhinorrhea, erythematous nasal mucosa, sneezing, nasal and sinus blockage, headache, sore throat, cough, and malaise.

Workup

The common cold is typically diagnosed on the basis of reported symptoms and signs.

Treatment

Supportive care is a standard treatment option for a common cold. In particular, management of a common cold requires rest, hydration, warm salt water gargles, and/or nasal irrigation, along with the use of steam or a humidifier. Oral decongestants have been shown to provide relief from rhinorrhea and nasal obstruction in some older children. Acetaminophen and ibuprofen are recommended for fever and pain. Aspirin is only recommended for adults due to the risk of Reye's syndrome in children.[10]

Pharyngitis/Tonsillitis

Overview

Pharyngitis and tonsillitis refer to inflammation of the pharynx or tonsils. Pharyngitis and tonsillitis are commonly caused by viral agents such as RSV, influenza A and B, and the Epstein-Barr virus (EBV).[47] Pharyngitis and tonsillitis may also be caused by bacterial agents, with group A beta-hemolytic streptococcus (GABHS) being of most concern, as it can lead to subsequent complications including rheumatic fever and glomerulonephritis.[10]

Presentation

Common signs and symptoms of viral pharyngitis and tonsillitis include an erythematous pharynx, rhinorrhea, cough, anterior cervical adenopathy, low-grade fever, sore throat, and maculopapular rash.[48] Clinical features most suggestive of GABHS pharyngitis are listed under the acronym "FLEA": fever over 100.4 °F (38 °C), lack of cough, pharyngo-tonsillar exudate, and anterior cervical adenopathy. Clinical features suggestive of EBV may include marked lymphadenopathy, shaggy, white-purple tonsillar exudate, and sometimes hepatosplenomegaly. Approximately one-third of all patients with mononucleosis have a secondary infection with streptococcus.[10]

Workup

A standard diagnostic procedure for pharyngitis and tonsillitis includes a rapid streptococcal antigen test, which is known for its efficiency and high sensitivity, or a single swab throat culture.[49] In addition, the Monospot test (i.e., heterophil agglutination test), elevated anti-EBV titer, and complete blood count (CBC) with a differential may also be used to help diagnose pharyngitis and tonsillitis.

Treatment

Standard treatment options for pharyngitis and tonsillitis include rest, hydration, salt water gargles, and analgesic medication (e.g., ibuprofen, acetaminophen, or aspirin). In addition, antibiotics (e.g., Penicillin VK, erythromycin) are ordered for streptococcal infections, whereas ceftriaxone is the treatment for gonococcal infections.[47]

Influenza ("flu")

Overview

Influenza (popularly known as the flu) is an acute illness that is typically febrile in nature and stems from infection by influenza type A and B viruses.

Presentation

The clinical presentation of influenza often consists of an abrupt onset of fever, headache, myalgias, coryza, anorexia, malaise, and coughing.[50]

Workup

The rapid diagnostic test for influenza involves viral isolation from nasal swabs, throat swabs, or sputum specimens.[51] Rapid immunofluorescence assays and enzyme immunoassays are available to distinguish between types A and B, but the results of these tests should be interpreted with caution due to limited sensitivity.[10]

Treatment

Supportive care for influenza often involves the use of antipyretics and, in cases of bacterial infection, antibiotics. Neuraminidase inhibitors such as zanamivir (Relenza), which is contraindicated in asthmatic patients due to risk of bronchospasm, and oseltamivir (Tamiflu) are known to shorten the duration of symptoms by up to 2 days and can effectively treat both influenza A and B.[52] These drugs must be initiated within 48 hours of the onset of flu symptoms, however.

Mononucleosis

Overview

Mononucleosis is a symptomatic infection caused by the Epstein-Barr virus. It is particularly common among people 15–24 years of age.[32]

Presentation

The incubation period of mononucleosis averages 1–2 months. Common signs and symptoms following the incubation period include fever, chills, malaise, fatigue, anorexia, white tonsillar exudates, and lymphadenopathy of the posterior cervical region.[53] Pharyngitis is often considered to be the most severe finding in mononucleosis. Furthermore, splenomegaly can be present during the second week of illness. Mononucleosis is usually self-limiting; however, symptoms of malaise and fatigue may pervade for months after the illness wanes. A maculopapular or occasionally a petechial rash occurs in less than 15% of all patients, unless they are treated with ampicillin, which increases the risk of a rash to more than 90%.[10]

Workup

A diagnosis of mononucleosis is usually made using the Monospot, which is the most rapid and sensitive test for the condition.[54] In addition, lymphocytosis and neutropenia are usually detected acutely by means of a CBC.

Treatment

Mononucleosis rarely requires more than supportive therapy. Prednisone or a steroid taper may be used for severe pharyngitis with severely enlarged tonsils. Furthermore, contact sports should be avoided for 3 weeks to several months since splenic rupture may occur even in the absence of clinically detectable splenomegaly.[54] Secondary bacterial infections with GABHS should be considered.

Sinusitis (Rhinosinusitis)

Overview

Sinusitis or rhinosinusitis is an inflammation of one or more of the paranasal sinuses, manifesting in the mucous membranes; inflammation of the nasal mucosa almost always accompanies this initial inflammation. The majority of cases are caused by a viral infection. The most common causes of bacterial sinusitis are *S. pneumoniae*, *H. influenzae*, and less commonly *S. aureus* and *M. catarrhalis*.[10]

Presentation

Patients diagnosed with sinusitis or rhinosinusitis often have a history of recent upper respiratory illness; these patients typically show some improvement, which is then followed by a recurrence of symptoms. Patients with sinusitis or rhinosinusitis usually present with red nasal mucosa, nasal obstruction or congestion, post-nasal drainage, and pain or pressure over the face.[10]

Workup

The diagnosis of acute rhinosinusitis is usually made on clinical grounds alone. Decreased light transmission with transillumination is often suggestive of sinusitis. Routine radiographs are not recommended for adults and are typically reserved for patients not responding to appropriate therapy. Coronal CT often provides more information and is more cost effective than conventional sinus films.[10,55]

Treatment

Patients with sinusitis or rhinosinusitis require rest, sufficient hydration, and supportive care. In addition, treatment of sinusitis or rhinosinusitis may consist of analgesics, oral decongestants, or antihistamines. Antibiotics such as amoxicillin/clavulanate (Augmentin) and clarithromycin (Biaxin) are considered only for bacterial cases.[56] Patients who do not respond to treatment should be referred to an otorhinolaryngolotist.

Nose Bleeds

Overview

Most nosebleeds originate at the anterior septum at Kiesselbach's plexus and are caused by trauma (e.g., nose picking).[57] Posterior septum nosebleeds are more complicated and originate from an artery in the back of the nose. Posterior septum nosebleeds are characterized by more profuse bleeding and are refractory to basic management.

Presentation

Patients with nosebleeds usually experience bleeding from one nostril only. Blood may drip down the back of the throat and into the stomach, causing nausea and vomiting. Signs of excessive blood loss may include dizziness, weakness, confusion, and fainting.[58]

Workup

The diagnosis of a nosebleed is typically self-evident and is based upon appearance. A nurse practitioner, however, is expected to locate the source of bleeding and ascertain whether the patient has an anterior or posterior nosebleed.[59] If excessive blood loss is suspected, a CBC should be ordered. If the patient experiences intractable bleeding, prothrombin time/international normalized ratio should be considered.

Treatment

Nosebleeds are generally easy to control. Patients experiencing nosebleeds should sit upright, apply constant pressure (minimum of 5 minutes) to the bridge of the nose, and apply ice to the upper portion of the nose. If an anterior bleeding source can be visualized, chemical or electrical cautery is often recommended as a standard treatment option.[58] If bleeding does not stop, patients should be referred to an emergency room.

References

1. Fundoscopic exam. Stanford Medicine 25 Web site. http://stanfordmedicine25.stanford.edu/the25/fundoscopic.html. Accessed March 13, 2015.

2. Gelb D. The detailed neurologic examination in adults. In: Basow DS, ed. *UpToDate*. Waltham, MA: UpToDate; 2015. http://www.uptodate.com/contents/the-detailed-neurologic-examination-in-adults?source=preview&anchor=H21&selectedTitle=1~150#H21. Updated September 7, 2012. Accessed March 13, 2015.

3. Normal optic disc. American Academy of Ophthalmology Web site. http://www.aao.org/theeyeshaveit/optic-fundus/normal-disc.cfm. Accessed March 13, 2015.

4. Kanski JJ, Bowling B. *Synopsis of Clinical Ophthalmology*. 3rd ed. Cambridge, MA: Elsevier Saunders; 2013.

5. Dahl, AA. Retinal abnormalities: 14 signs of systemic disease. In: Brady MP, ed. Medscape. http://reference.medscape.com/features/slideshow/retina. Updated September 23, 2013. Accessed April 13, 2015.

6. Mian SI. Visual impairment in adults: Refractive disorders and presbyopia. In: Basow DS, ed. *UpToDate*. Waltham, MA: UpToDate; 2015. http://www.uptodate.com/contents/visual-impairment-in-adults-refractive-disorders-and-presbyopia?source=preview&anchor= H7&selectedTitle=2~15#H7. Updated January 6, 2015. Accessed March 13, 2015.

7. Ghosh C, Ghosh T. Eyelid lesions. In: Basow DS, ed. *UpToDate*. Waltham, MA: UpToDate; 2015. http://www.uptodate.com/contents/eyelid-lesions?source=preview&anchor=H7&selectedTitle=1~17#H7. Updated September 27, 2013. Accessed March 13, 2015.

8. Khairallah M, Kahloun R. Infections of the eyelids. In: Tabbara KF, El-Asrar AMMA, Khairallah M, eds. *Ocular Infections*. Heidelberg, Germany: Springer-Verlag; 2014: 51–61.

9. Lindsley K, Nichols JJ, Dickersin K. Interventions for acute internal hordeolum. *Cochrane Database Syst Rev.* 2013; 4. doi: 10.1002/14651858.CD007742.pub2. http://www.researchgate.net/publication/46171569_Interventions_for_acute_internal_hordeolum/file/d912f510812d56a744.pdf

10. Papadakis M, McPhee SJ, Rabow MW, eds. *CURRENT Medical Diagnosis and Treatment 2015.* 54th ed. New York, NY: McGraw-Hill Medical; 2015.

11. Gerzevitz D, Porter BO, Dunphy LN. Eyes, ears, nose, and throat. In: Dunphy LM, Winland-Brown JE, Porter BO, Thomas DJ, eds. *Primary Care: The Art and Science of Advanced Practice Nursing.* 3rd ed. Philadelphia, PA: F.A. Davis Company; 2011: 245–330.

12. Deschênes J, Fansler JL, Plouznikoff A. Chalazion treatment & management. In: Roy H Sr, ed. Medscape. http://emedicine.medscape.com/article/1212709-treatment. Updated October 31, 2014. Accessed March 13, 2015.

13. Bope ET, Kellerman RD, eds. *Conn's Current Therapy 2014.* 66th ed. Philadelphia, PA: Elsevier Saunders; 2014.

14. Shtein RM. Blepharitis. In: Basow DS, ed. *UpToDate.* Waltham, MA: UpToDate; 2015. http://www.uptodate.com/contents/blepharitis?detectedLanguage=en&source=search_result&search=blepharitis&selectedTitle=1~101&provider=noProvider. Updated March 3, 2015. Accessed March 13, 2015.

15. Jacobs DS. Conjunctivitis. In: Basow DS, ed. *UpToDate.* Waltham, MA: UpToDate; 2015. http://www.uptodate.com/contents/conjunctivitis?detectedLanguage=en&source=search_result&search=conjunctivitis&selectedTitle=1~150&provider=noProvider. Updated March 3, 2015. Accessed March 13, 2015.

16. Sambursky R, Raykovicz L. Acute conjunctivitis: treatment approach. Epocrates Web site. https://online.epocrates.com/noFrame/showPage?method=diseases&MonographId=68&ActiveSectionId=41. Updated October 16, 2014. Accessed March 13, 2015.

17. Jacobs DS. Open-angle glaucoma: Epidemiology, clinical presentation, and diagnosis. In: Basow DS, ed. *UpToDate.* Waltham, MA: UpToDate; 2015. http://www.uptodate.com/contents/open-angle-glaucoma-epidemiology-clinical-presentation-and-diagnosis. Updated March 16, 2015. Accessed March 17, 2015.

18. Neuburger M, Großwendt J, Lautebach S, et al. Dynamic contour tonometry, Tono-Pen XL, and Goldmann applanation tonometry in comparison to intracameral intraocular pressure (IOP) measurements in patients with corneal pathologies. *Open J Ophthalmology.* 2014; 4(2): 46–55. doi: 10.4236/ojoph.2014.42009

19. Orme M, Collins S, Dakin H, Kelly S, Loftus J. Mixed treatment comparison and meta-regression of the efficacy and safety of prostaglandin analogues and comparators for primary open-angle glaucoma and ocular hypertension. *Curr Med Res Opin.* 2010; 26(3): 511–528. doi: 10.1185/03007990903498786

20. Khondkaryan A, Francis BA. Angle-closure glaucoma: treatment approach. Epocrates Web site. https://online.epocrates.com/noFrame/showPage?method=diseases&MonographId=372&ActiveSectionId=41. Updated September 29, 2014. Accessed March 13, 2015.

21. Pershing S, Kumar A. Phacoemulsification versus extracapsular cataract extraction: Where do we stand? *Curr Opin Ophthalmology.* 2011; 22(1): 37–42. doi: 10.1097/ICU.0b013e3283414fb3

22. Pascolini D, Mariotti SP. Global estimates of visual impairment: 2010. *Br J Ophthalmol.* 2012; 96(5): 614–618. doi: 10.1136/bjophthalmol-2011-300539

23. Nernet AY, Vinker S, Levartovsky S, Kaiserman I. Is cataract associated with cardiovascular morbidity? *Eye.* 2010; 24(8): 1352–1358. http://www.medscape.com/viewarticle/728163_4

24. Churchill A, Graw, J. Clinical and experimental advances in congenital and paediatric cataracts. *Philos Trans R Soc Lond B Biol Sci.* 2011; 366(1568): 1234–1249. doi: 10.1098/rstb.2010.0227

25. Wong SC, Ramkissoon YD, Charteris, DG. Rhegmatogenous retinal detachment. In: Besharse JC, Bok D, eds. *The Retina and its Disorders.* Oxford, UK: Academic Press; 2011: 801–810.

26. William son TH. Posterior vitreous detachment. In *Vitreoretinal Surgery.* Heidelberg, Germany: Springer-Verlag; 2013: 89–100.

27. Arroyo JG. Retinal detachment. In: Basow DS, ed. *UpToDate.* Waltham, MA: UpToDate; 2015. http://www.uptodate.com/contents/retinal-detachment?detectedLanguage=en&source=search_result&search=retinal+detachment&selectedTitle=1~118&provider=noProvider#H14. Updated December 5, 2013. Accessed March 13, 2015.

28. Comer GM. Detached retina (retinal detachment). University of Michigan Kellogg Eye Center Web site. http://www.kellogg.umich.edu/patientcare/conditions/detached.retina.html#treatment. Accessed March 13, 2015.

29. Hui CPS, Canadian Paediatric Society Infectious Diseases and Immunization Committee. Acute otitis externa. *Paediatr Child Health.* 2013; 18(2); 96–98. http://www.ncbi.nlm.nih.gov/pmc/articles/PMC3567906/

30. Goguen LA. External otitis: Pathogenesis, clinical features, and diagnosis. In: Basow DS, ed. *UpToDate*. Waltham, MA: UpToDate; 2015. http://www.uptodate.com/contents/external-otitis-pathogenesis-clinical-features-and-diagnosis?detectedLanguage=en&source=search_result&search=Otitis+externa&selectedTitle=2~64&provider=noProvider#H191116177. Updated September 19, 2014. Accessed March 13, 2015.

31. Jensen D, Hirose K. Otitis media. In: Pensak ML, Choo DI, eds. *Clinical Otology*. 4th ed. New York, NY: Thieme; 2014: Ch. 18.

32. Barkley TW Jr. *Adult-Gerontology Primary Care Nurse Practitioner*. West Hollywood, CA: Barkley & Associates; 2015.

33. Hoberman A, Paradise JL, Rockette HE. Acute otitis media treatment research: Choosing outcome measures, adhering to protocol, and reporting results. *Ann Emerg Med*. 2012; 60(3): 393–394. doi: 10.1016/j.annemergmed.2012.02.031

34. Amsden GW. Tables of antimicrobial agent pharmacology. In: Bennett JE, Dolin R, Blaser MJ, eds. *Principles and Practice of Infectious Diseases*. 7th ed. Philadelphia, PA: Churchill Livingstone Elsevier; 2010: 705–763.

35. Roland PS. Cholesteatoma. In: Meyers AD, ed. Medscape. http://emedicine.medscape.com/article/860080-overview. Updated January 21, 2015. Accessed March 13, 2015.

36. Corrales CE, Blevins NH. Imaging for evaluation of cholesteatoma: Current concepts and future directions. *Curr Opin Otolaryngol Head Neck Surg*. 2013; 21(5), 461–467. doi: 10.1097/MOO.0b013e328364b473

37. Bansal M. *Diseases of Ear, Nose, & Throat*. New Delhi: Jaypee Brothers Medical Publishing; 2012.

38. Karatas, M. Vascular vertigo: Epidemiology and clinical syndromes. *Neurologist*. 2011; 17(1): 1–10. doi: 10.1097/NRL.0b013e3181f09742

39. Samy HM, Hamid MA, Friedman M. Dizziness, vertigo, and imbalance clinical presentation. In: Egan RA, ed. Medscape. http://emedicine.medscape.com/article/2149881-clinical#showall. Updated October 15, 2014. Accessed March 13, 2015.

40. Zaidi SH, Sinha A. *Vertigo: A Clinical Guide*. Heidelberg, Germany: Springer-Verlag; 2013.

41. Brandt, T. *Vertigo: Its Multisensory Syndromes*. 2nd ed. New York, NY: Springer-Verlag; 2003.

42. Saliba I, Abela A, Arcand P. Tympanic membrane perforation: Size, site and hearing evaluation. *Int J Pediatr Otorhinolaryngol*. 2011; 75(4): 527–531. doi: 10.1016/j.ijporl.2011.01.012

43. Chandrasekhar SS, Saunders J, Vambutas A, Schwartz SR. Sudden hearing loss: Evidence-based management and the latest in research. *Otolaryngol Head Neck Surg*. 2014; 151(1 Suppl): P22. doi: 10.1177/0194599814538403a65

44. Weber PC. Evaluation of hearing loss in adults. In: Basow DS, ed. *UpToDate*. Waltham, MA: UpToDate; 2015. http://www.uptodate.com/contents/evaluation-of-hearing-loss-in-adults?source=related_link#H6. Updated January 9, 2015. Accessed March 13, 2015.

45. Önerci TM. *Diagnosis in Otorhinolaryngology: An Illustrated Guide*. Heidelberg, Germany: Springer-Verlag; 2010.

46. Yueh B, Collins MP, Souza PE, et al. Long-term effectiveness of screening for hearing loss: The screening for auditory impairment – which hearing assessment test (SAI-WHAT) randomized trial. *J Am Geriatr Soc*. 2010; 58(3): 427–434. doi: 10.1111/j.1532-5415.2010.02738.x

47. Bartlett JG. Pharyngitis, acute. In: Bartlett JG, Auwaerter PG, Pham PA, eds. *Johns Hopkins ABX Guide 2010: Diagnosis and Treatment of Infectious Diseases*. 2nd ed. Burlington, MA: Jones & Bartlett Learning; 2010: 130–131.

48. Kociolek LK, Shulman ST. Pharyngitis. *Ann Intern Med*. 2012; 157(5), ITC3-1–ITC3-16. doi: 10.7326/0003-4819-157-5-20129040-01003

49. Shulman ST, Bisno AL, Clegg HW, et al. Clinical practice guideline for the diagnosis and management of group A streptococcal pharyngitis: 2012 update by the Infectious Diseases Society of America. *Clin Infect Dis*. 2012. doi: 10.1093/cid/cis629

50. Clark NM, Lynch JP III. Influenza: Epidemiology, clinical features, therapy, and prevention. *Semin Respir Crit Care Med*. 2011; 32(4): 373–392. doi: 10.1055/s-0031-1283278

51. Leonardi GP, Wilson AM, Zuretti AR. Comparison of conventional lateral-flow assays and a new fluorescent immunoassay to detect influenza viruses. *J Virol Methods*. 2013; 189(2), 379–382. doi: 10.1016/j.jviromet.2013.02.008

52. Michiels B, Van Puyenbroeck K, Verhoeven V, Vermiere E, Coenen S. The value of neuraminidase inhibitors for the prevention and treatment of seasonal influenza: A systematic review of systematic reviews. *PLoS One*. 2013; 8(4): e60348. doi: 10.1371/journal.pone.0060348.

53. Luzuriaga K, Sullivan JL. Infectious mononucleosis. *N Engl J Med*. 2010; 362(21): 1993–2000. doi: 10.1056/NEJMcp1001116

54. Hockenberry MJ, Wilson D. *Wong's Essentials of Pediatric Nursing*. 9th ed. St. Louis, MO: Elsevier Mosby: 2013.

55. Kormos WA. Approach to the patient with sinusitis. In: Goroll AH, Mulley AG, eds. *Primary Care Medicine: Office Evaluation and Management of the Adult Patient.* 6th ed. Philadelphia, PA: Lippincott Williams & Wilkins; 2011: 1402–1407.

56. Chow AW, Benninger MS, Brook I, et al. IDSA clinical practice guideline for acute bacterial rhinosinusitis in children and adults. *Clin Infect Dis.* 2012; 54(8): e72–e112. doi: 10.1093/cid/cir1043

57. Barnes ML, Spielmann PM, White PS. Epistaxis: A contemporary evidence based approach. *Otolaryngol Clin North Am.* 2012: 45(5); 1005–1017. doi: 10.1016/j.otc.2012.06.018

58. Fried MP. Nosebleeds. In: Porter RS, Kaplan JL, eds. The Merck Manual Online. http://www.merckmanuals.com/home/ear_nose_and_throat_disorders/symptoms_of_nose_and_throat_disorders/nosebleeds.html. Updated July 2012. Accessed March 13, 2015.

59. Doerr S. Nosebleeds. In: Stöppler MC, ed. eMedicineHealth. http://www.emedicinehealth.com/nosebleeds/page6_em.htm. Updated October 23, 2014. Accessed March 13, 2015.

Chapter 4
Integumentary Disorders

1. The practitioner knows that which of the following agents is <u>least</u> effective in the treatment of candida balanitis?

   a. Griseofulvin

   b. Clotrimazole

   c. Steroids

   d. Miconazole

2. Which of the following types of skin cancer has the highest mortality rate?

   a. Seborrheic keratosis

   b. Basal cell carcinoma

   c. Squamous cell carcinoma

   d. Malignant melanoma

3. A 27-year-old female presents with a ring-shaped skin lesion with a central clearing on her left leg. The skin lesion would most accurately be charted as which of the following?

   a. Target

   b. Zosteriform

   c. Annular

   d. Confluent

4. A 19-year-old female presents with the following rash and describes the itchy sensation as intense. Additionally, she says that she has been experiencing occasional itchy flare-ups since childhood, yet her symptoms last no more than a few days. Which condition do her complaints most likely indicate?

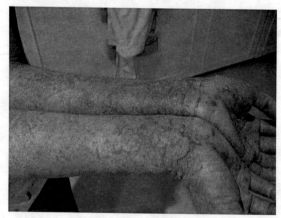

Figure 4.1

   a. Eczema

   b. Allergic contact dermatitis

   c. Psoriasis

   d. Pityriasis rosea

5. Which of the following skin conditions is usually <u>not</u> caused by Staphylococci?

   a. Erysipelas

   b. Impetigo

   c. Paronychia

   d. Hidradenitis suppurativa

6. The practitioner knows that the peak age of onset for xanthelasma is:

    a. From 20–30 years of age

    b. From 30–40 years of age

    c. From 40–50 years of age

    d. From 60–70 years of age

7. What would be the best classification for this lesion?

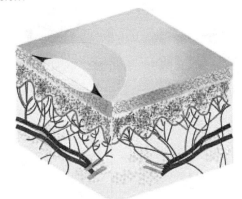

Figure 4.2

    a. Nodule

    b. Plaque

    c. Pustule

    d. Vesicle

8. Based on the image below, which of the following is the most likely diagnosis?

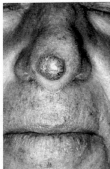

Figure 4.3

    a. Seborrheic keratosis

    b. Squamous cell carcinoma

    c. Actinic keratosis

    d. Basal cell carcinoma

9. Tretinoin cream is specifically used as first-line treatment for which two kinds of warts?

    a. Common and filiform

    b. Filiform and flat

    c. Flat and plantar

    d. Plantar and genital

10. The practitioner knows that when a smallpox rash appears, the lesion usually turns into small blisters filled with clear fluid:

    a. Within 12 hours

    b. Within 2 days

    c. Within 5 days

    d. Within 1 woek

11. As a nurse practitioner, you know that the most common cause of cellulitis in outpatients is which of the following?

    a. *Escherichia coli*

    b. *Klebsiella*

    c. *Staphylococcus aureus*

    d. *Streptococcus pyogenes*

12. Which of these is not a typical finding of malignant melanoma?

    a. Asymmetry

    b. Border irregularity

    c. Radius larger than 6 mm

    d. Elevation

13. Which of these management strategies is commonly ordered to treat severe cases of allergic contact dermatitis?

    a. Biopsy

    b. Soap and water

    c. Topical selenium sulfide

    d. Prednisone taper

14. Which of these choices would best treat a *Rickettsia rickettsii* disease that results in your patient having a maculopapular rash, abdominal pain, joint pain, and flu-like symptoms?

    a. Amoxicillin

    b. Doxycycline

    c. Ciprofloxacin

    d. Penicillin

15. In smallpox cases, initial lesions classically appear on the oral mucosa, face, or forearms. Which form does the distribution of lesions usually take as the lesions continue to spread?

    a. Centrifugal

    b. Linear

    c. Grouped

    d. Gyrate

16. A female patient presents to the clinic with the following lesion on her eye. Which treatment would you be <u>least</u> likely to recommend?

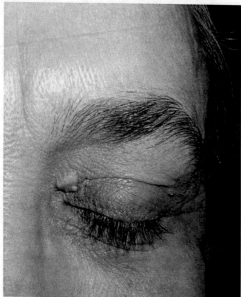

Figure 4.4

    a. Chemical cauterization

    b. Carbon dioxide laser ablation

    c. Cryotherapy

    d. Steroid injection

17. A patient presents to the clinic with the following lesion. Based on the presentation, which is the most likely diagnosis?

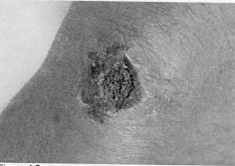

Figure 4.5

    a. Anthrax

    b. Psoriasis

    c. Smallpox

    d. Eczema

18. Which of the following treatments is a priority when treating for frostbite?

    a. Treat for pain

    b. Soak in water above 100 °F

    c. Assess for hyperthermia

    d. Apply moisturizing lotions and massage area

19. Ant bites, elevated nevi, and common skin warts are examples of which type of skin lesion?

    a. Macule

    b. Patch

    c. Papule

    d. Pustule

20. Sharon, age 45, comes to your office with asymmetrical skin lesions that are elevated and are larger than 6 mm. The color of the lesions varies from brown to purple, and the borders are irregular. Which of the following is the most likely diagnosis?

    a. Malignant melanoma

    b. Squamous cell carcinoma

    c. Basal cell carcinoma

    d. Kaposi's sarcoma

21. A 22-year-old male comes to the clinic complaining of pain in the groin area. Upon examination of his groin area, you identify abscess formations. Based on the patient's presentation, what is the best diagnosis for his skin condition?

    a. Erysipelas

    b. Candidiasis

    c. Impetigo

    d. Hidradenitis suppurativa

22. An otherwise healthy, 28-year-old male presents with fever, chills, and joint pain. The patient says he went on a hiking trip in a wooded area 2 weeks prior. Upon examination, you notice a circular pattern resembling a bull's eye on his back. Which test would you initially order to narrow the differential diagnosis of the patient's most likely condition?

    a. Western blot

    b. Polymerase chain reaction

    c. ELISA

    d. Indirect immunofluorescence assay

23. Which of these would not be considered a first-line treatment for inflammation of the glans penis caused by *Candida albicans*?

    a. Miconazole

    b. Ketoconazole

    c. Clotrimazole

    d. Fluconazole

24. A young adult presents with the following lesion on his face. This rash is most characteristic of which condition?

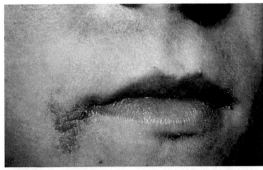

Figure 4.6

    a. Erysipelas

    b. Hidradenitis suppurativa

    c. Paronychia

    d. Impetigo

25. Which of the following best describes the appearance of Auspitz sign when psoriasis scales are removed?

    a. Erythematous, warm, indurated areas

    b. Rough skin that is either flesh-colored, pink, or hyperpigmented

    c. Droplets of blood

    d. Honey-colored crusts at the edges

26. Which acne treatment would not be recommended to a patient who is going on a 3-month backpacking trip in the desert and will not have access to electricity?

    a. Benzoyl peroxide

    b. Clindamycin

    c. Erythromycin-benzoyl peroxide

    d. Clindamycin-benzoyl peroxide gel

27. A fair-skinned 47-year-old woman undergoing a periodic health assessment presents with pink patches on her upper chest. She says that the patches appeared about a year ago. Within the past couple of weeks, though, the patches have started to itch. Which of the following would best treat the patient's most likely condition?

   a. Topical antibiotics

   b. Liquid nitrogen

   c. Topical steroids

   d. UVB light exposure

28. Which of the following would a nurse practitioner be most likely to prescribe for a minor bacterial skin infection?

   a. Topical corticosteroid

   b. Oral antibiotics

   c. Topical antimicrobial

   d. Antihistamines

29. A 25-year-old female presents with the following lesions. Which of these would most effectively treat the patient's condition?

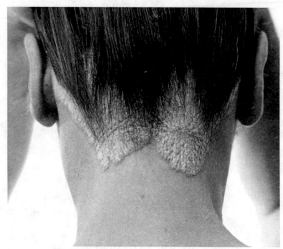

Figure 4.7

   a. Miconazole

   b. Clindamycin

   c. Betamethasone

   d. Doxycycline

30. If a patient experiences a painful, blistering eruption in a dermatomal distribution that resembles the following, which is the most likely diagnosis?

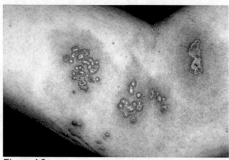

Figure 4.8

   a. Erysipelas

   b. Eczema

   c. Xanthelasma

   d. Herpes zoster

31. Which of the following is not a dermatophyte infection?

   a. Candida balanitis

   b. Tinea capitus

   c. Ringworm

   d. Onychomycosis

32. The image below illustrates which bacterial issue?

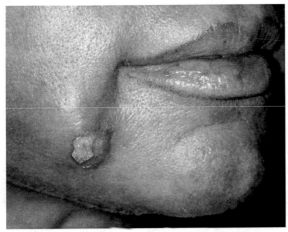

Figure 4.9

   a. MRSA

   b. Carbuncle

   c. Impetigo

   d. Furuncle

33. The practitioner knows that all of the following agents are commonly used to treat candida intertrigo <u>except</u>:

   a. Ciclopirox

   b. Itraconazole

   c. Selenium sulfide

   d. Cornstarch

34. A patient arrives at your clinic after camping in the woods of Connecticut over a week ago. He says he had a fever and nausea last week but didn't think it was serious enough to go to the doctor. This morning he noticed purple spots on his legs. Upon examination, you identify a petechial rash around his ankles. You immediately prescribe an antibiotic. Which of the following is the most likely diagnosis?

   a. Allergic contact dermatitis

   b. Lyme disease

   c. Pityriasis rosea

   d. Rocky Mountain spotted fever

35. Which of the following is the best description of trephination?

   a. Removing a fingernail with a scalpel and forceps

   b. Using a razor to scrape the surface of the skin or fingernail

   c. Heating the end of a needle and pushing it into the fingernail

   d. Debridement of the fingernail bed

36. If a patient presents with a xanthoma, how would you best describe the skin configuration?

   a. Nodule

   b. Papule

   c. Macule

   d. Pustule

37. A 24-year-old male presents with the following skin rash on the torso. This presentation is most indicative of which condition?

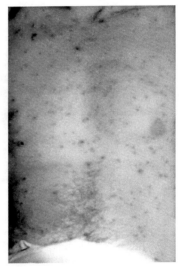

Figure 4.10

   a. Varicella zoster

   b. Atopic dermatitis

   c. Herpes zoster

   d. Molluscum contagiosum

38. The practitioner teaches the patient that an eruption of pityriasis rosea typically lasts for how long?

    a. One to 2 weeks

    b. Two to 3 weeks

    c. Four to 8 weeks

    d. Eight to 12 weeks

39. A positive purified protein derivative test would produce which lesion?

    a. Macule

    b. Wheal

    c. Papule

    d. Pustule

40. Of the following, which type of cancer usually develops from actinic keratosis?

    a. Squamous cell carcinoma

    b. Seborrheic keratoses

    c. Basal cell carcinoma

    d. Malignant melanoma

RATIONALES

1. a

The use of griseofulvin has not been shown to be effective in the treatment of candida balanitis. Griseofulvin is more likely to see use in treating skin infections (e.g., tinea capitis, tinea corporis, tinea cruris), and fungal infections of the scalp, fingernails, and toenails. Miconazole, clotrimazole, and steroids are common forms of management for candida balanitis.

2. d

Malignant melanoma has the highest mortality rate among all skin cancers. A seborrheic keratosis is a benign form of keratosis. Basal cell carcinoma is the most common form of skin cancer; however, it is very rarely life-threatening. Squamous cell carcinoma is fatal in about 1% of cases.

3. c

A ring-shaped skin lesion with a central clearing is an annular skin lesion. Target lesions may be circular but have concentric rings of color around the center. Zosteriform lesions are linear and follow nerve routes. Confluent lesions are groups of lesions that run together.

4. a

A history of inflamed forearms presenting with red, intensely itchy patches, as seen in Figure 4.1, is indicative of eczema, a chronic condition. Pityriasis rosea, allergic contact dermatitis, and psoriasis do not typically present with intense pruritus. Furthermore, allergic contact dermatitis and pityriasis rosea are not chronic skin conditions. Although psoriasis can be either acute or chronic, it most commonly presents with plaques with silvery scales.

5. a

Erysipelas is typically caused by the *Streptococcus* bacterium, rather than the *Staphylococcus* bacterium. Impetigo, paronychia, and hidradenitis suppurativa are commonly caused by *Staphylococcus*.

6. c

Although xanthelasma may appear at any age, the peak age of onset is 40–50 years. Xanthelasma is more common in older individuals than in younger individuals. The appearance of xanthelasma at a young age usually indicates familial hypercholesterolemia.

7. d

Figure 4.2 depicts a vesicle, which is a circumscribed elevation of the skin less than 1 cm in diameter that typically contains serous fluid. A pustule is best described as a visible accumulation of purulent, rather than clear, fluid underlying the skin. A nodule is an elevated, palpable solid mass of skin that may extend into the dermis. Plaques are elevations of skin that are usually greater than 1 cm in diameter.

8. d

The lesion appearing in Figure 4.3, which has a waxy appearance with a red shine and telangiectatic vessels, would most likely be diagnosed as basal cell carcinoma. Seborrheic keratoses, on the other hand, typically present with benign, painful lesions or beige, brown or black plaques, which are 3–20 mm in diameter. An actinic keratosis usually presents with small patches on sun-exposed parts of the body, premalignant lesions, tender patches, and rough hyperpigmentation. Lastly, squamous cell carcinoma normally presents with firm, irregular papules and scaly bleeding.

9. b

Tretinoin cream is a first-line treatment for filiform and flat warts. Common warts can be managed with salicylic acid, and plantar warts are frequently managed with salicylic acid and Compound W Freeze Off. Podophyllum (Pododerm, Podofilox) would be used to treat genital warts.

10. b

Smallpox lesions turn into blisters with clear fluid within 2 days of the initial onset of the smallpox rash. Blisters are not expected to develop within 12 hours because the rash is still spreading to all parts of the body at that time. Because signs and symptoms of smallpox occur rapidly, lesions would not be expected to turn into blisters after 5 days or a week. By around day 6 or 7 of onset, smallpox blisters turn into firm pustules.

11. d

The most common cause of cellulitis for outpatients is *Streptococcus pyogenes*. *Escherichia coli* and *Klebsiella* are gram-negative organisms that typically cause cellulitis for inpatients. *Staphylococcus aureus* also causes cellulitis for outpatients, but it is less common than *Streptococcus pyogenes*.

12. c

When assessing early signs of malignant melanoma, a radius larger than 6 mm is not a typical finding of this condition. Rather, a diameter larger than 6 mm is more common. Asymmetry, border irregularity, color variation, elevation, and enlargement are all common features of malignant melanoma.

13. d

Prednisone, in the form of a tapered dosing regimen, is commonly used to treat severe cases of allergic contact dermatitis. Biopsy is commonly used to manage a potential actinic keratosis and skin cancers rather than allergic contact dermatitis. Scrubbing the affected area with soap and water is not advised, as soap is one of the most common skin irritants. Lastly, topical selenium sulfide is an anti-infection agent and is frequently recommended for patients with tinea versicolor.

14. b

Doxycycline is often used to treat Rocky Mountain spotted fever (RMSF), a *Rickettsia rickettsii* disease characterized by a maculopapular rash. Abdomen and joint pain and flu-like symptoms also are common findings of RMSF. Doxycycline should be used as a 7-day prophylaxis after the tick has been removed. Amoxicillin and doxycycline are both frequently used to treat Lyme disease for a 14-day regimen, but amoxicillin is not usually used to treat RMSF. Lastly, ciprofloxacin and penicillin are commonly used in postexposure prophylaxis of anthrax for 60 days.

15. a

In smallpox cases, the spreading of lesions classically takes the form of centrifugal distribution, with the greatest concentration of lesions generally occurring on the face and distal extremities. Smallpox lesions do not typically spread according to linear, grouped, or gyrated patterns of distribution.

16. d

Although steroid injections are often used to treat inflammatory conditions, steroid injections would generally not be effective in treating the xanthelasma seen in Figure 4.4, a condition frequently characterized by yellow plaques on the upper eyelid. Because xanthelasma normally presents with benign lesions, intervention is typically employed for cosmetic reasons and can include cauterization, laser ablation, or cryotherapy.

17. a

Anthrax lesions, such as the one in Figure 4.5, are typically cutaneous and appear on the arms and hands. These lesions originate as pruritic papules that develop into black necrotic central eschar with edema. Psoriasis, on the other hand, often presents with itchy, red plaques that are clearly demarcated and have silvery scales. Smallpox lesions are typically blister-like and filled with clear fluid. Eczema usually presents with red, shiny patches or inflamed lesions with scaling.

18. a

Patients with frostbite should initially be treated for pain and assessed for hypothermia, not hyperthermia. Additionally, the affected area should be soaked in water at 100 °F for 15–30 minutes. Any temperature higher than that can damage the skin. Moisturizing lotions and massages are beneficial treatments for allergic reactions, but are not helpful for frostbite.

19. c

Ant bites, elevated nevi, and warts are all common examples of papules. A papule is usually palpable and typically remains less than 1 cm in diameter. Examples of macules include freckles, petechiae, and flat nevi. Patches are commonly presented as Mongolian spots or café au lait spots. Pustules are exemplified by acne and impetigo.

20. a

The findings of malignant melanoma include skin lesions that are asymmetrical, elevated, and larger than 6 mm. These skin lesions are typically brown or multi-colored and have notched borders. Squamous cell carcinoma typically presents with scaly patches and sharp margins that are larger than 1 cm. Basal cell carcinoma usually presents as a papule and then generally progresses into a red ulcer with rounded borders. Kaposi's sarcoma is characterized by patches, lesions, or papules that are pink, violet, or brown.

21. d

A patient presenting with an abcess formation in the groin is most likely to be diagnosed with hidradenitis suppurativa. Erysipelas typically presents as a rapid progression of an erythematous, warm, indurated area. Candidiasis is not an abscess, although it may be located in the groin. Lastly, impetigo typically presents with a thin-walled vesicle and honey-colored crusts at the edge.

22. c

An ELISA is the initial diagnostic test for Lyme disease, which is suggested by the patient's flu-like symptoms and circular pattern on his back. A Western blot may follow this initial diagnostic to confirm the condition. A polymerase chain reaction and indirect immunofluorescence assay are not generally used to diagnose Lyme disease, but when used, these tests are not initial diagnostic tests. These tests are more commonly used to diagnose Rocky Mountain spotted fever though.

23. b

Ketoconazole is not a first-line treatment for candida balanitis caused by a *Candida albicans* infection. According to the U.S. Food and Drug Administration, ketoconazole tablets should not be prescribed to treat any fungal infection due to the potential of serious liver injury. Miconazole, clotrimazole, and fluconazole are antifungals that may be used for different applications as well, but all have the commonality of treating *Candida albicans* infections.

24. d

The lesions seen in figure 4.6 are characteristic of impetigo. Fragile, thin-walled vesicles are generally not characteristic of erysipelas, hidradenitis suppurativa, or paronychia. Erysipelas is typically characterized by a warm, indurated area. Abscess formation is common in hidradenitis suppurativa and paronychia is an infection around the nail fold.

25. c

Auspitz sign is marked by the appearance of droplets of blood when psoriasis scales are removed. Erythematous, warm, indurated areas are normally indicative of erysipelas. Rough skin that is either flesh-colored, pink, or hyperpigmented is generally a sign of actinic keratosis. Honey-colored crusts at the edges frequently indicate impetigo.

26. c

Erythromycin-benzoyl peroxide is an acne treatment that requires refrigeration; therefore, it would not usually be recommended to a patient in a hot climate without electricity. Comedolytic agents, such as benzoyl peroxide, and topical antibiotics, such as clindamycin, typically do not require refrigeration. Further, clindamycin-benzoyl peroxide gel generally does not require refrigeration either.

27. b

The recommended treatment for actinic keratosis, the condition indicated by the hyperpigmented spots on the sun-exposed parts of the patient's body, is liquid nitrogen. Topical antibiotics would not effectively treat actinic keratosis because this condition does not have a bacterial etiology. An actinic keratosis develops as a result of repeated ultraviolet (UV) light exposure, so repeated exposure with treatments, such as UVB light, would not be effective. Although photodynamic therapy is sometimes used to treat actinic keratosis, UVB light exposure is not a recommended treatment for the condition.

28. c

A topical antimicrobial, such as clindamycin, is often recommended to treat minor bacterial skin infections. Antihistamines are typically prescribed as a topical steroid or oral treatment to treat other skin conditions, such as pityriasis rosea. Oral antibiotics are often prescribed to treat acne. Lastly, topical corticosteroids are commonly prescribed to treat insect bites and stings.

29. c

Betamethasone, a topical steroid, would be the most effective medication for treating plaque psoriasis, the condition indicated in figure 4.7. Plaque psoriasis is an inflammatory disease that may present with multiple red, scaly patches that consist of oval-shaped lesions. Miconazole is an antifungal medication used to treat candidiasis and tinea versicolor and is not an effective treatment for psoriasis. Topical antibiotics, such as clindamycin and doxycycline, are not typically used in treating plaque psoriasis but may be prescribed if the outbreak is due to an infection, like streptococcal pharyngitis.

30. d

Herpes zoster presents with pain and a dermatomal distribution of blisters, such as the blisters seen in figure 4.8. Although erysipelas also presents as a rapid progression of erythema, it does not typically involve pain along a dermatomal distribution. A common symptom of eczema is erythema; however, eczema does not usually present with pain along a dermatomal distribution. Xanthelasma are yellow plaques that develop as a result of fat build-up under the skin.

31. a

Dermatophyte infections are generally categorized as fungal infections in the skin and nails; candida balanitis is a fungal inflammation in the superficial tissues of the penile head and, thus, would not be classified as a dermatophyte infection. Examples of dermatophyte infections include tinea capitus, which affects the scalp; ringworm, which affects the body; and onychomycosis, which affects the nails.

32. b

Figure 4.9 best illustrates a carbuncle, a cluster of furuncles connected subcutaneously. Furuncles are pus-discharging nodules. Cellulitis, which can be caused by MRSA, is a generalized classification of a breach in the skin from inflammation of the surrounding skin and tissues. Lastly, impetigo is a skin infection typically characterized by a thin-walled vesicle surrounded by honey-colored crusts.

33. c

Topical selenium sulfide is often used to treat tinea versicolor, not candida intertrigo. Candida intertrigo is commonly treated with drying agents (e.g., talc or cornstarch), topical antifungals (e.g., ciclopirox), and oral antifungals (e.g., itraconazole).

34. d

Although Lyme disease and Rocky Mountain spotted fever are both transmitted by tick bites, which cause rashes and flu-like symptoms, a petechial rash is more indicative of Rocky Mountain spotted fever. Lyme disease, on the other hand, commonly presents with a "bull's eye" shaped rash. Allergic contact dermatitis, which could derive from poison ivy in a patient who has been camping, would likely itch and be contained to only those areas where contact was made. Pityriasis rosea occurs more often during the spring and fall and does not derive from a tick bite. These lesions present as a herald patch and do not manifest for 1–2 weeks.

35. c

Trephination, which is the process of drilling a hole through the fingernail into the hematoma, is the best way to release the pressure of a fingernail hematoma. Typically, a heated instrument, such as a needle, is used. Removing the fingernail with a scalpel and forceps may be used, but this is not the definition of trephination. Using a razor to scrape the surface of the skin or fingernail is a shave biopsy. Debridement of the fingernail bed removes dead or infected tissue.

36. a

A xanthoma is clinically characterized by the appearance of a nodule, which is a solid mass of skin larger than 1 cm in diameter. These types of lesions typically extend into the dermis. The appearance of papules, on the other hand, is typically indicative of ant bites, elevated nevi, and verrucae. Macules are often characteristic of tinea versicolor rather than xanthoma. Lastly, pustules often present in cases of acne and bacterial infections, among others.

37. a

The image is most indicative of varicella, a virus that results in small macules on the scalp, face, trunk, and limbs that eventually progresses to clear vesicles that crust over. Atopic dermatitis results in red, shiny patches or erythematic scaling. Herpes zoster commonly results in grouped vesicle eruption with a dermatomal distribution. Molluscum contagiosum usually causes pink, waxy papules.

38. c

An eruption of pityriasis rosea typically lasts 4–8 weeks. In most cases, a herald patch first appears and then more patches appear a week or two later. The rash begins to heal after 2–4 weeks and is completely healed within 6–14 weeks. Pityriasis rosea is most common in adolescents and young adults, but when it appears in individuals over 60 years old, the rash may last for several months.

39. b

A positive purified protein derivative (PPD) test would produce a wheal. A PPD test would not produce macules, papules, or pustules. Macules are a typical presentation of tinea versicolor. Papules can be seen in various skin disorders, such as basal cell carcinoma or acne. Pustules, however, may be a sign of acne or a bacterial infection.

40. a

Squamous cell carcinoma may develop from actinic keratosis. Seborrheic keratoses and malignant melanoma are not associated with actinic keratoses. Squamous cell carcinomas may turn into basal cell carcinomas.

DISCUSSION

Morphology

Primary/Secondary Skin Lesions

Primary lesions develop on previously unaltered skin and are a direct result of trauma, insult, or disease. A secondary skin lesion is a modification of a primary lesion, resulting from either a change in impression over time or insult to the lesion (e.g., scratching, infection, etc.).[1]

Macule (see figure 4.11)

A macule is a circumscribed, discolored, flat area of skin that is smaller than 1 cm in size.[1] Ephelides (freckles), flat moles, and petechiae are all examples of macules.[2]

Patch (see figure 4.12)

A patch is a macule measuring greater than 1 cm in diameter.[3] Examples of patches include Mongolian spots and café-au-lait spots.[2]

Papule (see figure 4.13)

Papules are solid, elevated lesions with distinct borders that measure smaller than 1 cm in diameter.[1] Examples of papules include elevated moles, warts, and ant bites.[4]

Plaque (see figure 4.14)

Plaques are solid elevations of skin that have a flattened surface and are greater than 1 cm in diameter.[1] Plaques are palpable and oval-shaped with well-defined boundaries. Examples of plaques include psoriasis lesions, in addition to seborrheic and actinic keratoses.[2,5]

Pustule (see figure 4.15)

Pustules are visible subdermal collections of purulent fluid that measure smaller than 1 cm in diameter. Examples of pustules include acne and impetigo.[6]

Vesicle (see figure 4.16)

A vesicle is a circumscribed elevation of the skin that is smaller than 1 cm in diameter and contains serous fluid. Herpes simplex, herpes zoster (shingles), and varicella zoster (chicken pox) are all conditions that present with vesicles.[7]

Nodule (see figure 4.17)

A nodule is a solid mass of tissue greater than 1 cm in diameter. Nodules often extend into the dermis and can be palpated or observed by the practitioner. Examples of nodules include xanthomas, fibromas, erythema nodosum, and lipomas.[2,4]

Bulla (see figure 4.18)

Bullae, commonly known as blisters, are circumscribed, fluid-filled elevations that measure greater than 1 cm in diameter and extend only into the epidermis. Examples of bullae include burns, superficial blisters, and contact dermatitis.[1,4]

Wheal

A wheal is an itchy elevation of skin that is reddish in color. Wheals are slightly irregular in shape due to swelling.[4,8] Wheals are commonly associated with allergic reactions, reactions to purified protein derivative (PPD) tests, and insect bites.[9]

Cyst (see figure 4.19)

A cyst is any closed cavity or sac that contains fluid or semisolid material located in the dermis or subcutaneous layer.[2] Cysts may present with normal or abnormal epithelia. Examples of cysts include sebaceous cysts and cystic acne.[4]

Abscess

An abscess is a localized collection of purulent fluid that measures greater than 1 cm in size in a cavity that results from necrosis. Abscesses are red, elevated, and often painful.[10]

Tumor

Tumors are firm or soft masses that extend more than a few centimeters into the dermis. Tumors may be benign or malignant.[11]

Configurations of Lesions (see figures 4.20–4.28)

Annular skin lesions are circular formations that begin in the center and spread to the periphery. When multiple annular lesions merge, they are known as polycyclic lesions.[12] Confluent configurations are characterized by lesions that run together, whereas grouped lesions form in a cluster. Solitary, or discrete, lesions remain distinct and do not merge with other lesions. Gyrate lesions are twisted, coiled, spiral, or snake-like in appearance.

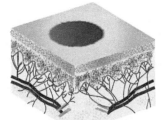

Figure 4.11. Macule

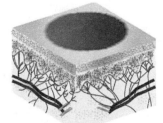

Figure 4.12. Patch

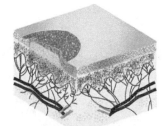

Figure 4.13. Papule

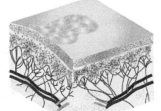

Figure 4.14. Plaque

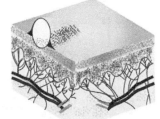

Figure 4.15. Pustule

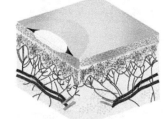

Figure 4.16. Vesicle

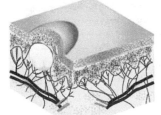

Figure 4.17. Nodule

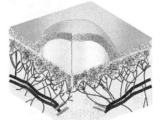

Figure 4.18. Bulla

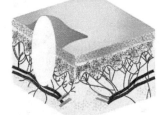

Figure 4.19. Cyst

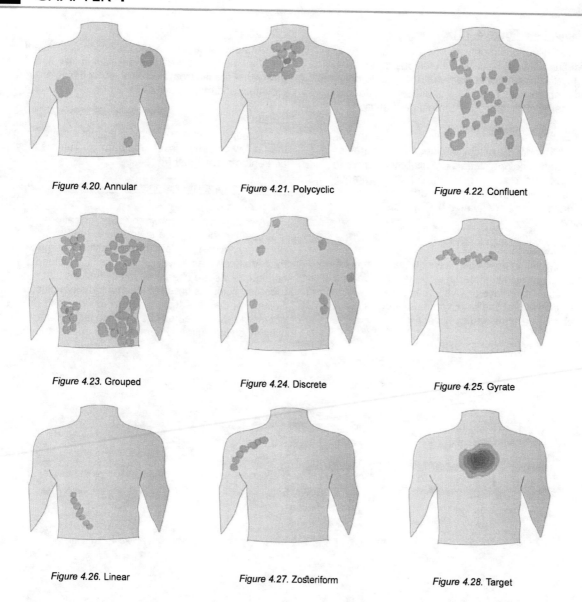

Figure 4.20. Annular

Figure 4.21. Polycyclic

Figure 4.22. Confluent

Figure 4.23. Grouped

Figure 4.24. Discrete

Figure 4.25. Gyrate

Figure 4.26. Linear

Figure 4.27. Zosteriform

Figure 4.28. Target

Linear lesions may appear to resemble scratches, streaks, lines, or stripes. Zosteriform lesions form in a linear arrangement along a dermatomal pathway. Lastly, target lesions present with concentric rings of color, oftentimes resembling the iris of an eye.[1]

Acne

Overview

Acne vulgaris, popularly known as acne, is the most common skin disorder in the United States, affecting approximately 80% of all Americans at some point during their lives.[13] Factors that contribute to the development of acne include the buildup of dead skin cells, the presence and activity of bacteria (e.g., *Propionibacterium acnes*), excess sebum production, and possibly genetics, among others.[13]

Presentation

Acne usually presents in areas where sebaceous follicles are particularly dense, such as the face, upper chest, and back.[13] Comedonal acne is characterized by open and closed comedones. Open comedones, known as blackheads, are openings in the skin that are capped with blackened skin debris. Closed comedones, known as whiteheads, present as obstructed openings topped with white skin debris.[4] Depending on the severity of acne, patients may have papules, pustules, nodules, or a combination of the three; depending on severity, scarring may result.[13]

Workup

Diagnosis of acne is based on examination of the skin, with signs such as comedones helping to rule out other skin disorders, such as rosacea and folliculitis.[13,14] After a diagnosis of acne is confirmed, the severity of the patient's acne is classified as mild, moderate, or severe, based on the number and type of lesions.[14]

Management

Non-prescription regimens are the first-line method of management for many patients with acne.[15] For example, affected areas should be washed once or twice per day with a mild soap; antibacterial or abrasive soaps should be avoided, as they may further irritate the skin.[14] It is also recommended that patients avoid topical oil-based products and use oil-free cleansers and moisturizers.[9,15] If a patient with mild or moderate acne does not respond to non-prescription products after several months, then a clinical evaluation is warranted.[15]

Comedonal acne is treated with a topical retinoid (e.g., tretinoin). Topical retinoids treat blackheads and whiteheads, but tretinoin may cause skin irritation and sunlight sensitivity. Adapalene (Differin) may be used as an alternative to tretinoin, and tends to cause less skin irritation.[16] Tazarotene (Tazorac) and azelaic acid (Azelex) are two other alternatives to tretinoin and adapalene.[14,17] For nurse practitioners (NPs) treating patients who are pregnant, acne drugs should be prescribed with caution; tretinoin and adapalene are both Pregnancy Category C drugs, whereas tazarotene is Pregnancy Category X.

In addition to topical retinoids, treatment of mild acne often includes an antimicrobial (e.g., benzoyl peroxide) for papulopustules. Antimicrobials decrease the number of *P. acnes* microbes colonizing the skin, thus reducing inflammation.[14,18] When using benzoyl peroxide and tretinoin in combination, the benzoyl peroxide should be applied in the morning and the tretinoin in the evening.[18] Topical antibiotics (e.g., erythromycin, clindamycin) may also be prescribed in cases of mild inflammatory acne. These antibiotics should be used in combination with retinoids or benzoyl peroxide for increased efficacy. All topical antibiotics may cause skin irritation.[18]

Moderate acne is treated with topical retinoids, topical benzoyl peroxide, and oral antibiotics (e.g., tetracycline, doxycycline). Oral antibiotics work faster than topical antibiotics but have increased side effects, such as vaginal candidiasis and gastrointestinal distress.[14,18] If oral antibiotics do not result in improvement, referral is warranted.

Oral isotretinoin is used to treat severe acne and milder acne that is resistant to other treatments.[18] The oral antibiotic, which should be used as monotherapy, can cure acne but can have very severe side effects.[14,18] For NPs treating patients who are pregnant, oral isotretinoin is contraindicated, as it is a Pregnancy Category X drug. Women must be enrolled in the "iPLEDGE" registry and have frequent lab tests and follow-up visits.[19]

Females with acne may also be treated with oral contraceptives, such as Ortho Tri-Cyclen and Estrostep; these drugs exhibit particular benefits in patients with evidence of hyperandrogenism, but may also help patients with moderate or severe acne.[20,21] Among other side effects, some oral contraceptives may cause brownish blotches or melasma.[9] Effects from oral contraceptives are typically seen around six months after the start of treatment.[14]

Intralesional triamcinolone (Kenalog-10) and dermabrasion may also be used in treatment of acne.[22,23]

Bacterial Infections

Folliculitis

Folliculitis is an inflammation of the hair follicles caused by a superficial bacterial infection with purulent material in the epidermis.[24] Folliculitis is usually caused by *Staphylococcus aureus* bacteria.[9]

Furuncle

Furuncles, commonly known as boils, are localized infections originating in the hair follicle.[25] These infections are predominantly caused by *S. aureus* bacteria.[25]

Carbuncle

Carbuncles occur when several inflamed follicles produce purulent drainage, thus resulting in a single inflammatory mass.[25] Carbuncles, like furuncles, are typically caused by *S. aureus*.[25] Carbuncles, however, are larger in size.

Cellulitis

Cellulitis is a spreading bacterial infection of the skin and subcutaneous tissues that causes inflammation, swelling, and redness of the affected skin.[26] Cellulitis typically occurs in the extremities, especially the lower legs, and may be caused by damage to the skin from an insect bite or wounds.[26] The most common pathogens responsible for cellulitis are beta-hemolytic *Streptococci* (groups A, B, C, G, and F) and *S. aureus*.[27] Patients with cellulitis should be treated with empiric antibiotic therapy.[28]

Erysipelas

Erysipelas is a type of cellulitis that most commonly involves the face, arm, and upper thigh, and manifests as rapid development of an erythematous, indurated area. Erysipelas typically has more distinctive anatomic features than cellulitis, such as well-defined borders and raised lesions.[29] A common cause of erysipelas is group A *Streptococci*.[29]

Hidradenitis suppurativa

Hidradenitis suppurativa is a *S. aureus* infection that causes red, swollen, painful abscesses, often in places where the skin rubs together such as the armpits or the groin.[30] The abscesses may rupture after becoming inflamed, leaking pus.[31] Hidradenitis suppurativa typically begins after puberty.

Impetigo

Impetigo is a bacterial skin infection often caused by *S. aureus*, but may also be caused by *Streptococci* bacteria. The infection is characterized by thin-walled vesicles that can easily rupture. Honey-colored crusts at the edges of the primary lesion are one of the hallmark signs of impetigo.[32] Satellite lesions commonly spread to remote areas of the skin.[9]

Paronychia

Paronychia is inflammation of the lateral and proximal finger folds.[33] This condition is caused by a superficial infection of epithelium lateral to the nail plate. The most common bacterial cause of paronychia is *Staphylococci*, but mixed aerobic and anaerobic flora may also be present.[33,34]

Presentation

Signs and symptoms of inflammation due to bacterial infections include warmth, swelling, redness, and pain. The initial findings are followed by pustular discharge and the formation of tiny, rounded masses of infected tissue.[35] Systemic bacterial infections frequently present with fever, malaise, and chills.[36]

Workup

Although cultures may be performed on patients suspected of having bacterial infections, no additional laboratories or diagnostics are typically required.[9]

Treatment

Depending on the size and location of the infected area, treatment of bacterial infections includes the use of topical or systemic antibiotics such as amoxicillin, clindamycin, and cephalexin.[2] Minor infections may be treated with topical antimicrobials (e.g., bacitracin and mupirocin), first-generation cephalosporins (e.g., cephalexin), or penicillinase-resistant penicillins (e.g., dicloxacillin).[2,9,37] Some infections, such as furuncles and carbuncles, may require incision and drainage.[2,9]

Fingernail Hematomas (Subungual Hematoma)

Overview

Fingernail hematomas (i.e., subungual hematomas) are caused by an accumulation of blood that collects in the space between the fingernail and nail bed. Subungual hematomas result from blunt or sharp trauma to the fingers or toes.[38]

Presentation (see figure 4.29)

Bleeding from the nail bed causes increased pressure under the nail, which results in significant discomfort and intense pain.[38,39]

Treatment

The recommended treatment for subungual hematoma is trephination, a process where pressure is relieved by drilling a hole into the hematoma through the nail.[39] Trephination is generally performed using a heated instrument, such as a surgical blade, needle, small drill, or laser.[40]

Candida Balanitis

Overview

Candida balanitis is the inflammation of the glans penis and the superficial tissues of the penile head due to *Candida albicans*.[41] Although diabetes is the most common underlying cause of adult balanitis, candida balanitis often affects uncircumcised men with poor hygiene.[42]

Presentation

Clinical features of candida balanitis include itching, burning, and white patches on the penis.[43] In severe cases, patients may have difficulty urinating or controlling their urine stream.[42] Additional physical examination findings may include lymphadenopathy, erythema, and edema.[42]

Workup

A physical examination and patient history should be sufficient to diagnose balanitis.[42]

Treatment

Balanitis is treated with long courses of topical antifungals, such as miconazole, clotrimazole, and fluconazole. Occasionally, topical steroids may be necessary.[26]

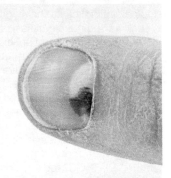

Figure 4.29. Subungual hematoma.

Candida Intertrigo

Overview

Candida intertrigo is an irritation in the skin folds in areas where two skin surfaces rub together.[44] This condition occurs in warm, moist areas of the body.[44]

Presentation

Intertrigo presents with erythematous, macerated plaques and erosions.[45] Additional findings include itching, burning, and stinging in the affected skin folds.[46]

Workup

Diagnosis of intertrigo is based on the location and appearance of the affected skin as well as the typical appearance and distribution of lesions.[44,45] Skin scrapings may be cultured or observed under a microscope to confirm the diagnosis.[44]

Treatment

Candida intertrigo is treated with topical antifungals, such as ciclopirox (Loprox). If topical antifungals do not result in improvement, oral antifungals, such as fluconazole (Diflucan) or itraconazole (Sporanox), may be prescribed. Preventative measures, such as using drying agents to eliminate friction, heat, and maceration, should be taken to lower the risk of recurrence.[46]

Tinea Capitis

Overview

Tinea capitis is a dermatophytic infection of the scalp, eyebrows, and eyelashes.[47] Tinea capitis is commonly caused by *Microsporum* and *Trichophyton* fungi.[44]

Presentation (see figure 4.30)

Tinea capitis is characterized by pale red, scaly papules. As the condition progresses, the lesions form a ring pattern and hair may easily detach from the scalp. Mild pruritus, accompanied by inflammation, is common. [47]

Workup

Tinea capitis is diagnosed by evaluating the patient's scalp and taking samples of hair or scales.[44] A potassium hydroxide preparation or fungal culture can be used to confirm the diagnosis.[48]

Treatment

The traditional choice of treatment for tinea capitis is griseofulvin. Oral terbinafine, itraconazole, and fluconazole are newer therapeutic options with shorter courses of treatment than griseofulvin.[48] Selenium 2.5% shampoo may help stop the spread of tinea capitis in the early stages, but is usually ineffective in treating the later stages.[7,47]

Tinea Corporis (ringworm)

Overview

Tinea corporis, commonly known as ringworm, is a dermatophyte infection that affects the head, neck, and arms.[49] Like tinea capitis, tinea corporis is caused by the genera *Microsporum* or *Trichophyton*.[44]

Presentation (see figure 4.31)

Tinea corporis is characterized by an erythematous, scaly plaque that rapidly enlarges. Inflammation may result in scales, crusts, papules, vesicles, or bullae. Although some patients are asymptomatic, most experience burning and itching.[49,50] Patients with tinea corporis who are HIV-positive or immunocompromised may also experience severe pruritus or pain.[49]

Workup

Tinea corporis is diagnosed by visual examination or collecting skin scrapings.[44] These scrapings can be examined under a microscope in a potassium hydroxide test, which shows segmented hyphae and arthrospores indicative of all dermatophyte infections.[51]

Treatment

Topical antifungals, such as miconazole, clotrimazole, naftifine, and econazole, are recommended for treatment of tinea corporis. In severe cases, tinea corporis may require a systemic course of antifungal agents, such as ketoconazole.[44]

Tinea Cruris (jock itch)

Overview

Commonly known as jock itch, tinea cruris is a dermatophyte infection of the groin stemming from the genera *Trichophyton*, *Epidermophyton*, and *Microsporum*.[9]

Presentation (see figure 4.32)

Tinea cruris presents with an erythematous patch that begins in the skinfolds of the genital area and spreads to the upper, inner thighs.[44] Additional signs and symptoms include abnormally dark or light skin and itching in the groin, thigh, or anus.[52]

Workup

Tinea cruris is diagnosed through a physical examination, but a potassium hydroxide test may be used for confirmation.[53,54]

Treatment

Uncomplicated cases of tinea cruris are treated with topical antifungals, such as imidazole and allylamine.[54] Oral antifungals may be prescribed in severe cases.[44]

To prevent recurrence, patients should keep the affected area dry by applying desiccant powders (e.g., talcum powder).[44]

Tinea Pedis (athlete's foot)

Overview

Tinea pedis (i.e., athlete's foot) is a dermatophyte infection of the foot.[55] The infection is most commonly caused by *Trichophyton rubrum*.[56]

Presentation (see figure 4.33)

Tinea pedis can affect any portion of the foot, but infections most often occur in the space between the toes.[57] The infection causes mild scaling; in severe cases, this scaling can cause a breakdown and fissuring of the skin.[44] Patients may also present with redness, itching, burning, or stinging, as well as blisters that leak or crust over.[58]

Workup

Although tinea pedis is traditionally diagnosed by the patient's history and clinical picture, scrapings may also be examined.[56] Fungal cultures can also serve to confirm a diagnosis.[56]

Treatment

Treatment consists of topical (e.g., miconazole, clotrimazole) or oral (e.g., itraconazole, terbinafine) antifungals.[56]

Tinea Manuum (hand/palm)

Overview

Tinea manuum is a dermatophyte infection of the hand, usually caused by the same types of fungi as tinea pedis.[59]

Presentation

Tinea manuum presents with itching, scaling, and redness. Severe cases can present with fissuring of the skin.[59]

Workup

Tinea manuum can be diagnosed by clinical observation.[59]

Treatment

Treatment for tinea manuum consists of aluminum subacetate solution soaks and topical antifungals. The same topical antifungals used in the treatment of tinea pedis may be used to treat tinea manuum as well.[59]

Tinea Unguium (onychomycosis)

Overview

Tinea unguium, also known as onychomycosis, is a persistent fungal infection that manifests in the toenails and fingernails. Onychomycosis may involve any part of the nail unit, including the matrix, bed, or plate.[60] Most cases of onychomycosis are caused by dermatophytes, but other fungi, such as *Candida*, can produce the condition.[60] Additionally, most patients with onychomycosis either currently have or have had tinea pedis.[61]

Presentation

Initially, patients with onychomycosis may complain about the appearance of the affected nail but may not present with any other symptoms.[60] In mild cases of onychomycosis, the patient's nails frequently present with white or yellow discolored patches with a slow-spreading chalky, white scale underneath the nail's surface. As the condition progresses, it can cause significant discomfort.[62] In severe cases, the nails thicken and detach from the nail bed.[63]

Onychomycosis may interfere with standing, walking, and exercising.[60] Moreover, onychomycosis can increase the risk of bacterial infections in diabetic or immunocompromised patients.[64]

Workup

A clinical diagnosis of onychomycosis is made based on the appearance of the patient's nails.[63] However, a potassium hydroxide test is useful in ruling out the presence of fungi, and polymerase chain reaction can help detect fungal DNA from infected nails.[60] Infected fingernails may also be cultured to establish the causative organism.[60]

Treatment

Oral antifungals such as itraconazole and terbinafine are typically prescribed for tinea unguium. Topical antifungals may be used as well, although these medications are generally less effective.[55,60]

Tinea Versicolor

Overview

Tinea versicolor is a fungal infection of the chest and back that causes hypopigmented or hyperpigmented macules and patches.[65] Tinea versicolor is caused by yeasts in the genus *Malassezia*, formerly known as *Pityrosporum*.[65]

Presentation

Patients with tinea versicolor present with hypopigmented or hyperpigmented macules on the limbs and scaly patches of skin.[53] Mild pruritus may accompany the macules as well.[65]

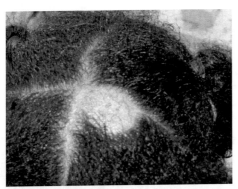

Figure 4.30. Tinea capitus.

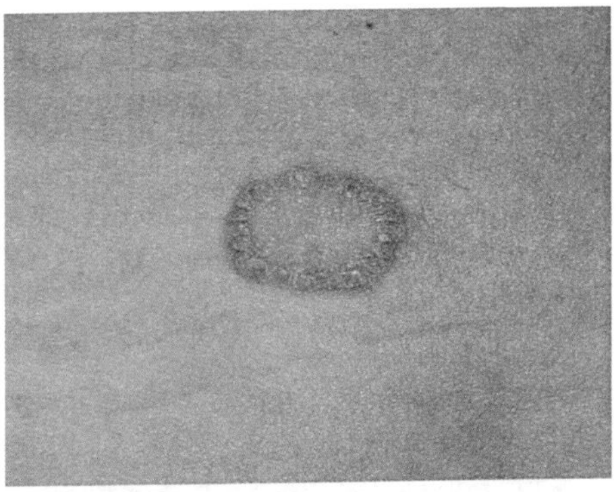

Figure 4.31. Tinea corporis

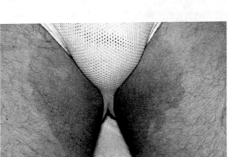

Figure 4.32. Tinea cruris

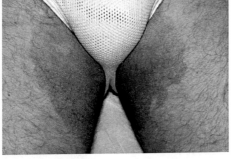

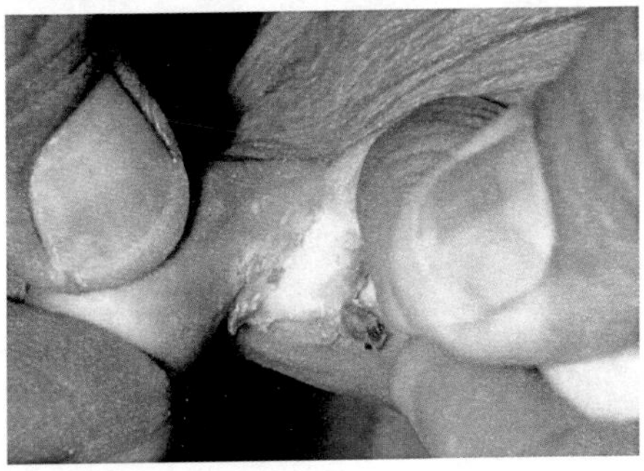

Figure 4.33. Tinea pedis

Workup

A diagnosis of tinea versicolor is based on clinical presentation without any laboratory findings.[65] However, the diagnosis can be confirmed with a potassium hydroxide test.[66] Additionally, an ultraviolet light can be used to show the infection more clearly.[53]

Treatment

Tinea versicolor is treated with topical selenium sulfide or topical antifungals such as miconazole, ciclopirox, and clotrimazole. Many patients with tinea versicolor prefer oral antifungals; these agents are less time-consuming but do not prevent recurrence.[65]

Herpes Zoster (Shingles) (see figure 4.8)

Overview

Herpes zoster is an acute vesicular eruption that appears as a painful, blistering skin rash.[67] Commonly known as shingles, herpes zoster is caused by varicella zoster virus infection. This condition most frequently presents in patients over 50 years of age and may be life-threatening in immunocompromised adults.[9,68]

Presentation

Herpes zoster presents with pain that manifests in a dermatomal distribution; this pain most commonly manifests along the thorax, but may present in the face and hands, among other sites. Patients may also complain of itching, burning, and tingling. After these preliminary symptoms, a painful rash develops, characterized by grouped vesicle eruptions of erythema and exudate along the dermatomal pathway.[69] Regional lymphadenopathy may also present.[68]

Workup

A diagnosis of herpes zoster is usually based on the characteristic dermatomal rash.[70] However, a skin sample and Tzanck stain may be taken to help confirm a diagnosis.[67,70]

Treatment

Antiviral drugs are the standard of care in the treatment of herpes zoster. Acyclovir is the most common choice for treatment, but famciclovir and valacyclovir may also see use. These agents must be started as soon as possible after the rash appears, ideally within 72 hours after onset.[67,71] If ocular involvement is suspected, patients should be referred immediately to an ophthalmologist.[9] Gabapentin (Neurontin) and pregabalin (Lyrica) are agents approved by the Food and Drug Administration for management of post-herpetic neuralgia. The herpes zoster vaccine (Zostavax) is approved for the prevention of herpes zoster in patients 50 years of age and older.[71]

Actinic Keratoses

Overview

Actinic keratoses present as small patches on sun-exposed parts of the body.[69] Premalignant lesions may progress to squamous cell carcinoma if left untreated.

Presentation

Actinic keratoses are asymptomatic, but findings of the condition include rough pink or hyperpigmented spots that may be tender. Over time, the patient's lesions tend to enlarge and become red and scaly.[73]

Workup

Actinic keratoses are diagnosed by examining the patient's skin.[72] A skin biopsy may be used to rule out invasive squamous cell carcinoma.[73]

Treatment

Common treatment options for actinic keratoses include topical agents such as 5-fluorouracil, imiquimod, ingenol mebutate, and diclofenac sodium 3%.[73] Actinic keratoses may also be treated with photodynamic therapy and liquid nitrogen.[74]

Squamous Cell Carcinoma

Overview

Squamous cell carcinoma is most common in fair-skinned individuals who have experienced prolonged sun exposure. This skin cancer usually develops over a few months and may metastasize in 3%–7% of all patients.[75,76]

Presentation (see figure 4.34)

The earliest form of squamous cell carcinoma is a scaly, crusted, and large reddish patch.[75] As the condition develops, squamous cell carcinoma presents with firm, irregular papules or nodules as well as scaly, keratotic patches that may bleed when scratched.[77]

Workup

A biopsy is essential in diagnosing squamous cell carcinoma.[76] The differential diagnosis varies based on the lesion's appearance and helps to rule out other skin conditions with similar signs, such as actinic keratoses and bowenoid papulosis.[78]

Treatment

Squamous cell carcinoma is treated with surgical excision using the Mohs procedure.[75] Topical treatments, such as imiquimod and 5-fluorouracil, may also be used.[79] Photodynamic therapy can also be used to manage the condition, and radiation therapy may be warranted in cases with recurrences or larger tumors.[76]

Seborrheic Keratoses

Overview

Seborrheic keratoses are benign skin lesions. The cause of seborrheic keratoses is unknown; however, the condition tends to run in families, suggesting a genetic link.[80] Seborrheic keratoses are the most common benign tumor in older adults.[80,81]

Presentation (see figure 4.35)

Seborrheic keratoses characteristically present as benign, painless lesions and beige, brown, or black plaques. These growths vary in size from 3 to 20 mm in diameter, and appear to be "stuck on" the patient's skin.[82]

Workup

Seborrheic keratoses are diagnosed through a clinical exam. Although a skin biopsy may be needed to confirm a diagnosis, additional laboratory tests are only indicated if the patient displays the Leser-Trélat sign, which is the sudden appearance of multiple pruritic seborrheic keratoses.[80,81]

Treatment

Although liquid nitrogen may be used as a treatment for seborrheic keratoses, treatment is generally unnecessary. If removal is desired, the patient may be referred to a dermatology specialist, as needed.[81]

Basal Cell Carcinoma

Overview

The most common type of skin cancer, basal cell carcinoma arises from the basal layer of the epidermis and occurs mainly on skin that is regularly exposed to sunlight or other ultraviolet radiation.[83,84] Basal cell carcinoma is most common among fair-skinned patients with a history of sun exposure.[76]

Presentation (see figure 4.36)

Basal cell carcinoma presents with slow-growing lesions that may eventually grow to 1–2 cm in diameter.[9] These lesions are characterized by a waxy, pearly appearance with a central depression or rolled edge, and may exhibit a shiny red color and telangiectatic vessels.

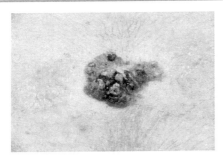

Figure 4.34. Squamous cell carcinoma

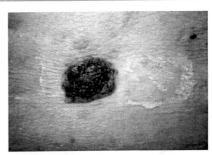

Figure 4.35. Seborrheic keratoses

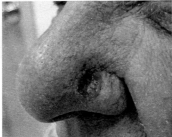

Figure 4.36. Basal cell carcinoma

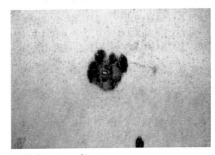

Figure 4.37. Malignant melanoma

Workup

A diagnosis of basal cell carcinoma is based upon clinical examination, with a shave/punch biopsy and histological examination typically used to confirm the diagnosis.[83,85]

Treatment

Surgical excision is the most common and most effective treatment for basal cell carcinoma.[85,86] In cases where surgery is not recommended, alternative treatments include radiation therapy, photodynamic therapy, or topical antineoplastic agents.[85]

Malignant Melanoma

Overview

Malignant melanoma is a type of skin cancer that develops from melanocytes and may metastasize to any organ. This cancer has the highest mortality rate of all skin cancers, as well as a median age of diagnosis of 40 years.[87]

Presentation (see figure 4.37)

Malignant melanoma presents with lesions that can be described by the mnemonic ABCDEE, which stands for asymmetry, border irregularity, color variation, diameter greater than 6 mm, elevation, and enlargement.[9] This condition is also suggested if a preexisting mole exhibits color changes, possesses an irregular shape, or grows bigger over time.[88]

Workup

A diagnosis of malignant melanoma is confirmed with a biopsy. Once confirmed, the progression of the melanoma is staged using the TNM classification system.[76,89]

Treatment

Surgical excision is the treatment for malignant melanoma.[76] Adjuvant therapy using agents such as interferon alfa is recommended for high-risk patients and patients with advanced melanoma.[88]

Eczema (Atopic Dermatitis) (see figure 4.1)

Overview

Eczema, also known as atopic dermatitis, is a chronic skin condition characterized by intense pruritus. Although eczema may appear in children, adult cases may have a genetic component and are exacerbated by stress.[90,91,92]

Presentation

In addition to pruritus, atopic dermatitis presents with acute flare-ups that include red, shiny, or thickened patches on the patient's skin.[90] Patients also exhibit inflamed or scabbed lesions with erythema and scaling, followed by dry, leathery lichenification.

Workup

The diagnosis of atopic dermatitis is made by clinical evaluation.[76] If necessary, a skin biopsy can be used to confirm the diagnosis and to rule out other causes.[90,93]

Treatment

Atopic dermatitis is treated by topical steroids, such as clobetasol cream or lotion. Other treatment options include supportive care, immune modulators, and ultraviolet therapy.[93]

Allergic Contact Dermatitis

Overview

Allergic contact dermatitis is an acute or chronic condition characterized by inflammation at the site of contact with an allergen.[94]

Presentation

Allergic contact dermatitis presents with a variety of findings that include redness, pruritus, and scabbing. Lesions with sharp, defined borders may also appear on the patient's skin.[95]

Workup

Diagnosis of allergic contact dermatitis is made by clinical evaluation and, sometimes, by patch testing.[96,97]

Treatment

Allergic contact dermatitis is treated with topical steroids and, in severe cases, a prednisone taper. Patients are advised not to scrub the affected areas with soap or water, as doing so may further irritate the skin.[95]

Psoriasis

Overview

Psoriasis is a benign hyperproliferative inflammation of the skin that can be either acute or chronic. Although most cases do not affect general health, psoriasis can, in rare cases, be life-threatening.[98] An explosive onset of psoriasis may be the first sign of HIV.[9]

Presentation (see figures 4.38–4.39)

Psoriasis is characterized by erythematous papules, as well as itchy, red, precisely defined plaques with silvery scales.[98] Psoriasis may also present with fine pitting of the nails, among other findings. Auspitz sign is another common finding, consisting of droplets of blood that appear when the patient's scales are removed.[99]

Workup

The diagnosis of psoriasis is clinical and is based on the appearance and distribution of the patient's lesions.[9]

Treatment

When treating psoriasis, topical agents containing tar and salicylic acid may be used.[59] Topical steroids, such as betamethasone, may also be ordered for patients. In moderate or severe cases, ultraviolet light therapy may be part of treatment.[100,101]

Pityriasis Rosea

Overview

Pityriasis rosea is a self-limiting inflammatory skin disease characterized by oval lesions on the trunk and extremities.[102] Pityriasis rosea presents at a slightly higher rate in females than males and commonly occurs during the spring and fall.[9]

Presentation (see figure 4.40)

In most presentations of pityriasis rosea, the initial finding is a "herald patch" that measures 2–10 cm in diameter.[103] A generalized rash then develops within 1–2 weeks, which can last up to 4–8 weeks. The patient's lesions often follow a Christmas tree pattern, with cleavage lines on the trunk and pruritic rashes on the trunk and proximal extremities.

Workup

A diagnosis of pityriasis rosea is made by considering the clinical distribution and appearance

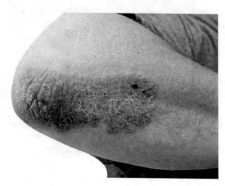

Figure 4.38. Psoriasis on elbow.

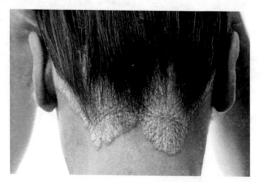

Figure 4.39. Psoriasis on neck.

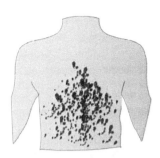

Figure 4.40. Pityriasis rosea

of the patient's lesions.[103] A serologic test for syphilis should also be performed if the patient's lesions are small in number, perfectly-shaped, not pruritic, or located on the palmar or plantar surfaces.[9]

Treatment

Because pityriasis rosea usually remits within weeks and often confers lifelong immunity after one episode, supportive treatment is indicated. Treatment may involve oral antihistamines, topical steroids, and topical antipruritics. Oral erythromycin may see use if infection occurs due to scratching of lesions. Exposure to ultraviolet light may also be recommended.[104]

Xanthelasma (see figure 4.4)

Overview

Xanthelasma is a condition in which yellow plaques develop as a result of adipose tissue buildup beneath the skin, usually accumulating close to the inner canthus. The condition is more common in women than in men, with peak onset between the ages of 40 and 50. Hyperlipidemia is the most common underlying cause of xanthelasma.[9]

Presentation

Xanthelasma presents with soft, yellowish lesions that form plaques across the upper eyelids, generally on the medial side.[105] Although eyelid function remains unaffected in most cases, ptosis has been known to occur.[105]

Workup

When diagnosing xanthelasma, a lipid panel is necessary for patients suspected of having hyperlipidemia.[105] A biopsy should also be performed as needed to rule out other conditions.[105]

Treatment

Treatments for xanthelasma are purely cosmetic. The condition may be treated through surgical excision, argon and carbon dioxide laser abrasion, chemical cauterization, electro-desiccation, or cryotherapy.[105]

Lyme Disease

Overview

Lyme disease, the most common vector-born disease in the United States, is spread by infected blacklegged ticks or deer ticks (*Ixodes scapularis*), who transmit the disease through bites.[106,107] Patients who live in wooded and grassy areas are at increased risk; this risk is especially increased between May and November, when ticks are most active. After a patient is bitten, it usually takes 36–48 hours for a tick to transmit the infecting organism—*Borrelia burgdorferi*—to the host via feeding.[108]

Presentation

Lyme disease typically presents with distinctive erythema migrans that appears as an expanding red lesion with a "bull's eye pattern" and central clearing. The rash usually appears 7 days after the host has been infected. Approximately half of all patients with Lyme disease also present with flu-like symptoms.[109]

Workup

Antibody detection tests are widely used to determine if a patient has been exposed to *B. burgdorferi*.[110] An ELISA test is used first; if the test is positive, a Western blot is used to confirm the diagnosis.[109]

Treatment

Patients with Lyme disease may need to be referred to an infectious disease specialist. In early cases, Lyme disease can be treated in an outpatient setting with oral antibiotics such as doxycycline and amoxicillin, among others.[110] Advanced cases may require hospitalization.

Rocky Mountain Spotted Fever

Overview

Rocky Mountain spotted fever is a potentially lethal bacterial infection transmitted by tick bites. After a patient is bitten, the tick normally takes 24 hours to transmit *Rickettsiae rickettsii*, the infecting organism, to the host.[111]

Presentation

A febrile illness is often the initial finding of Rocky Mountain spotted fever and occurs approximately two days after the patient is infected.[111] Subsequent petechial and maculopapular rashes typically appear, initially presenting on the wrists and ankles as spots that are 1–5 mm in diameter. These rashes then spread to the rest of the body. Patients with Rocky Mountain spotted fever may also present with flu-like symptoms and experience abdominal and joint pain.[111]

Workup

A diagnosis of Rocky Mountain spotted fever is based on clinical criteria such as fever, rash, and myalgia.[112] Laboratory tests that help confirm the diagnosis include polymerase chain reaction, immunohistochemical staining, and an indirect immunofluorescence assay with *R. rickettsii* antigens.[109]

Treatment

Patients with Rocky Mountain spotted fever may need to be referred to an infectious disease specialist.[109] To eliminate the infection, patients are prescribed antibiotics, namely doxycycline.[113]

Smallpox

Overview

Smallpox is caused by variants of the variola virus and takes root in blood vessels in the skin, mouth, and throat.[114] Although preventative measures have been established to prevent smallpox outbreaks in the event of a bioterror attack, the last naturally occurring case was reported in 1977.[115]

Presentation

The hallmark sign of smallpox is the distribution and progression of lesions. Patients with smallpox initially present with rashes that appear as flat, red spots or lesions. Within 2 days, these rashes develop into small blisters, which are initially filled with clear fluid and later with pus. These lesions first appear on the face, forearms, or oral mucosa and palate then undergo centrifugal distribution, with the greatest concentration appearing on the face and distal extremities. On any one part of the body, all lesions will exhibit the same stage of development. The scabs from these lesions characteristically lead to deep, pitted scars. Finally, patients may experience excruciating pain.[116]

Smallpox also presents with a sudden onset of flu-like symptoms, such as fever and headache. Other findings may include fatigue, back pain, vomiting, and diarrhea.[116]

Workup

A diagnosis of smallpox is confirmed via polymerase chain reaction of samples from the patient's pustules or vesicles. Electron microscopy or a viral culture of a scraped skin lesion may also be used to confirm the presence of the smallpox virus.[117]

Treatment

All cases of smallpox should be reported to the health department. As there is no cure for smallpox, patients should be vaccinated for the disease if the risk of infection presents. Infected patients should be isolated to prevent the spread of smallpox to others.[116]

Anthrax (see figure 4.5)

Overview

Anthrax is an acute disease stemming from infection by the bacterium *Bacillus anthracis.* The disease affects both humans and animals and is mostly lethal. Anthrax spores are transported by clothing, shoes, and bodies of dead animals that have died of anthrax. Moreover, anthrax spores can be produced in vitro; as such, the disease has a history of use as a biological weapon.[118]

Presentation

Anthrax predominantly occurs on exposed areas of the arms and hands, but can occur on the face and neck as well. The most common form of anthrax is cutaneous, which typically begins with pruritic papules that develop into vesicles and ulcers.[119,120] Subsequently, these lesions evolve into black necrotic central eschar with edema.[121] Regional lymphadenopathy may also be seen.

Inhalation anthrax is a less common form of anthrax that results from the inhalation of spore-bearing particles. This form clinically presents in a biphasic pattern. The prodromal phase is characterized by non-specific flu-like signs and symptoms, such as fever, dyspnea, malaise, and myalgia. Fever may also present in the fulminant phase, but this phase is distinguished by the development of diaphoresis and septic shock.[9]

Workup

A clinical diagnosis of anthrax may be made based on the appearance of the patient's skin lesions. A gram stain is used to confirm the diagnosis by isolating *B. anthracis* bacilli.[121] A chest x-ray or computerized tomography scan is ordered if pulmonary symptoms are present.[120]

Treatment

An anthrax vaccine is only recommended for those at a high risk of contracting the disease, such as military personnel. Patients with anthrax should also be reported to the health department, and those with serious cases should be hospitalized. The course of treatment focuses on oral antibiotics such as penicillin, ciprofloxacin, and doxycycline, among others.[118]

Warts

Overview

Warts are benign epidural neoplasms that are caused by the human papillomavirus (HPV) and transmitted via direct contact. Warts appear on the skin as raised, round, or oval growths.[122] These growths are generally painless and harmless, although some warts may cause itching and pain, especially on the feet.[123] Most warts resolve spontaneously without treatment.[124]

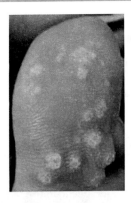

Figure 4.41. Common warts

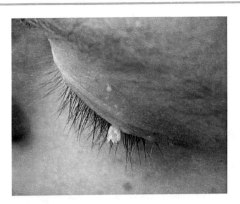

Figure 4.42. Filiform wart

Workup

A diagnosis of warts is made on the basis of the patient's clinical appearance.[123] A biopsy may also see use as needed.[124]

Common Warts (verrucae vulgaris)

Presentation (see figure 4.41)

Common warts (verrucae vulgaris) present as flesh- or dark-colored papules with a rough surface. Although these warts are usually asymptomatic, they may cause mild pain if they appear on a weight-bearing surface such as the bottom of the feet.[125] Common warts can appear anywhere on a patient's skin, but most often affect the fingers, hands, knees, and elbows.[122]

Treatment

Common warts are treated with salicylic acid, a first-line therapy in wart treatment.[124] Liquid nitrogen and electrocautery can also be used to remove the wart.

Filiform Warts (digitate)

Presentation (see figure 4.42)

Filiform warts (digitate) present with a finger-like appearance with various projections. This type of wart is usually asymptomatic and appears as long, narrow, and frondlike growths. Filiform warts tend to present on the eyelids, face, neck, or lips.[125]

Treatment

Filiform warts are treated with tretinoin cream.[124] Liquid nitrogen and electrocautery may also be recommended.[126] Salicylic acid may be used as an alternative treatment.

Flat Warts

Presentation

Flat warts appear as flat or slightly elevated papules that may be smooth or slightly hyperkeratotic.[124] These warts may be flesh-colored, pink, or light yellow, and are most often located on the face and along scratch marks.[125]

Treatment

Tretinoin cream, liquid nitrogen, and electrocautery are common treatment methods for flat warts.[126]

Plantar Warts

Presentation

Plantar warts are slightly raised with a roughened surface and are commonly found on the soles of the feet. These warts may be painful and tender, producing discomfort when the patient is walking, running, or standing.[123,125]

Treatment

Plantar warts are treated with salicylic acid (Occlusal-HP, Mediplast). Other treatments for plantar warts include blunt dissection, laser therapy, and Compound W Freeze Off.[126]

Genital Warts

Presentation

Genital warts are small, skin-colored or pink growths that form on the vulva, vagina, penis, or anus.[127] These growths present with several projections, a broad base, and a cauliflower-like distribution. Unlike other types of warts, genital warts are considered a sexually transmitted disease (STD).[128]

Treatment

Vaccines for HPV can prevent the occurrence of genital warts.[129] Common methods of wart removal include cryotherapy, electrocauterization, and laser or surgical incision.[127] Other agents include podofilox (Condylox), 20% podophyllin resin (Pododerm), bichloracetic acid, and trichloroacetic acid.[128,129]

Allergic Reactions

Overview

Allergic reactions involve a hypersensitive reaction to contact with a particular allergen. This contact may occur when allergens are inhaled into the lungs, swallowed, or injected.[130]

Presentation

Because allergic reactions may range from mild to severe, signs and symptoms can vary greatly in intensity. Common findings of mild allergic reactions include hives, rashes, and nasal congestion, among others. Patients with moderate or severe allergic reactions may present with difficulty breathing or swallowing, palpitations, hives, and abdominal pain.[130] Serious cases of allergic reactions may result in anaphylactic shock and, rarely, death.

Workup

When diagnosing a patient with an allergic reaction, it is crucial to obtain a history of the patient's exposure and reaction.[26]

Treatment

Mild cases of allergic reactions are treated with antihistamines (e.g., diphenhydramine). Moderate to severe cases may require intramuscular diphenhydramine or subcutaneous epinephrine.[26,129]

Senile Pruritus

Overview

Senile pruritus is an idiopathic type of pruritus common in the elderly that is precipitated by circumstances that result in skin dryness and irritation.[131,132]

Presentation

Senile pruritus results in a tingling or burning skin sensation.[26] Itching may occur over the patient's entire body or in a single location.

Workup

In a physical examination for senile pruritus, a patient's skin should be examined for lesions and secondary infections. Furthermore, the patient's history may help identify potential causative factors for senile pruritus, such as certain medications.[131]

Treatment

Treatments that are often beneficial for patients with senile pruritus include bath oils, moisturizing lotions, and massage, among others. Additionally, antihistamines and topical steroids may see use.[133]

Frost Bite

Overview

Frostbite is a type of tissue damage resulting from exposure to cold, which causes the interstitial and cellular spaces to freeze. This exposure results in a loss of color and feeling in the affected areas and may cause permanent tissue damage.[134,135]

Presentation

Frostbite may affect any area of the patient's body. Affected areas are typically cold, white, hard, and numb.[136,137] The patient may complain of stinging or burning, in addition to loss of muscle control. After the affected areas thaw, the patient's skin may become red and painful, with potential development of bullae.[134]

Workup

A diagnosis of frostbite is based on clinical findings.[137]

Treatment

Management of frostbite includes warming the patient and immediate transport to an emergency care facility.[138]

Insect stings and bites

Overview

Insect bites and stings can potentially produce toxic reactions that range from local and mild irritation to life-threatening complications. Severe medical problems, such as transmission of insect-borne illnesses and severe allergic reactions, can result from insect bites.[139]

Presentation

Insect bites and stings cause swelling, pain, and itching. Patients may also complain of burning, numbness, and tingling.[140,141]

Workup

A diagnosis of insect stings and bites is made clinically and includes checking the patient for the stinger and assessing the patient's airways for allergic reactions.[141] Identification of the offending insect can potentially be made by examining the location, size, and pattern of the bite or sting. Moreover, it may be necessary to rule out other conditions that present with papules similar to insect bites.[139]

Treatment

Antihistamines such as diphenhydramine may be ordered for hives, and subcutaneous epinephrine may be necessary if the patient exhibits stridor or respiratory distress. Any stingers found should be removed.[141] Topical anesthetics are recommended for treatment of insect bites and stings in general; topical or intralesional corticosteroids may also be prescribed. Ice packs may minimize swelling and should be applied with a cloth barrier for no more than 15 minutes at a time.

Figures

Figure 4.1. Jambula. Eczema. http://commons.wikimedia.org/wiki/File:Eczema-arms.jpg. Published 2006. Accessed April 2015. Reproduced with permission.

Figure 4.2. Pustule. Barkley & Associates, Inc. Published 2015.

Figure 4.3. Sand M, Sand D, Thrandorf C, Paech V, Altmeyer P, Bechara FG. Basal cell carcinoma. http://commons.wikimedia.org/wiki/File:BCC_Nodular_type.jpg. Published 2010. Accessed April 2015. Reproduced with permission.

Figure 4.4. Peter KD. Xanthelasma palpebrarum. http://commons.wikimedia.org/wiki/File:Xanthelasma.jpg. Published 2005. Accessed April 2015. Reproduced with permission.

Figure 4.5. Steele J. Anthrax. CDC. http://commons.wikimedia.org/wiki/File:Anthrax_PHIL_2033.png. Published 1962. Accessed April 2015. Reproduced with permission.

Figure 4.6. Harris DA. Impetigo. Phototake. Reproduced with permission.

Figure 4.7. Farina2000. Psoriasis on scalp. By Farina2000. iStock.com. Reproduced with permission.

Figure 4.8. Jerjian J. Herpes zoster. Phototake. Reproduced with permission.

Figure 4.9. ISM. Furuncle. Phototake. Reproduced with permission.

Figure 4.10. Camiloaranzales. Varicella. http://commons.wikimedia.org/wiki/File:Varicela_Aranzales.jpg. Published 2010. Accessed April 2015. Reproduced with permission.

Figures 4.11-4.28. Barkley & Associates, Inc. Published 2015.

Figure 4.29. Claudiodivizia. Subungal hematoma. iStock. Reproduced with permission.

Figure 4.30. Oger GD. Tinea capitus. http://commons.wikimedia.org/wiki/File:Teigne_-_Tinea_capitis.jpg. Accessed April 2015. Reproduced with permission.

Figure 4.31. Camazine S. Tinea corporis. Phototake. Reproduced with permission.

Figure 4.32. Harris A. Tinea cruris. Phototake. Accessed April 2015. Reproduced with permission.

Figure 4.33. Marazzi P. Tinea pedis. Science Source. Reproduced with permission.

Figure 4.34. Craig B. Squamous cell carcinoma. CDC. http://phil.cdc.gov/phil/details.asp. Published 1965. Accessed April 2015. Reproduced with permission.

Figure 4.35. Kraus S. Seborrheic keratosis. CDC. http://phil.cdc.gov/phil/details.asp. Published 1981. Accessed April 2015. Reproduced with permission.

Figure 4.36. Hellman J. Basal cell carcinoma. http://commons.wikimedia.org/wiki/File:Basal_cell_carcinoma2.JPG. Published 2009. Accessed April 2015. Reproduced with permission.

Figure 4.37. Harris A. Malignant melanoma. Phototake. Accessed April 2015. Reproduced with permission.

Figure 4.38. Jacobson J. Psoriasis on elbow. iStock. Accessed April 2015. Reproduced with permission.

Figure 4.39. Farina2000. Psoriasis on neck. iStock. Accessed April 2015. Reproduced with permission.

Figure 4.40. Pityriasis rosea. Barkley & Associates, Inc. Published 2015.

Figure 4.41. Common warts. http://commons.wikimedia.org/wiki/File:Dornwarzen.jpg. Accessed April 2015. Reproduced with permission.

Figure 4.42. Schweintechnik. Filiform wart. http://commons.wikimedia.org/wiki/File:Wart_filiform_eyelid.jpg. Accessed April 2015. Reproduced with permission.

References

1. Macnab M. Approach to skin lesions. University of British Columbia. Web site. http://learnpediatrics.com/body-systems/general-pediatrics/aproach-to-skin-lesions/. Last updated March 11, 2012. Accessed March 11, 2015.

2. Nicol NH, Huether SE. Structure, function, and disorders of the integument. In: Huether SE, McCance KL, eds. *Understanding Pathophysiology.* 5th ed. St. Louis, MO: Elsevier Mosby; 2012: 1038–1069.

3. Patches. MedlinePlus Web site. http://www.nlm.nih.gov/medlineplus/ency/article/003231.htm. Updated November 4, 2012. Accessed March 11, 2015.

4. Jarvis C. *Physical Examination & Health Assessment.* 6th ed. St. Louis, MO: Saunders Elsevier; 2012.

5. Lui H, Mamelak AJ. Plaque psoriasis. In: Elston DM, ed. Medscape. http://emedicine.medscape.com/article/1108072-overview. Updated January 22, 2015. Accessed March 11, 2015.

6. Acne: Symptoms. Mayo Clinic Web site. http://www.mayoclinic.com/health/acne/DS00169/DSECTION=symptoms. Updated January 20, 2015. Accessed March 11, 2015.

7. Vesicles. MedlinePlus Web site. http://www.nlm.nih.gov/medlineplus/ency/article/003939.htm. Updated April 14, 2013. Accessed March 11, 2015.

8. Definition of wheal. MedicineNet Web site. http://www.medicinenet.com/script/main/art.asp?articlekey=9539. Updated September 20, 2012. Accessed March 11, 2015.

9. Barkley TW Jr. Diagnosis and management of integumentary disorders. In: Barkley TW Jr, ed. *Adult-Gerontology Primary Care Nurse Practitioner Certification Review/Clinical Update Continuing Education Course.* West Hollywood, CA: Barkley and Associates; 2015: 39–51.

10. Abscess. MedlinePlus Web site. http://www.nlm.nih.gov/medlineplus/ency/article/001353.htm. Updated August 31, 2014. Accessed March 11, 2015.

11. Tumor. MedlinePlus Web site. http://www.nlm.nih.gov/medlineplus/ency/article/001310.htm. Updated August 17, 2014. Accessed March 11, 2015.

12. Sharma A, Lambert PJ, Maghari A, Clark W. Arcuate, annular, and polycyclic inflammatory and infectious lesions. *Clin Dermatol.* 2011; 29(2): 140–150. doi: 10.1016/j.clindermatol.2011.02.001

13. Rao J. Acne vulgaris. In: James WD, ed. Medscape. http://emedicine.medscape.com/article/1069804-overview. Updated January 23, 2013. Accessed March 11, 2015.

14. McKoy K. Acne. In: Porter RS, Kaplan JL. The Merck Manual Online. http://www.merckmanuals.com/home/skin_disorders/acne_and_related_disorders/acne.html?qt=acne&alt=sh. Updated April 2013. Accessed March 11, 2015.

15. Dover JS, Batra P. Light-based, adjunctive, and other therapies for acne vulgaris. In: Basow DS, ed. *UpToDate.* Waltham, MA; UpToDate; 2015. http://www.uptodate.com/contents/light-based-adjunctive-and-other-therapies-for-acne-vulgaris?source=search_result&search=Light-based%2C+adjunctive%2C+and+other+therapies+for+acne+vulgaris&selectedTitle=1~150. Updated July 7, 2014. Accessed March 11, 2015.

16. Adapalene. MedlinePlus Web site. http://www.nlm.nih.gov/medlineplus/druginfo/meds/a604001.html. Updated September 1, 2010. Accessed March 11, 2015.

17. Epstein EL, Gold LS. Safety and efficacy of tazarotene foam for the treatment of acne vulgaris. *Clin Cosmet Investig Dermatol.* 2014; 6: 123–125. doi: 10.2147/CCID.S34054

18. Graber E. Treatment of acne vulgaris. In: Basow DS, ed. *UpToDate.* Waltham, MA: UpToDate; 2015. http://www.uptodate.com/contents/treatment-of-acne-vulgaris?source=search_result&search=treatment+of+acne+vulgaris&selectedTitle=1~150. Updated February 18, 2015. Accessed March 11, 2015.

19. Isotretinoin (oral route). Mayo Clinic Web site. http://www.mayoclinic.org/drugs-supplements/isotretinoin-oral-route/proper-use/drg-20068178. Updated April 1, 2015. Accessed April 3, 2015.

20. Graber E. Hormonal therapy for women with acne vulgaris. In: Basow DS, ed. *UpToDate.* Waltham, MA: UpToDate; 2015. http://www.uptodate.com/contents/hormonal-therapy-for-women-with-acne-vulgaris?source=search_result&search=hormonal+therapy+for+women+with+acne+vulgaris&selectedTitle=1~150. Updated March 30, 2015. Accessed April 3, 2015.

21. Arowojolu AO, Gallo MF, Lopez LM, Grimes DA, Garner SE. Cochrane review: Combined oral contraceptive pills for treatment of acne. *Evid-Based Child Health.* 2011; 6(5): 1340–1433. doi: 10.1002/ebch.841

22. Kenalog injection. WebMD Web site. http://www.webmd.com/drugs/drug-9275-Kenalog+Inj.aspx. Accessed March 11, 2015.

23. Poinier AC, Denkler KA. Dermabrasion. WebMD Web site. http://www.webmd.com/beauty/dermabrasion/dermabrasion-21085. Updated March 12, 2014. Accessed March 11, 2015.

24. Baddour LM. Folliculitis. In: Basow DS, ed. *UpToDate.* Waltham, MA: UpToDate; 2015. http://www.uptodate.com/contents/folliculitis?source=search_result&search=folliculitis&selectedTitle=1~150. Updated February 3, 2014. Accessed March 11, 2015.

25. Baddour LM. Skin abscesses, furuncles, and carbuncles. In: Basow DS, ed. *UpToDate.* Waltham, MA: UpToDate; 2015. http://www.uptodate.com/contents/skin-abscesses-furuncles-and-carbuncles?source=search_result&search=Skin+abscesses%2C+furuncles%2C+and+carbuncles&selectedTitle=1~150. Updated March 9, 2015. Accessed March 11, 2015.

26. *Taber's Cyclopedic Medical Dictionary.* 21st ed. Philadelphia, PA: F. A. Davis Company; 2013.

27. Baddour LM. Cellulitis and erysipelas. In: Basow DS, ed. *UpToDate.* Waltham, MA: UpToDate; 2015. http://www.uptodate.com/contents/cellulitis-and-erysipelas?source=search_result&search=cellulitis+and+erysipelas&selectedTitle=1~150. Updated March 20, 2015.

28. Cellulitis treatment & management. Medscape Web site. http://emedicine.medscape.com/article/214222-treatment. Updated August 19, 2014.

29. Herchline TE, Chandrasekar PH, Swaminathan S. Erysipelas. In: Bronze MS, ed. Medscape. http://emedicine.medscape.com/article/1052445-overview#showall. Updated August 15, 2014. Accessed March 11, 2015.

30. Patient information: Hidradenitis suppurativa (the basics). In: Basow DS, ed. *UpToDate*. Waltham, MA: UpToDate; 2015. http://www.uptodate.com/contents/hidradenitis-suppurativa-the-basics?source=search_result&search=Patient+information%3A+Hidradenitis+suppurativa&selectedTitle=1~40. Accessed March 11, 2015.

31. United States Department of Health and Human Services, National Institutes of Health, United States National Library of Medicine, Lister Hill National Center for Biomedical Communication. Hidradenitis suppurativa. http://ghr.nlm.nih.gov/condition/hidradenitis-suppurativa. Updated December 2013. Accessed March 11, 2015.

32. Baddour LM. Impetigo. In: Basow DS, ed. *UpToDate*. Waltham, MA: UpToDate; 2015. http://www.uptodate.com/contents/impetigo?source=search_result&search=impetigo&selectedTitle=1~96. Updated February 26, 2015. Accessed March 11, 2015.

33. Billingsley EM, Vidimos AT. Paronychia. In: James WD, ed. Medscape. http://emedicine.medscape.com/article/1106062-overview#showall. Updated November 17, 2014. Accessed March 11, 2015.

34. Ritting AW, O'Malley MP, Rodner CM. Acute paronychia. *J Hand Surg [Am]*. 2012; 37(5): 1068–1070. doi: 10.1016/j.jhsa.2011.11.021

35. Nordqvist C. Inflammation: Causes, symptoms and treatment. Medical News Today Web site. http://www.medicalnewstoday.com/articles/248423.php. Updated May 25, 2015.

36. Cassoobhoy A. Sepsis (blood infection) and septic shock. WebMD Web site. http://www.webmd.com/a-to-z-guides/sepsis-septicemia-blood-infection. Updated January 21, 2015.

37. Nicol NH, Huether SE. Alterations of the integument in children. In: Huether SE, McCance KL, eds. *Understanding Pathophysiology*. 5th ed. St. Louis, MO: Elsevier Mosby; 2012: 1070–1082.

38. Subungual hematoma drainage. Medscape Web site. http://emedicine.medscape.com/article/82926-overview. Updated September 11, 2014.

39. Fastle RK, Bothner J. Subungual hematoma. In: Basow DS, ed. *UpToDate*. Waltham, MA: UpToDate; 2015. http://www.uptodate.com/contents/subungual-hematoma?source=search_result&search=Subungual+hematoma&selectedTitle=1~9. Updated January 6, 2015. Accessed March 11, 2015.

40. Dean B, Becker G, Little C. The management of the acute traumatic subungual haematoma: A systematic review. *Hand Surg*. 2012; 17(151). doi: 10.1142/S021881041230001X

41. Rosenblatt A, De Campos Guidi HG, Belda W Jr. Nonsexually transmitted diseases. In *Male Genital Lesions: The Urological Perspective*. Heidelberg, Germany: Springer-Verlag; 2013: 167–212.

42. Leber MJ, Tirumani A. Balanitis. In: Schraga ED, ed. Medscape. http://emedicine.medscape.com/article/777026-overview#showall. Updated October 22, 2014. Accessed March 11, 2015.

43. Kauffman CA, Campbell JR. Candida infections in children: An overview. In: Basow DS, ed. *UpToDate*. Waltham, MA: UpToDate; 2015. http://www.uptodate.com/contents/candida-infections-in-children-an-overview?source=search_result&search=Candida+infections+in+children%3A+An+overview&selectedTitle=1~150. Updated January 22, 2014. Accessed March 11, 2015.

44. Aaron DM. Fungal skin infections. In: Porter RS, Kaplan JL, eds. The Merck Manual Online. http://www.merckmanuals.com/home/skin_disorders/fungal_skin_infections/intertrigo.html?qt=candidaintertrigo&alt=sh. Updated June 2013. Accessed March 11, 2015.

45. Parker ER. Candidal intertrigo. In: Basow DS, ed. *UpToDate*. Waltham, MA: UpToDate; 2015. http://www.uptodate.com/contents/candidal-intertrigo?source=search_result&search=Candidal+intertrigo&selectedTitle=1~150. Updated October 21, 2013. Accessed March 11, 2015.

46. Selden ST. Intertrigo. In: James WD, ed. Medscape. http://emedicine.medscape.com/article/1087691-overview. Updated September 3, 2014. Accessed March 12, 2015.

47. Kao GF. Tinea capitis. In: Elston DM, ed. Medscape. http://emedicine.medscape.com/article/1091351-overview#showall. Updated July 21, 2014. Accessed March 12, 2015.

48. Goldstein AO, Goldstein BG. Dermatophyte (tinea) infections. In: Basow DS, ed. *UpToDate*. Waltham, MA: UpToDate; 2015. http://www.uptodate.com/contents/dermatophyte-tinea-infections?source=search_result&search=dermatophyte&selectedTitle=1~50. Updated April 1, 2015. Accessed April 3, 2015.

49. Lesher JL Jr. Tinea corporis. In: Elston DM, ed. Medscape. http://emedicine.medscape.com/article/1091473-overview. Updated July 21, 2014. Accessed March 12, 2015.

50. Tinea corporis. MedlinePlus Web site. http://www.nlm.nih.gov/medlineplus/ency/article/000877.htm. Updated November 20, 2012. Accessed March 12, 2015.

51. Abdel-Rahman SM, Farrand N, Schuenemann E, et al. The prevalence of infections with *Trichophyton tonsurans* in schoolchildren: the CAPITIS study. *Pediatrics*. 2010; 125(5): 966–973. doi: 10.1542/peds.2009-2522

52. Jock itch. MedlinePlus Web site. http://www.nlm.nih.gov/medlineplus/ency/article/000876.htm. Updated May 15, 2013. Accessed March 12, 2015.

53. Aaron DM. Introduction to benign skin tumors, growths, and vascular lesions. In: Porter RS, Kaplan JL, ed. The Merck Manual Online. http://www.merckmanuals.com/professional/dermatologic_disorders/benign_skin_tumors_growths_and_vascular_lesions/introduction_to_benign_skin_tumors_growths_and_vascular_lesions.html. Updated September 2013. Accessed March 12, 2015.

54. Wiederkehr M, Schwartz RA. Tinea cruris. In: Elston DM, ed. Medscape. http://emedicine.medscape.com/article/1091806-overview. Updated July 21, 2014. Accessed March 12, 2015.

55. Aaron DM. Athlete's foot: Fungal skin infections. In: Porter RS, Kaplan JL, eds. The Merck Manual Online. http://www.merckmanuals.com/home/skin_disorders/fungal_skin_infections/athletes_foot.html?qt=athlete%27s%20food&alt=sh. Updated June 2013. Accessed March 12, 2015.

56. Robbins CM, Elewski BE. Tinea pedis. In: Elston DM, ed. Medscape. http://emedicine.medscape.com/article/1091684-overview. Updated December 10, 2014. Accessed March 12, 2015.

57. United States Department of Health and Human Services, Centers for Disease Control and Prevention. Symptoms of ringworm infections. http://www.cdc.gov/fungal/diseases/ringworm/symptoms.html. Updated September 30, 2014. Accessed March 12, 2015.

58. Athlete's foot. MedlinePlus Web site. http://www.nlm.nih.gov/medlineplus/ency/article/000875.htm. Updated May 15, 2013. Accessed March 12, 2015.

59. Ely JW, Rosenfeld S, Seabury Stone M. Diagnosis and management of tinea infections. *Am Fam Physician*. 2014; 90(10): 702–711. http://www.aafp.org/afp/2014/1115/p702.html

60. Tosti A. Onychomycosis. In: Elston DM, ed. Medscape. http://emedicine.medscape.com/article/1105828-overview. Updated January 21, 2015. Accessed March 12, 2015.

61. Onychomycosis. ClinicalKey Web site. https://www.clinicalkey.com/topics/dermatology/onychomycosis.html. Accessed March 12, 2015.

62. Moreno-Coutiño G, Arenas R, Reyes-Terán G. Clinical presentation of onychomycosis in HIV/AIDS: a review of 280 Mexican cases. *Indian J Dermatol*. 2011; 56(1): 120–121. doi: 10.4103/0019-5154.77577

63. Rehmus WE. Fingernail and toenail injury. In: Porter RS, Kaplan JL, eds. The Merck Manual Online. http://www.merckmanuals.com/home/skin_disorders/nail_disorders/fingernail_and_toenail_infections.html?qt=onychomycosis&alt=sh. Updated August 2014. Accessed March 12, 2015.

64. Ghannoum M, Isham N. Fungal nail infections (onychomycosis): a never-ending story? *PLoS Pathog*. 2014; 10(6): e1004105. doi:10.1371/journal.ppat.1004105

65. Burkhart CG. Tinea versicolor. In: Elston DM, ed. Medscape. http://emedicine.medscape.com/article/1091575-overview. Updated July 21, 2014. Accessed March 12, 2015.

66. Dourmishev LA. Pediatric tinea versicolor workup. In: Elston DM, ed. Medscape. http://emedicine.medscape.com/article/911138-workup. Updated November 4, 2014. Accessed March 12, 2015.

67. Shingles. MedlinePlus Web site. http://www.nlm.nih.gov/medlineplus/ency/article/000858.htm. Updated June 6, 2013. Accessed March 12, 2015.

68. Stevens DL, Bisno AL, Chambers HF, et al. Practice guidelines for the diagnosis and management of skin and soft tissue infections: 2014 update by the Infectious Diseases Society of America. *Clin Infect Dis*. 2014; 59(2), 147–159. doi: 10.1093/cid/ciu296

69. United States Department of Health and Human Services, Centers for Disease Control and Prevention. Shingles (herpes zoster). http://www.cdc.gov/shingles/index.html. Updated May 1, 2014.

70. Kaye KM. Herpes zoster. In: Porter RS, Kaplan JL, eds. The Merck Manual Online. http://www.merckmanuals.com/professional/infectious_diseases/herpesviruses/herpes_zoster.html?qt=shingles&alt=sh. Updated May 2013. Accessed March 12, 2015.

71. Lichtenstein R. Varicella-zoster (shingles) organism-specific therapy. In: Bronze MS, ed. Medscape. http://emedicine.medscape.com/article/1966889-overview. Updated March 6, 2013. Accessed March 12, 2015.

72. Patient information: Actinic keratosis (the basics). UpToDate Web site. http://www.uptodate.com/contents/actinic-keratosis-the-basics?source=search_result&search=Patient+information%3A+Actinic+keratosis+%28the+basics%29&selectedTitle=1~150. Accessed March 12, 2015.

73. Spencer JM, Henry M. Actinic keratosis. IN: James WD, ed. Medscape. http://emedicine.medscape.com/article/1099775-overview. Updated September 10, 2014. Accessed March 12, 2015.

74. Wiegell SR, Wulf HC, Szeimies RM, et al. Daylight photodynamic therapy for actinic keratosis: an international consensus. *J Eur Acad Dermatol Venereol*. 2012; 26(6): 673–679. doi: 10.1111.j.1468-3083.2011.04386.x

75. Squamous cell skin cancer. MedlinePlus Web site. http://www.nlm.nih.gov/medlineplus/ency/article/000829.htm. Updated August 9, 2013. Accessed March 12, 2015.

76. Wells GL. Squamous cell carcinoma. In: Porter RS, Kaplan JL, eds. The Merck Manual Online. http://www.merckmanuals.com/professional/dermatologic_disorders/cancers_of_the_skin/squamous_cell_carcinoma.html?qt=squamous%20cell%20carcinoma&alt=sh. Updated November 2013. Accessed March 12, 2015.

77. Squamous cell carcinoma. Skin Cancer Foundation Web site. http://www.skincancer.org/skin-cancer-information/squamous-cell-carcinoma. Accessed March 12, 2015.

78. Monroe MM. Cutaneous squamous cell carcinoma differential diagnosis. In: Meyers AD, ed. Medscape. http://emedicine.medscape.com/article/1965430-differential. Updated January 14, 2015. Accessed March 12, 2015.

79. Stockfleth E, Rosen T, Shumack S, eds. *Managing Skin Cancer*. New York, NY: Springer Heidelberg Dordrecht; 2010.

80. Seborrheic keratosis. MedlinePlus Web site. http://www.nlm.nih.gov/medlineplus/ency/article/000884.htm. Updated November 20, 2012. Accessed March 12, 2015.

81. Balin AK. Seborrheic keratosis. In: James WD, ed. Medscape. http://emedicine.medscape.com/article/1059477-overview. Updated May 19, 2012. Accessed March 12, 2015.

82. Seborrheic keratoses. American Academy of Dermatology Web site. https://www.aad.org/dermatology-a-to-z/diseases-and-treatments/q---t/seborrheic-keratoses. Accessed March 12, 2015.

83. Epidemiology and clinical features of basal cell carcinoma. UpToDate Web site. http://www.uptodate.com/contents/epidemiology-and-clinical-features-of-basal-cell-carcinoma?source=search_result&search=Epidemiology+and+clinical+features+of+basal+cell+carcinoma&selectedTitle=1~140. Updated August 21, 2014.

84. Basal cell carcinoma. MedlinePlus Web site. http://www.nlm.nih.gov/medlineplus/ency/article/000824.htm. Updated August 9, 2013.

85. Bader RS, Kennedy AS, Santacroce L, Diomede L. Basal cell carcinoma workup. In: Harris JE, ed. Medscape. http://emedicine.medscape.com/article/276624-workup. Updated October 24, 2014. Accessed March 12, 2015.

86. Rimoin DL, Pyeritz RE, Korf BR, eds. *Emery and Rimoin's Principles and Practice of Medical Genetics*. 6th ed. Waltham, MA: Elsevier Science; 2013: 1–8.

87. What is melanoma skin cancer? American Cancer Society Web site. http://www.cancer.org/cancer/skincancer-melanoma/detailedguide/melanoma-skin-cancer-what-is-melanoma. Updated September 5, 2014. Accessed March 12, 2015.

88. Tan WW. Malignant melanoma. In: Harris JE, ed. Medscape. http://emedicine.medscape.com/article/280245-overview. Updated October 3, 2014. Accessed March 12, 2015.

89. Staging. American Cancer Society Web site. http://www.cancer.org/treatment/understandingyourdiagnosis/staging. Updated June 7, 2012. Accessed March 12, 2015.

90. Kim BS. Atopic dermatitis. In: James WD, ed. Medscape. http://emedicine.medscape.com/article/1049085-overview. Updated December 8, 2014. Accessed March 12, 2015.

91. Kim BE, Leung DYM. Epidermal barrier in atopic dermatitis. *Allergy Asthma Immunol Res*. 2011; 4(1): 12–16. doi: 10.4168/aair.2012.4.1.12

92. Jaliman D. Detecting and dealing with eczema. WebMD Web site. http://www.webmd.com/skin-problems-and-treatments/eczema/treatment-11/eczema-stress?page=1. Reviewed June 11, 2015. Accessed June 14, 2015.

93. McKoy K. Contact dermatitis. In: Porter RS, Kaplan JL, eds. The Merck Manual Online. http://www.merckmanuals.com/professional/dermatologic_disorders/dermatitis/contact_dermatitis.html?qt=dermatitis&alt=sh. Updated October 2014. Accessed March 12, 2015.

94. Hogan DJ. Allergic contact dermatitis. In: James WD, ed. Medscape. http://emedicine.medscape.com/article/1049216-overview#aw2aab6b2b2. Updated March 19, 2014. Accessed March 12, 2015.

95. Usatine RP, Riojas M. Diagnosis and management of contact dermatitis. *Am Fam Physician*. 2010; 82(3): 249–255.

96. McKoy K. Atopic dermatitis. In: Porter RS, Kaplan JL, eds. The Merck Manual Online. http://www.merckmanuals.com/professional/dermatologic_disorders/dermatitis/atopic_dermatitis_eczema.html?qt=atopic%20dermatitis&alt=sh. Updated October 2014. Accessed March 12, 2015.

97. McKoy K. Atopic dermatitis. In: Porter RS, Kaplan JL, eds. The Merck Manual Online. http://www.merckmanuals.com/home/skin_disorders/itching_and_dermatitis/atopic_dermatitis.html. Updated October 2012. Accessed March 12, 2015.

98. About psoriasis. National Psoriasis Foundation Web site. https://www.psoriasis.org/about-psoriasis. Accessed March 12, 2015.

99. Raychaudhuri SK, Maverakis E., Raychaudhuri SP. Diagnosis and classification of psoriasis. *Autoimmunity Rev*. 2014; 13(4–5): 490–495. doi: 10.1016/j.autrev.2014.01.008

100. Schalock PC. Psoriasis. In: Porter RS, Kaplan JL, eds. The Merck Manual Online. http://www.merck-manuals.com/professional/dermatologic_disorders/psoriasis_and_scaling_diseases/psoriasis.html?qt=psoriasis&alt=sh. Updated December 2014. Accessed March 12, 2015.

101. Position Statement for maintenance therapy for psoriasis patients. American Academy of Dermatology and AAD Association. https://www.aad.org/forms/policies/Uploads/PS/PS-Maintenance%20Therapy%20for%20Psoriasis%20Patients.pdf. Published 2012. Accessed March 12, 2015.

102. Goldstein BG, Goldstein AO. Tinea versicolor. In: Basow DS, ed. *UpToDate*. Waltham, MA: UpToDate; 2015.http://www.uptodate.com/contents/tinea-versicolor?source=search_result&search=Tinea+versicolor&selectedTitle=1~38. Updated May 4, 2014. Accessed March 12, 2015.

103. Schwartz RA. Pityriasis rosea. In: Elston DM, ed. Medscape. http://emedicine.medscape.com/article/1107532-overview. Updated September 15, 2014. Accessed March 12, 2015.

104. Davis D, Litin S, Bundrick JB. Clinical pearls in dermatology 2013. *Dis Mon*. 2014; 60(7): 332–344. doi: 10.1016/j.disamonth.2014.04.010

105. Roy H Sr. Xanthelasma. In: Roy H Sr, ed. Medscape. http://emedicine.medscape.com/article/1213423-overview. Updated September 18, 2014. Accessed March 12, 2015.

106. United States Department of Health and Human Services, Centers for Disease Control and Prevention. Lyme disease. http://www.cdc.gov/lyme/. Updated September 18, 2014. Accessed March 12, 2015.

107. Lyme disease. American Lyme Disease Foundation Web site. http://aldf.com/lyme-disease/. Updated 2015. Accessed March 12, 2015.

108. United States Department of Health and Human Services, Centers for Disease Control and Prevention. Transmission. http://www.cdc.gov/lyme/Transmission/. Updated March 4, 2015. Accessed March 12, 2015.

109. United States Department of Health and Human Services, Centers for Disease Control and Prevention. Tickborne diseases of the United States: a reference manual for health care providers. http://www.uphs.upenn.edu/bugdrug/antibiotic_manual/TickborneDiseasesCDC2013.pdf. Published 2013. Accessed March 12, 2015.

110. Meyerhoff JO, Zaidman GW, Steele RW. Lyme disease. In: Diamond HS, ed. Medscape. http://emedicine.medscape.com/article/330178-overview. Updated January 22, 2015. Accessed March 12, 2015.

111. United States Department of Health and Human Services, Centers for Disease Control and Prevention. Rocky Mountain spotted fever (RMSF). http://www.cdc.gov/rmsf/. Updated November 21, 2013. Accessed March 12, 2015.

112. Cunha BA. Rocky Mountain spotted fever. In: Bronze MS, ed. Medscape. http://emedicine.medscape.com/article/228042-overview. Updated December 9, 2014. Accessed March 12, 2015.

113. Rocky Mountain spotted fever. MedlinePlus Web site. http://www.nlm.nih.gov/medlineplus/ency/article/000654.htm. Updated May 19, 2013. Accessed March 12, 2015.

114. Hussain AN, Hussain F, Alam M, Cleri DJ. Smallpox. In: Wallace MR, ed. Medscape. http://emedicine.medscape.com/article/237229-overview. Updated December 19, 2013. Accessed March 12, 2015.

115. United States Department of Health and Human Services, Centers for Disease Control and Prevention. Course: "Smallpox: disease, prevention, and intervention." http://www.bt.cdc.gov/agent/smallpox/training/overview/. Updated August 25, 2014. Accessed March 12, 2015.

116. Global alert and response (GAR): Frequently asked questions and answers on smallpox. World Health Organization Web site. http://www.who.int/csr/disease/smallpox/faq/en/. Accessed March 12, 2015.

117. Caserta MT. Smallpox (Variola). In: Porter RS, Kaplan JL, eds. The Merck Manual Online. http://www.merckmanuals.com/professional/infectious_diseases/pox_viruses/smallpox.html?qt=smallpox&alt=sh. Updated October 2014. Accessed March 12, 2015.

118. United States Department of Health and Human Services, Centers for Disease Control and Prevention. Anthrax: Treatment. http://www.cdc.gov/anthrax/medicalcare/treatment/index.html. Updated April 30, 2014. Accessed March 12, 2015.

119. Wilson KH. Clinical manifestation and diagnosis of anthrax. In: Basow DS, ed. *UpToDate*. Waltham, MA: UpToDate; 2015. http://www.uptodate.com/contents/clinical-manifestations-and-diagnosis-of-anthrax?source=search_result&search=Clinical+manifestation+and+diagnosis+of+anthrax&selectedTitle=1~70. Updated June 5, 2013. Accessed March 12, 2015.

120. Perez MT, Bush LM. Anthrax. In: Porter RS, Kaplan JL, eds. The Merck Manual Online. http://www.merckmanuals.com/professional/infectious_diseases/gram-positive_bacilli/anthrax.html?qt=anthrax&alt=sh. Updated September 2013. Accessed March 12, 2015.

121. Cunha BA. Anthrax. In: Bronze MS, ed. Medscape. http://emedicine.medscape.com/article/212127-overview. Updated July 16, 2014. Accessed March 12, 2015.

122. Patient information: Skin warts (the basics). UpToDate Web site. http://www.uptodate.com/contents/skin-warts-the-basics?source=-search_result&search=Patient+information%3A+Skin+warts+%28the+basics%29&selectedTitle=1~150. Accessed March 12, 2015.

123. Warts. PubMed Health Web site. http://www.ncbi.nlm.nih.gov/pubmedhealth/PMH0001888/. Accessed March 12, 2015.

124. Shenefelt PD. Nongenital warts. In: James WD, ed. Medscape. http://emedicine.medscape.com/article/1133317-overview. Updated December 9, 2014. Accessed March 12, 2015.

125. Dinulos JGH. Warts (Verrucae vulgaris). In: Porter RS, Kaplan JL, eds. The Merck Manual Online. http://www.merckmanuals.com/professional/dermatologic_disorders/viral_skin_diseases/warts.html?qt=warts&alt=sh. Updated January 2014. Accessed March 12, 2015.

126. Warts. American Academy of Dermatology Web site. https://www.aad.org/dermatology-a-to-z/diseases-and-treatments/u---w/warts. Accessed March 12, 2015.

127. Patient information: Anogenital warts (the basics). UpToDate Web site. http://www.uptodate.com/contents/anogenital-warts-the-basics?source=search_result&search=Patient+information%3A+Genital+warts+%28the+basics%29.&selectedTitle=1~150. Accessed March 12, 2015.

128. Ghadishah D. Genital warts in emergency medicine. In: James WD, ed. Medscape. http://emedicine.medscape.com/article/763014-overview. Updated November 4, 2014. Accessed March 12, 2015.

129. United States Department of Health and Human Services, Centers for Disease Control and Prevention. http://www.cdc.gov/std/treatment/2010/genital-warts.htm. Updated August 15, 2014. Accessed March 12, 2015.

130. Allergic reactions. MedlinePlus Web site. http://www.nlm.nih.gov/medlineplus/ency/article/000005.htm. Updated May 10, 2014. Accessed March 12, 2015.

131. MacNeal RJ. Itching (pruritus). In: Porter RS, Kaplan JL, eds. The Merck Manual Online. http://www.merckmanuals.com/professional/dermatologic_disorders/approach_to_the_dermatologic_patient/itching.html?qt=pruritus&alt=sh. Updated November 2013. Accessed March 12, 2015.

132. Fazio SB, Yosipovitch G. Pruritus: Etiology and patient evaluation. In: Basow DS, ed. *UpToDate*. Waltham, MA: UpToDate; 2015. http://www.uptodate.com/contents/pruritus-etiology-and-patient-evaluation?source=search_result&search=Pruritus%3A+Etiology+and+patient+evaluation&selectedTitle=1~150. Updated January 21, 2015. Accessed March 12, 2015.

133. Reich A, Stander S, Szepietowski JC. Pruritus in the elderly. *Clin Dermatol*. 2011; 29(1): 15–23. doi: 10.1016/j.clindermatol.2010.07.002

134. Zafren K, Mechem CC. Frostbite. In: Basow DS, ed. *UpToDate*. Waltham, MA: UpToDate; 2015. http://www.uptodate.com/contents/frostbite?source=search_result&search=frostbite&selectedTitle=1~40. Updated September 18, 2014. Accessed March 12, 2015.

135. United States Department of Health and Human Services, Centers for Disease Control and Prevention. Emergency preparedness and response: Frostbite. http://emergency.cdc.gov/disasters/winter/staysafe/frostbite.asp. Updated December 3, 2012. Accessed March 12, 2015.

136. Frostbite. MedlinePlus Web site. http://www.nlm.nih.gov/medlineplus/ency/article/000057.htm. Updated January 13, 2014. Accessed March 12, 2015.

137. Danzl DF. Frostbite. In: Porter RS, Kaplan JL, eds. The Merck Manual Online. http://www.merckmanuals.com/professional/injuries_poisoning/cold_injury/frostbite.html?qt=frostbite&alt=sh. Updated January 2014. Accessed March 12, 2015.

138. News and resources—frostbite and hypothermia. The National Safety Council Web site. http://www.nsc.org/learn/safety-knowledge/Pages/news-and-resources-frostbite-and-hypothermia.aspx. Accessed March 12, 2014.

139. Castells MC. Insect bites. In: Basow DS, ed. *UpToDate*. Waltham, MA: UpToDate; 2015. http://www.uptodate.com/contents/insect-bites?source=search_result&search=insect+bite&selectedTitle=1~150 . Updated October 14, 2014. Accessed March 12, 2015.

140. Insect bites and stings. MedlinePlus Web site. http://www.nlm.nih.gov/medlineplus/ency/article/000033.htm. Updated January 13, 2014. Accessed March 12, 2015.

141. Barish RA, Arnold T. Insect stings. In: Porter RS, Kaplan JL, eds. The Merck Manual Online. http://www.merckmanuals.com/professional/injuries_poisoning/bites_and_stings/insect_stings.html?qt=insect%20bites&alt=sh. Updated October 2014. Accessed March 12, 2015.

Chapter 5

Endocrine Disorders

QUESTIONS

1. Your patient, Franklin, age 64, has the following lab values: elevated TSH, low T4, and decreased T3. Which of the following drugs should be prescribed to treat his condition?

   a. Propranolol

   b. Levothyroxine

   c. Propylthiouracil

   d. Methimazole

2. Which of the following conditions involving damage to the adrenal glands includes metastatic cancer as a possible etiology?

   a. Addison's disease

   b. Hyperosmolar hyperglycemic non-ketosis

   b. Cushing's syndrome

   d. Hypothyroidism

3. You are seeing a diabetic patient who regularly monitors her blood glucose levels. She says that she has noticed a spike in her levels when she wakes up in the morning. You tell her to record her levels at 3 a.m. over the next 3 days. During the follow-up, the patient reports that her glucose is slightly elevated at 3 a.m. Based on this information, which treatment plan would be most beneficial in managing the patient's early morning hyperglycemia?

   a. Advise the patient to eat a carbohydrate or protein snack prior to going to sleep.

   b. Increase the patient's at-bedtime dose of insulin.

   c. Omit the patient's at-bedtime dose of insulin.

   d. Increase the patient's morning dose of insulin.

4. Which of the following would most likely result from a breakdown in the body's ability to either produce or utilize insulin in type 1 diabetic patients?

   a. Severe dehydration without ketone production

   b. High triglycerides

   c. Low high-density lipoprotein levels

   d. Inappropriate hyperglycemia

5. A female presents to the urgent care unit with complaints of constant nausea, weakness, and fatigue. She reports that she has been feeling extremely thirsty since her symptoms began 2 days ago, and she also has been "urinating a lot," which she attributes to constantly drinking water. The physical exam reveals that the patient has a normal blood pressure and heart rate. A urine test indicates ketones. For which condition should the patient be further evaluated?

   a. Diabetic ketoacidosis

   b. Type 2 diabetes

   c. Hyperosmolar hyperglycemic non-ketosis

   d. Type 1 diabetes

6. Which of the following processes is most commonly associated with type 2 diabetes mellitus?

   a. Hypersecretion of ACTH from the pituitary gland

   b. Intracellular dehydration resulting from hyperglycemia

   c. Secretory defect causing a resistance to insulin

   d. Ketone development

7. What is the traditionally recommended morning dose of a conventional split-dose mixture for type 1 diabetes mellitus patients?

   a. Approximately 1/2 neutral protamine Hagedorn insulin (NPH), 1/2 regular insulin

   b. Approximately 2/3 regular insulin, 1/3 NPH

   c. Approximately 0.1 U/kg regular insulin IV bolus, followed by 0.1 U/kg/hr

   d. Approximately 2/3 NPH, 1/3 regular insulin

8. Which of these is often the first sign of type 2 diabetes mellitus in females?

   a. Amenorrhea

   b. Cramps

   c. Vaginitis

   d. Hirsutism

9. Which of the following lab values would most likely confirm a diagnosis of hyperthyroidism?

   a. Low TSH, low free T3, low free T4

   b. Normal TSH, increased free T3, increased free T4

   c. Elevated TSH, normal free T3, normal free T4

   d. Low TSH, increased free T3, normal free T4

10. All of these findings are components of metabolic syndrome except:

   a. Waist circumference > 40 inches in men

   b. Blood pressure > 130/85 mmHg

   c. Fasting blood glucose > 100 mg/dl

   d. High-density lipoprotein < 50 mg/dl in men

11. A 25-year-old female patient presents with increased sweating, fatigue, tremors, and weight loss. Upon examination, you note that she has moist, velvety skin and fine hair. Based on the most likely condition, which of the following findings would you least likely expect?

   a. Puffy eyes

   b. Heat intolerance

   c. Anxiety

   d. Increased appetite

12. Patients diagnosed with hyperthyroidism face a variety of treatment options, depending on etiology, severity, and other factors. Radioactive iodine therapy is one such option that should be specifically considered in which of the following patients?

   a. A male diagnosed with Hashimoto's thyroiditis

   b. A female diagnosed with Graves' disease

   c. A female with hyperthyroidism who is in her third week of pregnancy

   d. A male diagnosed with toxic adenoma with a normal thyroid stimulating hormone level

13. Nick, a 39-year-old patient diagnosed with hyperthyroidism, complains of frequent hand tremors. Lab results indicate that the patient presents with subacute thyroiditis. Which of the following medications would be the preferred symptomatic treatment in this case?

   a. Amiodarone

   b. Levothyroxine

   c. Propranolol

   d. Propylthiouracil

14. You are seeing a patient who was diagnosed with hyperthyroidism and had treatment for thyroid storm. When reviewing the patient's medical history for any medications that the patient takes either regularly or as needed, you advise the patient that which of the following should be avoided to decrease the risk of developing another thyroid crisis?

   a. Acetaminophen

   b. Ibuprofen

   c. Naproxen

   d. Aspirin

15. Kussmaul's breathing is a finding most commonly associated with which condition?

   a. Hyperthyroidism

   b. Diabetic ketoacidosis

   c. Hypothyroidism

   d. Hyperosmolar hyperglycemic non-ketosis

16. What complication usually occurs as a result of type 2 diabetes mellitus, causing patients to produce insufficient amounts of insulin to prevent severe hyperglycemia, osmotic diuresis, and extracellular fluid depletion?

    a. Addison's disease

    b. Hyperosmolar hyperglycemic non-ketosis

    c. Cushing's syndrome

    d. Diabetic ketoacidosis

17. A 45-year-old patient comes to your office presenting with nausea and a fever of 104.4°F. He said the fever appeared earlier in the day, and that he has vomited more than once prior to arriving at your office. During the examination, he states that he feels dizzy and lightheaded whenever he stands up. His vitals indicate that he has low blood pressure. Based on these findings, which of these is the most likely diagnosis?

    a. Cushing's syndrome

    b. Type 1 diabetes mellitus

    c. Addison's disease

    d. Type 2 diabetes mellitus

18. Which of the following methods would be most helpful in counteracting the Somogyi effect in a diabetic patient?

    a. Increase the patient's morning dose of insulin.

    b. Switch the patient's insulin from human insulin to animal insulin.

    c. Tell the patient that eating breakfast may help normalize insulin levels.

    d. Decrease the patient's at-bedtime dose of insulin.

19. Which of the following is not an expected cause of Cushing's syndrome?

    a. Chronic administration of glucocorticoids

    b. Adrenocorticotropic hormone hypersecretion

    c. Autoimmune destruction of the adrenal gland

    d. Adrenal tumors

20. Jonathan, a 49 year-old-patient, complains of frequent dizzy spells. His lab tests yield an elevated erythrocyte sedimentation rate, normal iodine uptake, normal thyroid stimulating hormone levels, and low plasma cortisol. In addition, you note the appearance of hyperpigmentation on the patient's skin, particularly in skin creases. What would be the most likely diagnosis?

    a. Graves' disease

    b. Hashimoto's thyroiditis

    c. Cushing's syndrome

    d. Addison's disease

21. Lactic acidosis is a potential side effect of what treatment for type 2 diabetes mellitus?

    a. Nateglinide

    b. Rosiglitazone

    c. Acarbose

    d. Metformin

22. You are treating a 55-year old male who is at risk of developing diabetes. When making recommendations about diet, what should you tell the patient about carbohydrate intake?

    a. Advise to take 40%–50% of carbohydrate caloric intake.

    b. Advise to take 55%–60% of carbohydrate caloric intake.

    c. Advise to take 60%–65% of carbohydrate caloric intake

    d. Advise to take 65%–75% of carbohydrate caloric intake.

23. As a nurse practitioner, you know that all of the following are insulin analogs that can be used to manage diabetes mellitus except:

    a. Lispro

    b. Glargine

    c. Sitagliptin

    d. Aspart

24. You are treating Jake, a 50-year old patient diagnosed with type 2 diabetes mellitus. You know that the patient's blood glucose levels tend to surge following the consumption of a meal. Which of the following agents would help decrease hepatic glucose production and intestinal absorption of glucose, while improving sensitivity by increasing peripheral glucose utilization and uptake?

    a. Metformin

    b. Acarbose

    c. Glyburide

    d. Insulin lispro

25. Which of the following is not a common component of the pathology for type 1 diabetes mellitus?

    a. Human leukocyte antigens

    b. Islet cell antibodies

    c. Peripheral insulin resistance

    d. Ketone development

26. The metabolic syndrome, also known as syndrome X, is associated with the risk of type 2 diabetes mellitus. It is characterized by a group of predisposing factors that include obesity and hypertension. What additional risk factors are associated with syndrome X?

    a. High total cholesterol and high LDL levels

    b. High triglyceride levels and high LDL levels

    c. High total cholesterol and low HDL levels

    d. High triglyceride levels and low HDL levels

27. In the United States, type 2 diabetes mellitus comprises approximately what percentage of diabetic cases?

    a. Approximately 90%

    b. Approximately 80%

    c. Approximately 70%

    d. Approximately 60%

28. A 45-year-old male recently diagnosed with type 1 diabetes mellitus has been monitoring his blood sugar over a 2-week period. Although he has been administering the recommended dose of insulin to himself at night, his blood sugar levels are low around 3:00 a.m. and high around 7:00 a.m. Which of the following complications do the patient's blood sugar levels most likely indicate?

    a. The Dawn phenomenon

    b. Hyperosmolar hyperglycemic non-ketosis

    c. The Somogyi effect

    d. Diabetic ketoacidosis

29. Your patient has just been diagnosed with hyperthyroidism. When looking at her chart, you also note that she has a long-standing history of severe asthma. Which of the following medications would you be least likely to prescribe to the patient unless absolutely necessary?

    a. Propranolol

    b. Methimazole

    c. Propylthiouracil

    d. Lugol's solution

30. What is the preferred diagnostic test for visualizing Graves' ophthalmopathy?

    a. Thyroid radioactive iodine uptake

    b. Magnetic resonance imaging

    c. Serum anti-nuclear antibody

    d. Thyroid-stimulating hormone assay

31. What would be your most likely reason for prescribing Lugol's solution to a patient?

    a. Destroy goiters

    b. Visualize Graves' ophthalmopathy

    c. Reduce vascularity of the gland

    d. Determine how effectively the thyroid gland absorbs from the bloodstream

32. A 36-year-old patient presents to your office with concerns over experiencing uncontrollable fine tremors in her hands. When you ask her about other concerns, she tells you that she's been feeling anxious and nervous, and that her emotions seem to have been fluctuating "up and down" over the past 2 weeks. Her complaints are most likely associated with which of the following endocrine conditions?

a. Iodine deficiency

b. Hashimoto's thyroiditis

c. Hypothalamic deficiency of TRH

d. Graves' disease

33. Which of the following is most true regarding the treatment of hypothyroidism with levothyroxine?

a. The dosage is 50–100 mg.

b. The dosage should be given every day.

c. The dosage is typically tapered down every 2 weeks.

d. The dosage is standardized for all patients regardless of age.

34. A nurse practitioner is slowly and cautiously rewarming a patient with blankets to avoid circulatory collapse. Which of the following conditions is the nurse practitioner most likely trying to prevent?

a. Addison's disease

b. Thyroid crisis

c. Myxedema coma

d. Cushing's syndrome

35. Which of these statements is true regarding hyperthyroidism?

a. The incidence of hyperthyroidism is higher in women than in men.

b. The most common presentation of hyperthyroidism is subacute thyroiditis.

c. Hyperthyroidism causes bradycardia.

d. Hyperthyroidism is most commonly caused by a toxic adenoma.

36. A patient diagnosed with hyperthyroidism is about to undergo thyroid surgery. Which of the following factors would be most reliable as an indicator of a euthyroid state?

a. T4 is normal

b. T3 is normal

c. Thyroid stimulating hormone is normal

d. Thyroid resin uptake is normal

37. During a routine examination, a diabetic patient reports that he has felt extreme thirst over the last 2 days, and that he has been drinking more water and urinating more frequently. You observe that he appears lethargic, and that his skin is warm to the touch and displays poor turgor. His breathing pattern appears to be normal, and he does not report nocturia. Vitals include a resting heartbeat of 112 bpm, a blood pressure of 88/52, and a serum glucose level of 649 mg/dl. For which of the following conditions should the patient be further evaluated?

a. Diabetic ketoacidosis

b. Cushing's syndrome

c. Hyperthyroidism

d. Hyperosmolar hyperglycemic non-ketosis

38. Which of the following lab results is typically present in diabetic ketoacidosis but not in hyperosmolar hyperglycemic non-ketosis?

a. Hyperosmolality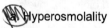

b. Decreased sodium

c. Relatively low pH

d. Elevated BUN and Cr

39. Susan, age 25, presents to the clinic with an altered level of consciousness, Kussmaul's breathing, polyuria, and fruity breath. Upon looking at her medical file, you note that she has type 1 diabetes mellitus. You immediately direct the patient to an emergency room for treatment and further evaluation. Which of the following lab results would you least expect Susan to have?

a. Hyperglycemia

b. Ketonuria

c. Alkalosis

d. Hyperkalemia

40. With regards to pathology of diabetes mellitus (DM), which of the following factors plays a principal role in causing type 1 DM?

    a. Obesity

    b. Toxic environmental insult to pancreatic beta cells

    c. Insulin secretory defects resulting in resistance

    d. Intracellular dehydration due to elevated blood glucose levels

RATIONALES

1. b

A patient with an elevated TSH level, low T4 level, and decreased T3 level, is most likely to be diagnosed with hypothyroidism. When treating a patient with hypothyroidism, levothyroxine should be prescribed 50–100 mcg daily; dosage should be increased by 25 mcg every 1–2 weeks until the patient's symptoms stabilize. Propranolol would be prescribed for symptomatic relief of hyperthyroidism as opposed to hypothyroidism. Methimazole and propylthiouracil are both types of thiourea drugs, which are commonly given to patients with hyperthyroidism, not hypothyroidism.

2. a

Metastatic cancer is a possible etiology of Addison's disease. Adrenal tumors in Cushing's syndrome are typically noncancerous, and both hyperosmolar hyperglycemic non-ketosis and hypothyroidism are not commonly associated with any form of cancer.

3. b

The patient is most likely experiencing the effects of the Dawn phenomenon as indicated by blood glucose becoming slightly elevated throughout the night and resulting in hyperglycemia in the morning. Therefore, the most beneficial recommendation to manage this patient's morning hyperglycemia would be to increase the patient's at-bedtime dose of insulin. Insulin treatment should not be eliminated as it is needed to manage high blood glucose in the patient with hyperglycemia. Increasing the morning dose of insulin would not help prevent the patient's morning hyperglycemia since the latter is characterized by blood glucose levels gradually increasing throughout the night. Advising the patient to eat a snack containing either carbohydrate or protein would not be beneficial, as it could lead to a higher increase in the patient's blood glucose.

4. d

Type 1 diabetes mellitus (DM) and, to some extent, type 2 DM, results from a breakdown in the body's ability to either produce or utilize insulin, resulting in inappropriate hyperglycemia. High triglycerides and low high-density lipoproteins are abnormal lipid profiles associated with syndrome X and type 2 DM. Although type 1 DM patients may experience excessive thirst, they also typically present with high ketone levels that build up due to insufficient insulin. Severe dehydration without ketone production is associated with hyperosmolar hyperglycemic non-ketosis and is not a finding of type 1 DM.

5. d

Of the conditions, the patient should receive further evaluation for type 1 diabetes mellitus (DM). The patient is reporting polyuria, polydipsia, and ketonuria. Polyuria and polydipsia occur in both type 1 and type 2 DM, but ketones are not a finding indicative of type 2 DM. Ketones, however, are present in cases of diabetic ketoacidosis (DKA). Although additional diagnostic tests would be required to rule out DKA, the patient does not display poor skin turgor, which is a characteristic finding of DKA. Additionally, DKA and hyperosmolar hyperglycemic non-ketosis both typically present with tachycardia and hypotension; the patient's vitals, however, indicate normal blood pressure and heart rate.

6. c

A secretory defect that causes insulin resistance is associated with type 2 diabetes mellitus (DM). The hypersecretion of ACTH from the pituitary gland is a process that occurs in Cushing's syndrome, which is not associated with type 2 DM. Intracellular dehydration resulting from hyperglycemia is associated with diabetic ketoacidosis and, in some cases, type 2 DM; however, it is a condition that commonly involves ketone development and primarily affects type 1 DM patients.

7. d

The recommended morning dose of conventional split-dose regimen for type 1 diabetes mellitus (DM) patients is 2/3 neutral protamine Hagedorn (NPH) insulin and 1/3 regular insulin, not 2/3 regular insulin and 1/3 NPH. A dose of 1/2 NPH insulin and 1/2 regular insulin is the recommended evening dose for type 1 DM patients. Administering 0.1 U/kg of regular insulin intravenously, followed by 0.1 U/kg/hr, is used for immediate treatment of patients experiencing diabetic ketoacidosis.

8. c

Recurrent vaginitis is often the first symptom of type 2 diabetes mellitus (DM) among females. Amenorrhea and hirsutism are both symptoms that may occur in Cushing's syndrome, and cramps are a symptom that may accompany hypothyroidism; these symptoms are not commonly associated with type 2 DM.

9. d

A diagnosis of hyperthyroidism can usually be determined with lab values indicating subnormal TSH levels and elevated values of either free T3 or free T4. Lab findings indicating elevated TSH and subnormal T4 values typically indicate hypothyroidism. Cases in which free T3 is elevated may indicate T3 thyrotoxicosis if TSH is subnormal; however, if TSH is normal, then elevated T3 could be a result of other conditions such as pregnancy or liver disease, among others.

10. d

A low HDL cholesterol level is one component of metabolic syndrome (i.e., syndrome X), commonly used for predicting the risk of type 2 diabetes, and is also beneficial in predicting the risk of heart disease. Among males, HDL less than or equal to 40 mg/dl is considered low; 50 mg/dl is within the normal range for HDLs. The HDL level in females is considered low if it falls below 50 mg/dl. The components of metabolic syndrome that typically increase the risk of type 2 diabetes include a waist circumference of 40 inches or greater in men, blood pressure that is 130/85 mmHg or higher, and fasting blood glucose of 100 mg/dl or higher.

11. a

A patient with hypothyroidism is likely to present with puffy eyes, whereas a patient with hyperthyroidism is more likely to have lid lag. Heat intolerance, anxiety, and increased appetite are all signs and symptoms of hyperthyroidism.

12. b

Radioactive iodine treatment is commonly considered as the preferred method of treatment for Graves' disease. Hashimoto's thyroiditis is associated with hypothyroidism and usually treated with replacement of thyroid hormone. Radioactive iodine treatment may be administered as an alternative to patients with toxic adenoma who are at an increased risk of developing complications associated with worsening hyperthyroidism, but it is not the primary treatment for toxic adenoma. Moreover, caution should be exercised in patients with a normal or elevated TSH levels and patients already receiving antithyroid therapy. Radioactive therapy can be administered to females with hyperthyroidism but is contraindicated in pregnancy. The gender of the patient does not necessarily determine the preferred treatment.

13. c

Propranolol is the preferred symptomatic treatment for tremors in hyperthyroidism patients who present with subacute thyroiditis. Patients with hyperthyroidism due to excess exposure to high-dose amiodarone treatment may be advised to reduce or omit the dosage of amiodarone. Levothyroxine is commonly used to treat hypothyroidism, rather than hyperthyroidism. Lastly, although propylthiouracil may be prescribed to patients with hyperthyroidism, it is not specifically used to treat tremors in cases of subacute thyroiditis; furthermore, this medication is not considered the preferred symptomatic treatment since it may cause severe liver damage.

14. d

Use of acetylsalicylic acid (i.e., aspirin) should be avoided in hyperthyroid patients. Aspirin use is known to induce thyroid storm by increasing T3 and T4 levels in hyperthyroid patients via displacement of thyroid hormone binding from thyroid binding globulin. Although aspirin, naproxen, and ibuprofen are all non-steroidal anti-inflammatory drugs (NSAIDs), aspirin is the only NSAID known to induce thyroid storm. Acetaminophen is also not known to affect hormone levels and, therefore, would not induce thyroid storm in a patient with hyperthyroidism.

15. b

Kussmaul's breathing, which is characterized by deep, rapid breaths, is a typical finding of diabetic ketoacidosis (DKA). This type of breathing pattern serves to expel carbon dioxide produced as a result of metabolic acidosis. Kussmaul's breathing is not a sign of hyperthyroidism, hypothyroidism, or hyperosmolar hyperglycemic non-ketosis.

16. b

Hyperosmolar hyperglycemic non-ketosis (HHNK) normally occurs as a result of type 2 diabetes mellitus (DM). Patients with HHNK are unable to produce enough insulin to prevent hyperglycemia, osmotic diuresis, and extracellular fluid depletion. Cushing's syndrome and Addison's disease are not commonly indicated as complications of type 2 DM. Cushing's syndrome is a result of the pituitary gland producing too much adrenocorticotropic hormone, and is most commonly caused by administration of glucocorticosteroid medication. On the other hand, Addison disease usually results from autoimmune destruction of the adrenal gland, which causes production of insufficient levels of cortisol, androgens, and aldosterone. Diabetic ketoacidosis is often an acute complication of type 1 DM, not type 2 DM.

17. c

Based on the patient's presentation of an acute fever, orthostasis, and hypotension, as well as symptoms of nausea and vomiting, the most likely diagnosis is Addison's disease. Characteristic signs of diabetes include polyuria and polydipsia, both of which are absent in this patient. Moreover, acute fever is characteristic of Addison's disease, and does not occur in either type of diabetes except for cases involving diabetic ketoacidosis or hyperosmolar hyperglycemic non-ketosis. Cushing's syndrome is also less likely to be a suspected diagnosis, as it commonly presents with polyuria. Furthermore, patients with Cushing's syndrome typically present with hypertension, not hypotension.

18. d

When advising a diabetic patient on how to manage the effects of post-hypoglycemic hyperglycemia (i.e., the Somogyi effect), the nurse practitioner should recommend decreasing the at-bedtime doses of insulin. Transitioning the patient from human insulin to animal insulin is not beneficial, particularly because the peak activity time of animal insulin may occur 3 to 4 hours after injecting, thus complicating timing of meals in relation to injections. Advising the patient to either increase the morning dose of insulin or to eat breakfast to normalize insulin levels may be beneficial to managing the effects of the dawn phenomenon, and not the Somogyi effect.

19. c

Autoimmune destruction of the adrenal gland commonly results in deficient cortisol, androgens, and aldosterone, thereby causing Addison's disease. Cushing's syndrome is typically caused by excessive adrenocorticotropic hormone (ACTH) levels, which may in turn be caused by ACTH hypersecretion of the pituitary gland, adrenal tumors, or chronic administration of glucocorticoids.

20. d

Frequent dizzy spells are usually indicative of orthostatic hypotension, which commonly presents in Addison's disease. The plasma cortisol of a patient with Addison's disease would most likely be less than 5 mg/dl at 0800 h while the erythrocyte sedimentation rate would typically be elevated. Hyperpigmentation in skin creases is a common sign of Addison's disease and is typically considered in the course of differential diagnosis. Although hyperpigmentation may also present in cases of Graves' disease, this condition is characterized by a high iodine uptake, which is not present in this case. Hashimoto's thyroiditis is an autoimmune disease that may lead to hypothyroidism; it is usually diagnosed through a TSH test, which reveals high TSH levels. Lastly, patients with Cushing's syndrome present with elevated plasma cortisol in the morning and do not commonly exhibit hyperpigmentation that is characteristic of Addison's disease.

21. d

Lactic acidosis is a potential side effect of metformin. This condition may arise because metformin promotes conversion of glucose into lactate and inhibits hepatic gluconeogenesis from lactate, pyruvate, and alanine, resulting in additional lactate and substrate for lactate production. The mechanisms of action for the other diabetic treatments are not likely to produce lactic acidosis because they do not affect lactate levels. Nateglinide is a non-sulfonylurea insulin-release stimulator used to treat type 2 diabetes mellitus (DM). Also used in the treatment of type 2 DM are rosiglitazone, which is a thiazolidinedione used to decrease gluconeogenesis, and acarbose, which is an alpha-glucosidase inhibitor.

22. b

To prevent an onset of diabetes, the patient should be advised that total carbohydrate intake should be 55%–60% of total caloric intake. Diabetic diets generally call for a limited carbohydrate intake because foods high in carbs may adversely affect blood sugar.

23. c

Sitagliptin is not an insulin analog used in the management of diabetes mellitus (DM); rather, it is a dipeptidyl peptidase-4 inhibitor used to break down incretins in type 2 DM patients. Insulin analogs used to manage DM include aspart, glargine, and lispro.

24. a

Metformin is considered to be a first-line therapy for type 2 diabetes mellitus (DM); it works by suppressing hepatic glucose production and internal absorption of glucose, while increasing insulin sensitivity and enhancing peripheral glucose uptake. Alpha-glucosidase inhibitors, such as acarbose, work by delaying the absorption of carbohydrates and lowering postprandial glucose levels in patients with type 2 DM. Sulfonylureas, such as glyburide and glipizide, stimulate insulin release from pancreatic beta cells. Insulin lispro (Humalog) is an insulin analog that mimics the effects of rapidly acting insulin in the body.

25. c

Peripheral insulin resistance, which refers to the body's reduced response to insulin within skeletal muscle and organs, is a finding commonly attributed to type 2 diabetes mellitus (DM). Type 1 DM is strongly associated with the presence of human leukocyte antigens. Furthermore, ketone build-up in blood and urine typically takes place in diabetic ketoacidosis, which predominantly occurs in patients with type 1 DM. Lastly, islet cell antibodies are found in approximately 90% of patients with type 1 DM within the first year of diagnosis.

26. d

High levels of triglycerides and low levels of HDL are considered as a part of syndrome X, which refers to a group of predisposing factors for type 2 diabetes. Although high total cholesterol and LDL levels are often counted among predisposing factors to other conditions, such as heart disease, they do not comprise a part of syndrome X.

27. a

Type 2 diabetes mellitus makes up approximately over 90% of all cases of diabetes in the United States. Approximately 5% of diabetes patients have type 1 diabetes, and the other 5% have rare and atypical types of diabetes.

28. c

The patient's blood sugar data—low blood sugar at night and high blood sugar in the morning—most likely indicate that the patient is experiencing the Somogyi effect, which stimulates a surge of regulatory hormones to counter nocturnal hypoglycemia. Similar to the Somogyi effect, the dawn phenomenon causes glucose levels to be elevated in the morning, which is due to tissue insensitivity to insulin that typically occurs between the hours of 5 a.m. and 8 a.m. Diabetic ketoacidosis (DKA) commonly results from a lack of insulin at multiple enzymatic locations within the body, while elevated levels of other hormones, catecholamines, and glucagon all contribute to the development of DKA. A hyperglycemic hyperosmolar state is initiated by a relative or absolute deficiency of insulin and reduced utilization of glucose by body tissues, which usually results in hepatoglucogenesis and profound dehydration.

29. a

Although propranolol is used to treat symptoms associated with hyperthyroidism, beta blockers are contraindicated in patients with chronic obstructive pulmonary disease, bronchospasm, severe heart failure, or asthma. The mechanism of action of propranolol on beta 2 receptors may exacerbate asthma symptoms, increase airway reactivity, and promote bronchoconstriction. Methimazole, propylthiouracil, and Lugol's solution are commonly used in the treatment of hyperthyroidism and may be used in patients with asthma.

30. b

The preferred diagnostic test for visualizing Graves' ophthalmopathy is magnetic resonance imaging of the orbits, which reveals the degree and activity of eye muscle inflammation. A thyroid radioactive iodine uptake on the other hand, is typically used along with a thyroid scan to establish the etiology of hyperthyroidism, which may include conditions other than Graves' disease. The serum anti-nuclear antibody test is usually used to find evidence of lupus or other collagen diseases. Lastly, the thyroid-stimulating hormone assay test is often considered to be the most sensitive test to diagnose hyperthyroidism; it is not a diagnostic test for visualizing Graves' ophthalmopathy.

31. c.

Lugol's solution may be prescribed to patients with hyperthyroidism to reduce the vascularity of the gland, which may temporarily lower serum thyroid hormone concentrations. Although Lugol's solution may have historically been used as a treatment for goiters, it is not currently used. Radioactive iodine 131-I would most likely be implemented to destroy goiters. Magnetic resonance imaging is used to visualize Graves' ophthalmopathy and a thyroid radioactive iodine uptake test is used to determine how effectively the thyroid gland is working.

32. d

Graves' disease, which is the most common presentation of hyperthyroidism, is likely to be associated with fine tremors in the hands, psychological symptoms that include anxiety and nervousness, and emotional lability. Iodine deficiency, Hashimoto's thyroiditis, and hypothalamic deficiency of thyrotropin-releasing hormone are all associated with hypothyroidism. Although hypothyroidism may also cause emotional symptoms, fine tremors are not known to occur with conditions associated with hypothyroidism and are more often associated with Graves' disease.

33. b

A typical regimen of levothyroxine may be 50–100 mcg every day, rather than 50–100 mg. The dosage is typically increased by 25 mcg every 1–2 weeks until symptoms become stabilized; it is not tapered down every 2 weeks. Patients over 60 years of age and those who have cardiovascular disease should receive half the recommended adult dosage, which is usually 25–50 mcg/day.

34. c

A patient with severe hypothermia is most likely
    experiencing a myxedema crisis, which is a
    life-threatening event with a high mortality rate.
    When treating a patient in a myxedema coma, a
    nurse practitioner should slowly and cautiously
    rewarm the patient with blankets to avoid
    circulatory collapse. Addison's disease, thyroid
    crisis, and Cushing's syndrome do not typically
    require rewarming with blankets as a treatment.

35. a

The incidence of hyperthyroidism is higher in women
    than in men, with a ratio of approximately 8
    to 1. Graves' disease, rather than subacute
    thyroiditis, is the most common presentation.
    Although toxic adenoma is a common cause of
    hyperthyroidism, other causes include subacute
    thyroiditis, a thyroid stimulating hormone tumor,
    and high dose amiodarone. A characteristic
    symptom of hyperthyroidism is tachycardia;
    bradycardia is more likely to be a presentation
    of hypothyroidism.

36. c

A TSH assay is considered to be the most sensitive
    test for evaluating thyroid function with
    normal TSH levels indicating euthyroid state
    and patients with hyperthyroidism should be
    euthyroid prior to surgery of the thyroid gland. A
    euthyroid patient typically has normal serum T3,
    T4, and thyroid resin uptake. However, these
    tests are not as sensitive as TSH assay since
    patients with hyperthyroidism do not necessarily
    present with consistently high levels of all
    thyroid hormones.

37. d

The patient should be further evaluated for
    hyperosmolar hyperglycemic non-ketosis
    (HHNK) because the patient's serum glucose is
    higher than 600 mg/dl and the patient displays
    signs of dehydration. The patient's symptoms
    of hypotension, tachycardia, polyuria, and an
    altered level of consciousness typically present
    in both HHNK and diabetic ketoacidosis (DKA);
    however, the patient's serum glucose level of
    649 mg/dl is too high for DKA, and the patient
    does not present with characteristic signs of
    DKA—Kussmaul's breathing and fruity breath.
    Cushing's syndrome would not be considered
    because it's usually accompanied with
    hypertension, not hypotension. Hyperthyroidism
    would also be ruled out because the patient
    does not exhibit signs of nervousness, anxiety,
    or other characteristic symptoms of this
    condition.

38. c

A pH level lower than 7.3 indicates acidosis, which
    is a common finding of diabetic ketoacidosis
    (DKA) and not hyperosmolar hyperglycemic
    non-ketosis (HHNK). HHNK is a condition that
    typically presents with relatively normal pH
    levels. Findings of hyperosmolality, decreased
    sodium, elevated blood urea nitrogen, and
    elevated creatinine may manifest in both DKA
    and HHNK.

39. c

Based on the presentation of an altered level of
    consciousness, Kussmaul's breathing, and fruity
    breath in a patient with type 1 diabetes mellitus,
    the patient is most likely experiencing diabetic
    ketoacidosis (DKA), which does not typically
    result in alkalosis. More often, DKA results in
    metabolic acidosis characterized by pH levels
    lower than 7.30. Hyperglycemia, ketonuria, and
    hyperkalemia are lab findings that are consistent
    with DKA. Other lab results that typically
    occur in a patient with DKA include glycosuria,
    hyperosmolality, elevated hematocrit, elevated
    blood urea nitrogen, and elevated creatinine.

40. b

Type 1 diabetes mellitus (DM) is believed to be
    the result of the autoimmune destruction
    of pancreatic beta cells due to genetic
    predisposition or an environmental trigger.
    Type 2 DM is typically attributed to decreased
    sensitivity to insulin or insulin secretory
    defects resulting in resistance and impaired
    insulin production. Neither of these causes
    is commonly associated with type 1 DM.
    Intracellular dehydration due to elevated blood
    glucose levels is a common cause of diabetic
    ketoacidosis, not type 1 or type 2 DM. Obesity
    is more often associated with type 2 DM, rather
    than type 1.

DISCUSSION

Diabetes Mellitus

Overview

Diabetes mellitus (DM) is a group of diseases
characterized by elevated blood glucose levels due
to the body's inability to produce or utilize insulin.
This rise in blood glucose results in findings that
include polyuria, polydipsia, and polyphagia, among
others.[1,2,3]

Approximately 29 million Americans have
diabetes; of those cases, approximately 27% are
undiagnosed.[4] Of the types of diabetes, the two most
prevalent are type 1 and type 2 DM. Type 1 DM

accounts for about 5%–10% of all diabetics, while type 2 DM accounts for more than 90% of all cases.

Patients diagnosed with either type of DM are at risk of developing further complications, including hyperosmolar hyperglycemic non-ketosis (HHNK), diabetic ketoacidosis (DKA), the Somogyi effect, and the dawn phenomenon. Furthermore, diabetes is linked to secondary conditions such as hypertension, renal failure, and stroke. Some complications, such as heart disease, can be fatal. Diabetes ranks among the top ten leading causes of death in the United States.[2]

The severity of a diabetic patient's condition is affected by various factors that include obesity, diet, and overall health, but diabetes can be managed through healthy lifestyle changes and medication. When assessing diabetic patients, it is always important to consider the type of diabetes, as well as the patient's health, lifestyle, diet, and overall well-being.

Diabetes Mellitus (Type 1 DM)

Overview

Type 1 DM is an inflammatory autoimmune disease of insulin-producing beta cells found in the islet of Langerhans region of the pancreas. This condition causes a lack of insulin production, resulting in high glucose levels in the blood.[5]

Type 1 DM was previously known as insulin-dependent diabetes because treatment involved insulin therapy to counter rising glucose levels in the blood. However, type 2 DM can sometimes also require insulin treatment, rendering this name for type 1 DM a misnomer.

The etiology of type 1 DM is unclear; however, genetic factors such as polymorphisms of class II human leukocyte antigen (HLA) genes are strongly associated with type 1 DM, as 95% of all type 1 DM patients have either HLA-DR3 or HLA-DR4.[6] Autoimmunity is also considered a major factor, as the prevalence is increased in patients diagnosed with comorbid autoimmune diseases.

Type 1 DM is usually diagnosed in children and adolescents, but can be diagnosed at any age. Type 1 DM accounts for approximately 5% of all diagnosed cases of diabetes in adults.[2]

Presentation

The predominant findings of type 1 DM in undiagnosed patients are polyuria, polydipsia, and polyphagia, which are characteristic of uncontrolled hyperglycemia. Additional findings include nocturnal enuresis, nausea, blurred vision, weakness, and fatigue.[6] Weight loss regularly occurs in patients with type 1 DM who are undiagnosed.[6] Hypotension and tachycardia are findings associated with DKA, as are gastrointestinal (GI) signs and symptoms such as nausea, abdominal discomfort or pain, and change in bowel movements.[6,7]

Workup

Several diagnostic methods exist to diagnose type 1 DM.[8] The fasting plasma glucose (FPG) test measures glucose levels after the patient has fasted for 6–8 hours. Normal values are generally 100 mg/dl or lower, and a reading of 126 mg/dl or higher on two separate occasions is necessary for diagnosis of DM.[8]

The glycated hemoglobin (Hgb A1C) diagnostic, also known as the A1C test, is currently used for routine diagnosis. This test provides an indication of average blood glucose over the last 2 to 3 months. The following table applies to current guidelines:

Patient	Hemoglobin A1C
Those without diabetes	4%–5.6%
Increased risk of diabetes	5.7%–6.4%
Diabetes	6.5% or more
The goal for those without diabetes is to especially maintain values of < 7%, with values ≤ 6% indicating adequate/good control.	

The oral glucose tolerance test (OGTT) is rarely used today as a diagnostic method. Still, normal readings are 140 mg/dl or below, and a reading of 200 mg/dl or higher suggests diabetes.[8]

The random plasma glucose test may be conducted when the patient is displaying severe diabetic findings associated with hyperglycemia, such as polyuria, polydipsia, and weight loss. Blood glucose measuring 200 mg/dl or higher, along with the patient's clinical presentation of hyperglycemic findings, suggests DM.[6]

If diagnosis is unclear by clinical presentation, the patient may be referred to an endocrinologist for autoantibody testing to differentiate between type 1 and type 2 DM.[6]

DKA, which results from excessive ketone production, is a common complication seen in type 1 DM patients that can lead to coma or death. DKA develops over time as the body begins burning fat for energy, producing ketones, and results in either ketonuria, ketonemia, or both.[7] In cases where hyperglycemia is found and DKA is suspected, the patient will be further managed and evaluated at an acute care facility.[9]

Treatment (see tables 5.1–5.2)

Patients initially diagnosed with type 1 DM may need to be referred to an endocrinologist. The condition requires lifelong insulin therapy, and dosages must be individualized for each patient. This requires an analysis of baseline studies that includes the age of onset and risk factors. Lifestyle risk factors, such as obesity and cardiac risk, should also be taken into consideration when creating a treatment plan for patients. The American Diabetes Association notes that hypertension and dyslipidemia control significantly assist in lowering a diabetic's 10-year coronary heart disease risk.[8] The baseline physical exam also includes an evaluation of peripheral pulses and neurological function. Additionally, type 1 DM patients should be screened within 5 years of diagnosis to assess for any evidence of diabetic retinopathy.[8]

Patients with type 1 DM should be educated on how to perform frequent self-monitoring and documentation of glucose levels to adjust insulin dosage as required. Also, it is important that patients be able to recognize signs and symptoms of hypoglycemia.

Examples of various insulin management strategies may include conventional split dose mixtures, intensive insulin therapy, and insulin analogs, among others (see table 5.1).

A Medical Nutritional Therapy plan (MNT) is a crucial aspect in developing a treatment plan, and requires a referral to a dietitian to address individual needs, cultural practices and constraints, health literacy, and barriers to change, among other factors.[10] The goal is to move away from a "one size fits all" approach and develop more comprehensive, individualized plans of treatment.

Diabetic Ketoacidosis (DKA)

Overview

DKA is one of two serious complications associated with diabetes. This complication is a state of intracellular dehydration characterized by a triad of hyperglycemia, ketonemia, and metabolic acidosis. DKA is a classic complication of type 1 DM.[5]

DKA occurs when the body produces deficient levels of insulin. As a result, glucose accumulates and does not get converted into fuel for the cells; the body then begins to break down protein and fats to be converted into energy. This process produces ketones as a byproduct, leading to an accumulation of ketones in the body. Because the glucose entering the body is not being processed into fuel, the unprocessed glucose enters the circulatory system, which then obstructs the kidneys' ability to reabsorb water from the blood. Excess amounts of ketones and glucose are expelled from the body through urine, which causes dehydration and ketonuria, in addition to hyperglycemia due to elevated glucose levels.[11]

The leading causes of DKA include an underlying or concurrent infection (40%), failure to administer insulin treatments (25%), and newly-diagnosed or unknown diabetes (15%).[12]

Causes for the other 20% of all cases may include poor compliance with insulin, insulin infusion catheter blockage, or mechanical failure if an insulin pump is used to deliver insulin doses. Bacterial infections and intercurrent illness, in addition to medical, surgical, or emotional distress, can also trigger an onset of DKA.[12]

Presentation

Hypotension, tachycardia, tachypnea, and hypotension are all strong indicators for DKA in diabetic patients. Because the onset of DKA is characterized by signs of hyperglycemia, ketonemia, and normal anion gap metabolic acidosis, typical findings include polydipsia and polyuria associated with hyperglycemia.

A characteristic sign associated with metabolic acidosis is Kussmaul's breathing, which is characterized by rapid, shallow breaths in mild cases of acidosis, or a deep, labored breathing pattern in severe cases of acidosis.

Other potential findings of DKA include an ill appearance, dry mucous membranes, decreased skin turgor, dry tongue and skin, decreased reflexes, and a characteristic acetone breath odor (i.e., fruity smelling breath). Vital signs should be assessed, as findings of tachycardia, hypotension, tachypnea, or hypothermia may further suggest a state of DKA.[12] In severe cases, DKA can present with confusion, abdominal tenderness, and fatigue or weakness. In some cases, patients may enter into a coma.

Precipitating factors for DKA include infections (e.g., urinary tract infections, pneumonia), myocardial infarction, and abscesses.[12]

Workup

Diagnostics for DKA are performed in emergency care.

Treatment

Patients experiencing an onset of DKA are immediately hospitalized to prevent serious life-threatening complications. Critical care will include close monitoring, fluid resuscitation, and IV insulin.[12,13,14]

Diabetes Mellitus (Type 2 DM)

Overview

Type 2 DM develops mainly in adults, with a particularly higher incidence noted among the overweight and obese populations. This variant is the most prevalent form of diabetes, accounting for more than 90% of all diabetes cases.[15]

This condition occurs when the pancreas produces insufficient levels of insulin, or when the body develops a resistance to insulin.[16] As peripheral tissues become resistant to insulin, blood glucose levels rise. However, the pancreas produces enough circulating insulin throughout the body to prevent a buildup of ketones, which prevents the potential occurrence of DKA.[15] The most life-threatening complication of type 2 DM is HHNK. The causes of type 2 DM can be attributed to insulin secretory defects that may cause resistance, impaired insulin production, and excessive or inappropriate glucagon secretion.[17] The leading long-term complication

Table 5.1	Common Types of Insulin		
Insulin	**Onset**	**Peak**	**Duration**
Rapid-acting: covers insulin needs for meals eaten at the same time as the medication is administered; used in combination with longer-acting insulins			
Humalog (Lispro)	15–30 minutes	~30–90 minutes	3–5 hr
Novolog (Aspart)	10–20 minutes	~40–50 minutes	3–5 hr
Apidra (Glulisine)	20–30 minutes	~30–90 minutes	1–1.5 hr
Short-acting: covers insulin needs for meals between 30 and 60 minutes after administration			
Regular (Humulin R, Novolin R),	30–60 minutes	2–6 hr	5–8 hr
Humulin R U-500	30 minutes	1.7–4 hr	Up to 12 hr if given in high doses
Intermediate-acting: covers insulin needs overnight or at least for half of the night; usually combined with rapid- or short-acting preparations			
NPH (Humulin N, Novolin N)	2–4 hr	6–8 hr	12–15 hr
Long-acting: covers insulin needs throughout an entire day/24-hour period; often combined with rapid- or short-acting preparations, but do not mix in same syringe. Do not exceed greater than 50 units long acting per injection site. Levemir and/or Lantus can be split in to b.i.d. dosing. Humulin R U-500 can be potentiated by oral hypoglycemics.			
Levemir (Detemir)	1–2 hr	Maximal effect at 4–6 hr	Up to 24 hr
Lantus (glargine)	1–1.5 hr	Maximal effect at 4–6 hr	24+ hr
Pre-mixed: combinations of intermediate- and short-acting preparations in a bottle or in an insulin pen; usually taken BID before meals			
NPH/Regular 70/30 or 50/50	~30 minutes	Varies	18–24 hr
NPL/Humalog 75/25, 50/50	10–15 minutes	Varies	12–15 hr
Novolog 70/30	10–20 minutes	1–4 hr	Up to 24 hr

Note. B.I.D. = Bis in die (bid); NPH = neutral protamine hagedorn; NPL = neutral protamine lispro.

Used with permission from Barkley TW Jr., Appel SJ. Diabetes mellitus In: Barkley TW Jr, Myers CM, eds. *Practice Considerations for the Adult-Gerontology Acute Care Nurse Practitioner.* West Hollywood, CA: Barkley and Associates; 2015: 427–441.

of type 2 DM is cardiovascular disease. Type 2 DM patients have twice the risk of developing cardiovascular disease compared to non-diabetic patients.[16]

Presentation

Although many undiagnosed patients appear asymptomatic, an insidious onset of hyperglycemia is the standard initial presentation of type 2 DM. Regardless, classic clinical manifestations of type 2 DM include polyuria, polydipsia, and polyphagia.

Other clinical findings of the disease eventually include blurred vision, peripheral neuropathies, and paresthesias of the lower extremities. Recurrent vaginal yeast infections are common in female patients, sometimes serving as the first sign of type 2 DM. Some of the standard indicators that suggest an increased risk of developing type 2 DM include obesity, hypertension, and abnormal lipid

profiles, previously known as syndrome X.[17] Today, metabolic syndrome is used as the indicator for type 2 DM, and is heralded by these five findings: a waist circumference equal to or greater than 40 inches (101.6 cm) in men and 35 inches (88.9 cm) in women, a blood pressure equal to or greater than 130/85, triglycerides equal to or greater than 150 mg/dl, fasting blood glucose of 100 mg/dl or higher, and high-density lipids under 40 mg/dl in men and under 50 mg/dl in women.[1] The presence of at least three of these five findings in a patient indicates metabolic syndrome.

In some patients, HHNK may be the initial presentation of type 2 DM.[18] Signs and symptoms of HHNK include marked hypotension, tachycardia, poor skin turgor, dehydration, and focal or global neurological signs, including delirium and seizures. Some findings, such as polyuria, present with both HHNK and normal cases of type 2 DM.[18]

Oral agent	Duration	Starting dose	Daily dosage	Comment(s)
Table 5.2 Oral Hypoglycemic Agents				
Biguanides				
Metformin HCl (Glucophage) Oral Solution: Riomet 500 mg/5 ml	12–24 hr	500, 800, or 1000 mg	500 mg–2.55 grams 1–3 times a day	"Insulin-sparing" agent that does not cause weight gain in patients with diabetes; therefore, extremely popular with obese patients and in combination with a sulfonylurea
Metformin, Extended Release (Glucophage XL)	Half-life: 6 hr	500 mg	500–2000 mg 1 time daily with evening meal	Dosage may be increased from starting dose by 500 mg weekly GI-related side effects are less severe with extended release
Sulfonylureas				
Glipizide (Glucotrol)	10–24 hr	5, 10 mg	5–40 mg per day single dose or in 2 divided doses	Should be taken on an empty stomach 30 minutes before meals
Glipizide Extended Release (Glucotrol XL)	Half-life, 2.5 hr	2.5, 5, 10 mg with meal	20 mg per day	
Glyburide (Diabeta, Micronase, Glynase)	24 hr	1.25, 2.5, or 5 mg	0.75–20 mg per day (Administered in single or 2 divided doses)	Use lower initial dose in the elderly, those with hepatic or renal impairment, and those at serious risk for hypoglycemia (may cause prolonged hypoglycemia); should not be taken on an empty stomach, or severe hypoglycemia may occur
Glimepiride (Amaryl)	24 hr	1, 2, or 4 mg	1–8 mg per day	Prescribed once each day as monotherapy or in combination with insulin
α-Glucosidase Inhibitors				
Acarbose (Precose)	6–12 hr	25, 50, 100 mg once or TID	In patients weighing greater than 60 kg: 50 mg 3 times a day In patients weighing greater than 60 kg: 100 mg 3 times a day	May cause flatulence; dosage should be increased slowly to reduce GI adverse effects; take with first bite of meal. Do not use in patients with significant renal dysfunction (serum creatinine greater than 2 mg/dl)

Table 5.2	Oral Hypoglycemic Agents			
Oral agent	**Duration**	**Starting dose**	**Daily dosage**	**Comment(s)**
α-Glucosidase Inhibitors				
Miglitol (Glyset)	2–4 hr	25, 50, 100 mg 3 times a day at the first bite of each meal; if severe GI adverse effects occur, may start at 25 mg each day	100 mg 3 times a day	Increases risk of hypoglycemia if taken with certain foods (e.g., garlic, celery, juniper berries, ginseng); contraindicated in type 1 diabetes. Do not use in patients with significant renal dysfunction (serum creatinine greater than 2 mg/dl). Take with first bite of meal.
Meglitinides				
Repaglinide (Prandin)	Half-life, 1 hr	0.5, 1, 2 mg 30 minutes or less before meals, 2–4 times a day	Maximum dose, 16 mg per day	Use cautiously in patients with hepatic or renal impairment; contraindicated in patients with type 1 diabetes; preferably taken less than 15 minutes prior to meal; omit if no meal eaten
Nateglinide (Starlix)	Half-life, 1 hr	60, 100 mg 3 times a day	480 mg/day	Preferably taken less than 15 minutes prior to meal; omit if no meal eaten. Use cautiously in patients with hepatic or renal impairment.
Thiazolinediones				
Rosiglitazone maleate (Avandia)	Half-life, 3–4 hr	2, 4, 8 mg BID	8 mg, may take 4 mg BID or an 8-mg tablet once daily	Contraindicated in patients with established New York Heart Association Class III or IV heart failure. May be taken with or without food; after 12 weeks of therapy, may increase dosage to 8 mg; may be used with metformin and/or insulin
Pioglitazone hydrochloride (Actos)	Half-life, 3–7 hr	15, 30, 45 mg daily	45 mg once daily	Contraindicated in patients with established New York Heart Association Class III or IV heart failure. May be used as monotherapy or in combination with metformin and/or insulin; minor GI upset may occur; monitor liver enzymes. May increase risk of bladder cancer.
Dipeptidyl Peptidase-4 Inhibitor (DPP-4)				
Linagliptin (Tradjenta)	8–14 hr	5 mg	5 mg once per day	
Saxagliptin (Onglyza)	8–14 hr	2.5, 5 mg	5 mg once per day	Contraindicated in end-stage renal disease; dose adjustment required for renal impairment

Table 5.2	Oral Hypoglycemic Agents			
Oral agent	**Duration**	**Starting dose**	**Daily dosage**	**Comment(s)**
Dipeptidyl Peptidase-4 Inhibitor (DPP-4)				
Sitagliptin (Januvia)	8–14 hr	25, 50, or 100 mg	100 mg once per day	Contraindicated in end-stage renal disease; dose adjustment required for renal impairment
Combination Preparations				
Actoplus met: pioglitazone (Actos) + metformin (Glucophage)		15 mg/500 mg, 15 mg/850 mg	Maximum dose is pioglitazone 45 mg or metformin 2550 mg daily	
Avandaryl: rosiglitazone (Avandia) 4 mg +glimepiride (Amaryl)		4 mg/1, 2, 4 mg once daily titrated carefully	Maximum dose is 8 mg rosiglitazone and 4 mg glimepiride	Given once daily with the first meal
Avandamet: metformin (Glucophage) + rosiglitazone (Avandia)		2 mg/500 mg once or BID	Maximum daily dose is 8 mg/2000 mg in divided doses	
Glucovance: glyburide (Diaβ) + metformin (Glucophage)		1.25, 2.5, 5 mg/250 or 500 mg once or BID with meals	Maximum dose is 20 mg/2000 mg daily in single or divided doses	Dosage may be increased every 2 weeks from initial dose to maximum dose
Metaglip: glipizide (Glucotrol) + metformin (Glucophage)		2.5, 5 mg/250 or 500 mg	20 mg glipizide/2000 mg metformin	May cause profound hypoglycemia; caution recommended if used in patients with cardiovascular heart disease risk
Linagliptin + metformin (Jentadueto)		2.5 mg/500, 850, or 1000 mg	2.5 mg/1000 mg twice a day	
Saxagliptin + Metformin (ext-rel) (Kombiglyze XR)		2.5, 5 mg/500 or 100 mg	5 mg/2 grams per day	
Sitagliptin + metformin (Janumet or Janumet XR)		50 mg/500 or 100 mg For XR: 50, 100 mg/500 or 1000 mg	100 mg/2 grams per day	
Pioglitazone + glimepride (Duetact)		30 mg/2 or 4 mg	30 mg/4 mg per day	
Rosiglitazone + glimepride (Avandaryl)		4 mg/1, 2, or 4 mg	8 mg/4 mg per day	

Table 5.2	Oral Hypoglycemic Agents			
Oral agent	**Duration**	**Starting dose**	**Daily dosage**	**Comment(s)**
Other Agents for Type 2 Diabetes				
Amylin Receptor Agonist				
Pramlintide (Symlin)	2–3 hr	Diabetes mellitus type 1: 15 mcg SQ immediately prior to major meals Diabetes mellitus type 2: 60 mcg SQ immediately prior to major meals	Diabetes mellitus type 1: titrate at 15 mcg increments to 30–60 mcg SQ as tolerated Diabetes mellitus type 2: 120 mcg SQ as tolerated	Adjunct therapy for type 1 and type 2 diabetes mellitus. Contraindicated in patients with hypoglycemic unawareness or gastroparesis. Black box warning for individuals while driving. Severe hypoglycemia with concurrent insulin or oral hypoglycemic agent. When initiating pramlintide, reduce dose of any secretagogues; reduce insulin dose by at least 50%
Glucagon-Like Peptide-1 Receptor Agonist				
Liraglutide (Victoza)		6 mg/ml	Initially 0.6 mg/day x 1 week, then 1.2 mg/day and may increase to 1.8 mg/day	Several drug-drug interactions. Contraindicated in severe renal dysfunction, pancreatitis, or thyroid cancer
Exenatide (Byetta) for type 2 diabetes with oral agents such as metformin, a sulfonylurea, or both	9 hr	5-mcg and 10-mcg injection pen doses SQ	10 mcg twice a day SQ	Contraindicated in severe renal dysfunction, pancreatitis. Taken within 1 hr before meals. Administer as an SQ dose in the thigh, abdomen, or upper arm. Major side effects N/V/D. Warning: has been associated with acute pancreatitis
Exenatide Extended -Release (Bydureon		2 mg/vial	2 mg once every 7 days (weekly) SQ	Contraindicated in severe renal dysfunction, pancreatitis
Sodium-Glucose Co-Transporter 2 Inhibitors (SGLT-2 Inhibitor)				
Canaglifozin (Invokana)	10–13 hr	100, 300 mg	300 mg Take prior to first meal	Renal dosing advised Major side effect urinary infections

Note. HCl = hydrochloride; GI = gastrointestinal; XL, XR = extended release; SQ = subcutaneous; N/V/D = nausea, vomiting, diarrhea.

Used with permission from Barkley TW Jr., Appel SJ. Diabetes mellitus In: Barkley TW Jr, Myers CM, eds. *Practice Considerations for the Adult-Gerontology Acute Care Nurse Practitioner.* West Hollywood, CA: Barkley and Associates; 2015: 427–441.

Workup

The diagnosis of type 2 DM requires much of the baseline data that also provides a diagnosis of type 1 DM. Possible diagnostic findings of type 2 DM may include a fasting blood glucose reading of 126 mg/dl or higher, a random plasma glucose reading of 200 mg/dl or higher, an elevated Hgb A1C, and rarely, an oral glucose tolerance test revealing elevations of 200 mg/dl or higher.[8]

Patients with suspected HHNK and with characteristic findings such as dehydration, increased serum osmolality, and extremely high blood glucose levels should be transported to the emergency department, where they will undergo additional tests. Unlike with DKA, there is no presence of anion gap metabolic acidosis in HHNK.[5]

Treatment (see tables 5.1–5.2)

Because type 2 DM patients are at increased risk of developing cardiovascular disease, lifestyle changes are recommended to prevent further complications. Smoking cessation, exercise, hypertension and lipid control, and diet are all recommended measures. An added benefit of regular exercise is that it can improve how the body responds to insulin.[16] Just as those with type 1 DM, patients with type 2 DM should see an ophthalmologist within the first 5 years of diagnosis, if not earlier, to assess for any evidence of diabetic retinopathy.[8]

Early use of oral antidiabetic therapy is recommended to improve glycemic control and to reduce the chance of long-term complications. The most regularly prescribed oral antidiabetics include the following: biguanides, sulfonylureas, alpha-glucosidase inhibitors, thiazolidinediones, and meglitinide derivatives (see table 5.2).

Hyperosmolar Hyperglycemic Non-ketosis (HHNK)

Overview

HHNK is a serious, acute, metabolic complication primarily associated with type 2 DM that can lead to coma or death in severe or untreated cases. Emergency intervention is warranted, as the condition has an associated mortality rate of approximately 30%–50%.[5]

This condition is characterized by greatly elevated serum glucose levels that occur when the body is unable to produce enough insulin to prevent severe hyperglycemia, osmotic diuresis, and extracellular fluid depletion. This results in hyperosmolality and severe dehydration without ketone production.

HHNK occurs in previously undiagnosed diabetic patients or patients who are unable to effectively manage their diabetes. A common precipitating factor for HHNK is a concomitant illness in type 2 diabetics that leads to reduced fluid intake.[15] Medications that lower glucose tolerance may also cause HHNK.[19]

Presentation

Patients with HHNK may complain of experiencing thirst, polydipsia, polyuria, and weakness. Physical examination findings of HHNK include dehydration and signs and symptoms suggestive of possible underlying causes (e.g., infection). In patients with HHNK, tachycardia serves as an indicator for the early stages of dehydration. Profound dehydration would be suggested by hypotension.[18]

Many patients may also exhibit an altered level of consciousness, characterized as decreased or degrading. Patients may also present with poor skin turgor. Additionally, hemoconcentration and volume depletion can cause focal and global neurological findings, such as sensory or motor impairments, delirium, visual changes or disturbances, and possible risk of seizures.

Workup

Diagnostics for HHNK are performed in emergency care.

Treatment

Just as with DKA patients, patients with HHNK should be immediately hospitalized to prevent life-threatening complications.[15] Fluid resuscitation and restoration of normal glucose levels are the key elements of the plan of care.[19,20]

Problems with Early Morning Hyperglycemia

Diabetic patients may experience early morning hyperglycemia as a result of blood glucose rising at night or during sleep. The majority of patients with this problem have type 1 DM. Two of the processes responsible for triggering early morning hyperglycemia are the Somogyi effect and the dawn phenomenon.

The Somogyi effect occurs in patients who experience nocturnal hypoglycemia. A diabetic patient's blood glucose drops overnight, which causes the body to stimulate a surge of regulatory hormones to counter it. Patients should be aware that triggers for nocturnal hypoglycemia include alcohol consumption, eating too little, and taking too much insulin.[21] Patients experiencing the Somogyi effect should consult with their nurse practitioner (NP) to either reduce or omit the bedtime dose of insulin.[1] Patients can also eat a snack that is high in protein and carbohydrates before they go to bed.[17]

The dawn phenomenon occurs in patients who develop a nocturnal resistance to insulin; it is normally attributed to tissue insensitivity. The rise in glucose occurs in the early morning hours, usually between 3 a.m. and 6 a.m. in patients with a normal sleeping schedule. The body stimulates a predawn increase in hormone levels that signals an increase in glucose. Without sufficient insulin, the glucose does not get processed, which causes morning hyperglycemia. Eating breakfast can help normalize blood glucose levels, and treatment involves either including or increasing the bedtime dose of insulin.[1,21]

Hyperthyroidism

Overview

Hyperthyroidism is a metabolic disorder with multiple etiologies, manifestations, and potential treatment options. This condition is characterized by an overactive thyroid gland that synthesizes and secretes excess thyroid hormones—thyroxine (T4), triiodothyronine (T3), or both—throughout the body.[22]

Hyperthyroidism can cause prominent cardiovascular manifestations and aggravate pre-existing cardiac disease.[23] The disorder can also lead to a potentially fatal complication known as thyrotoxicosis, which develops when thyroid hormone levels in the bloodstream get too high, resulting in a severe hypermetabolic condition.[24]

The three predominant causes of hyperthyroidism are Graves' disease, toxic multinodular goiter, and toxic adenoma.[22] Graves' disease, the leading cause of hyperthyroidism, occurs when antibodies in the blood attack the thyroid, causing the entire thyroid gland to produce excess thyroid hormone.[25] Toxic multinodular goiters, the second most common cause, are characterized by one or more nodules in the thyroid that gradually grow, increasing activity and releasing excess thyroid hormone into the bloodstream.[26] Toxic adenoma, the third most common cause, mainly appears in younger patients and is characterized by a single hyperfunctioning follicular thyroid adenoma. A benign monoclonal tumor secretes excess thyroid hormone, which suppresses levels of thyroid-stimulating hormone (TSH).[22]

A common cause of hyperthyroidism includes a genetic predisposition to the condition. Non-genetic causes include subacute thyroiditis, a TSH-secreting tumor of the pituitary, and factitial hyperthyroidism. High amounts of iodine in the body, either through diet or high doses of amiodarone (Cordarone), can also cause hyperthyroidism.[27] In addition to the various etiologies, hyperthyroidism occurs more often in women than men by an 8:1 ratio, and usually manifests between 20 and 40 years of age.[28]

Presentation

Signs and symptoms of hyperthyroidism vary according to the severity of the condition, the patient's age, and etiology. Patients with mild cases of hyperthyroidism tend to appear asymptomatic. Those with moderate to severe cases present with more pronounced indications that can overlap with the underlying cause.[27]

Common findings of hyperthyroidism include nervousness, anxiety, and increased sweating. Further neurological signs and symptoms may include fatigue, emotional lability, fine tremors, and hyperreflexia of deep tendon reflexes. A physical exam may reveal fine and/or thin hair, lid lag, and smooth, warm, moist velvety skin. In severe cases, standard findings include weakness, nervousness, and dyspnea, with weight loss presenting as well in many cases.[25,27] Signs and symptoms associated with heart failure may also be common, with atrial fibrillation being the predominant cardiac manifestation.[23]

Certain variants of hyperthyroidism present with distinguishing findings. Characteristic findings of Graves' disease may include bilateral exophthalmos, also known as Graves' ophthalmopathy.[29,30] Toxic multinodular goiters are indicated by a swollen thyroid gland that may exert pressure on the trachea and esophagus, producing respiratory symptoms.[22,24,31] Patients with toxic adenoma may present with signs and symptoms associated with thyrotoxicosis, as well as a single, palpable thyroid nodule that is visible at the front of the neck.[24,32]

Some patients with hyperthyroidism also experience an onset of thyrotoxicosis. In this case, overlapping clinical manifestations include nervousness, palpitations, fatigue, weakness in the upper arms and thighs, and fine or brittle hair.[22,25] In cases of thyroid storm, which is a severe form of thyrotoxicosis, patients may present with a high fever and a hypermetabolic state, appearing agitated or nauseous. Tachycardia, psychosis, and vomiting are standard findings, and patients experience coma if thyrotoxicosis advances.[25]

Workup

The best initial test to screen for hyperthyroidism is a TSH assay. In the majority of cases, a single serum TSH assessment is enough to confirm hyperthyroidism.[22,33] Patients with primary hyperthyroidism have typical lab findings that include a low TSH level, as well as elevated T3, T4, thyroid resin uptake, and FTI.[33] In some cases, T4 levels may be normal, but T3 levels will be elevated. An antinuclear antibody (ANA) test may also be ordered, as Graves' disease is autoimmune in nature and will present with elevated ANAs.

A radioactive iodine scan may be ordered to help determine the etiology, particularly in cases where the etiology is unclear. A high iodine uptake is consistent with Graves' disease, whereas a low iodine uptake is consistent with subacute thyroiditis. An MRI of the orbits may also be ordered in suspected cases of Graves' disease to confirm the presence of Graves' ophthalmopathy.[22,33]

Treatment

Treatment options for hyperthyroidism are vast. Several factors determine which treatment options are available depending on the cause, severity, age of the patient, comorbid conditions, goiter size, and patient preference for the type of treatment. Because treatment depends on etiology and patient-related factors, patients should be referred to a specialist for treatment and may require immediate hospitalization if they experience severe symptoms.[25]

Because Graves' disease is the predominant cause of hyperthyroidism, general treatment options for patients include antithyroid medications, radioactive iodine therapy, and removal of the thyroid gland (either partially or completely).[22,34]

Thiourea drugs, such as methimazole (Tapazole) and propylthiouracil (PTU), are recommended for patients with mild cases of hyperthyroidism or small goiters, as well as patients who are adverse to radioactive therapy. Methimazole is prescribed at 30–60 mg per day taken orally in four divided doses, whereas propylthiouracil is prescribed at 300–600 mg taken orally in four divided doses per day.[35,36,37] Propranolol (Inderal) and other beta blockers may be used for symptomatic treatment of hyperthyroidism, and are recommended for treatment of subacute thyroiditis. Treatment with propranolol should begin with 10 mg administered orally, but may be increased to 80 mg administered orally four times per day, as needed.[22]

In the United States, radioactive iodine therapy is the preferred treatment for patients with Graves' disease, and can also be prescribed to patients with toxic multinodular goiter and toxic adenoma.[34] Dosage is determined by thyroid activity based on the size and ability to trap iodine.[22,34]

A thyroidectomy may be required for patients with either toxic multinodular goiters or toxic adenoma.[36] Patients should reach a euthyroid state before undergoing surgery. Before surgery, a regimen of Lugol's solution at 2–3 drops taken orally every day for 10 days is recommended to reduce the vascularity of the gland.[38]

Patients exhibiting findings suggestive of thyroid storm should be transported to the emergency department for acute management. Management of this crisis begins with a course of propylthiouracil or methimazole, paired with either Lugol's solution or a regimen of sodium iodide, propranolol, and hydrocortisone. Acetylsalicylic acid should be avoided in patients experiencing a crisis, as it may lead to increased T3 and T4 levels.[25]

Hypothyroidism

Overview

Hypothyroidism is a thyroid disorder with several etiologies. The disorder is characterized by an underactive thyroid that produces deficient thyroid hormone, resulting in increased TSH levels, decreased levels of T3 and T4, and slower basal metabolism. If left untreated or undiagnosed, hypothyroidism can adversely affect the cardiovascular and respiratory systems, as well as gastrointestinal function. In severe cases, hypothyroidism can lead to myxedema coma.[39]

Hypothyroidism is more prevalent among women than men, and the risk of developing hypothyroidism increases with age.[40] Autoimmune diseases, such as Hashimoto's thyroiditis, are the leading cause of hypothyroidism. Iodine deficiency is associated with the condition, but is not a common cause in the United States. Other causes include thyroidectomy or damage to part or all of the gland due to certain medications, such as amiodarone or radioactive iodine treatment.[41] Hypothyroidism can also result from decreased production of TSH by the pituitary gland or decreased secretion of thyrotropin-releasing hormone (TRH) from the hypothalamus.[42]

Presentation

The signs and symptoms of hypothyroidism are often subtle and nonspecific, varying among individuals according to a number of factors that include etiology, duration of the condition, and severity of the hypothyroid state. Patients may originally appear asymptomatic; however, standard clinical indications include slowing of physical activity, mental activity, and metabolic functions.[39,40,42]

Some of the signs and symptoms of hypothyroidism can be ascribed to slower metabolism, such as fatigue, weakness, cold intolerance, weight gain, slow reflexes, slower heart rate, and dry skin. Forgetfulness and depression may also present, as well as signs and symptoms of hypertension or high cholesterol.[39,42] Other findings can include arthralgias, cramps, constipation, bradycardia, and hypoactive bowel sounds. Some patients may also present with puffy eyes, brittle nails, hair loss, and edema of the hands and face.[39]

Findings that are specific to Hashimoto's thyroiditis include painless thyroid enlargement, exhaustion, and transient pain or fullness in the neck or throat.[39] Rapid precipitation of existing findings of hypothyroidism and the rapid onset of altered level of consciousness suggest myxedema coma.[40]

Workup

Expected findings in a patient with hypothyroidism include elevated TSH levels and low to low-normal T4 levels. A resin T3 uptake may show decreased T3 levels; however, this is not a reliable metric for diagnosing hypothyroidism. Other laboratory findings suggestive of hypothyroidism include hyponatremia and hypoglycemia.[40]

Treatment

Hypothyroidism cannot be cured; however, treatment and management should primarily be handled by an endocrinologist and focus should consist of T4 replacement to normalize thyroid hormone levels.[42]

The standard treatment for hypothyroidism is levothyroxine (Synthroid), which is a synthetic form of T4. Generally, patients are initially prescribed 50–75 µg daily for mild to moderate cases, with dosage increased by 25 µg every 1–2 weeks until symptoms stabilize; in most cases, the dosage does not exceed 100 µg. The initial dose may need to be reduced in patients older than 60 years of age.[39] For all patients, TSH should be checked every 6–10 weeks following an adjustment to dosage.[42]

Patients presenting with myxedema coma should be transported to the emergency department for immediate care.[39]

Cushing's Syndrome

Overview

Cushing's syndrome is caused by prolonged and inappropriately high exposure of tissue to either exogenous glucocorticoids or endogenous glucocorticoids, resulting in excess cortisol production.[43]

Most cases of Cushing's syndrome are caused by excessive glucocorticoid exposure from medically prescribed corticosteroids. Endogenous causes of Cushing's syndrome, however, are very uncommon and can stem from independent adrenal overproduction of cortisol or from hypersecretion of adrenocorticotropic hormone (ACTH) by either a pituitary tumor or other ectopic tumor. Adrenal tumors that ectopically secrete ACTH are rare, and tumors secreting corticotropin-releasing hormone (CRH) are extremely rare.[43,44]

Cushing's syndrome should be distinguished from Cushing's disease. Cushing's disease results from an ACTH-producing tumor in the pituitary gland that causes the adrenal glands to produce excess cortisol levels. With the exception of glucocorticoid-related complications, Cushing's disease is the predominant non-iatrogenic cause of Cushing's syndrome. ACTH levels are lower in Cushing's syndrome because the hypothalamus and anterior pituitary have increased negative feedback of cortisol.[43,44]

Presentation

Because Cushing's syndrome tends to be progressive, overt clinical features rarely present with onset. Findings of Cushing's syndrome include poor wound healing, weakness, amenorrhea, impotence, headache, polyuria, thirst, and frequent infections.[43] Patients may also exhibit psychological symptoms, which include cognitive defects, depression, sleep disturbances, and labile mood, among others.[43]

As Cushing's syndrome progresses, the characteristic signs become more noticeable, which include a round-shaped face, the development of a fatty mound at the base of the back of the neck, central obesity, and purple or pink striae. Acne, glucose intolerance, and hirsutism are also closely associated with the disease, as well as muscular atrophy and loss of subcutaneous fat, which can be seen as visible subcutaneous blood vessels. Patients may appear with ecchymoses or bruises and thin skin.[44]

Patients with signs and symptoms of Cushing's syndrome should undergo a full, comprehensive evaluation to determine if the syndrome is a primary or secondary cause of the condition and to either rule out or identify other conditions before determining a definitive diagnosis.

Workup

Patients with an initial suspected diagnosis of Cushing's syndrome should be referred to an endocrinologist.[43] However, prior to any biochemical testing, a thorough drug history of the patient should be obtained to exclude an exogenous etiology and to reduce the risk of drug interactions.[46]

A diagnosis of Cushing's syndrome due to an endogenous etiology is based upon lab findings that indicate inappropriately high levels of serum cortisol or urine cortisol. Initial diagnostic testing is done to determine the presence and severity of Cushing's syndrome, and follow-up testing is implemented to determine the etiology.[43,45,46]

Depending on which test is suitable for the patient, one of the following tests will be ordered as an initial diagnostic: at least two measurements of either 24-hour urinary free cortisol (UFC) or late-night salivary cortisol test; low-dose overnight dexamethasone suppression test (DST); or a longer low-dose DST (LDDST) of 2 mg/day for 48 hours.[43]

Laboratory findings associated with Cushing's syndrome include hyperglycemia, hypernatremia, hypokalemia, glycosuria, and leukocytosis.[1]

Treatment

Treatment for Cushing's syndrome depends on the etiology and should focus on reducing cortisol secretion. Electrolytes should also be regulated to sufficient levels.

Because the majority of cases of Cushing's syndrome are due to exogenous exposure to synthetic glucocorticoids, medications that are determined to be responsible should be discontinued. Adrenal tumors should be removed, and ACTH-secreting tumors can be resectioned. Transsphenoidal resection is used to remove tumors from the pituitary gland.[43]

Primary Adrenocortical Insufficiency (Addison's Disease)

Overview

Addison's disease, also known as chronic primary adrenal insufficiency, is a rare, chronic endocrine disorder in which the adrenal glands do not produce a sufficient amount of steroid hormones. This results in deficient levels of glucocorticoids (cortisol) and mineralocorticoids (androgen and aldosterone), which can cause various secondary conditions such as hypoglycemia and hypotension.[47]

Addison's disease applies only to primary adrenal insufficiency and should be distinguished from secondary and tertiary adrenal insufficiency.[48]

The leading cause of Addison's disease is autoimmune destruction of the adrenal cortex.[49] The disease is closely associated with other autoimmune disorders, such as type 1 DM and thyroiditis. Rare causes of Addison's disease include HIV and tuberculosis, among others.[47,50]

If left undiagnosed or untreated, Addison's disease can result in an acute adrenal crisis, also known as an Addisonian crisis.[47] An Addisonian crisis is brought about by a lack of cortisol, often triggered by serious infection.[51] Patients experiencing an Addisonian crisis should receive immediate emergency treatment in an acute care facility.

Presentation

Hyperpigmentation of the skin, a characteristic sign of Addison's disease, manifests in almost all cases and is especially evident in patients experiencing an acute adrenal crisis. This hyperpigmentation stems from the stimulation of melanocytes by excess ACTH production.[52] Hyperpigmentation occurs primarily on sun-exposed areas of the skin and particularly in skin creases, the buccal mucosa, and areas exposed to friction or pressure, such as the elbows and knees. Diffuse tanning and freckles can also appear on the skin.[50]

Frequent findings of Addison's disease include weakness, fatigue, body weight loss due to anorexia, and scant axillary or pubic hair.[50] Patients may also exhibit a craving for salt, stemming from loss of sodium. Orthostatic hypotension precedes an impending adrenal crisis.[51]

Shock is a sign of an acute adrenal crisis. Patients experiencing an acute adrenal crisis may complain of abdominal tenderness and fever, exhibit a change in level of consciousness, or demonstrate a rapid worsening of other characteristic manifestations of chronic Addison's disease, such as hypotension. These patients should be admitted immediately to an emergency department for treatment and diagnosis.[51]

Workup

Patients with an initial suspected diagnosis of adrenal insufficiency assessment should be referred to an endocrinologist.[53]

Expected findings for a patient with Addison's disease include hypoglycemia, hyponatremia, hyperkalemia, lymphocytosis, elevated ESR, and low serum cortisol.[48,50,54]

Treatment

An adrenal crisis should be treated as a life-threatening emergency, and treatment should focus on immediate therapeutic management that includes fluid resuscitation and stress dose hydrocortisone. Patients presenting with adrenal crisis should be transported to emergency care, where they may receive treatment over the course of several days aimed at restoring fluids, stimulating adrenaline, addressing the underlying cause of the condition, and managing low blood pressure.[50]

For long-term care of Addison's disease, a referral to an endocrinologist is recommended. Outpatient management of Addison's disease includes steroid replacement therapy to correct deficient steroid hormones, as well as lifestyle changes to manage the condition and prevent an adrenal crisis.

Steroid replacement involves glucocorticoid and mineralocorticoid replacement therapy.[49,50]

Non-pharmaceutical treatments include an increase in exercise. Increasing sodium intake is recommended for patients who are undergoing stress, participating in vigorous physical activity, exposed to high temperatures, or experiencing gastrointestinal distress.[55]

References

1. Barkley TW Jr. Diagnosis and management of endocrine disorders. In: Barkley TW Jr., ed. *Adult-Gerontology Primary Care Nurse Practitioner*. West Hollywood, CA: Barkley & Associates; 2015: 52–58.

2. United States Department of Health and Human Services, Centers for Disease Control and Prevention. National diabetes fact sheet, 2011. http://www.cdc.gov/diabetes/pubs/pdf/ndfs_2011.pdf. Published 2011. Accessed March 19, 2015.

3. McCulloch DK. Classification of diabetes mellitus and genetic diabetic syndromes. In: Basow DS, ed. *UpToDate*. Waltham, MA: UpToDate; 2015. http://www.uptodate.com/contents/classification-of-diabetes-mellitus-and-genetic-diabetic-syndromes. Last updated October 6, 2014. Accessed March 19, 2015.

4. Fast facts: Data and statistics about diabetes. American Diabetes Association web site. http://professional.diabetes.org/admin/UserFiles/0%20-%20Sean/14_fast_facts_june2014_final3.pdf. Revised July 2014. Accessed March 19, 2015.

5. Barkley TW Jr., Appel SJ. Diabetes-related emergencies. In: Barkley TW Jr, Myers CM, eds. *Practice Considerations for the Adult-Gerontology Acute Care Nurse Practitioner*. West Hollywood, CA: Barkley and Associates; 2015: 442–446.

6. Khardori R. Type 1 diabetes mellitus. In: Griffing GT, ed. Medscape. http://emedicine.medscape.com/article/117739-overview. Updated March 10, 2015. Accessed March 19, 2015.

7. DKA (Ketoacidosis) & Ketones. American Diabetes Association web site. http://www.diabetes.org/living-with-diabetes/complications/ketoacidosis-dka.html. Reviewed August 21, 2013. Edited March 18, 2015. Accessed March 19, 2015.

8. American Diabetes Association (ADA). Standards of medical care in diabetes—2013 [Supplemental material]. *Diabetes Care*. 2013; 37(Supplement 1): S14–S80. doi:10.2337/dc14-S014

9. Kitabchi AE, Hirsch IB, Emmett M. Diabetic ketoacidosis and hyperosmolar hyperglycemic state in adults: Clinical features, evaluation, and diagnosis. In: Basow DS, ed. *UpToDate*. Waltham, MA: UpToDate; 2015. http://www.uptodate.com/contents/clinical-features-and-diagnosis-of-diabetic-ketoacidosis-and-hyperosmolar-hyperglycemic-state-in-adults. Last updated July 2, 2014. Accessed March 19, 2015.

10. Evert AB, Boucher JL, Cypress M, et al. Nutrition therapy recommendations for the management of adults with diabetes. *Diabetes Care*. 2013; 36: 3821–3824.

11. Gebel E. How to avoid DKA. Diabetes Forecast. http://www.diabetes forecast.org/2013/mar/how-to-avoid-dka.html. Published March 2013. Accessed March 19, 2015.

12. Hamdy O. Diabetic ketoacidosis. In: Khardori R, ed. Medscape. http://emedicine.medscape.com/article/118361-overview#showall. Updated October 29, 2014. Accessed March 19, 2015.

13. Hamdy, O. Diabetic ketoacidosis treatment and management. In: Khardori R, ed. Medscape. http://emedicine.medscape.com/article/118361-treatment. Updated October 29, 2014. Accessed March 19, 2015.

14. Goguen J, Gilbert J. Hyperglycemic emergencies in adults. Canadian Diabetes Association Clinical Practice Guidelines. http://guidelines.diabetes.ca/browse/Chapter15. Published 2013. Accessed March 19, 2015.

15. ADA. Diagnosis and classification of diabetes mellitus [Supplemental material]. *Diabetes Care*. 2013; 36(Supplement 1): S67–S74. doi:10.2337/dc13-S067

16. McCulloch DK. Patient information: Diabetes mellitus type 2: Treatment (beyond the basics). In: Basow DS, ed. *UpToDate*. Waltham, MA: UpToDate; 2015. http://www.uptodate.com/contents/diabetes-mellitus-type-2-treatment-beyond-the-basics. Last updated March 14, 2014. Accessed March 19, 2015.

17. Khardori R. Type 2 diabetes mellitus. In: Griffing GT, ed. Medscape. http://emedicine.medscape.com/article/117853-overview. Updated March 10, 2015. Accessed March 19, 2015.

18. Hemphill RR. Hyperosmolar hyperglycemic state. In: Griffing GT, ed. Medscape. http://emedicine.med scape.com/article/1914705-overview. Updated April 30, 2014. Accessed March 19, 2015.

19. Diabetic hyperglycemic hyperosmolar syndrome. A.D.A.M. Medical Encyclopedia. http://www.nlm.nih.gov/medlineplus/ency/article/000304.htm. Updated May 10, 2014. Accessed March 19, 2015.

20. Kitabchi AE, Hirsch IB, Emmett M. Diabetic ketoacidosis and hyperosmolar hyperglycemic state in adults: Treatment. In: Basow DS, ed. *UpToDate*. Waltham, MA: UpToDate; 2015. http://www.uptodate.com/contents/treatment-of-diabetic-ketoacidosis-and-hyperosmolar-hyperglycemic-state-in-adults. Last updated October 17, 2014. Accessed March 19, 2015.

21. Gebel E. Handling morning highs in blood glucose. Diabetes Forecast. http://www.diabetesforecast.org/2012/mar/handling-morning-highs-in-blood-glucose.html. Published March 2012. Accessed March 19, 2015.

22. Lee SL, Ananthakrishnan S. Hyperthyroidism. In: Khardori R, ed. Medscape. http://emedicine.med scape.com/article/121865-overview. Updated September 4, 2014. Accessed March 19, 2015.

23. Sabatino L, Iervasi G, Pingitoire A. Thyroid hormone and heart failure: From myocardial protection to systemic regulation. *Expert Rev Cardiovasc Ther*. 2014; 12(10): 1227–1236. doi: 10.1586/14779072.2014.957674,

24. Kopp P. Thyrotoxicosis of other etiologies. In: De Groot LJ, ed. *Thyroid Disease Manager*. South Dartmouth, MA: Endocrine Education Inc; 2015. http://www.thyroidmanager.org/wp-content/uploads/chapters/thyrotoxicosis-of-other-etiologies.pdf. Document last updated December 1, 2010. Accessed March 19, 2015.

25. Schraga ED. Hyperthyroidism, thyroid storm, and Graves' disease. In: Khradori R, ed. Medscape. http://emedicine.medscape.com/article/767130-overview. Updated May 30, 2014. Accessed March 20, 2015.

26. Stock J. Severe hyperthyroidism: Cause, patient features and treatment outcomes. *Clinical Thyroidology for Patients*. 2010; 3(1): 5–6. http://www.thyroid.org/patient-thyroid-information/ct-for-patients/volume-3-issue-1/vol-3-issue-1-p-5-6/

27. Hyperthyroidism. American Thyroid Association web site. http://www.thyroid.org/wp-content/uploads/patients/brochures/ata-hyperthyroidism-brochure.pdf. Published 2014. Accessed March 20, 2015.

28. Dello Stritto R, Barkley TW Jr. Thyroid disease. In: Barkley TW Jr., Myers CM, eds. *Practice Considerations for the Adult-Gerontology Acute Care Nurse Practitioner*. West Hollywood, CA: Barkley and Associates; 2015:447–451.

29. De Groot LJ. Diagnosis and treatment of Graves' disease. In: De Groot, LJ, ed. *Thyroid Disease Manager*. South Dartmouth, MA: Endocrine Education Inc; 2015. http://www.thyroidmanager.org/wp-content/uploads/chapters/diagnosis-and-treatment-of-graves-disease.pdf. Revised September 20, 2012. Accessed March 20, 2015.

30. Davies TF. Pretibial myxedema (thyroid dermopathy) in autoimmune thyroid disease. In: Basow DS, ed., *UpToDate*. Waltham, MA: UpToDate; 2015. http://www.uptodate.com/contents/pretibial-myxedema-thyroid-dermopathy-in-autoimmune-thyroid-disease#H57417960. Last updated February 13, 2014. Accessed March 20, 2015.

31. Medeiros-Neto G. Multinodal goiter. In: De Groot LJ, ed. *Thyroid Disease Manager*. South Dartmouth, MA: Endocrine Education Inc; 2015. http://www.thyroidmanager.org/chapter/multinodular-goiter/#toc-pathology. Last updated February 12, 2013. Accessed March 20, 2015.

32. Thyroid nodules. New York Thyroid Center web site. http://columbiasurgery.org/node/1048. Accessed March 20, 2015.

33. Ross DS. Diagnosis of hyperthyroidism. In: Basow DS, ed. *UpToDate*. Waltham, MA: UpToDate; 2015. http://www.uptodate.com/contents/diagnosis-of-hyperthyroidism. Last updated December 15, 2014. Accessed March 20, 2015.

34. Bahn RS, Burch HB, Cooper DS, et al. Hyperthyroidism and other causes of thyrotoxicosis: Management guidelines of the American Thyroid Association and American Association of Clinical Endocrinologists. *Thyroid*. 2011; 21(6): 593–646. doi:10.1089/thy.2010.0417

35. Institute for Quality and Efficiency in Health Care. Research studies: What are the advantages and disadvantages of combined treatment with anti-thyroid drugs and radioiodine? PubMed Health. http://www.ncbi.nlm.nih.gov/pubmedhealth/PMH0005044/. Last updated October 9, 2014. Accessed March 20, 2015.

36. United States Department of Health and Human Services, United States Food and Drug Administration. FDA drug safety communication: New boxed warning on severe liver injury with propylthiouracil. http://www.fda.gov/Drugs/DrugSafety/PostmarketDrugSafetyInformationforPatientsandProviders/ucm209023.htm#ds. Published April 21, 2010. Last updated May 6, 2010. Accessed March 20, 2015.

37. Propylthiouracil: Dosing & uses. Medscape web site. http://reference.medscape.com/drug/ptu-propylthiouracil-342735. Accessed March 20, 2015.

38. Hyperthyroidism. New York Thyroid Center web site. http://columbiasurgery.org/node/992. Accessed March 20, 2015.

39. Orlander PR, Varghese JM, Freeman LM. Hypothyroidism. In: Griffing GT, ed. Medscape. http://emedicine.medscape.com/article/122393-overview. Updated February 20, 2015. Accessed March 20, 2015.

40. Wiersinga, WM. Adult hypothyroidism. In: De Groot LJ, ed. *Thyroid Disease Manager*. South Dartmouth, MA: Endocrine Education Inc; 2015. http://www.thyroidmanager.org/wp-content/uploads/chapters/adult-hypothyroidism.pdf. Last updated December 12, 2013. Accessed March 20, 2015.

41. Ross DS. Patient information: Hypothyroidism (underactive thyroid) (beyond the basics). In: Basow DS, ed. *UpToDate*. Waltham, MA: UpToDate; 2015. http://www.uptodate.com/contents/hypothyroidism-underactive-thyroid-beyond-the-basics. Last updated December 5, 2013. Accessed March 20, 2015.

42. Hypothyroidism. American Thyroid Association web site. http://www.thyroid.org/what-is-hypothyroidism. Published May 21, 2012. Accessed March 20, 2015.

43. Adler G. Cushing syndrome. In: Khardori R, ed. Medscape. http://emedicine.medscape.com/article/117365-overview. Updated April 4, 2014. Accessed March 20, 2015.

44. Chrousos GP, Lafferty A. Glucocorticoid therapy and Cushing syndrome. In: Kemp S, ed. Medscape. http://emedicine.medscape.com/article/921086-overview. Updated March 13, 2014. Accessed March 20, 2015.

45. Healthwise, Inc. Information and resources: Cortisol in blood. WebMD. http://www.webmd.com/a-to-z-guides/cortisol-14668. Updated June 20, 2012. Accessed March 20, 2015.

46. Nieman L. Pitfalls in the diagnosis and differential diagnosis of Cushing's syndrome. *Clin Endocrinol*. 2014; 80(3): 333–334. doi: 10.1111/cen.12362.

47. Nieman LK. Causes of primary adrenal insufficiency (Addison's disease). In: Basow DS, ed. *UpToDate*. Waltham, MA: UpToDate; 2015. http://www.uptodate.com/contents/causes-of-primary-adrenal-insufficiency-addisons-disease. Last updated February 1, 2013. Accessed March 20, 2015.

48. Nieman LK. Treatment of adrenal insufficiency in adults. In: Basow DS, ed. *UpToDate*. Waltham, MA: UpToDate; 2015. http://www.uptodate.com/contents/treatment-of-adrenal-insufficiency-in-adults. Last updated December 18, 2014. Accessed March 20, 2015.

49. Falorni A, Minarelli V, Moreli S. Therapy of adrenal insufficiency: An update. *Endocrine*. 2013; 43(3): 514–528. doi:10.1007/s12020-012-9835-4

50. Mascarenhas JV, Jude EB. Delayed diagnosis of Addison's disease: An approach to management. *BMJ Case Rep*. 2014. doi: 10.1136/bcr-2014-204005.

51. Nieman LK. Clinical manifestations of adrenal insufficiency in adults. In: Basow DS, ed. *UpToDate*. Waltham, MA: UpToDate; 2015. http://www.uptodate.com/contents/clinical-manifestations-of-adrenal-insufficiency-in-adults. Last updated February 1, 2013. Accessed March 20, 2015.

52. Griffing GT, Odeke S, Nagelberg SB. Addison disease. In: Khardori R, ed. Medscape. http://emedicine.medscape.com/article/116467-overview. Updated November 10, 2014. Accessed March 20, 2015.

53. Nieman LK. Diagnosis of adrenal insufficiency in adults. In: Basow DS, ed. *UpToDate*. Waltham, MA: UpToDate; 2015. http://www.uptodate.com/contents/diagnosis-of-adrenal-insufficiency-in-adults?detected. Last updated December 17, 2014. Accessed March 20, 2015.

54. Mayo Clinic Staff. Addison's disease: Test and diagnosis. Mayo Clinic. http://www.mayoclinic.com/health/addisons-disease/DS00361/DSECTION=-tests-and-diagnosis. Reviewed December 4, 2012. Accessed March 20, 2015.

55. Mayo Clinic Staff. Addison's disease: Treatment and drugs. Mayo Clinic. http://www.mayoclinic.com/health/addisons-disease/DS00361/DSECTION=treatments-and-drugs. Reviewed December 4, 2012. Accessed March 20, 2015.

Chapter 6
Musculoskeletal Disorders

1. Of the following, which medical imaging technique is most routinely used to rule out other bone or joint conditions in patients with suspected cases of bursitis?

   a. Magnetic resonance imaging

   b. Plain x-rays

   c. Electromyography

   d. Computed tomography

2. All of the following musculoskeletal disorders affect women at a higher rate than men except:

   a. Rheumatoid arthritis

   b. Carpal tunnel syndrome

   c. Morton's neuroma

   d. Plantar fasciitis

3. Jerry, age 64, has a history of a herniated disk. He comes to your practice complaining of pain that radiates from his lower back down through the left side of his calf. He is also experiencing numbness in his back and left foot. During the examination, he has difficulty dorsiflexing his great toe. Given his most likely injury, which of the following would be best to have Jerry perform for a proper assessment?

   a. Standing on toes for 5 seconds

   b. Walking on toes

   c. Walking on heels

   d. Squatting and rising

4. Which of the following choices is least likely to cause costochondritis?

   a. Injury to the chest

   b. Physical strain

   c. Giant cell arteritis

   d. Fibromyalgia

5. Which of the following choices best describes the proper order of steps for performing the Lachman's test?

   a. Bend the knee 20°, apply pressure to proximal tibia, and stabilize the thigh.

   b. Stabilize the thigh, bend the knee 20°, and apply pressure to the proximal tibia.

   c. Apply pressure to the proximal tibia, stabilize the thigh, and bend the knee 20°.

   d. Bend the knee 20°, stabilize the thigh, and apply pressure to the proximal tibia.

6. An obese patient is usually at an increased risk of developing all of the following except:

   a. Osteoarthritis

   b. Plantar fasciitis

   c. Low back pain

   d. Polymyalgia rheumatica

7. Among patients experiencing knee injuries, which type of tear is typically the most common?

   a. Medial meniscus

   b. Anterior cruciate ligament

   c. Lateral meniscus

   d. Posterior cruciate ligament

8. Tyler, age 20, fell during a basketball game and injured his left quadricep. In addition to recommending rest and immobilization, you want to help him with the pain. Which of these medications is least likely to see use in the initial treatment of Tyler's injury?

   a. Naproxen

   b. Celecoxib

   c. Metaxalone

   d. Tramadol

9. Positive radiographic findings are most instrumental in diagnosing which of these conditions?

   a. Plantar fasciitis

   b. Bursitis

   c. Carpal tunnel syndrome

   d. Osteoarthritis

10. Morton's neuroma is a benign neuroma that causes a compression neuropathy on an intermetatarsal nerve, most commonly on which two intermetatarsal spaces?

    a. First or second intermetatarsal spaces

    b. Second or third intermetatarsal spaces

    c. Third or fourth intermetatarsal spaces

    d. Fourth or fifth intermetatarsal spaces

11. A woman comes to your practice with complaints of stiffness in her shoulder and "this terrible ache" in her hips. You also find that she has anemia and a mild fever. Which of the following is the patient most likely experiencing?

    a. Rheumatoid arthritis

    b. Costochondritis

    c. Polymyalgia rheumatica

    d. Osteoarthritis

12. A professional male hockey player presents with pain around the sternum that worsens whenever he takes a deep breath. He says his symptoms began nearly a week ago after receiving a hard blow to the chest during a game, and that the pain has been getting progressively worse. For which condition should the patient most likely be first evaluated?

    a. Costochondritis

    b. Muscle strain

    c. Bursitis

    d. Osgood-Schlatter disease

13. A 71-year-old male with an active lifestyle presents to your practice with complaints of pain in his right shoulder. Which of these statements from the patient would most strongly indicate bursitis?

    a. "It hurts when I move my arms over my head."

    b. "Sometimes it feels like I can't move it, no matter how hard I try."

    c. "My biggest problem is this discomfort I feel when I sleep on that side."

    d. "It feels really warm, sometimes even hot, on the inside."

14. Which of the following areas is not a common site of bursitis?

    a. Postpatellar

    b. Olecranon

    c. Subdeltoid

    d. Ischial

15. Which of these tests would provide the best assessment for carpal tunnel syndrome?

    a. McMurray's test

    b. Hirschberg's test

    c. Phalen's test

    d. Allen's test

16. "Locking" of the knee usually indicates loose bodies in the affected area. What other type of knee injury would this presentation most likely suggest?

    a. Ligament tear

    b. Knee sprain

    c. Soft tissue injury

    d. Meniscal tear

17. Which of the following musculoskeletal disorders would most likely compel a referral for cryogenic neuroablation?

    a. Low back pain

    b. Morton's neuroma

    c. Osgood-Schlatter disease

    d. Carpal tunnel syndrome

18. A 42-year-old secretary is diagnosed with carpal tunnel syndrome, and you are advising her on proper forms of management. Which of the following medications would be best for early treatment of her symptoms?

    a. Celecoxib

    b. Betamethasone

    c. Hydroxychloroquine

    d. Methotrexate

19. For swollen, painful knees, what is the easiest, most sensitive test to assess for anterior and posterior cruciate ligament tears?

    a. Straight leg raise test

    b. Lachman's test

    c. McMurray's test

    d. Apley's grind test

20. A 74-year-old patient presents with fatigue, as well as pain, stiffness, and some diminished motion in her shoulders and hip. The patient is given an initial diagnosis of polymyalgia rheumatica. Which of the following tests would best assist in initially confirming this diagnosis?

    a. Computed tomography scan

    b. Erythrocyte sedimentation rate

    c. Synovial aspirate

    d. Radiography

21. A "heavy-set" dock worker in his late 30s presents with pain in his back. The patient says that the pain has recently increased and has begun spreading to his legs. His posture is slightly twisted to the right, and he appears to be stooped forward, indicating that he may have radiating or sciatic pain. Given the most likely condition, which of these test results would best confirm the initial diagnosis?

    a. Positive straight leg raise test

    b. Negative pelvic rock test

    c. Positive McMurray's test

    d. Negative Lachman's test

22. In order to correctly perform the pelvic rock test, the practitioner must place his or her hands on the:

    a. Anterior superior iliac spine

    b. Posterior inferior iliac spine

    c. Anterior inferior iliac spine

    d. Posterior superior iliac spine

23. Joshua, age 35, comes to your practice with pain in his back and legs. You ask him to describe his recent history of symptoms. Which of these symptoms would be least indicative of lower back pain?

    a. Numbness along inner surface of thighs

    b. Ataxic gait

    c. Heightened proprioception

    d. Bladder problems

24. Common concerns regarding musculoskeletal changes in the gerontologic population often include all of the following except:

    a. Thickened skin

    b. Unstable gait and muscle strength

    c. Increased percentage of body fat

    d. Height reduction

25. A patient comes to your practice with a severely swollen knee. He says that he was training for a marathon and attempted to run at a faster pace than he usually runs. Almost as soon as he sat down to rest, he noticed swelling, inflammation, and pain upon knee movement. Which of the following would not be a standard form of treatment for the patient's symptoms at this time?

    a. Splinting

    b. Aspirin

    c. Oral steroids

    d. Heat application

26. A patient presents to your practice with pain and loss of movement in his right knee. As you are performing the physical exam, you notice a loss of the patellar tendon reflex and difficulty moving his quadriceps. The patient's pain most likely stems from which of the following?

    a. L3–L4 disk compression

    b. Bursal inflammation

    c. L4–L5 disk compression

    d. Tibial tuberosity rupture

27. Jason, age 18, comes to your practice with deep purple marks under his skin; however, the skin and bone are not broken and a quick physical exam does not detect any dislocation in the underlying joint. Which of the following would best describe Jason's injury?

    a. Abrasion

    b. Contusion

    c. Laceration

    d. Subluxation

28. Of the following, which musculoskeletal disorder would most likely present with symmetrical inflammation?

    a. Osteoarthritis

    b. Plantar fasciitis

    c. Rheumatoid arthritis

    d. Costochondritis

29. A female presents with an ankle sprain. She is unable to walk unassisted, and egg-shaped swelling is identified around the affected area. The patient's ankle sprain should be classified as which of the following?

    a. Grade 1

    b. Grade 2

    c. Grade 3

    d. Grade 4

30. A patient comes to your practice with a knee that keeps "locking," making it difficult for him to walk. You perform the Apley's grind test on the patient to determine the presence of soft tissue damage. What would be the best method for carrying out this test?

    a. Applying pressure to the heel while rotating the lower leg, and then flexing the knee 90°.

    b. Rotating the lower leg while flexing the knee 90°, and then applying pressure to the heel.

    c. Rotating the lower leg while applying pressure to the heel, then flexing the knee 90°.

    d. Flexing the knee 90°, and then applying pressure to the heel while rotating the lower leg.

31. A 26-year-old male was recently diagnosed with plantar fasciitis. He says he experiences sharp pain and stiffness in the affected foot each morning; however, this pain usually fades by the time he's ready for work. Which of the following treatments would have the lowest priority at this time?

    a. Orthotics

    b. Physical therapy

    c. Night splints

    d. Opioids

32. An adolescent has experienced a tibial tubercle apophyseal traction injury as a result of stress on the patellar tendon. In educating the patient on the resulting condition, which of these statements would you most likely make?

    a. "The pain may be worse in the morning but may subside as the day progresses."

    b. "The pain may be insignificant in the morning but may get progressively worse as the day progresses."

    c. "You will most likely require surgical treatment."

    d. "The pain will often be worsened by running, jumping, and climbing stairs."

33. A 20-year-old patient is brought to the clinic after crushing his finger in a door. The blow has caused throbbing in the finger, blue and black discoloration of the nail, and bleeding from the nail bed. Which of the following methods of management would be least appropriate at this time?

    a. Hydrocodone and acetaminophen

    b. Naproxen

    c. Triamcinolone hexacetonide

    d. Ibuprofen

34. After identifying the possibility of Osgood-Schlatter disease during a physical exam, what test would best confirm the diagnosis?

    a. X-ray

    b. Magnetic resonance imaging scan

    c. Computed tomography scan

    d. Electromyography

35. Ollie, age 45, presents to the clinic with swelling and redness in her wrists. She says the pain is the worst in the morning and gets better as the day progresses. Suspecting rheumatoid arthritis, you order an x-ray. Which of the following findings would you least expect to see?

    a. Joint swelling

    b. Juxta-articular sclerosis

    c. Cortical thinning

    d. Joint space narrowing

36. When performing an x-ray on a patient with osteoarthritis, which of the following findings would be least expected?

    a. Osteophytes

    b. Narrowing of joint space

    c. Cortical thinning

    d. Juxta-articular sclerosis

37. Your male patient says that he experiences severe, sharp pain in the bottom of his right foot when he wakes up in the morning, which subsides throughout the day. He describes a dull pain in the heel and a throbbing ache in the arch of his foot. Which of the following would be the most likely diagnosis?

    a. Morton's neuroma

    b. Osteoarthritis

    c. Plantar fasciitis

    d. Bursitis

38. For which of these musculoskeletal disorders would antimalarial agents most likely be indicated?

    a. Rheumatoid arthritis

    b. Costochondritis

    c. Polymyalgia rheumatica

    d. Bursitis

39. Of the following, when is an antinuclear antibody examination of a knee injury most often indicated?

    a. If rheumatoid arthritis is suspected

    b. If there is a positive Lachman's test

    c. If osteoarthritis is suspected

    d. If a meniscal tear is present

40. The following methods of management are recommended for both plantar fasciitis and Morton's neuroma except:

    a. Corticosteroids

    b. Orthotics

    c. Cryosurgery

    d. Night splints

RATIONALES

1. b

Plain x-rays are typically used to rule out other bone or joint conditions in the diagnosis of patients with bursitis. While magnetic resonance imaging, electromyography, and computed tomography may be used, these imaging techniques are not the most routinely used to rule out other bone or joint conditions in patients with bursitis.

2. d

Plantar fasciitis is a particularly common skeletal disorder among runners, but there is no higher prevalence in a specific gender. Rheumatoid arthritis affects women three times more than men, and carpal tunnel syndrome affects women two to five times more than men. Morton's neuroma is more common in women because it is often caused by wearing high-heeled shoes.

3. c

Weakness while dorsiflexing the big toe, numbness of the foot, and pain in the lateral calf suggests a pinched nerve in L4-L5; the screening exam to support this diagnosis consists of asking the patient to walk on his or her heels. Complications with the L5-S1 disks, which are assessed by having the patient walk on his or her toes, may present pain in the lateral leg, numbness of the foot, and weakness of the big toe; however, said weakness usually presents in plantar flexion, not dorsiflexion. Asking a patient to stand on his or her toes is not one of the standard criteria for assessing nerve damage in the lower back. Asking the patient to squat and rise is a way to assess nerve damage in the L3-L4 disks, which would typically be necessary if the patient presented with weak quadriceps or pain and numbness in the medial knee.

4. c

Giant cell arteritis is not likely to cause costochondritis, but may be associated with polymyalgia rheumatica. Additionally, giant cell arteritis affects the blood vessels that supply blood to the head. Typical causes for costochondritis include physical strain, injury to the chest, and fibromyalgia.

5. a

To accurately perform the Lachman's test, the nurse practitioner (NP) must first bend the knee 20°–30°. Then, the NP must grab and apply pressure to the proximal tibia with one hand, which places stress on the anterior cruciate ligament and posterior cruciate ligament. The other hand is used to stabilize the thigh. Any other order of steps would not accurately gauge the extent of a cruciate ligament tear, which is graded on a 1+ to 3+ scale of displacement.

6. d

The etiology of polymyalgia rheumatica is unknown, but development of the condition is believed to derive from giant cell arteritis, not weight gain and obesity. The risk of developing osteoarthritis, plantar fasciitis, and low back pain is increased with weight gain and obesity.

7. a

Medial meniscus tears are the most common type of tear in patients experiencing knee injuries; moreover, these tears are ten times more common than lateral meniscus tears. Tears in the anterior or posterior cruciate ligament are not as common as those in the medial meniscus.

8. b

COX-2 inhibitors, such as celecoxib, are not typically the first agent of choice in treating soft muscle injury, as these drugs may have deleterious effects on fracture and tendon healing. Preferred agents for treatment of soft muscle injury include other NSAIDs, such as naproxen, and muscle relaxants, such as metaxalone. Tramadol and other narcotics may also see short-term use for pain relief.

9. d

The findings of osteophytes, juxta-articular sclerosis, and subchondral bone on an x-ray would most strongly indicate that a patient has osteoarthritis. X-rays do not show bursae, but may be helpful in excluding other conditions. X-rays can be used to rule out other causes of heel pain, but ligaments, which cause the heel pain in plantar fasciitis, are not visible in x-rays. X-rays are not used to diagnose carpal tunnel syndrome.

10. c

Morton's neuroma causes a compression neuropathy on an intermetatarsal nerve, most commonly on the third or fourth intermetatarsal spaces. The first, second, and fifth intermetatarsal spaces may be affected, but are not the most commonly affected by Morton's neuroma.

11. c

Polymyalgia rheumatica often presents with pain and stiffness in the hip and shoulder that is often accompanied by anemia and a mild fever. Rheumatoid arthritis more typically presents with pain in the proximal interphalangeal joints, the metacarpophalangeal joints, and the wrists, not the hips and shoulders. Osteoarthritis may present with pain in the hips, but would usually present with pain in other weight-bearing joints, such as the knees, instead of the shoulders. Costochondritis presents with pain in the sternum, not the shoulders and hips.

12. a

The patient should most likely be evaluated for costochondritis, as the pain he is experiencing in the sternum manifested after he received a blow to the chest, possibly causing inflammation of the cartilage and resulting in pain with deep breathing. Muscle strain and bursitis would more likely present with pain during range of motion, not during deep breathing, and would typically present with visible manifestations such as edema. Osgood-Schlatter disease involves the tibial tuberosity, not the chest.

13. a

Pain from bursitis most commonly presents when the affected joint moves. Although warmth in the shoulder may indicate septic bursitis, this finding may also present in cases of polymyalgia rheumatica. Likewise, stiffness in the affected joint is more indicative of polymyalgia rheumatica than bursitis. Joints affected by bursitis may be tender, but pain due to motion would be more indicative of the condition.

14. a

One of the most common sites for bursitis is the prepatellar, not postpatellar, area. Other common sites for bursitis include the olecranon, subdeltoid, and ischial areas.

15. c

In Phalen's test, a patient with suspected carpal tunnel syndrome is asked to hold his or her wrist in complete flexion for 1 minute; the test is considered positive if symptoms reproduce during that time. McMurray's test is typically used to assess the nature and grade of knee injury, whereas the Hirschberg's test assesses for strabismus. Allen's test is used to check for abnormal circulation in the hand, not carpal tunnel syndrome.

16. d

Knee "locking" usually indicates either a meniscal tear or loose bodies in the affected area. Ligament tears more often present with increased translational movement on a Lachman's test, rather than "locking" of the knee. Lastly, locking of the knee would not typically indicate either a soft tissue injury or knee sprain.

17. b

A case of Morton's neuroma may warrant referral for cryogenic neuroablation. Low back pain, Osgood-Schlatter disease, and carpal tunnel syndrome may require referral for surgery, but not for cryogenic neuroablation.

18. a

Celecoxib, a COX-2 inhibitor, and other NSAIDs may see use as the first step in pain management for carpal tunnel syndrome. Injected corticosteroids, such as betamethasone, may also be used to manage carpal tunnel syndrome, but usually see use after treatment with anti-inflammatory drugs has failed to properly manage pain. Methotrexate and antimalarials such as hydroxychloroquine would more likely see use in the management of rheumatoid arthritis.

19. b

The easiest, most sensitive test on swollen, painful knees is Lachman's test, which assesses for anterior and posterior cruciate ligament tears. McMurray's test is often used to assess for medial meniscal injuries, whereas Apley's grind test usually assesses for medial or lateral collateral ligament damage or meniscus injury. Lastly, the positive straight leg raise test is most often used for assessing lower back pain.

20. b

An erythrocyte sedimentation rate would usually assist in initially confirming a diagnosis of polymyalgia rheumatica. Computed tomography scans are more likely to be recommended for a patient being evaluated for lower back pain. Synovial aspirates are typically used to evaluate and distinguish between osteoarthritis and rheumatoid arthritis. Radiography is more often used to rule out other conditions in patients with suspected cases of polymyalgia rheumatica, rather than to confirm a diagnosis.

21. a

A straight leg raise test would best help to confirm a diagnosis of low back pain, and would present with radiating or sciatic pain as a positive finding when the patient's legs are elevated off the exam table. Pelvic rock tests are also used to confirm or rule out low back pain, but negative findings would typically rule out injury to the lower back as the primary cause of symptoms. McMurray's test and Lachman's test are more often used to assess for knee injuries and pain, not for lower back pain.

22. a

A pelvic rock test is typically confirmed if the patient feels pain in either, or both, sacroiliac joints while the practitioner assesses the pelvis via the anterior superior iliac spine. Assessment of the posterior inferior, anterior inferior, or posterior superior iliac spines are not part of the standard pelvic rock test.

23. c

Patients with lower back pain typically experience a loss, rather than a heightened sense, of proprioception; as a result, sense of movement and awareness of the limbs is likewise diminished. Pain in the back also often results in numbness along dermatomes—for the lower back, specifically, this may include a loss of sensation in the thighs or lower legs. An ataxic gait, which is indicated by limping or bending forward while walking, and bladder problems are also consistent with lower back pain.

24. a

Although bruising is more common in elderly patients, this is usually due to thinning, not thickened, skin as a result of aging. Other common physiologic changes that come with aging include decreased muscle mass and strength, which may produce unstable gait; redistribution of body fat, which may result in an increased percentage of body fat; and intervertebral disc degeneration, which may lead to height reduction.

25. c

Swelling and inflammation of the joint structure of the knee would strongly indicate bursitis; although bursitis may be managed through steroid injections, oral steroids are not typically recommended for management of this condition. More common first-line treatments for bursitis include splinting the joint to prevent excessive movement, aspirin or other NSAIDs to manage pain and inflammation, and applying heat for 30 minutes, after applying ice to reduce the swelling, about three to four times a day.

26. a

Low back pain in the L3–L4 disks often presents with loss of patellar reflexes and weak quadriceps muscles, as well as pain and numbness in the medial malleolus. Bursal inflammation may limit movement in the knee because of pain; however, bursal inflammation would not typically cause a loss of the patellar reflex and would likely be noticeable during a physical exam. Weakness with toe and foot movement, as well as pain in the lateral calf or dorsum of the foot, would more strongly indicate L4–L5 disk involvement. A rupture in the tibial tubercle is most indicative of Osgood-Schlatter disease, which presents with pain below the kneecaps that increases upon exertion; although Osgood-Schlatter disease may limit movement of the quadriceps, it does not typically affect flexibility of the knee.

27. b

Contusions are often characterized by injury to the body in which skin and bone are not broken, but damage is done to tissues under the skin, thus causing a bruise. Abrasions are typically characterized by the scraping away of skin or mucous membrane, as a result of injury or by mechanical means. Lacerations are classified as cuts of the skin, rather than bruising. Further, subluxations may present with bruising but are characterized by partial dislocation, which has not occurred in this patient.

28. c

In rheumatoid arthritis, inflammation usually presents symmetrically, whereas osteoarthritis usually presents with asymmetrical inflammation. Inflammation may be present in plantar fasciitis and costochondritis, but typically is not symmetrical.

29. c

Inability to walk unassisted and an egg-shaped swell around the affected area are signs of a grade 3 ankle sprain. Patients presenting with a grade 1 ankle sprain are typically able to walk with normal range of motion in the ankle, and mild tenderness is often localized around the affected area. Grade 2 ankle sprains present with moderate pain when bearing weight, causing difficulty to walk, along with swelling and ecchymosis. Grade 4 ankle sprains do not exist.

30. d

To properly perform the Apley's grind test, the nurse practitioner (NP) must first flex the patient's knee 90° while the patient is lying face down. Then the NP must put pressure on the patient's heel with one hand while using the other hand to rotate the leg internally and externally. If done accurately, pain or a click may result if the patient has ligament damage or meniscal injury. Performing these steps in any other order will not provide a proper assessment for damage to the knee.

31. d

Opioids would not be standard treatment for plantar fasciitis at this time, as the patient's pain, though sharp and persistent, fades away shortly after waking. A patient diagnosed with plantar fasciitis should typically be referred to physical therapy to improve the condition via physical training. Other typical methods of treatment include orthotics and night splints to reduce early morning foot pain.

32. d

Osgood-Schlatter disease is a tibial tubercle apophyseal traction injury, which typically causes pain in the area of the knee when one engages in activities such as running, jumping, and climbing stairs. Pain that is worse in the morning but subsides as the day progresses is often a symptomatic presentation of rheumatoid arthritis, which does not present in adolescents. Likewise, osteoarthritis is indicated by pain that gets progressively worse throughout the day and does not present in adolescents. Only rare cases of Osgood-Schlatter disease require surgery; more common interventions include the R-I-C-E method and NSAIDs.

33. c

The crushing of a finger or toe that results in bleeding from the nail bed is referred to as a subungual hematoma; although corticosteroid injections may be used to treat soft tissue injuries, low-solubility corticosteroids such as triamcinolone hexacetonide are indicated for joint injuries, as these preparations may produce atrophy when injected into soft tissue. Corticosteroid injections are more often a form of treatment for carpal tunnel syndrome and are not first-line management for simple musculoskeletal disorders. Soft tissue injuries, which include hematomas, are usually managed with NSAIDs, such as ibuprofen and naproxen, and narcotics, which include hydrocodone and acetaminophen. Other forms of management may include the R-I-C-E method, muscle relaxants, immobilization, and physical therapy.

34. a

In diagnosing Osgood-Schlatter disease, an x-ray would typically be used to confirm the disease and simultaneously rule out other conditions, as the x-ray would confirm the presence of the hallmark rupture of the growth plate at the tibial tuberosity that defines the condition. A magnetic resonance imaging scan, electromyography, or computed tomography scan would be more useful in ruling out other conditions than in confirming the presence of Osgood-Schlatter disease.

35. b

Rheumatoid arthritis does not commonly present with juxta-articular sclerosis on an x-ray; rather, juxta-articular sclerosis is more often associated with osteoarthritis. Joint swelling that results in the narrowing of the joint space, as well as cortical thinning and osteopenia, are common x-ray findings in patients with rheumatoid arthritis.

36. c

Progressive cortical thinning is a typical x-ray finding of rheumatoid arthritis, not osteoarthritis. After performing x-rays on a patient with osteoarthritis, a nurse practitioner can typically expect to find narrowing of the joint space, osteophytes, and juxta-articular sclerosis, as well as subchondral bone.

37. c

As the patient experiences severe, sharp pain in the bottom of his right foot, which is most severe in the morning, plantar fasciitis is the most likely condition. Osteoarthritis typically presents with pain which is less intense in the morning and progresses throughout the day, contrary to the patient's symptoms. Morton's neuroma affects the intermetatarsal plantar nerve and often causes numbness in the toes, not pain that radiates from heel to toe. Bursitis usually presents with pain that is dependent on movement, not time of day, as well as inflammation and erythema.

38. a

Rheumatoid arthritis may be treated with antimalarials such as hydroxychloroquine and chloroquine; these drugs fall into the category of disease-modifying antirheumatic drugs, otherwise unrelated drugs that serve to slow the progression of rheumatoid arthritis. Antimalarial agents are not indicated for the treatment of polymyalgia rheumatica, costochondritis, or bursitis.

39. a

An antinuclear antibody (ANA) examination for a knee injury is typically indicated if rheumatoid arthritis is suspected. A positive Lachman's test is usually present in cases of anterior and posterior cruciate ligament tears, and would not specifically indicate an ANA test. Suspicion of meniscal tears would more typically indicate an x-ray, whereas synovial aspirate tests would confirm a suspected case of septic osteoarthritis.

40. d

Although night splints are often recommended for management of plantar fasciitis, these splints do not serve appreciable use in treating Morton's neuroma. Plantar fasciitis and Morton's neuroma may both be treated through corticosteroid injections, orthotics, or cryosurgery.

DISCUSSION

Soft Tissue Injuries

Overview

Soft tissue injuries result from either direct or indirect trauma to non-osseous elements in the musculoskeletal system, such as the muscles, bursa, ligaments (i.e., the fibrous tissue connecting bone to bone), tendons (i.e., the fibrous tissue connecting muscle to bone), or cartilage (i.e., dense connective tissue with no blood supply).

Most types of soft tissue injuries are classified as abrasions, contusions, hematomas, lacerations, tears, strains, or sprains.[1] In addition to the type of injury, soft tissue injuries are classified according to phases that correspond to the time frame since the injury occurred. These include the acute/protection phase, subacute/repair phase, late stage/remodeling phase, and chronic phase.

Presentation

Patients with soft tissue injuries may present with mild to severe signs and symptoms, depending on the degree and type of injury. Mild to moderate cases may include indications of pain, edema, effusion, and bruising. Moderate to severe injuries may be accompanied by impaired or lost function in the injured area.

Workup

A clinical assessment determines the severity and location of the injury. Imaging studies, including plain radiographs, are used to identify any fractures but rarely provide sufficient evidence for most soft tissue injuries. Magnetic resonance imaging (MRI) and computerized tomography scans, on the other hand, identify certain types of soft tissue injury such as damage to the meniscus, ligaments, or tendons.[2]

Additional diagnostic tests may include a complete blood count (CBC) and an erythrocyte sedimentation rate (ESR) test to rule out infection or gouty arthritis.

Treatment

Management for all types of soft tissue injuries involves implementation of the R-I-C-E method, which consists of Rest, Ice, Compression, and Elevation of the injured parts.[3]

Immobilization of the injured body part depends on location, severity, and the type of injury. Casts, splints, immobilizers, or slings may be used.[4]

Pharmacologic management for pain and inflammation includes non-steroidal anti-inflammatory drugs (NSAIDs), muscle relaxants, or narcotics. NSAIDs that are used with mild to moderately severe injuries include ibuprofen ordered at 600–800 mg three to four times a day. Narcotic regimens, which are typically for short-term use, include tramadol (Ultram), a narcotic-like drug; hydrocodone plus acetaminophen (Vicodin, Lortab, Lorcet); acetaminophen plus codeine (Tylenol #3); and oxycodone and/or acetaminophen (Percocet, Tylox). For chronic pain related to arthritis, naproxen 250–500 mg every day in divided doses may be used. For patients with continued and severe pain, COX-2 inhibitor or celecoxib (Celebrex) may be employed.[4]

Knee Injury/Pain

Overview

Knee injuries or knee pain arise from mechanical, inflammatory, and/or degenerative problems. Causes may be due to trauma or exercise, as well as arthritis and age-related wear and tear. The incidence of medial meniscus tears is ten times more common than lateral tears and most often associated with sports-related injury.[5]

Presentation

Presentation varies according to several factors. Pain may be either acute or chronic. Effusion, erythema, warmth, and edema at the site of knee injury may accompany fractures, dislocation, ligament tears, or meniscal damage. Other findings may include ecchymosis, masses, and evidence of local trauma.

The patient may also complain of joint instability or display limited range of motion (ROM). Signs include "locking," which usually indicates a tear in the meniscus. Complaints that the knee is "giving way" also indicate instability. Crepitus may be described as a grating sensation, or the sound of "popping" or "crackling" near the joint.[6]

Workup

An initial assessment of knee injury or pain should include a review of the patient's history of knee pain, focusing on origin, duration, and association with trauma or specific activities. Typically, the uninjured knee is observed and used to determine baseline values to compare against the injured knee. If the patient is able to bear weight on the injured knee, the patient's stance and gait should be observed. Onset and degree of knee effusion should be noted if present. An assessment that involves palpation and stress testing of the injured knee joint should be performed to assess the stability and mobility of the joint, as well as determine the type and location of pain.[2,5]

One method to assess a knee injury is McMurray's test, which is conducted while the patient is in the supine position. The nurse practitioner (NP) places the distal hand on the foot and raises the knee slowly, keeping the foot and tibia externally rotated with the proximal hand resting on the joint line. The knee is flexed and then quickly straightened. If an audible or palpable click occurs during this test, the outcome is positive for medial meniscal injuries.[7]

The Lachman's test is a drawer test to assess for tears in the anterior and/or posterior cruciate ligament. It is the most sensitive and easiest test to perform on a swollen, painful knee. The Lachman's test is done by flexing the knee 20°–30°. Then, as one hand stabilizes the thigh, the NP grasps the leg with the other hand and applies anterior force to the proximal tibia, stressing the anterior cruciate ligament and/or posterior cruciate ligament. If the knee has 1+ to 3+ grade of displacement, the test is positive.[8]

Lastly, Apley's grind test is performed by flexing the patient's knee 90° with the patient in the prone position. The NP places pressure on his or her heel with one hand while using the other to rotate the patient's lower leg internally and externally. If there is pain or a click at the knee, the test either is positive for damage to the medial or is positive for damage to the lateral collateral ligament and/or injury to the meniscus.[4]

An x-ray is performed initially to assess for damage, and referral for an MRI may be considered for further assessment of soft tissue damage. Lab examination for knee injuries is indicated if rheumatoid arthritis is suspected, especially if synovial effusion is present.[4]

Treatment

Symptomatic treatment includes rest and application of the R-I-C-E method to the patient's knee. Therapy should also focus on increasing the patient's ROM. More severe knee injuries may require immobilization. NSAIDs may help to reduce inflammation and accumulation of fluid, and effusions of aspirate should be performed as needed. Because treatment and management depend on the type of knee injury sustained, consultation and/or referral to an orthopedic specialist may be necessary.[9]

Ankle Sprain

Overview

Ankle sprains are stretched, partially torn, or completely ruptured ligaments. Lateral sprains are the most frequent type of sports-related injury and most commonly involve injury to the anterior talofibular and fibulocalcaneal ligaments.[10]

Presentation

Physical exam findings for ankle sprains are graded from 1 to 3. Grade 1 ankle sprains involve slight stretching or tearing of the ligament. These types of ankle sprains present with mild, localized tenderness, as well as swelling and stiffness. Normal ROM is seen as patients are able to walk with minimal pain. Pain is immediate after injury with a grade 2 sprain, which involves partial tearing of the ligament. This type of sprain may cause the patient to have difficulty walking and may be accompanied by moderate or severe pain during weight bearing. Moderate swelling and tenderness, ecchymosis, and limited ROM are also typical findings of grade 2 ankle sprains. Grade 3 ankle sprains involve the complete rupture or tear of the injured ligament or ligaments, resulting in the impossibility to ambulate and the resistance of any motion of the feet. Significant swelling (i.e., an "egg-shaped" swelling) within 2 hours of injury is usually seen, in addition to significant tenderness, ecchymosis, and instability.[10]

Workup

A clinical diagnosis determines if additional tests are necessary. An x-ray may be ordered to rule out fractures. An MRI may be ordered if unusual features (e.g., extensive swelling or ecchymosis) continue.[11]

Treatment

General treatment and management of ankle sprains includes high doses of NSAIDs and implementation of the R-I-C-E method.

Specific management of grade 1 injuries includes weight bearing as tolerated and isometric exercises in addition to ROM and stretching/strengthening exercises. It may be necessary to refer patients with grade 2 and grade 3 ankle sprains for physical therapy in addition to ROM and stretching/strengthening exercises. Immobilization is usually required for grade 2 and grade 3 injuries; however, grade 3 sprains may be referred for possible casting or surgery, as needed.[12]

Muscle Strain

Overview

Muscle strains are injuries that result in the

tearing or stretching of a muscle or tendon. This type of injury is caused by fatigue, overuse, or improper use of a muscle, and is commonly seen after a traumatic or sports-related injury.[13]

Presentation

Presentations for mild muscle strains include pain during rotation of movement. Edema and ecchymosis are usually indicative of moderate strains. Patients with severe muscle strains may show weakness and deformity of the strained muscle.[13]

Workup

In most cases, a diagnosis is determined with a physical examination and a review of the patient's history. X-rays may be ordered if a fracture is suspected. MRIs may be necessary to detect soft tissue damage.[14]

Treatment

Initial treatment and management involves ice and rest. Severe muscle strains may require an orthopedist consult. Assistive devices are used as needed. Analgesics and NSAIDs are used as initial treatment, and the patient should receive education about how to prevent injury. If required, physical therapy may be initiated once pain and swelling subside.[15]

Bursitis

Overview

Bursitis is the inflammation of bursae, which are closed sacs lined with a synovial-like membrane that act as cushions in areas subject to friction or pressure. Most cases of bursitis are due to repetitive motions, such as weight lifting, or repetitive positions, such as sitting on a hard surface for a prolonged period of time. Bursitis can also be caused by trauma and either sepsis or infection in a joint space. Conditions such as rheumatoid arthritis and gout are also known to cause bursitis. The most common locations of these injuries are the olecranon, the subdeltoid bursa, the ischial area of the back, and the prepatellar.[16]

Presentation

Signs and symptoms for bursitis include pain with movement of the affected joint, decreased ROM, swelling, tenderness, and erythema. Patients may also have a history of trauma, repetitive movement, or inflammatory disease.[17]

Workup

A diagnosis can usually be determined with a physical exam and review of the patient's history.

Referral for an ultrasound or MRI may be helpful if a physical exam is unable to confirm a diagnosis. If a bacterial infection is suspected, laboratory tests would include aspiration with a culture and sensitivity test, as well as a Gram stain. Elevated ESR and white blood cells (WBC) are also indicative of septic bursitis. Plain x-rays may be used to rule out other bone or joint conditions.[18]

Treatment

Conservative measures to treat bursitis include application of the R-I-C-E method and medication. A splint or other assistive device may also be necessary. Applying heat for 30 minutes TID or QID may also be recommended. Aspirin or high-dose NSAIDs help to relieve pain and reduce inflammation. Injections of corticosteroids into the bursa can provide immediate relief of inflammation. Treatment for a septic infection may involve the use of parenteral antibiotics, aspiration, or surgical incision and drainage. Lastly, physical therapy may be recommended to ease pain and prevent future occurences.[17]

Osteoarthritis (OA)

Overview

Osteoarthritis (OA) is a degenerative joint disease characterized by gradual degeneration of the articular cartilage in the synovial joints, resulting in asymmetrical inflammation.[19] The condition occurs in 85% of all patients between the ages of 53 and 64. Although the incidence of OA is equal among men and women, women are more severely affected by the disease than men.[20]

Presentation

Signs and symptoms of OA usually present at the joints of the knees, hips, fingers, hands, and wrists. The primary symptom of the disease is deep, aching joint pain that is exacerbated after extensive use. Additional findings may include swelling, edema, reduced ROM, and crepitus. Patients may also complain of stiffness and joint pain that worsen throughout the day, or the joint may become aggravated with activity.[19]

Signs of OA in the hands include Heberden's nodes, which present as osteophytes at the distal interphalangeal joints, and Bouchard's nodes, which are osteophytes located at the proximal interphalangeal (PIPs) joints.[21] Obesity is also an exacerbating factor of OA.[22]

Workup

X-ray findings may show narrowing of the joint space, osteophytes, juxta-articular sclerosis, and subchondral bone.[23]

Treatment

Acute treatment includes high-dose NSAIDs while chronic treatment includes naproxen. Severe cases are treated with a COX-2 inhibitor.[24]

Supportive care includes weight loss, using a cane on the opposite side of the affected area, applying ice to improve ROM, and using moist heat to decrease muscle spasms and relieve stiffness. Physical or occupational therapy, as well as referral for joint replacement, may be necessary throughout the course of the disease.[19]

Rheumatoid Arthritis (RA)

Overview

Rheumatoid arthritis (RA) is a chronic, systemic autoimmune disease that causes symmetrical inflammation of connective tissue. The disease is characterized by destruction of the synovial joints, which can lead to disability and, in some cases, premature death. Although the disease primarily affects the joints, tissues of the lung, heart, and kidneys may also be involved. Approximately 80% of all RA cases are reported in patients between 35 and 50 years of age, and incidence is much higher in women than in men. Although the exact cause of RA is unclear, the etiology is associated with a genetic predisposition to the disease, hormonal involvement, and various environmental risk factors.[25]

Presentation

Presentations typically have an insidious onset but are known to have an acute onset in a small minority of cases. Joint swelling, redness, and tenderness are typical findings of RA. The patient may also complain of stiffness and "heat" in the joints.[26] The most frequently affected joints are in the PIPs, metacarpophalangeal joints, and the wrist. Signs and symptoms that may appear prior to joint complaints include fever, fatigue, weakness, malaise, anorexia, and weight loss. Unlike OA, RA stiffness and joint pain are worse in the morning but improve as the day progresses.[27,28]

Workup

A referral to a rheumatologist may be required, but diagnosis relies on a combination of a clinical evaluation of joint swelling, lab studies, and imaging. Typical lab studies include an assessment of ESR, which is usually elevated, and C-reactive proteins to assess disease activity. A CBC may provide evidence of anemia or thrombocytopenia. A rheumatoid factor (RF) assay indicates the presence of RF in most cases. An antinuclear antibody (ANA) assay shows evidence of ANAs in 1 out of 5 patients suspected of having RA.[29]

A synovial aspirate may be necessary. Usually, a synovial aspirate reveals elevated WBCs, indicating inflammation.[30]

X-rays are the initial imaging test to find evidence of joint swelling, progressive cortical thinning, osteopenia, and joint space narrowing. Other imaging studies, such as an MRI, may provide a more accurate assessment but are usually not required.[31]

Treatment

Treatment for RA includes medication-based therapy to reduce inflammation, relieve pain, and prevent or decelerate the rate of joint damage. Drug options include high doses of salicylates and NSAIDs, but biologic disease-modifying antirheumatic drugs (DMARDs) serve as the standard of care in early therapeutic regimens. Such DMARDs include corticosteroids, methotrexate, antimalarials (e.g., hydroxychloroquine), and gold salt injections.[32]

Supportive care for RA includes a combination of stress reduction, exercise, dietary modifications, rest, and occupational and physical therapy. Early detection of the disease should include a referral to a rheumatologist.[33]

Carpal Tunnel Syndrome

Overview

Carpal tunnel syndrome is a median nerve compression occurring beneath the transverse carpal ligament of the wrist. Causes are believed to be idiopathic and typically linked to repeated flexion of the wrist (e.g., job-related overuse). This condition frequently affects the dominant hand and is two to five times more prevalent in women.[34]

Presentation

Symptoms of carpal tunnel syndrome include numbness, tingling, "burning" along the median nerve, nocturnal pain, and pain exacerbated with dorsiflexion of the wrist.[34]

There are several tests to assess for carpal tunnel syndrome. Testing for Tinel's sign involves tapping the flexor surface of the wrist in the area over the median nerve. The test is positive if it produces a tingling sensation or pain that radiates from the wrist to the hand. A positive Phalen's test is indicated when the reproduction of symptoms occurs after 1 minute of wrist flexion. The carpal compression test requires pressure on the patient's carpal tunnel, with the examiner applying his or her thumb for 30 seconds to elicit symptoms of carpal tunnel syndrome.[35]

Workup

A diagnosis for carpal tunnel syndrome is often based on a history of the patient's signs and symptoms, as well as the results of testing for signs of the conditions during the physical exam. An assessment for muscle damage may require a referral for an electromyography to document motor involvement of the wrists. An x-ray may be ordered to rule out other causes of wrist pain, such as arthritis or a bone fracture.[34]

Treatment

Early non-surgical treatment includes elevation, occupational or nighttime splinting or bracing, and NSAIDs for pain. Corticosteroid injections into the carpal tunnel are often required to reduce pain, inflammation, and swelling. A referral for surgical intervention may be required if non-surgical interventions do not improve the condition.[35]

Low Back Pain (LBP)

Overview

Low back pain (LBP) is any pain that the patient recognizes as stemming from the lumbosacral region of the spinal column. LBP and headaches are two of the most common causes of pain presenting in primary care.[4] Common causes of LBD include mechanical strain, obesity, poor body mechanics, trauma, repetitive twisting (e.g., bending or lifting), and herniated lumbar disks, among others.[36,37]

Presentation

LBP comes with many different signs and symptoms, which may depend on disk pathology and severity. The pain in the lower back region may be localized or radiating to the feet. Numbness along specific dermatome areas may also accompany pain. Some patients may display decreased muscle strength; actual atrophy of the muscle may occur in some cases. Other findings include decreased or absent reflexes, an ataxic gait (i.e., a limp that is twisted to one side and bent forward), and decreased position sense (i.e., proprioception). Systemic symptoms may include fever, weight loss, or bowel, bladder, or sexual dysfunction.

Some tests can be performed to reproduce symptoms indicative of LBP. A straight leg raise test assesses for radiating or sciatic pain by having the patient's legs elevated off of the exam table while lying supine. Pain indicates a positive test result.[37,38,39]

The pelvic rock test also screens for sacroiliac joint pain. This test is performed by placing a hand on both anterior superior iliac spines and attempting to "open and close" the pelvis. Pain in either or both sacroiliac joints indicates a positive test result.[40]

Some indications are specific of lumbar nerve root pathology. An L3–L4 disk pathology involves gradual weakness and atrophy of the quadriceps muscles. Additionally, pain radiating into the medial malleolus may cause numbness in the same areas, especially the medial aspect of the knee; diminished or absent patellar reflexes may also be seen. Having the patient squat and rise to illicit pain helps screen for L3–L4.[41]

An L4–L5 disk pathology involves weakness of the dorsiflexion mechanism of the great toe and foot. Pain often radiates into the lateral calf, causing numbness of the dorsum of the foot and the lateral calf. Screening for L4–L5 disk pathology involves having the patient walk on the heels of his or her feet.[41]

An L5–S1 disk pathology may produce weakness of plantar flexion of the great toe and foot. Also, pain often runs along the buttocks, lateral leg, and lateral malleolus, which may cause numbness to the lateral aspect of the foot and in the posterior calf. A diminished or absent Achilles' reflex may also be present. Screening for this pathology can be performed by having the patient walk on his or her toes.[41]

Workup

X-rays are initially used to rule out fractures in the lumbar region of the coccyx. If findings are negative, the patient may be referred for an MRI to ascertain any disk or soft tissue pathology.[7]

Treatment

Patients with LBP are typically referred to a specialist. The treatment and management for LBP should focus on six areas: control of pain and inflammation; restoration of joint ROM and extensibility of soft tissue; improvement of muscular strength and endurance; coordination retraining; improving the patient's cardiovascular conditioning; and exercise programs for maintenance.[39] These goals may be achieved through a combination of physical therapy, functional bracing with an orthotic device, rest with limited activities that could increase pain, and alternating heat and ice therapy. Weight loss is recommended in obese patients. The patient should also receive education in proper body mechanics. A psychosocial assessment with stress management strategies may be beneficial. Physical therapy, including therapeutic ultrasound and transcutaneous electric nerve stimulation, can help reduce pain and inflammation. NSAIDs, such as ibuprofen (600–800 mg three to four times per day), in addition to acetaminophen and corticosteroids, may be included as part of pharmacologic therapy.[37]

Morton's Neuroma

Overview

Morton's neuroma is a benign neuroma that causes nerve compression syndrome of an intermetatarsal plantar nerve. This condition is usually seen in the third or fourth intermetatarsal spaces of the foot. The usual cause of Morton's neuroma is injury of the nerve caused by wearing high-heeled shoes, particularly shoes with narrow toe boxes that affect the toes and balls of the feet by applying extra pressure. Heavy impact activities, flat feet, bunions, and hammertoes are also considered to be contributing factors.[42]

Presentation

Episodes of pain are common complaints of Morton's neuroma; the patient may describe the discomfort as feeling as though he or she is "standing on a pebble" inside the shoe. A shooting pain is typically described along the contiguous halves of two toes. Pain may also be accompanied by a sensation of tingling or numbness in the toes.[43]

Workup

Lab studies are not indicated for Morton's neuroma. X-rays may be used to rule out other causes of pain, such as a fracture. An ultrasound is the standard diagnostic to identify the neuroma. MRIs are rarely used because of their high expense.[39,42]

Treatment

Orthotics and corticosteroid injections may be included as part of treatment. Referral for physical therapy is usually the initial step in conservative treatment plans. For more severe cases, cryogenic neuroablation or neurectomy may be required.[42]

Plantar Fasciitis

Overview

Plantar fasciitis is the inflammation of the plantar fascia, the thick tissue connecting the heel bone to the toes on the bottom of the foot, creating the arch of the foot. The etiology is often unclear and may include several factors. Common contributing factors include structural risk factors (e.g., flat-footedness, high arch, prolonged foot pronation), obesity, and sudden weight gain. The incidence of this condition is particularly high among runners, and is more commonly seen in men between the ages of 40 and 70 years.[44,45]

Presentation

Plantar fasciitis commonly presents with pain and stiffness along the bottom of the heel. The pain in the heel may be dull or sharp and can radiate from the heel to the toes. Aching or burning sensations may also present in the bottom of the foot. Typically, the pain is worse in the morning with the first few steps but gradually decreases after ambulation or warm up exercises. Pain may also develop after long periods of inactivity, such as after standing or sitting.[44,45]

Workup

A physical exam and review of the patient's history is typically sufficient to diagnose plantar fasciitis. X-rays may be considered to rule out other problems.[44,45]

Treatment

Implementation of the R-I-C-E method is the first-line treatment in treating plantar fasciitis, particularly applying ice after strenuous activity or exercise. Pharmacologic treatment for plantar fasciitis may include NSAIDs and corticosteroids. Physical therapy for long-term relief, as well as the use of orthotics and night splints, are recommended. Surgery may be necessary if the patient does not respond to traditional therapy.[44,45]

Osgood-Schlatter Disease

Overview

Osgood-Schlatter disease is a rupture in the tibial tuberosity, primarily affecting the growth plate and resulting from stress on the patellar tendon. The condition is also known as "tibial tubercle apophyseal traction injury." The disease manifests in late childhood to early adolescence as a result of growth spurts during puberty.[46,47]

Presentation

The characteristic presentation of Osgood-Schlatter disease is painful inflammation with swelling just below the kneecap. Calcification may also occur where the tendon attaches to the tibia. The condition can occur in one or both legs. Patients complain of pain that is exacerbated by running, jumping, and climbing stairs. Furthermore, although the disease typically resolves on its own by adulthood, some adults may have a "knobby" appearance at the front of the knee.[46,47]

Workup

A physical exam is usually sufficient to diagnose Osgood-Schlatter disease. X-rays are used to rule out other conditions.[46]

Treatment

Mild pain relievers and physical therapy, in addition to the R-I-C-E method, are the general treatment for Osgood-Schlatter disease prior to adulthood. If the problem has not resolved by adulthood, a referral for surgery may be indicated.[46]

Costochondritis

Overview

Costochondritis is the inflammation of the cartilage that connects the ribs to the sternum. Most cases have an unknown etiology; known causes include minor trauma or injury (e.g., a blow to the chest), physical strain, upper respiratory illness or infection, and fibromyalgia.

Presentation

Pain and tenderness at the costosternal joints that attach the breastbone to the ribs are characteristic findings for costochondritis. The pain may be described as sharp or aching, and may also worsen while the patient is taking a deep breath or coughing.[48]

Workup

A physical exam and history are sufficient to diagnose costochondritis. X-rays and bloodwork may be ordered to rule out other causes.[49,50]

Treatment

Costochondritis usually resolves on its own. The use of NSAIDs, as well as the administration of ice or heat, may be helpful in reducing inflammation.[50,51]

Polymyalgia Rheumatica

Overview

Polymyalgia rheumatica is a chronic inflammatory disorder characterized by stiffness and pain in the shoulder and, usually, the hip. Although the etiology of polymyalgia rheumatica is unknown, the condition almost always occurs in people older than 50 years of age and occurs in about 50% of people with giant cell arteritis.[52,53,54]

Presentation

Presentations of polymyalgia rheumatica include stiffness and pain in the neck, shoulders, and hips.[53] Patients may also show a loss of ROM in the affected areas. General symptoms include fatigue, anemia, and mild fever.[52,55]

Workup

When diagnosing polymyalgia rheumatica, onset after the age of 50 should be taken into consideration, as well as pain in more than two areas (e.g., neck, shoulder, pelvic girdle) that persists for longer than a month and morning stiffness that lasts for more than an hour. Lab findings include an elevated ESR. Typically, a CBC shows evidence of mild normocytic, normochromic anemia.[52] An x-ray may be ordered to rule out other conditions.

Treatment

Oral corticosteroids or glucocorticoid are the first line of treatment for polymyalgia rheumatica. A referral for physical therapy or further consult with a specialist may be required.[52]

References

1. Sprains and strains. Better Health Channel web site. http://www.betterhealth.vic.gov.au/bhcv2/bhcarticles.nsf/pages/Sprains_and_strains?open. Last reviewed February 2014. Accessed March 24, 2015.

2. Levy DB, Dickey-White HI. Soft tissue knee injury workup. In: Mills TJ, ed. Medscape. http://emedicine.medscape.com/article/826792-workup#a0721. Reviewed April 28, 2014. Accessed March 24, 2015.

3. Bleakley CM, Glasgow PD, Phillips P, et al. Guidelines on the Management of Acute Soft Tissue Injury Using Protection Rest Ice Compression and Elevation. London: ACPSM; 2011.

4. Barkley TW Jr. Musculoskeletal disorders. In: Barkley TW Jr., ed. *Adult-Gerontology Primary Care Nurse Practitioner*. West Hollywood, CA: Barkley & Associates; 2015: 59–69.

5. Anderson BC. General evaluation of the adult with knee pain. In: Basow DS, ed. *UpToDate*. Waltham, MA: UpToDate; 2015. http://www.uptodate.com/contents/general-evaluation-of-the-adult-with-knee-pain. Last updated November 21, 2014. Accessed March 24, 2015.

6. Hergenroeder AC. Approach to the child or adolescent athlete with chronic knee pain or injury. In: Basow DS, ed. *UpToDate*. Waltham, MA: UpToDate; 2015. http://www.uptodate.com/contents/approach-to-the-child-or-adolescent-athlete-with-acute-knee-pain-or-injury. Last updated January 6, 2014. Accessed March 24, 2015.

7. Teh J, Kambouroglou G, Newton J. Investigation of acute knee injury. *BMJ*. 2012; 344: e3167. doi: 10.1136/bmj.e3167

8. Gammons M. Anterior cruciate ligament injury. In: Ho SSW, ed. Medscape. http://emedicine.medscape.com/article/89442-overview. Reviewed October 6, 2014. Accessed March 24, 2015.

9. Common knee injuries. American Academy of Orthopaedic Surgeons web site. http://orthoinfo.aaos.org/topic.cfm?topic=a00325. Last reviewed March 2014. Accessed March 25, 2015.

10. Young CC. Ankle sprain. In: Ho SSW, ed. Medscape. http://emedicine.medscape.com/article/1907229-overview. Reviewed December 16, 2014. Accessed March 24, 2015.

11. Sprained ankle. American Academy of Orthopaedic Surgeons web site. http://orthoinfo.aaos.org/topic.cfm?topic=a00150. Last reviewed September 2012. Accessed March 24, 2015.

12. Kemler E, van de Port I, Backx F, van Dijk CN. A systematic review on the treatment of acute ankle sprain. *Sports Med*. 2011; 41(3): 185–197. doi:10.2165/11584370-000000000-00000

13. Biundo JJ. Bursitis, tendinitis, and other periarticular disorders and sports medicine. In: Goldman L, Schafer AI, eds. *Goldman's Cecil Medicine*. 24th ed. Philadelphia, PA: Saunders Elsevier; 2011: 1676–1680.

14. Kirkendall DT, Garrett WE. Muscle strain injuries: Research findings and clinical applicability. Medscape Multispeciality. http://www.medscape.com/viewarticle/715533_4. Accessed March 25, 2015.

15. Strains. A.D.A.M. Medical Encyclopedia. http://www.nlm.nih.gov/medlineplus/ency/article/000042.htm. Updated April 13, 2013. Accessed March 25, 2015.

16. Silverstein JA, Moeller JL, Hutchinson MR. Common issues in orthopedics. In: Rakel RE, Rakel DP, eds. *Textbook of Family Medicine.* 8th ed. Philadelphia, PA: Saunders Elsevier; 2011: 601–630.

17. Sheon RP. Patient information: Bursitis (Beyond the Basics). In: Basow DS, ed. *UpToDate.* Waltham, MA: UpToDate; 2015. http://www.uptodate.com/contents/bursitis-beyond-the-basics. Last updated November 7, 2012. Accessed March 25, 2015.

18. Mayo Clinic Staff. Bursitis: Tests and diagnosis. Mayo Clinic web site. http://www.mayoclinic.org/diseases-conditions/bursitis/basics/tests-diagnosis/con-20015102. Reviewed August 20, 2014. Accessed March 25, 2015.

19. Sinusas K. Osteoarthritis: Diagnosis and treatment. *Am Fam Physician.* 2012; 85(1): 49–56. http://www.aafp.org/afp/2012/0101/p49.html

20. Prieto-Alhambra D, Judge A, Javaid MK, et al. Incidence and risk factors for clinically diagnosed knee, hip, and hand osteoarthritis: Influences of age, gender, and osteoarthritis affecting other joints. *Ann Rheum Dis.* 2014; 73(9): 1659–1664. doi: 10.1136/annrheumdis-2013-203355

21. Grainger AJ. Arthritis. In: Davies AM, Grainger AJ, James SJ, eds. *Imaging of the Hand and Wrist: Techniques and Applications.* Heidelberg, Germany: Springer; 2013: 233–262.

22. Teeple E, Jay GD, Elsaid KA, Fleming BC. Animal models of osteoarthritis: Challenges of model selection and analysis. *AAPS J.* 2013; 15(2): 438–446. doi: 10.1208/s12248-013-9454-x.

23. Sanford SO. Arthrocentesis. In: Roberts JR, Custalow CB, Hedges JR, et al., eds. *Roberts and Hedges' Clinical Procedures in Emergency Medicine.* 6th ed. Philadelphia, PA: Elsevier Saunders; 2013: 1075–1094.

24. American College of Rheumatology Communications and Marketing Committee. NSAIDs: Nonsteroidal anti-inflammatory drugs. American College of Rheumatology web site. http://www.rheumatology.org/Practice/Clinical/Patients/Medications/NSAIDs__Nonsteroidal_Anti-inflammatory_Drugs. Updated August 2012. Accessed March 25, 2015.

25. Mayo Clinic Staff. Rheumatoid arthritis. Mayo Clinic web site. http://www.mayoclinic.org/diseases-conditions/rheumatoid-arthritis/basics/definition/con-20014868. Reviewed October 29, 2014. Accessed March 25, 2015.

26. Tsou IYY. Rheumatoid arthritis hand imaging. In: Chew FS, ed. Medscape. http://emedicine.medscape.com/article/401271-overview#showall. Updated July 28, 2014. Accessed March 25, 2015.

27. Having RA: What to expect. Arthritis Foundation web site. http://www.arthritistoday.org/about-arthritis/types-of-arthritis/rheumatoid-arthritis/what-to-expect. Accessed March 25, 2015.

28. Mayo Clinic Staff. Rheumatoid arthritis: Symptoms. Mayo Clinic web site. http://www.mayoclinic.org/diseases-conditions/rheumatoid-arthritis/basics/symptoms/con-20014868. Reviewed October 29, 2014. Accessed March 25, 2015.

29. Venables PJW, Maini RN. Diagnosis and differential diagnosis of rheumatoid arthritis. In: Basow DS, ed. *UpToDate.* Waltham, MA: UpToDate; 2015. http://www.uptodate.com/contents/diagnosis-and-differential-diagnosis-of-rheumatoid-arthritis?source=see_link. Last updated March 3, 2015. Accessed March 25, 2015.

30. Horowitz DL, Katzap E, Horowitz S, Barilla-LaBarca ML. (2011). Approach to septic arthritis. *Am Fam Physician.* 2011; 84(6): 653–660.

31. Mayo Clinic Staff. Rheumatoid arthritis: Test and diagnosis. Mayo Clinic web site. http://www.mayoclinic.org/diseases-conditions/rheumatoid-arthritis/basics/tests-diagnosis/con-20014868. Reviewed October 29, 2014. Accessed March 25, 2015.

32. Bingham C III, Ruffing V. Rheumatoid arthritis treatment. Johns Hopkins Arthritis Center web site. http://www.hopkinsarthritis.org/arthritis-info/rheumatoid-arthritis/ra-treatment. Updated September 24, 2013. Accessed March 25, 2015.

33. Mayo Clinic Staff. Rheumatoid arthritis: Treatments and drugs. Mayo Clinic web site. http://www.mayoclinic.org/diseases-conditions/rheumatoid-arthritis/basics/treatment/con-20014868. Reviewed October 29, 2014. Accessed March 25, 2015.

34. United States Department of Health and Human Services, National Institutes of Health (NIH), National Institute of Neurological Disorders and Stroke (NINDS). Carpal tunnel syndrome fact sheet. http://www.ninds.nih.gov/disorders/carpal_tunnel/detail_carpal_tunnel.htm#236423049. Published July 2012. Accessed March 25, 2015.

35. Ashworth NL. Carpal tunnel syndrome treatment and management. In: Meier RH III, ed. Medscape. http://emedicine.medscape.com/article/327330-treatment#showall. Updated August 25, 2014. Accessed March 25, 2015.

36. United States Department of Health and Human Services, NIH, NINDS. Low back pain fact sheet. http://www.ninds.nih.gov/disorders/backpain/detail_backpain.htm. Published December 2014. Accessed March 25, 2015.

37. Bronfort G, Haas M, Evans R, Kawchuk G, Dagneais S. Spinal manipulation and mobilization. In: Dagenais S, Haldeman S, eds. *Evidence-Based Management of Low Back Pain.* St. Louis, MO: Elsevier Mosby; 2011: 229–247.

38. Dubin A, Lalani I, Argoff CE. History and physical examination of the pain patient. In: Benzon HT, Rathmell JP, Wu CL, Turk DC, Argoff CE, Hurley RW, eds. *Practical Management of Pain*. 5th ed. Philadelphia, PA: Elsevier Mosby; 2014: 151–161.

39. Hills EC. Mechanical low back pain clinical presentation. In: Kishner S, ed. Medscape. http://emedicine.medscape.com/article/310353-clinical. Updated August 4, 2014. Accessed March 25, 2015.

40. Ajakwe R, Ferrante FM. Sacroiliac joint injections and sacroiliac joint denervation techniques. In: Gupta A, ed. *Interventional Pain Medicine*. Oxford, UK: Oxford University Press; 2012: 185–192.

41. Casazza BA. Diagnosis and treatment of acute low back pain. *Am Fam Physician*. 2012; 85(4): 343–350. http://www.aafp.org/afp/2012/0215/p343.html.

42. Jain S, Mannan K. The diagnosis and management of Morton's neuroma: A literature review. *Foot Ankle Spec*. 2013; 6(4): 307–317. doi:10.1177/1938640013493464

43. Mayo Clinic Staff. Morton's neuroma: Overview. Mayo Clinic web site. http://www.mayoclinic.org/diseases-conditions/mortons-neuroma/basics/definition/con-20026482. Reviewed May 16, 2013. Accessed March 25, 2015.

44. Goff JD, Crawford R. Diagnosis and treatment of plantar fasciitis. *Am Fam Physician*. 2011; 84(6): 676–682. http://www.aafp.org/afp/2011/0915/p676.html

45. Plantar fasciitis. A.D.A.M. Medical Encyclopedia. http://www.nlm.nih.gov/medlineplus/ency/article/007021.htm. Updated March 8, 2014. Accessed March 25, 2015.

46. Atanda A, Shah SA, O'Brien K. Osteochondrosis: Common causes of pain in growing bones. *Am Fam Physician*. 2011; 83(3): 285–291. Retrieved from http://www.aafp.org/afp/2011/0201/p285.html

47. Mayo Clinic Staff. Osgood-Schlatter disease. Mayo Clinic web site. http://www.mayoclinic.com/health/osgood-schlatter-disease/DS00392. Reviewed February 28, 2014. Accessed March 25, 2015.

48. Flowers L. Costochondritis clinical presentation. In: Brenner BE, ed. Medscape. http://emedicine.medscape.com/article/808554-clinical. Updated October 7, 2014. Accessed March 25, 2015.

49. Flowers L. Costochondritis workup. In: Brenner BE, ed. Medscape. http://emedicine.medscape.com/article/808554-workup. Updated October 7, 2014. Accessed March 25, 2015.

50. Ohri S, Fields SA. Costochondritis. In: Domino FJ, Baldor RA, Golding J, Grimes JA, eds. *The 5-Minute Clinical Consult 2014*. 22nd ed. Philadelphia, PA: Wolters Kluwer Health/Lippincott Williams & Wilkins; 2014: 290–291.

51. Flowers L. Costochondritis medication. In: Brenner BE, ed. Medscape. http://emedicine.medscape.com/article/808554-medication. Updated October 7, 2014. Accessed March 25, 2015.

52. Polymyalgia rheumatica. A.D.A.M. Medical Encyclopedia. http://www.nlm.nih.gov/medlineplus/ency/article/000415.htm. Updated February 21, 2013. Accessed March 25, 2015.

53. Docken WP. Polymyaglia rheumatica. American College of Rheumatology web site. https://www.rheumatology.org/Practice/Clinical/Patients/Diseases_And_Conditions/Polymyalgia_Rheumatica. Updated February 2013. Accessed March 25, 2015.

54. Hunder GG. Patient information: Polymyalgia rheumatica and giant cell (temporal) arteritis (Beyond the Basics). In: Basow DS, ed. *UpToDate*. Waltham, MA: UpToDate; 2015. http://www.uptodate.com/contents/polymyalgia-rheumatica-and-giant-cell-temporal-arteritis-beyond-the-basics?source=search_result&search=polymalgia+rheumatica+and+giant+cell+arteritis&selectedTitle=3~150. Last updated November 14, 2013. Accessed June 29, 2015.

55. Serrate-Sztein S, Gretz L, Hunder GG, Weyland CM, Healey LA; U.S. Department of Health and Human Services, National Institutes of Health, National Institute of Arthritis and Musculoskeletal and Skin Diseases. Questions and answers about polymyalgia rheumatica and giant cell arteritis. http:/ /www.niams.nih.gov/Health_Info/ Polymyalgia. Published August 2012. Accessed March 25, 2015.

Chapter 7
Sexually Transmitted Infectious Diseases

QUESTIONS

1. All of the following sexually transmitted diseases are paired with a pathogen commonly responsible for the condition <u>except</u>:

   a. Pelvic inflammatory disease—*Neisseria gonorrhoeae*

   b. Lymphogranuloma venereum—*Chlamydia trachomatis*

   c. Chancroid—*Haemophilus ducreyi*

   d. Condyloma acuminata—*Treponema pallidum*

2. Sharyl, a 25-year-old female, says that she experiences pain whenever she urinates, bleeds after she has intercourse, and experiences vaginal discharge. Which diagnostic test would help to confirm the most likely diagnosis?

   a. Erythrocyte sedimentation rate

   b. Enzyme immunoassay

   c. Western blot

   d. Viral load

3. What is the estimated rate of male-to-female transmission of gonorrhea following initial exposure?

   a. A rate of 20%–30%

   b. A rate of 40%–50%

   c. A rate of 60%–70%

   d. A rate of 80%–90%

4. Luis, a 42-year-old male, presents with a painless, indurated ulcer on his anus. An inspection of his body reveals no other lesions, and he cannot recall any recent illness. You prescribe the patient benzathine intramuscularly in a single dose. Which stage of syphilis are you most likely treating?

   a. Primary

   b. Secondary

   c. Latent

   d. Tertiary

5. You have just diagnosed your male patient with chancroid. You order a second battery of tests, knowing that other conditions are commonly associated with the presentation of chancroid. Which of the following conditions would you <u>least</u> expect to find?

   a. Syphilis

   b. Herpes simplex virus

   c. Molluscum contagiosum

   d. HIV

6. A male patient presents to you with flu-like symptoms and a rash on his palmar surfaces. The rash itself is characterized by rough, reddish-brown dots. Further examination shows enlarged lymph nodes. Following a diagnostic, you want to prescribe him medication, but his records show that he is allergic to penicillin. Based on the most likely condition, which two antibiotics would serve as suitable treatment alternatives?

   a. Doxycycline or erythromycin

   b. Erythromycin or ciprofloxacin

   c. Ciprofloxacin or doxycycline

   d. Acyclovir or erythromycin

7. Upon examining a 23-year-old patient, you identify pearly-white papules around her anogenital region. The papules are about 2 mm wide and are round, smooth, and firm. The patient does not exhibit any other signs or symptoms. You would most strongly suspect which of the following conditions?

   a. Genital warts

   b. Molluscum contagiosum

   c. Chancroid

   d. Herpes

8. Which finding from a patient's cervical cytology results would best confirm condyloma acuminata?

   a. Squamous intraepithelial lesions

   b. Multinucleated giant cells

   c. Infection

   d. Parabasal cells

9. Which of these STDs is caused by a parasitic pathogen?

   a. Chancroid

   b. Molluscum contagiosum

   c. Condyloma acuminata

   d. Chlamydia

10. What is the primary role of a polymerase chain reaction (PCR) in the treatment of a patient with HIV?

   a. The PCR helps quantitate the viral count of HIV in an infected person.

   b. The PCR confirms HIV-positive status following a positive result on an ELISA test.

   c. The PCR helps determine the number of CD4 cells in a patient with confirmed HIV.

   d. The PCR helps determine when a person will undergo seroconversion.

11. Which statement most accurately reflects the relationship between the human immunodeficiency virus (HIV) and CD4 cells?

   a. HIV infects CD4 cells and maintains the compromised cell for virus spreading.

   b. HIV uses CD4 cells as receptors and reservoirs.

   c. HIV causes an excessive increase in CD4 cells.

   d. HIV causes CD4 cells to attack the body.

12. A patient made an appointment with your clinic to be evaluated for a possible sexually transmitted infection. When the patient misses the appointment, you follow up and learn that the patient has been admitted to a hospital with a case of meningitis. Which of the following STDs would you most likely expect the patient to have?

   a. Gonorrhea

   b. Syphilis

   c. Chancroid

   d. Chlamydia

13. Your patient has an L3 immunotype of *Chlamydia trachomatis*. Which sign or symptom would be most expected from the suspected condition?

   a. Painful ulcers

   b. Green-yellow discharge

   c. Regional adenopathy

   d. Dysmenorrhea

14. Trimethoprim-sulfamethoxazole (Bactrim) is given to AIDS patients as a prophylaxis for which disease?

    a. Pneumocystis pneumonia

    b. Progressive multifocal leukoencephalopathy

    c. Coccidioidomycosis

    d. Histoplasmosis

15. A male presents to the clinic complaining of a painful ulcer on his genitals. A close examination reveals that the ulcer is surrounded by an erythematous halo. Given the most likely condition, which of the following antibiotics would not be prescribed?

    a. Doxycycline

    b. Ceftriaxone

    c. Azithromycin

    d. Ciprofloxacin

16. Melissa, a 25-year-old female, comes into the clinic after noticing "yellow-green" vaginal discharge. She also reports pain and swelling "down there"; a physical examination reveals labial swelling. Based on these findings, which is the most likely diagnosis?

    a. Chancroid

    b. Lymphogranuloma venereum

    c. HIV

    d. Gonorrhea

17. A woman comes into the clinic stating that she thinks she has a sexually transmitted disease because she has pain in the general groin area. Upon examination, you identify genital ulcers on her labia that she confirms are painful, as well as tender inguinal lymphadenopathy. You suspect chancroid but know that a definitive diagnosis is difficult. Which statement regarding a morphological diagnosis is true?

    a. The Gram stains for chancroid and gonorrhea identify the same bacteria.

    b. Absence of herpes simplex virus is part of a definitive diagnosis for chancroid.

    c. The bacteria that cause chancroid cannot be identified in a Gram stain.

    d. Diagnosis requires identification of chancroid-causing bacteria, but sensitivity is less than 80%.

18. Which of the following diagnostic tests is used to confirm HIV?

    a. ELISA

    b. CD4 lymphocyte count

    c. Western blot

    d. Viral load

19. You inform your patient Jack, a 25-year-old male, that he is in the latent stage of syphilis. Which sign or symptom would best characterize this stage of the disease?

    a. Mucous patches

    b. Indurated ulcers

    c. Skin rash on palmar and plantar surfaces

    d. No signs or symptoms

20. An examination of Andrew, a 28-year-old male, reveals a non-indurated ulcer on his prepuce that he claims appeared 3 days ago. He states that he did some research online and believes it may be either chancroid or lymphogranuloma venereum (LGV). While you examine him, which finding would you tell him best distinguishes chancroid from LGV?

    a. Only LGV typically starts as a small papule.

    b. LGV is asymptomatic in men.

    c. Tender inguinal lymphadenopathy is generally indicative of LGV.

    d. Only LGV may present with buboes.

21. You are meeting with a patient who is HIV-positive. The patient's CD4 lymphocyte percentage has fallen below 20%. What would you most likely say when discussing this with your patient?

    a. "The lower lymphocyte percentage indicates seroconversion."

    b. "The risk of your HIV infection progressing to AIDS has increased."

    c. "As your CD4 lymphocyte percentage drops, your viral load usually drops."

    d. "Now that your CD4 lymphocyte percentage is below 20%, you can start antiretroviral therapy."

22. You are talking to your male patient about the importance of practicing safer sex. You mention that certain STDs can cause urethritis and, in rare cases, this can lead to epididymitis and male infertility. Which of the following STDs is most likely to predispose a male patient to urethritis and infertility?

a. Genital warts

b. Gonorrhea

c. Molluscum contagiosum

d. Chancroid

23. Which of the following would be most indicative of an initial herpes outbreak?

a. Pruritic ulcers lasting 12 days

b. Pruritic and exuding ulcers lasting 5 days

c. Ulcers surrounded by an erythematous halo

d. Painless ulcers

24. What are the two most common methods for diagnosing molluscum contagiosum?

a. Serologic tests and complete blood count (CBC)

b. Inspection and microscopic exam

c. CBC and inspection

d. Microscopic exam and serologic tests

25. You are teaching a nurse practitioner class about a recurrent, viral sexually transmitted disease that can either be associated with infection of the face or infection of the genitalia. There is no cure for this condition and it typically presents with painful lesions. What is the most definitive test for this condition?

a. ELISA

b. Culture

c. Papanicolaou stain

d. Tzanck stain

26. A patient with the following lesions presents to the clinic. A diagnosis of syphilis would most likely be confirmed if the lesions are:

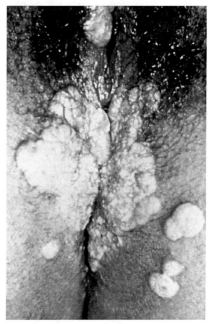

Figure 7.1

a. Mucous

b. Pearly-white

c. Soft

d. Painful

27. Of all these treatments for herpes, which is most useful for asymptomatic viral shedding of herpes simplex virus type 2?

a. Calamine lotion

b. Adefovir

c. Colloidal oatmeal baths

d. Valacyclovir

28. Which of the following lab results would best indicate that a patient's HIV is well controlled?

a. Viral load: detectable; CD4 lymphocyte count: 300 cells/μL

b. White blood cell count: 5,000 cells/mL

c. Viral load: undetectable; CD4 lymphocyte count: 700 cells/μL

d. White blood cell count: 10,000 cells/mL

29. An examination of a patient reveals a painful lesion on her cervix. She is also experiencing a fever and has been feeling extremely tired. You know that which of the following is the most likely diagnosis?

   a. Lymphogranuloma venereum

   b. Genital warts

   c. Chancroid

   d. Herpes

30. Robin, a 45-year-old female, presents to the clinic with rounded, firm, painless bumps along her lower abdomen and genital region. You note that the papules are about 3 mm and pearly-white. Which is the most common form of treatment for the most likely condition?

   a. Aspiration

   b. Antipruritic agents

   c. Laser therapy

   d. Cryoanesthesia with liquid nitrogen

31. Shaun, a 30-year-old male, presents to the clinic with yellow-green penile discharge, testicular pain, and nausea and vomiting. Given the most likely diagnosis, which of these drugs should you include in the regimen?

   a. Azithromycin

   b. Penicillin

   c. Erythromycin

   d. Valacyclovir

32. Which of the following is a commercially available vaccine that is implemented to prevent and protect against the hepatitis B virus?

   a. Kinrix-B

   b. Varivax-B

   c. Hiberix-B

   d. Engerix-B

33. All of the following keratolytic agents are routinely used to treat condyloma acuminata except:

   a. Podophyllin

   b. 5-fluorouracil

   c. Trichloroacetic acid

   d. Bichloroacetic acid

34. Which is the third most commonly reported sexually transmitted disease of bacterial etiology in the United States?

   a. Chlamydia

   b. Syphilis

   c. Human papillomavirus

   d. Gonorrhea

35. George, a 32-year-old male, comes to the clinic with swollen lymph nodes in his inguinal area. This finding is typically a sign of all of the following conditions except:

   a. Lymphogranuloma venereum

   b. Chancroid

   c. Syphilis

   d. Chlamydia

36. An examination of a patient diagnosed with an advanced case of lymphogranuloma venereum reveals buboes in the vulvovaginal area. Which treatment is recommended to prevent ulcerations?

   a. Drying agents

   b. Electrocautery

   c. Aspiration

   d. Cryotherapy

37. A patient presents to the clinic with purulent white discharge and six maculopapular lesions. He also complains of pain in his testicles and frequent nausea. Which of these is the most likely diagnosis?

   a. Herpes

   b. Chancroid

   c. Gonorrhea

   d. Syphilis

38. What is the typical window of time in which an infected person most commonly converts from HIV negative to HIV positive?

   a. Between 9 and 12 months

   b. Between 5 days and 6 weeks

   c. Between 3 weeks and 6 months

   d. Between 12 and 24 months

39. Henry, a 44-year-old male, is hospitalized and has an STD that is characterized by hemiparesis, hemiplegia, and cardiac insufficiency. Given the most likely stage of Henry's condition, which of the following signs or symptoms would you least expect to see?

   a. Chancre

   b. Aortic aneurysm

   c. Leukoplakia

   d. Meningitis

40. All of the following signs and symptoms are common indicators of an initial outbreak of herpes except:

   a. Fever

   b. Dysuria

   c. Malaise

   d. Urinary frequency

RATIONALES

1. d

Condyloma acuminata, or genital warts, are produced by the herpes simplex virus, not the bacterium *Treponema pallidum*. In turn, syphilis is caused by *T. pallidum*. Pelvic inflammatory disease is caused by several organisms, including *Neisseria gonorrhoeae* and, more commonly, *Chlamydia trachomatis*. Lymphogranuloma venereum is caused by *C. trachomatis*, and chancroid is caused by *Haemophilus ducreyi*.

2. b

Chlamydia, the most likely diagnosis based on pain during urination, bleeding after intercourse, and vaginal discharge, is often diagnosed through an enzyme immunoassay because it is quicker and less expensive than a chlamydia culture. The erythrocyte sedimentation rate is generally not affected by chlamydia. The Western blot and viral load tests are generally for assessing HIV, not chlamydia.

3. d

Male-to-female transmission of gonorrhea occurs at an estimated rate of 80%–90% after an initial exposure. A female has about a 50% risk of contracting the disease upon first contact. A male, however, has only about a 20% risk of contracting gonorrhea per episode of vaginal intercourse, but that number jumps to about 60%–80% chance of infection after four exposures.

4. a

The presence of an indurated ulcer without any pain or other symptoms suggests that the patient is in the primary stage of syphilis, which can be treated with a single dose of benzathine penicillin G. Secondary syphilis may be remedied with a single dose, but typically presents with flu-like symptoms, rash, and lymphadenopathy. Latent syphilis is asymptomatic but can be seropositive, and the tertiary stage is generally indicated by multi-system involvement.

5. c

There is no known correlation between the prevalence of chancroid and the prevalence of molluscum contagiosum, although both are genital infections. Furthermore, where chancroid typically presents with painful ulcers, molluscum contagiosum often presents with painless keratinized growths. Up to 10% of patients with chancroid have it concomitantly with syphilis and herpes simplex virus. Chancroid is also often a co-factor for HIV transmission.

6. a

In treating patients allergic to penicillin who present with secondary syphilis, as indicated by the patient's flu-like symptoms, palmar skin rash, and lymphadenopathy, prescribing doxycycline or erythromycin are possibilities for treatment. Ciprofloxacin, although a treatment for genital ulcers, is not recommended for treating syphilis, and neither is acyclovir, an antiviral medication commonly used to treat herpes.

7. b

The patient's presentation of small, round, white lesions on her anogenital region is suggestive of molluscum contagiosum. Genital warts present with growths as well; however, these are typically soft, fleshy, and keratinized in nature. The symptoms of chancroid include painful ulcers surrounded by an erythematous halo, if the condition presents with any symptoms at all. The first type of herpes is generally indicated by infection on the face or lips, whereas the second type of herpes typically affects the genitalia and may include painful ulcers.

8. a

A Pap smear that shows squamous intraepithelial lesions are consistent with a diagnosis of condyloma acuminata. Finding multinucleated giant cells from a cervical cytology smear generally indicates herpes simplex virus. If cytology results indicate infection, the patient should be further tested for trichomoniasis, vaginosis, herpes, and chlamydia, rather than condyloma acuminata. Parabasal cells are often confused with dysplastic cells, but parabasal cells are normal and occur most often prior to menarche or after menopause.

9. d

Chlamydia produces from *Chlamydia trachomatis*, a small Gram-negative bacterium that is an obligate intracellular parasite. Chancroid produces from *Haemophilus ducreyi*, a facultative anaerobic bacillus that is not parasitic in nature. Both molluscum contagiosum and condyloma acuminata are caused by viruses, with the former producing from the molluscum contagiosum virus and the latter producing from the human papillomavirus.

10. a

The polymerase chain reaction (PCR) test examines the viral load in a person who has confirmed HIV. Although the PCR test may detect HIV within 2–3 weeks of infection, the Western blot assay is more commonly used to confirm positive results following an ELISA test. Specifically examining the CD4 count is not done through a PCR test, and PCR results do not determine rate of seroconversion.

11. b

The human immunodeficiency virus uses CD4 cells as receptors and reservoirs and then subsequently destroys the cells, resulting in a dramatic decline, not increase, in the overall CD4 count. Although compromised CD4 cells transmit the virus through the body, the primary means of transmission is destroying the compromised cell to produce virus particles, not maintaining the cell to aid transmission.

12. b

Syphilitic aseptic meningitis is a type of meningitis that can result from tertiary syphilis. Cardiac insufficiency, aortic aneurysm, hemiplegia, and other signs of cardiovascular and central nervous system (CNS) involvement may also present with tertiary stage syphilis. Gonorrhea may also cause cardiovascular or CNS complications in rare cases, but meningitis from gonorrhea is extremely rare. Untreated chlamydia is not known to produce meningitis but may cause pelvic inflammatory disease, Reiter syndrome, and infertility in women. Complications of chancroid are typically limited to the genitals, and findings often include phimosis, balanoposthitis, and superinfection of ulcers.

13. c

Of the findings listed, regional adenopathy is most commonly associated with lymphogranuloma venereum (LGV). Although ulcers will typically present in LGV, ulcers in LGV are often painless; painful ulcers are a hallmark of chancroid. Discharge in advanced cases of LGV is bloody and purulent, not green-yellow; this color of discharge, as well as dysmenorrhea in females, is more often a symptom of gonorrhea.

14. a

Trimethoprim-sulfamethoxazole (TMP-SMZ) is given to AIDS patients as prophylaxis against *Pneumocystis jiroveci* pneumonia. The other choices do not use TMP-SMZ for prophylactic measures. Progressive multifocal leukoencephalopathy, caused by the John Cunningham (JC) virus, has no specific prophylactic treatment. Coccidioidomycosis is treated with antifungal drugs, not TMP-SMZ. In rare instances where prophylaxis is prescribed for coccidioidomycosis, fluconazole is generally prescribed. Although prophylaxis is rarely administered for histoplasmosis, itraconazole is usually the first choice for immunocompromised patients.

15. a

Doxycycline is not among the typical medications used to treat chancroid, a condition that often presents with by painful ulcers surrounded by erythematous halos. Doxycycline would more likely see use in treating other conditions, such as chlamydia or lymphogranuloma venereum. Patients with chancroid are often prescribed ceftriaxone, azithromycin, or ciprofloxacin.

16. d

Mucopurulent vaginal discharge and labial pain and swelling generally indicate gonorrhea. Other signs and symptoms of gonorrhea in females include dysuria, increased urinary frequency, lower abdominal pain, and abnormal menstrual periods. Chancroid typically does not cause mucopurulent vaginal discharge. Lymphogranuloma venereum may cause swelling in the rectal or inguinal region, but not commonly labial swelling, and is more often distinguished by painful ulcers. Women with HIV are more likely to get yeast infections, which typically result in odorless, white discharge.

17. d

Morphological diagnosis of chancroid is difficult because *Haemophilus ducreyi*, the bacteria that cause chancroid, must be identified on special culture media that is not widely available and has culture sensitivity of less than 80%. Absence of the herpes simplex virus is part of a probable, not definitive, diagnosis for chancroid, as is the absence of *Treponema pallidum*. The Gram stain for gonorrhea shows gram-negative diplococci; the Gram stain for chancroid shows gram-negative bacilli.

18. c

The Western blot test helps confirm a diagnosis of HIV after the initial screening with an ELISA test. A high viral load and low CD4 lymphocyte count indicates a high risk of progression to AIDS, but these tests are not typically used in the initial screening for HIV.

19. d

There are no distinguishing signs or symptoms of the latent clinical stage of syphilis, which is asymptomatic. Indurated ulcers are generally a finding of the primary stage of syphilis, while mucous patches and skin rashes on the palmar and plantar surfaces typically appear in the secondary stage.

20. c

Although inguinal lymphadenopathy may present in males with either chancroid or lymphogranuloma venereum (LGV), it is more commonly a feature of LGV, with only 50% of males with chancroid experiencing the condition. Both conditions often start with small papules that turn into ulcers. Painful buboes may present alongside lymphadenopathy in cases of chancroid and secondary LGV alike. Although both chancroid and LGV may be asymptomatic in women, men typically experience symptoms when infected with either condition.

21. b

A CD4 lymphocyte count below 20% indicates a high risk of progression from HIV to AIDS. Seroconversion is the process of converting from HIV negative to HIV positive; this would have already occurred in the patient and would not be indicated by the lower lymphocyte percentage. The viral load results closely correlate with the progression of HIV, but low CD4 lymphocyte percentages would most likely result in higher viral loads, not lower viral loads. When to start antiretroviral treatment is an important decision for each patient. Although patients start therapy at different times, the Centers for Disease Control and Prevention recommend starting at least by the time the CD4 count reaches 350/μL.

22. b

Of the choices, gonorrhea is the most likely to cause urethritis in males. In rare cases, urethritis may lead to epididymitis and male infertility. Genital warts, molluscum contagiosum, and chancroid are not commonly known to cause urethritis or male infertility.

23. a

An initial herpes outbreak typically presents with painful, pruritic ulcers that last approximately 12 days. Patients with recurrent herpes have pruritic ulcers that usually last for 5 days. Herpes ulcers do not typically exude. Ulcers surrounded by an erythematous halo are typical of chancroid, not genital herpes.

24. b

The two most common methods for diagnosing molluscum contagiosum are inspection and microscopic exams. Histologic exams may also prove beneficial. Serologic tests are more commonly used to diagnose syphilis, and a complete blood count would prove more useful in diagnosing gonorrhea.

25. b

The most definitive test for herpes, which is characterized by lesions on the face or genitals and an incurable nature, is a viral culture. Although herpes can be detected in a Papanicolaou smear or Tzanck stain, these tests do not provide a definitive diagnosis. There are also ELISA tests for herpes, but the ELISA test has a low sensitivity for herpes simplex virus type 2.

26. a

Syphilis most often results in mucous lesions, in addition to a rash that may show up after the initial sore has healed. Pearly-white papules are more commonly indicative of molluscum contagiosum; these lesions are often smooth and rounded. Initial sores from syphilis are typically firm and painless, rather than soft and painful.

27. d

Valacyclovir is especially useful for reducing asymptomatic viral shedding of herpes simplex virus type 2 (HSV2) in patients with herpes. Adefovir is used to treat hepatitis B, not herpes. Furthermore, calamine lotion and colloidal oatmeal baths are often given for symptomatic treatment of HSV2, not to reduce asymptomatic viral shedding.

28. c

A person's HIV status is well controlled if the CD4 count is at or near normal levels (normal is above 800 cells/μL) and if the viral load is undetectable. A CD4 count of 300 cells/μL indicates the patient is progressing towards AIDS. Lastly, even though the white blood cell counts (WBCs) are within normal ranges (normal blood cell count: 4,500–10,000 cells/mL), WBC counts are not a reliable indicator of a patient's HIV status; the counts are more useful in determining whether or not the patient has an opportunistic infection.

29. d

A patient who presents with a painful lesion on her cervix that is accompanied by fever and malaise is most likely experiencing herpes. Although lymphogranuloma venereum and genital warts also present with vesicles or ulcers, these lesions are painless. Lastly, chancroid is usually asymptomatic in women; men are more likely to develop painful ulcers surrounded by an erythematous halo.

30. d

Based on the patient's presentation, the patient's papules are most characteristic of molluscum contagiosum and cryoanesthesia with liquid nitrogen is the most common approved form of removal. Aspiration is more commonly used to lance buboes and prevent ulcerations associated with lymphogranuloma venereum. Antipruritic agents are frequently recommended for managing symptoms associated with herpes, and laser therapy is a treatment option more often used to remove genital warts. Laser therapy may remove molluscum contagiosum papules but is usually reserved for the extensive presentations seen in immunocompromised patients.

31. a

The first-line treatment for uncomplicated gonorrhea, as indicated by yellow-green penile discharge, testicular pain, and nausea and vomiting, is ceftriaxone plus either azithromycin or doxycycline to co-treat potential chlamydial coinfection. Penicillin and erythromycin are both recommended for treatment of syphilis, but not typically gonorrhea. Valacyclovir is a common treatment for herpes.

32. d

Engerix-B is a hepatitis B vaccine that uses noninfectious hepatitis B virus surface antigens so that the body can build immunity to the disease. Along with Recombivax-HB, it is one of the most widely used vaccines for the hepatitis B virus. There is no such thing as Kinrix-B, Hiberix-B, or Varivax-B; the vaccinations are called Kinrix, Hiberix, and Varivax. Kinrix is an inactivated combination vaccine that is used to prevent polio, diphtheria, tetanus, and pertussis. Varivax, a vaccine that prevents the contraction of varicella, is recommended for children over the age of 1. A booster shot of Hiberix, a bacterial meningitis vaccination, is given to children who have received previous *Haemophilus influenzae* type B vaccinations.

33. b

Although 5-fluorouracil may be used to treat condyloma acuminata, it is no longer recommended for routine use due to the risk of severe toxic reaction. Podophyllin, trichloroacetic acid, and chloracetic acid are all recommended treatments for condyloma acuminata.

34. b

Syphilis is the third most commonly reported sexually transmitted disease (STD) of bacterial etiology in the United States. Chlamydia is the most common bacterial STD in the United States, with gonorrhea being the second most common bacterial STD. The human papillomavirus is the most commonly reported viral STD in the United States.

35. d

Although the same genus of bacteria causes chlamydia and lymphogranuloma venereum, chlamydia does not typically present with lymphadenopathy, whereas lymphogranuloma venereum does. Chancroid and syphilis patients may also present with regional lymphadenopathy in the inguinal lymph nodes.

36. c

Needle aspiration may be needed to treat buboes in cases of lymphogranuloma venereum, as aspiration may relieve pain and prevent the formation of ulcers. Drying agents are recommended for symptomatic treatment of herpes simplex virus to keep sores from weeping. Electrocautery, as well as cryotherapy, laser therapy, and excision, are recommended for the removal of genital warts. Cryoanesthesia with liquid nitrogen is the preferred method of removing lesions produced by molluscum contagiosum.

37. c

Purulent penile discharge, testicular pain and nausea, and maculopapular and pustular lesions located peripherally to the site of infection are most indicative of gonorrhea. Gonorrhea does not always present with lesions; however, when lesions are present, they are often painful and may number anywhere from 5–40 lesions. Although herpes may also present with ulcers on the genitalia, the ulcers are more often pruritic. Additionally, purulent penile discharge is not commonly a sign of herpes. Chancroid often manifests with painful ulcers that are surrounded by an erythematous halo. Syphilis also commonly presents with flu-like symptoms and a painless chancre on the genitalia; however, purulent penile discharge is not a common finding.

38. c

Seroconversion, the process in which HIV antibodies develop and become detectable, generally takes approximately three weeks to six months after initial infection. During this process, the individual may report flu-like symptoms. Although seroconversion can occur sooner than 3 weeks, it generally does not occur within a period of 5 days, and a period of 9 or 12 months is abnormal.

39. a

A chancre, often the first sign that a person has entered the primary stage of syphilis, typically heals within 6 weeks. Hemiparesis, hemiplegia, and cardiac insufficiency all indicate the tertiary clinical stage of syphilis, which typically begins years after the initial infection. Leukoplakia, aortic aneurysms, and meningitis are also potential signs and symptoms of the tertiary stage of syphilis.

40. d

Although some patients experiencing an initial herpes outbreak may experience urinary frequency, it is more commonly an indicator of gonorrhea than herpes. Dysuria and urinary retention are common indications of an initial outbreak of herpes, as are fever and malaise.

DISCUSSION

Acquired Immune Deficiency Syndrome (AIDS)

Overview

Acquired Immune Deficiency Syndrome (AIDS) is an immunodeficiency disorder that comprises the final stage of HIV disease.[1] AIDS is caused by infection from two types of HIV, known as HIV-1 and HIV-2. HIV-2 infections are common in sections of West Africa, but the majority of infections worldwide are caused by HIV-1.[2]

HIV weakens the immune system by destroying CD4 cells (T cells), causing opportunistic infections to develop.[3,4] In order for HIV to be transmitted, patients must come into contact with body fluids that contain infected cells, such as blood, semen, vaginal secretions, and breast milk, among others.[2] Patients can come into contact with these infected fluids by sexual contact or by sharing injection equipment.[1] Moreover, there is a risk of HIV-positive mothers transmitting the condition to infants, either by shared blood circulation during pregnancy or by breast milk during the child's infancy.[3] HIV is not, however, transmitted by any form of casual contact.[5]

Presentation

HIV/AIDS often goes undetected due to the fact that patients can either be asymptomatic or present with a constellation of signs and symptoms rather than any single finding that raises suspicion of AIDS.[6] Many early findings of AIDS are flu-like, including fever, night sweats, and weight loss, among others.[1] These signs and symptoms could indicate seroconversion, the process by which an infected patient progresses from HIV-negative to HIV-positive, which lasts approximately three weeks to six months.[7] During seroconversion, antibodies first become detectable.[8]

Workup

The initial screening test for HIV/AIDS is the ELISA test, which is highly sensitive; however, because ELISA test results can return with a false-positive, a diagnosis of AIDS should be confirmed by the Western blot test, which is more specific.[2] Furthermore, HIV/AIDS patients should undergo regular blood tests to check their CD4 cell count, since the risk of infections increases when a patient's CD4 count is too low.[1] A CD4 count below 200 cells/µL is considered a diagnostic for AIDS. A count below 200 cells/µL likewise signifies an increased risk for opportunistic infections.[4] The risk of progression to AIDS is considered high when a patient's CD4 lymphocyte percentage is below 20%.[9] Along with CD4 count, the patient's viral load must also be monitored. Viral load is tested by polymerase chain reaction and based on compilation and measurement of HIV-branched DNA or RNA copies. The results of a viral load should correlate closely with the patient's progression of HIV, and treatment should aim to reach an undetectable viral load.[10]

Treatment

While there is no cure for AIDS, a variety of drugs and treatments can help control HIV, manage symptoms, and improve the patient's quality of life.[1,3] Treatment of AIDS is best determined by the stage of the patient's disease as well as the presence of opportunistic infections. To determine the best treatment goals, patients and health care providers must work together to create individualized strategies for management.[11] Furthermore, treating opportunistic infections is a critical part of AIDS treatment; prophylaxis for *Pneumocystis jiroveci* pneumonia is an especially important concern, as this infection commonly presents in AIDS patients with a CD4 count below 200 cells/µL. A common prophylactic agent used in the prevention of *Pneumocystis* pneumonia is sulfamethoxazole/trimethoprim (Bactrim).[4]

Furthermore, active antiretroviral therapy (AART) is standard and has greatly helped improve mortality rates of AIDS patients.[4] When to start AART, however, remains controversial, with some experts suggesting that patients start medications at the time of an HIV-positive diagnosis. The Centers for Disease Control and Prevention recommend that all individuals with HIV should begin AART before their CD4 count reaches below 350 cells/µL.[7] To achieve the goals of AART, it is important for patients to consistently adhere to their drug regimen.[2] Drugs must be taken exactly as prescribed, and patients should be monitored for the danger of drug resistance.

Chancroid

Overview

Chancroid is a sexually transmitted disease (STD) caused by *Haemophilus ducreyi*, a gram-negative bacillus. It is estimated that up to 10% of all chancroid patients in the United States are also infected with other STDs, such as syphilis or the herpes simplex virus (HSV).[12] Although chancroid is uncommon in the United States and much of the developed world, the condition is a major cause of genital ulcers in many developing countries.[13] Moreover, chancroid is well-established as a co-factor in the transmission of HIV. Although there are no predominant findings of chancroid in HIV-infected patients, an atypical presentation of chancroid can appear along with an HIV infection.[14]

Presentation

Women with chancroid are usually asymptomatic, which allows the condition to go undiagnosed.[14] However, dysuria and dyspareunia may be the main symptom in female chancroid patients with lesions of the vulva, vagina, or cervix.[15] Men with chancroid tend to present with one or more superficial, painful ulcers, surrounded by an erythematous halo. These ulcers can present as necrotic or severely erosive in nature, and tend to present on the penis. Male patients may often present with inguinal lymphadenopathy and a unilateral bubo.[14]

Workup

A definitive diagnosis of chancroid can be made morphologically using special culture media; however, sensitivity for the test is no greater than 80%.[16] Because of the challenges of diagnosing chancroid, a probable diagnosis of the condition is made on the basis of clinical findings.[17] The nurse practitioner should examine the patient's genital region and check for ulcers and swelling of any lymph nodes.[18] Furthermore, a diagnosis of chancroid is suggested if the patient's ulcer exudate tests negative for HSV or if there is no evidence of *T. pallidum* infection.[14,16]

Treatment

Treatment of chancroid should not be delayed for test results, but should instead begin immediately.[12] Chancroid is usually treated with a single dose of either azithromycin (Zithromax) 1 gram orally or ceftriaxone (Rocephin) 250 mg intramuscularly. Ciprofloxacin serves as an alternative treatment but is not favored due to the need for multiple doses.[12]

Chlamydia

Overview

Chlamydia is a parasitic STD caused by the bacteria *Chlamydia trachomatis*. Chlamydia is the predominant bacterial STD in the United States, as well as the leading bacterial cause of sexually transmitted infections (STIs).[7,19] The condition most commonly occurs among young women, but can affect males and females of any age group.[20]

Presentation

A large percentage of women with chlamydia have no signs or symptoms, and most male chlamydia patients are asymptomatic as well.[20] In symptomatic cases, dysuria can appear in both sexes. Discharge is also common, issuing from the penis in males and the vagina in females; this discharge can be white, yellow, or green. Furthermore, chlamydia often presents with other signs and symptoms that are specific either to males or females. Males may present with urethral pain and swelling of the scrotum, whereas females may present with dyspareunia and abnormal vaginal bleeding patterns, such as postcoital bleeding.[21]

Workup

Although the diagnosis of chlamydia is usually made without testing, routine screening for genital infections is recommended, as many cases are asymptomatic.[22] A diagnosis of chlamydia infections also involves a sampling of the urethral discharge in males or cervical secretions in females.[23] Of the diagnostic tests used for chlamydia, the most definitive test is a chlamydia culture; however, enzyme immunoassay methods are less expensive and produce results more quickly.[7]

Treatment

Patients with chlamydia should begin antibiotic treatment as soon as possible.[21] Uncomplicated infections are treated with azithromycin (Zithromax), prescribed as a single dose of 1 gram by mouth, or by doxycycline (Vibramycin), which is administered orally in 100 mg doses twice a day for 7 days.[22] Alternatives include erythromycin, which is recommended for pregnant women who cannot tolerate first-line therapies. Ofloxacin and levofloxacin, on the other hand, cannot be used in pregnancy and are recommended for nonpregnant patients who cannot tolerate first-line therapies.[24] Furthermore, in addition to antibiotic treatments, the majority of states hold that each incidence of chlamydia must be reported to the health department.

Genital Warts (Condyloma Acuminata)

Overview

Condyloma acuminata, also known as genital warts, is an STI caused by the human papillomavirus (HPV) that produces with soft growths on the skin and mucous membranes of the genitals.[25] Condyloma acuminata is the most commonly virally transmitted STI in the United States.[26,27]

Presentation

Genital warts present as a single or multiple painless keratinized growths, which are characterized as fleshy, papillary, or sessile in nature. These growths commonly occur on the penis or around the anus in men, and around the vulvovaginal area, perineum, or urethra in women.[27]

Workup

The standard diagnosis of genital warts is made by a visual inspection of the affected area.[26] Patients should, however, undergo laboratory tests based on their history and examination findings.[28] For instance, a Pap smear can detect squamous intraepithelial lesions or atypical squamous cells of undetermined significance. Furthermore, a colposcopy is useful in diagnosing flat lesions, and a biopsy may be performed in patients who are at risk for cervical intraepithelial neoplasia.[7]

Treatment

Prescription medications used to treat genital warts include keratolytic agents, such as imiquimod (Zyclara), podophyllin (Pododerm), bichloroacetic acid (BCA), and trichloroacetic acid (TCA), among others.[25] Genital warts can also be removed by laser therapy, cryotherapy, electrocauterization, or excision, all of which will require a referral to a dermatologist.[27] In pregnant patients, laser therapy is one of the preferred treatments for genital warts, as it is a drug-free process. Furthermore, the HPV quadrivalent vaccination is recommended to help protect against HPV types 6, 11, 16, and 18. The HPV quadrivalent vaccine is distributed under the brand name Gardasil. This vaccine is indicated for both females and males from 9 to 26 years of age. The HPV bivalent vaccination, distributed under the brand name Cervarix, is also a recommended measure for prevention of genital warts; however, unlike the HPV quadrivalent vaccination, it is indicated for females 10–25 years of age and protects only against HPV types 16 and 18. Both vaccines are administered in three injections; the second injection is given 1–2 months after the initial dose, whereas the third injection is given 6 months after the initial dose.[7,29]

Gonorrhea

Overview

Gonorrhea is a bacterial STD caused by the bacteria *Neisseria gonorrhoeae*, which is a gram-negative diplococci transmitted by sexual contact or by transmission during childbirth.[30,31] The risk of transmission of *N. gonorrhoeae* between males and females increases with each episode of exposure.[31] Gonorrhea is the second most frequently reported communicable disease in the United States as well as a major cause of urethritis and cervicitis in men and women, respectively.[32] The urethra and the cervix are predominantly affected in patients with gonorrhea because *N. gonorrhoeae* bacteria grow in warm, moist parts of the body.[33] Furthermore, bacteria can be isolated in and cultured from the anorectum, genitourinary tract, or oropharynx.[7]

Presentation

Gonorrhea infections tend to be asymptomatic in both men and women.[34] Patients of both genders may present with dysuria. Furthermore, males with gonorrhea can present with distinct findings such as testicular swelling and yellow/green penile discharge. Females, on the other hand, may present with fever and yellow/green vaginal discharge, among other findings.[33] Additional signs and symptoms specific to female gonorrhea patients include lower abdominal pain, abnormal menstrual periods, and labial pain and swelling.[7]

Workup

When performing diagnostics on patients with gonorrhea, a cervical culture for *N. gonorrhoeae* is performed using an appropriate medium such as modified Thayer-Martin media plates.[30] Gram stains of gonococcal discharge smears should show white blood cells and gram-negative diplococci, the latter of which is essential in establishing a diagnosis of gonorrhea.[7,31]

Treatment

Patients with gonorrhea should be prescribed a single 250 mg dose of ceftriaxone (Rocephin) intramuscularly, along with either a single 1 gram dose of azithromycin (Zithromax) orally or doxycycline prescribed as 100 mg doses twice a day for 7 days to cover potential concomitant cases of chlamydia.[30] Moreover, cases should be reported to the health department.

Hepatitis B

Overview

Hepatitis B is an inflammation of the liver caused by the hepatitis B virus, and is also the second leading cause of acute viral hepatitis.[35] Hepatitis B is transmitted through contact with any of the body fluids of a person who has the virus.[36]

Presentation

Hepatitis B often presents with physical examination findings such as low-grade fever, jaundice, hepatomegaly, and splenomegaly.[37] Moreover, hepatitis B is a leading risk factor for fulminant liver failure.[35]

Workup

Hepatitis B is commonly diagnosed by a series of blood tests called a hepatitis viral panel.[36] Additionally, liver enzyme tests see use in laboratory evaluation for hepatitis B disease, among other tests.[37]

Treatment

Recombivax HB and Energix-B, two hepatitis B preventative vaccines, are both available commercially; the recommended schedule for this vaccine is three doses at 0, 1, and 6 months. Additionally, hepatitis B immune globulin (HBIG) is administered to patients who have not been vaccinated but have been exposed to the virus, providing passive immunity. HBIG should be administered within 14 days of exposure; however, earlier administration is recommended.[7] When hepatitis B presents, it is regularly treated with supportive and symptomatic care, including bed rest, eating healthy foods, and drinking fluids.[37]

Herpes

Overview

Herpes is a recurrent viral STD that is transmitted by physical contact with active lesions or fluids that contain the virus, such as saliva or cervical secretions. There are two types of herpes, known as HSV types 1 and 2. These two types differ in epidemiology: HSV type 1 is associated with painful lesions of the lips and face, whereas HSV type 2 is associated with painful genital lesions.[38]

Presentation

Herpes can easily go unnoticed because many patients with the condition present with only mild signs and symptoms.[39] General symptoms in the initial presentation of genital herpes include fever, malaise, and dysuria. Painful and pruritic ulcers may also appear, with a standard duration of about 12 days in patients with initial herpes and about five days in patients with recurrent herpes.[7]

Workup

Although a diagnosis of herpes is made clinically, the diagnosis should be confirmed by laboratory tests, particularly if the patient is infected with HIV.[40]

A definitive diagnosis of herpes is best made through a viral culture.[41] Furthermore, a Papanicolaou or Tzanck stain can also be used to establish a diagnosis.

Treatment

Although there is no cure for herpes, antiviral treatment can help lesions heal more quickly and reduce pain and discomfort during outbreaks.[39] Acyclovir, famciclovir, and valacyclovir are the usual antiviral agents prescribed for patients with herpes.[41] Acyclovir (Zovirax) is recommended for topical, oral, and intravenous use. Valacyclovir is especially useful in cases of HSV type 2 to decrease transmission rates in patients with asymptomatic viral shedding.[7] Additionally, symptomatic treatment can be used for constitutional signs and symptoms such as fever.[38]

Lymphogranuloma Venereum (LGV)

Overview

Lymphogranuloma venereum (LGV) is an STD characterized by genital papules or ulcers and caused by immunotype serovars L1, L2, and L3 of *C. trachomatis*.[42] Without treatment, LGV can cause obstruction of the patient's lymph flow as well as chronic swelling of the genital tissues.[43]

Presentation

LGV often presents with painless vesicles, buboes, or non-indurated ulcers measuring 2–3 mm, which may result in a misdiagnosis of chancroid. The predominant finding of LGV is regional adenopathy, which follows in approximately one month. Patients may also present with stiffness and aching in the groin, as well as subsequent unilateral swelling of the inguinal region.

Workup

LGV and chancroid share a number of characteristics, leading to potential confusion between the two conditions; as such, a definitive diagnosis of LGV requires isolating *C. trachomatis* from an appropriate specimen. Additional tests for LGV include a biopsy of the lymph nodes and a blood test for *C. trachomatis*.[44]

Treatment

Doxycycline (Vibramycin) should be prescribed to patients with LGV in doses of 100 mg orally twice a day for 21 days. Erythromycin may likewise be used to treat the disease, and is given in doses of 500 mg orally four times a day for 21 days.[29,44] Additionally, aspiration of buboes may be needed to prevent ulcerations.

Molluscum Contagiosum

Overview

Molluscum contagiosum is a benign viral infection caused by the *Molluscum contagiosum* virus. This condition is characterized by the appearance of dome-shaped papules.[45] Furthermore, molluscum contagiosum has been reported worldwide and is particularly common in childhood.[46]

Presentation

Patients with molluscum contagiosum present with lesions that are 1–5 mm in diameter and appear as flesh-colored to pearly-white papules. These papules are generally smooth, rounded, firm, and shiny, and tend to produce on the trunk and anogenital region.

Workup

Diagnosis of molluscum contagiosum can be made through clinical appearance, and a skin biopsy or smear is only needed when diagnosis is uncertain.[47]

Treatment

Cryoanesthesia with liquid nitrogen is the most popular method of treatment for molluscum contagiosum, and the condition of patients receiving this treatment usually resolves without scarring.[48]

Syphilis

Overview

Syphilis is an STD involving multiple organ systems and caused by *Treponema pallidum*, a spirochete bacterium with six to 14 regular spirals. Syphilis is third amongst the most frequently reported infectious diseases in the United States.[7]

Presentation

There are four clinical stages of syphilis. In the first stage, known as the primary stage, the patient's chancre is painless, with an indurated ulcer located at the site of exposure.[49] The secondary stage of syphilis, on the other hand, presents with flu-like symptoms and lymphadenopathy.[50,51] Patients in the secondary stage often present with mucous patches and highly variable skin rashes on the palmar and plantar surfaces. Other signs and symptoms suggestive of the secondary stage include malaise, anorexia, alopecia, and arthralgias. Unlike the other stages of syphilis, the latent stage is seropositive but asymptomatic. Finally, the tertiary stage of syphilis presents with multisystem involvement, potentially including leukoplakia, cardiac insufficiency, aortic aneurysms, meningitis, hemiparesis, or hemiplegia.[51]

Workup

The first serologic test used to diagnose syphilis is the Venereal Disease Research Laboratory (VDRL) test or the rapid plasma reagin (RPR) test. Diagnosis is then confirmed by treponemal tests, such as the fluorescent treponemal antibody absorption test (FTA-ABS) or the microhemagglutination assay for antibody to *T. pallidum* (MHA-TP). The FTA-ABS is commonly used for confirmation purposes, and affirms a positive diagnosis in the majority of primary cases and all secondary and later cases.[51]

Treatment

The primary treatment for all stages of syphilis is benzathine penicillin G, prescribed as a dose of 2.4 million units intramuscularly. Early cases of the disease can be treated with one dose, whereas more developed cases will require multiple administrations.[49,51] Syphilis patients allergic to penicillin can be prescribed doxycycline 100 mg by mouth twice a day or tetracycline 500 mg orally four times a day.[29] Finally, syphilis cases must be reported to the health department.[51]

Figures

Figure 7.1. Lindsley S. Blisters on the vulva due to a recurring Herpes II (HSV-2) virus infection. CDC. http://phil.cdc.gov/phil/download. asp. Published 1978. Accessed April 2015. Reproduced with permission.

Figure 7.2. Secondary syphilis manifested as perineal wart-like growths. CDC. http://phil.cdc.gov/phil/download.asp. Accessed April 2015. Reproduced with permission.

References

1. Mayo Clinic Staff. HIV/AIDS. Mayo Clinic Web site. http://www.mayoclinic.com/health/hiv-aids/DS00005. Updated May 20, 2014. Accessed March 25, 2015.

2. McCutchan JA. Human immunodeficiency virus (HIV) infection. In: Porter RS, Kaplan JL, eds. *The Merck Manual Online*. http://www.merckmanuals.com/professional/infectious_diseases/human_immunodeficiency_virus_hiv/human_immunodeficiency_virus_hiv_infection.html?qt=aids&alt=sh. Updated September 2013. Accessed March 25, 2015.

3. HIV/AIDS. MedlinePlus Web site. http://www.nlm.nih.gov/medlineplus/ency/article/000594.htm . Updated May 12, 2014. Accessed March 25, 2015.

4. Bennett NJ, Gilroy SA. HIV disease. In: Bronze MS, ed. *Medscape*. http://emedicine.medscape.com/article/211316-overview#aw2aab6b2b3. Updated January 23, 2015. Accessed March 25, 2015.

5. Demberg T, Robert-Guroff M. Controlling the HIV/AIDS epidemic: Current status and global challenges. *Front Immunol*. 2012; 3: 250. doi: 10.3389/fimmu.2012.00250

6. Sax PE. Acute and early HIV infection: Clinical manifestations and diagnosis. In: Basow DS, ed. *UpToDate*. Waltham, MA: UpToDate; 2015. http://www.uptodate.com/contents/acute-and-early-hiv-infection-clinical-manifestations-and-diagnosis. Updated July 8, 2014. Accessed March 25, 2015.

7. Barkley TW Jr. *Adult-Gerontology Primary Care Nurse Practitioner Certification Review/Clinical Update Continuing Education Course*. West Hollywood, CA: Barkley and Associates; 2015.

8. Seroconversion. NAM aidsmap Web site. http://www.aidsmap.com/Seroconversion/page/1322973/. Accessed March 25, 2015.

9. CD4 cell counts. NAM aidsmap Web site. http://www.aidsmap.com/CD4-cell-counts/page/1254931/. Accessed March 25, 2015.

10. Viral load. NAM aidsmap Web site. http://www.aidsmap.com/Viral-load/page/1254932/. Accessed March 25, 2015.

11. Panel on Antiretroviral Guidelines for Adults and Adolescents. Guidelines for the use of antiretroviral agents in HIV-1-infected adults and adolescents. AIDSinfo Web site. http://aidsinfo.nih.gov/contentfiles/lvguidelines/adultandadolescentgl.pdf. Last updated May 1, 2014. Accessed March 25, 2015.

12. McCutchan JA. Chancroid. In: Porter RS, Kaplan JL, eds. *The Merck Manual Online*. http://www.merckmanuals.com/professional/infectious_diseases/sexually_transmitted_diseases_std/chancroid.html?qt=chancroid&sc=&alt=sh. Updated October 2013. Accessed March 25, 2015.

13. Hope-Rapp E, Anyfantakis V, Fouéré S, et al. Etiology of genital ulcer disease. A prospective study of 278 cases seen in an STD clinic in Paris. *Sex Transm Dis*. 2010; 37(3): 153–158. doi: 10.1097/OLQ.0b013e3181bf5a98

14. Hicks CB. Chancroid. In: Basow DS, ed. *UpToDate*. Waltham, MA: UpToDate; 2015. http://www.uptodate.com/contents/chancroid?source=search_result&search=chancroid&selectedTitle=1~46. Updated March 24, 2014. Accessed March 25, 2015.

15. Arsove P, Edwards B. Chancroid. In: Cunha BA, ed. *Medscape*. http://emedicine.medscape.com/article/214737-overview. Updated October 30, 2014. Accessed March 25, 2015.

16. Workowski KA, Berman S. Sexually transmitted diseases treatment guidelines. *MMWR Morb Mortal Wkly Rep*. 2010; 59(RR-12): 1–110. http://www.cdc.gov/mmwr/pdf/rr/rr5912.pdf 17. Tucker JD, Bien CH, Peeling RW. Point-of-care testing for sexually transmitted infections: Recent advances and implications for disease control. *Curr Opin Infect Dis*. 2014; 26(1): 73–79. doi: 10.1097/QCO.0b013e32835c21b0

18. Chancroid. MedlinePlus Web site. http://www.nlm.nih.gov/medlineplus/ency/article/000635.htm. Updated August 31, 2014. Accessed March 25, 2015.

19. United States Department of Health and Human Services, Centers for Disease Control and Prevention, National Center for HIV/AIDS, Viral Hepatitis, STD, and TB Prevention. Sexually transmitted disease surveillance, 2010. http://www.cdc.gov/std/stats10/surv2010.pdf. Published November 2011. Accessed March 25, 2015.

20. Mayo Clinic Staff. Chlamydia. Mayo Clinic Web site. http://www.mayoclinic.org/diseases-conditions/chlamydia/basics/definition/CON-20020807. Updated April 5, 2014. Accessed March 25, 2015.

21. Qureshi S. Chlamydial genitourinary infections. In: Bronze MS, ed. *Medscape.* http://emedicine.medscape.com/article/214823-overview. Updated February 3, 2015. Accessed March 25, 2015.

22. Hammerschlag MR. Chlamydia. In: Porter RS, Kaplan JL, ed. *The Merck Manual Online.* http://www.merckmanuals.com/professional/infectious_diseases/chlamydia_and_mycoplasmas/chlamydia.html?qt=chlamydia&alt=sh. Updated March 2014. Accessed March 25, 2015.

23. Chlamydia. MedlinePlus Web site. http://www.nlm.nih.gov/medlineplus/ency/article/001345.htm. Updated June 11, 2014. Accessed March 25, 2015.

24. Marrazzo J. Treatment of Chlamydia trachomatis infection. In: Basow DS, ed. *UpToDate.* Waltham, MA: UpToDate; 2015. http://www.uptodate.com/contents/treatment-of-chlamydia-trachomatis-infection?source=search_result&search=Treatment+of+Chlamydia+trachomatis+infection&selectedTitle=1~106 . Updated December 23, 2014. Accessed March 25, 2015.

25. Genital warts. MedlinePlus Web site. http://www.nlm.nih.gov/medlineplus/ency/article/000886.htm. Updated November 10, 2013. Accessed March 25, 2015.

26. Breen E, Bleday R. Condylomata acuminata (anogenital warts). In: Basow DS, ed. *UpToDate.* Waltham, MA: UpToDate; 2015. http://www.uptodate.com/contents/condylomata-acuminata-anogenital-warts-in-adults?source=search_result&search=Condylomata+acuminata+%28anogenital+warts%29&selectedTitle=1~112. Updated November 19, 2014. Accessed March 25, 2015.

27. McCutchan JA. Genital warts. In: Porter RS, Kaplan JL, eds. *The Merck Manual Online.* http://www.merckmanuals.com/professional/infectious_diseases/sexually_transmitted_diseases_std/genital_warts.html?qt=genital%20warts&sc=&alt=sh. Updated October 2013. Accessed March 25, 2015.

28. Ghadishah D. Condyloma acuminata. In: Brenner BE, ed. *Medscape.* http://emedicine.medscape.com/article/781735-overview. Updated December 16, 2014. Accessed March 25, 2015.

29. Workowski KA, Bolan GA. Sexually transmitted diseases treatment guidelines, 2015. *MMWR Morb Mortal Wkly Rep.* 2015; 64(3): 1–137. http://www.cdc.gov/std/tg2015/tg-2015-print.pdf

30. McCutchan JA. Gonorrhea. In: Porter RS, Kaplan JL, eds. *The Merck Manual Online.* http://www.merckmanuals.com/professional/infectious_diseases/sexually_transmitted_diseases_std/gonorrhea.html?qt=gonorrhea&sc=&alt=sh. Updated October 2013. Accessed March 25, 2015.

31. Wong B. Gonorrhea. In: Chandrasekar PH, ed. *Medscape.* http://emedicine.medscape.com/article/218059-overview. Updated April 16, 2014. Accessed March 25, 2015.

32. Leone PA. Epidemiology and pathogenesis of Neisseria gonorrhoeae infection. In: Basow DS, ed. *UpToDate.* Waltham, MA: UpToDate; 2015. http://www.uptodate.com/contents/epidemiology-and-pathogenesis-of-neisseria-gonorrhoeae-infection?source=search_result&search=Epidemiology%2C+pathogenesis%2C+and+clinical+manifestations+of+Neisseria+gonorrhoeae+infection&selectedTitle=3~150. Updated June 26, 2014. Accessed March 25, 2015.

33. Gonorrhea. MedlinePlus Web site. http://www.nlm.nih.gov/medlineplus/ency/article/007267.htm. Updated April 25, 2013. Accessed March 25, 2015.

34. Beck S, Ghazaryan L, Muse A. Characteristics of men with repeat gonorrhea and early syphilis case reports in New York state, excluding New York City, 2006–2012. In: Proceedings of the 2014 STD Prevention Conference; Jun 9–12, 2014; Atlanta, GA. WP 196.

35. Rutherford AE. Acute viral hepatitis. In: Porter RS, Kaplan JL, eds. *The Merck Manual Online.* http://www.merckmanuals.com/professional/hepatic_and_biliary_disorders/hepatitis/acute_viral_hepatitis.html?qt=hepatitis%20b&alt=sh#v900207. Updated March 2014. Accessed March 25, 2015.

36. Hepatitis B. PubMed Health Web site. http://www.ncbi.nlm.nih.gov/pubmedhealth/PMH0001324/. Accessed March 25, 2015.

37. Pyrsopoulos NT, Reddy KR. Hepatitis B. In: Anand BS, ed. *Medscape.* http://emedicine.medscape.com/article/177632-overview. Updated January 11, 2015. Accessed March 25, 2015.

38. Salvaggio MR, Lutwick LI, Seenivasan M, Kumar S. Herpes simplex. In: Bronze MS, ed. *Medscape.* http://emedicine.medscape.com/article/218580-overview. Updated November 14, 2014. Accessed March 25, 2015.

39. Genital herpes. MedlinePlus Web site. http://www.nlm.nih.gov/medlineplus/ency/article/000857.htm. Updated July 28, 2014. Accessed March 25, 2015.

40. Johnston C, Wald A. Epidemiology, clinical manifestations, and diagnosis of genital herpes simplex virus in HIV-infected patients. In: Basow DS, ed. *UpToDate*. Waltham, MA: UpToDate; 2015. http://www.uptodate.com/contents/epidemiology-clinical-manifestations-and-diagnosis-of-genital-herpes-simplex-virus-in-hiv-infected-patients?source=search_result&search=Epidemiology%2C+clinical+manifestations%2C+and+diagnosis+of+genital+herpes+simplex+virus+in+HIV-infected+patients&selectedTitle=1~150. Updated February 14, 2014. Accessed March 25, 2015.

41. Kaye KM. Herpes simplex virus (HSV) infections. *The Merck Manual Online*. http://www.merckmanuals.com/professional/infectious_diseases/herpesviruses/herpes_simplex_virus_hsv_infections.html?qt=herpes%20simplex&alt=sh. Updated July 2013. Accessed March 25, 2015.

42. Arsove P, Edwards B. Lymphogranuloma venereum. In: Cunha BA, ed. *Medscape*. http://emedicine.medscape.com/article/220869-overview. Updated October 30, 2014. Accessed March 25, 2015.

43. McCutchan JA. Lymphogranuloma venereum (LGV). In: Porter RS, Kaplan JL, eds. *The Merck Manual Online*. http://www.merckmanuals.com/professional/infectious_diseases/sexually_transmitted_diseases_std/chlamydia_trachomatis_lymphogranuloma_venereum_lgv.html. Updated October 2013. Accessed March 25, 2015.

44. Lymphogranuloma venereum. MedlinePlus Web site. http://www.nlm.nih.gov/medlineplus/ency/article/000634.htm. Updated August 31, 2014. Accessed March 25, 2015.

45. Bhatia AC. Molluscum contagiosum. In: Elston DM, ed. *Medscape*. http://emedicine.medscape.com/article/910570-overview#a0101. Updated November 4, 2014. Accessed March 25, 2015.

46. Isaacs SN. Molluscum contagiosum. In: Basow DS, ed. *UpToDate*. Waltham, MA: UpToDate; 2015. http://www.uptodate.com/contents/molluscum-contagiosum?source=search_result &search=molluscum+contagiosum&selectedTitle=1~38. Updated August 21, 2014. Accessed March 25, 2015.

47. Dinulos JGH. Molluscum contagiosum. In: Porter RS, Kaplan JL, eds. *The Merck Manual Online*. http://www.merckmanuals.com/professional/dermatologic_disorders/viral_skin_diseases/molluscum_contagiosum.html?qt=molluscum%20contagiosum&alt=sh. Updated January 2014. Accessed March 25, 2015.

48. Mayo Clinic Staff. Molluscum contagiosum. Mayo Clinic Web site. http://www.mayoclinic.org/diseases-conditions/molluscum-contagiosum/basics/treatment/con-20026391. Updated March 21, 2015. Accessed March 25, 2015.

49. Mayo Clinic Staff. Syphilis. Mayo Clinic Web site. http://www.mayoclinic.org/diseases-conditions/syphilis/basics/symptoms/con-20021862. Updated January 2, 2014. Accessed March 25, 2015.

50. United States Department of Health and Human Services, Centers for Disease Control and Prevention. Syphilis – CDC Fact Sheet. http://www.cdc.gov/std/syphilis/stdfact-syphilis.htm. Updated July 8, 2014. Accessed March 25, 2015.

51. Philip SS. Spirochetal infections. In: Papadakis MA, McPhee SJ, Rabow MW, eds. *CURRENT Medical Diagnosis & Treatment 2014*. 53rd ed. New York, NY: McGraw Hill Education; 2014:1456–1474.

Chapter 8
Gynecologic Concerns/ Men's Health Issues

QUESTIONS

1. A 16-year-old patient experiencing primary amenorrhea should be referred to a specialist and evaluated for various possible causes. The following are common known causes of primary amenorrhea except for:

   a. Turner syndrome

   b. Vaginal agenesis

   c. Resistant follicular stimulation

   d. Endocrine imbalance

2. Of the following, who is most likely to experience symptoms of premenstrual syndrome/premenstrual dysphoric disorder?

   a. A 17-year-old athlete on a strict vegan diet

   b. A fit, healthy 33-year-old with a high-stress job

   c. A 45-year-old who regularly practices yoga

   d. A 24-year-old artist who drinks caffeine

3. You order a referral to further evaluate your 19-year-old patient who reported symptoms of cramping, pain in her upper thighs, nausea, and fatigue during the first few days of her menstrual cycle. For which of the following do you make a referral?

   a. Primary dysmenorrhea

   b. Secondary dysmenorrhea

   c. Endometriosis

   d. Premenstrual dysphoric disorder

4. A 64-year-old male presents to your practice with complaints regarding urination. He says that he has trouble "getting started" when he wishes to void, and that the stream "keeps leaking" when he tries to terminate it. He also wakes frequently with the urge to urinate. Upon further discussion, he mentions with some embarrassment that he "let go" while celebrating a victory for his sports team. Which diagnostic test should the nurse practitioner order initially?

   a. Prostate-specific antigen

   b. Gram stain

   c. Urinalysis

   d. 24-hour urine collection

5. Of the available agents to prescribe for erectile dysfunction, which has the fastest onset and longest duration?

   a. Saw palmetto

   b. Sildenafil

   c. Tadalafil

   d. Vardenafil

6. The results of a patient's cervical cytology test indicate "atypical squamous cell of undetermined significance." Which test would you least likely order as a follow-up?

   a. Human papillomavirus testing

   b. A second Pap smear

   c. Ultrasound

   d. Colposcopy

7. Which patient has the most substantial signs for developing osteoporosis?

   a. A 5'2" African American female weighing 115 lb

   b. A 5'9" Caucasian male weighing 155 lb

   c. A 5'4" Asian female weighing 90 lb

   d. A 5'10" Latin female weighing 200 lb

8. A patient with pelvic inflammatory disease (PID) seeks outpatient treatment for her condition. As she is intolerant of fluoroquinolones, you decide to put her on a regimen that focuses on doxycycline. According to the most recent CDC recommendations for treating PID, which of the following drugs would not be paired with doxycycline?

   a. Cefoxitin

   b. Probenecid

   c. Metronidazole

   d. Butoconazole

9. You are seeing a 24-year-old female who states that she has been experiencing severe cramping pain during her last two menstrual cycles. Which of the following conditions is the patient experiencing?

   a. Pelvic inflammatory disease

   b. Secondary dysmenorrhea

   c. Premenstrual syndrome

   d. Primary dysmenorrhea

10. Your post-menopausal patient complains of "hot flashes all the time" and insists that her quality of life is poor. You consider hormone therapy (HT) with which fact in mind?

   a. She will definitely be at increased risk for a cerebrovascular accident.

   b. She will have less of a dietary need for red meats.

   c. Breast cancer has been linked to those taking HT.

   d. The development of hirsutism, especially hair on the face, is something to carefully consider.

11. A patient diagnosed with abnormal uterine bleeding is undergoing further evaluation to determine the etiology. Which condition is least likely to be the cause of the patient's abnormal uterine bleeding?

   a. Polycystic ovarian disease

   b. Primary dysmenorrhea

   c. Perimenopause

   d. Immature hypothalamic-pituitary-ovarian axis

12. A 79-year-old male presents to your practice stating, "I'm back today because I forgot to tell you last week that I'm having trouble with my urine. I go several times a night, feel like I have to go all of the time, and when I pee, it starts, stops and even dribbles sometimes." At his physical exam 1 week ago, his complete blood count, urinalysis, and vital signs, including temperature, were all normal. His prostate-specific antigen was noted to be 6.0 ng/ml. The nurse practitioner considers a referral for which of the following tests at this time?

   a. Magnetic resonance imaging

   b. Transrectal ultrasound

   c. Computed tomography of the pelvis

   d. X-ray of the kidney, ureters, and bladder

13. During a periodic health examination, your 19-year-old patient tells you that she normally experiences pain during the first few days of her menstrual cycle. She describes the pain as a cramp that radiates to her back and upper thighs, and states that the pain is usually accompanied by nausea and fatigue. Based on the patient's presentation, high levels of which hormone are most likely responsible for her symptoms?

   a. Estrogen

   b. Progesterone

   c. Prostaglandin

   d. Dopamine

14. The diagnosis of osteoporosis involves the dual-energy x-ray absorptiometry (DEXA) test to measure bone mineral density in four different parts of the skeletal system. The practitioner knows that all of the following types of bone tissue are typically measured by a DEXA except:

   a. Hip

   b. Tibia

   c. Spine

   d. Ankle

15. After performing an assessment on a 20-year-old female, you recommend that she significantly reduce her caffeine and salt intake. You also recommend that she eat more foods containing vitamins E and B6 to help reduce or manage symptoms associated with which condition?

   a. Fibrocystic breast disease

   b. Secondary dysmenorrhea

   c. Pelvic inflammatory disease

   d. Premenstrual syndrome

16. Which of the following drug therapies is associated with the rare complication of osteonecrosis of the jaw, especially in patients receiving cancer treatment?

   a. Alendronate (Fosamax)

   b. Trimethoprim-sulfamethoxazole (Bactrim)

   c. Ciprofloxacin (Cipro)

   d. Amoxicillin (Amoxil)

17. Which of the following classes of medications is least likely to contribute to erectile dysfunction?

   a. Macrolides

   b. H2 receptor blockers

   c. Antihypertensives

   d. Diuretics

18. Which of these represents the standard of care for men with a diagnosis of symptomatic benign prostatic hypertrophy?

   a. Terazosin (Hytrin)

   b. Saw palmetto

   c. Avanafil (Stendra)

   d. Dutasteride (Avodart)

19. George, a 46-year-old male, says that he feels a burning sensation every time he urinates. He also states that he urinates more frequently than usual, and that he often has to get up in the middle of the night to do so. Which of the following methods would yield the most sensitive but not specific lab results for the patient's suspected condition?

   a. Visual examination of the patient's urine sample

   b. Presence of nitrate by dipstick

   c. Esterase detection by dipstick

   d. Blood testing by dipstick

20. A nurse practitioner is most likely to inform a menopausal patient starting hormone therapy that she may not need as much daily intake of which supplement?

   a. Potassium

   b. Calcium

   c. Phosphorus

   d. Iron

21. Your patient complains that she has "gotten shorter over the years" and noticed a "hump" on the back of her neck. As she walks over to the exam table, you notice that she stoops forward. Based on the patient's condition, which of the following would you be most likely to recommend to help her manage her condition?

   a. Yogurt and green leafy vegetables

   b. Red meats and iron-fortified breads

   c. Salmon and beans

   d. Fruits and raw vegetables

22. You are performing a health check-up on a 47-year-old female. She tells you that she's recently been waking up at night to go to the bathroom. She mentions whenever she coughs or sneezes, she pees a little. She also says that she had to buy a bra with a smaller cup size the month prior and was surprised that her size had changed. Based on the patient's complaints, which of the following skin findings would you <u>least</u> expect to see?

    a. Thinning of the vagina

    b. Decreased skin elasticity

    c. Decreased melanin synthesis

    d. Dry skin

23. A 55-year-old patient going through menopause comes to your office with complaints of vaginal dryness. She also says she feels depressed and frequently experiences hot flashes. She then inquires about hormone therapy. As you go over her medical history, you know that which of the following conditions would <u>not</u> be a contraindication to hormone therapy?

    a. Breast cancer

    b. Infertility

    c. Myocardial infarction

    d. Uterine cancer

24. What proportion of osteoporotic bone loss stems from hypoestrogenic states?

    a. One-fourth

    b. One-half

    c. Three-fourths

    d. All bone loss

25. Which of these conditions is most closely associated with CIN 2?

    a. Carcinoma in situ

    b. Atypical squamous cells of undetermined significance

    c. Moderate dysplasia

    d. Human papillomavirus

26. A patient presents to your clinic with complaints of a fever and chills. While discussing the patient's history, she mentions that both urination and sex have been painful in the past few weeks, and that she keeps getting up in the middle of the night to urinate. You suspect that the patient may have pelvic inflammatory disease (PID); however, which of her complaints is <u>not</u> associated with PID?

    a. Chills

    b. Dysuria

    c. Nocturia

    d. Dyspareunia

27. Your patient's dual-energy x-ray absorptiometry scan reveals a value of -2.7. Based on this finding, your best course of action at this time would be to recommend which of these therapies?

    a. Alendronate

    b. Increase in dietary calcium

    c. Coumadin therapy once daily

    d. Calcium supplements daily

28. Which of the following findings is <u>not</u> a common somatic symptom of premenstrual syndrome?

    a. Tension

    b. Headaches

    c. Breast tenderness

    d. Poor coordination

29. Which of the following is <u>not</u> a finding of acute bacterial prostatitis?

    a. Fever

    b. Dysuria

    c. Scrotal edema

    d. Urgency

30. Which Tanner stage of breast development is characterized by the projection of the areola and nipple as a secondary mound?

    a. Tanner stage 1

    b. Tanner stage 2

    c. Tanner stage 3

    d. Tanner stage 4

31. Katie, a 17-year-old female, has a history of premenstrual syndrome (PMS). She comes to your clinic complaining of PMS symptoms that she says have gotten worse over the past few months. You consider pharmacological management for Katie's symptoms. Which of the following would not be effective in managing her concerns at this time?

    a. Selective serotonin reuptake inhibitors

    b. Corticosteroids

    c. Hormonal birth control

    d. Vitamin E

32. Which of the following would you least expect to occur during menopause?

    a. Loss of elasticity in the skin

    b. Changes in skin pigmentation

    c. Loss of muscle tone

    d. Increased sebaceous gland activity

33. A 64-year-old male presents to your practice with low back pain and fever and mentions that he wakes up at least four times a night with an urgent need to urinate. An examination indicates that the patient's prostate is boggy and tender to palpation. A urine culture returns positive results for a causative agent. Based on the patient's symptoms and clinical findings, which pathogen would be the most likely cause of the patient's condition?

    a. *Chlamydia trachomatis*

    b. *Mycoplasma genitalium*

    c. *Gardnerella vaginalis*

    d. *Escherichia coli*

34. Which of the following is the least definitive test in diagnosing pelvic inflammatory disease?

    a. Sexually transmitted disease screening

    b. Erythrocyte sedimentation rate test

    c. Ultrasound

    d. Thyroid-stimulating hormone test

35. Which of the following is the most accurate statement regarding the biological effects during menopause?

    a. The cervical mucus thickens, and the vagina becomes redder in tone.

    b. The vagina experiences decreased stimulation as the epithelium atrophies.

    c. Vaginal pH levels and vaginal secretions decrease.

    d. The decreased pH in the vaginal lactic acid increases susceptibility to urinary tract pathogens.

36. A patient presents with lower abdominal pain and vomiting. Her temperature is 40 °C. You perform a cervical exam, and your patient tests positive for cervical motion tenderness. Upon further testing, you identify *Chlamydia trachomatis*. Based on the likely diagnosis, which regimen would you most likely prescribe?

    a. Levofloxacin and probenecid

    b. Ofloxacin and ceftriaxone

    c. Cefoxitin and probenecid with or without ceftriaxone

    d. Ceftriaxone and doxycycline with or without metronidazole

37. You are treating four female patients who each exhibit predisposing factors for osteoporosis. Which patient is least likely to be at risk for osteoporosis?

    a. An overweight African American female with a family history of uterine cancer

    b. A Hispanic woman living a predominantly sedentary lifestyle

    c. An underweight Asian woman with a history of tobacco use

    d. A Caucasian woman experiencing early onset of menopause

38. A patient comes to your practice complaining of intense itching in her vaginal area and yellowish-green discharge that "smells like old garbage." Inspecting the patient's vulvovaginal region, you find erythema and red spots around the vagina. Based on your observations, you order a wet prep test to confirm the patient's condition and expect which of the following results?

    a. Clue cells

    b. Motile trichomonads

    c. Pseudo hyphae

    d. White blood cells

39. Which of the following drugs is <u>not</u> a phosphodiesterase inhibitor?

    a. Sildenafil

    b. Vardenafil

    c. Chlorophyllin

    d. Tadalafil

40. All of the following tests would be used to diagnose pelvic inflammatory disease <u>except</u> a:

    a. Venereal Disease Research Laboratory test

    b. Erythrocyte sedimentation rate test

    c. C-reactive protein test

    d. Ultrasound

RATIONALES

1. c

Resistant follicular stimulation is not generally considered a cause of primary amenorrhea, but is considered a possible cause of abnormal, heavy uterine bleeding. Primary amenorrhea is characterized by a lack of menarche by age 16. It may also cause an absence of sexual characteristics or abnormal growth and development. Diagnosis often requires a full examination from an endocrinologist to determine the proper etiology. Possible causes of primary amenorrhea include the following chromosomal disorders: Turner syndrome; anatomic abnormalities, such as vaginal agenesis; and hormonal imbalances due to endocrine abnormalities.

2. b

A fit, healthy 33-year-old with a high-stress job would be most likely to experience symptoms of premenstrual syndrome (PMS) and premenstrual dysphoric disorder (PDD) due to the combination of age and occupational stress. The incidence of PMS and PDD slowly increases during adolescence, peaks during the 30s, and declines in the 40s. Although adolescents should be monitored if following a strict vegan diet, a strict vegan diet is not known to increase incidence of PMS. A 45-year-old who regularly exercises would be less likely to experience symptoms of either PMS or PDD because incidence is more likely to decrease at her age. A 24-year-old who consumes caffeine may experience symptoms of PMS, but is less likely to experience those symptoms than a 33-year-old.

3. a

Because the patient's symptoms include nausea, fatigue, and severe radiating pain during her menstrual cycle, she should be evaluated for primary dysmenorrhea to determine if her body is producing too much prostaglandin. Secondary dysmenorrhea typically occurs in women age 20 or older and is most often associated with pelvic disease. Endometriosis may present with dysmenorrhea, but it typically presents with heavy or irregular bleeding, as opposed to the patient's regular flow. Premenstrual dysphoric disorder may produce with pain, but it begins prior to menses and ends when menses begins.

4. c

The nurse practitioner should initially order a urinalysis because the patient's symptoms of hesitancy, nocturia, dribbling, and incontinence may indicate urinary tract infection (UTI), benign prostatic hypertrophy (BPH), or prostate cancer. A Gram stain may also be helpful in determining causative pathogens, but it is labor intensive. A prostate-specific antigen test is primarily useful in diagnosing BPH and prostate cancer, and would typically come after a urinalysis rules out the possibility of UTI. Urine collection over 24 hours is typically a step in diagnosing kidney disorders, whereas the symptoms more strongly indicate urogenital involvement.

5. c

Of the various available agents for erectile dysfunction, tadalafil shows both the fastest onset at 15 minutes and longest efficacy at up to 36 hours. Sildenafil and vardenafil, on the other hand, generally require 30 minutes to take effect and may show effects for up to 4 hours. Saw palmetto may help in treating erectile dysfunction stemming from prostate issues, but is less helpful in treating erectile dysfunction resulting from other causes, such as stress or use of antidepressants.

6. c

An ultrasound is generally not recommended as a follow-up for a Papanicolaou test indicating atypical squamous cells of undetermined significance (ASCUS). An ultrasound is more likely to be used to scan for ovarian cysts in cases of pelvic inflammatory disease. A proper follow-up for ASCUS may include testing for human papillomavirus, repeating the Pap smear, and performing a colposcopy.

7. c

Females, individuals of white or Asian ethnicity, and individuals with small frames are at high risk for developing the most substantive signs of osteoporosis; therefore, a 5'4" Asian female weighing 90 lb would be at high risk for the development of osteoporosis. Females tend to develop osteoporosis at a 4:1 ratio to males, as women tend to have a sudden drop in estrogen levels. Hispanic and African American individuals are less likely to develop primary osteoporosis than Caucasian and Asian individuals.

8. d

Butoconazole, which is more commonly used to treat candidiasis, is not part of a pelvic inflammatory disease (PID) treatment regimen. One outpatient therapy regimen for PID that does not use fluoroquinolones pairs 2 grams intramuscular cefoxitin with 1 gram probenicid administered orally, followed by 100 mg doxycycline administered orally twice a day for 14 days. Metronidazole 500 mg orally twice a day for 14 days may also be added to treat bacterial vaginosis.

9. b

Severe cramping pain during menses occurs with secondary dysmenorrhea. Secondary dysmenorrhea is most likely to occur in women older than 20 years of age. In this case, the patient should undergo further evaluation to determine the etiology of her dysmenorrhea. Although both pelvic inflammatory disease and premenstrual syndrome can cause secondary dysmenorrhea, severe cramping during menses is not a finding in either condition. Primary dysmenorrhea may occur in adolescents due to excessive prostaglandin secretion and would not be considered in this case because the patient is not an adolescent.

10. c

Patients on hormone therapy (HT) are at increased risk of developing breast cancer; indeed, HT is contraindicated for those with a history of the disease. Although clinical trials suggest a potential increased risk of cerebrovascular accident (CVA) for those undergoing HT, the absolute findings are unclear, showing everything from increased risk to decreased risk of CVA. Diet is not a major concern in HT. HT is not known to cause hirsutism, but hirsutism may occur during menopause because of the decrease in estrogen.

11. b

Of the conditions listed, primary dysmenorrhea is not known to be a cause of abnormal uterine bleeding. Secondary dysmenorrhea may result in heavy or irregular bleeding, but primary dysmenorrhea does not usually affect uterine bleeding. Polycystic ovarian disease, perimenopause, and immature hypothalamic-pituitary-ovarian axis are known causes of abnormal uterine bleeding.

12. b

The patient's frequency, urgency, dribbling, nocturia, and prostate-specific antigen findings all indicate prostate cancer or benign prostatic hypertrophy; as such, the patient should be referred for a transrectal ultrasound, which will aid in identifying any solid nodules so that a needle biopsy can be performed. Magnetic resonance imaging and computed tomography of the pelvis are more useful in staging prostate cancer after the disease has been confirmed. Radiography of the kidney, ureters, and bladder is not typically used to diagnose prostate cancer.

13. c

The patient's nausea, fatigue, and cramping that radiates to the back and upper thighs are most indicative of primary dysmenorrhea, which occurs in younger women as a result of high prostaglandin levels. Estrogen or progesterone hormones may be found in oral contraceptives, which may be used in treating primary dysmenorrhea. Dopamine levels may be increased through the use of antidepressants, such as selegiline, which may produce dysmenorrhea as an adverse effect.

14. b

Tibial bone mineral density (BMD) is not measured when diagnosing osteoporosis. The dual energy x-ray absorptiometry test measures BMD in the hip, spine, wrist, and ankle because these sites are most effective at predicting osteoporotic fractures.

15. d

Patients experiencing emotional and psychological symptoms associated with premenstrual syndrome are generally advised to make dietary changes to alieve symptoms, such as reducing caffeine and salt and increasing intake of vitamins E and B6. A similar diet is recommended for patients with secondary dysmenorrhea, but these patients typically require further treatment options depending on etiology and would not generally be advised to increase intake of vitamin B6. Management of fibrocystic breast disease may include caffeine reduction and hormone therapy, among others, but does not generally include increased intake of vitamins E and B6. Patients with pelvic inflammatory disease are primarily treated with antibiotics.

16. a

Alendronate (Fosamax) belongs to the drug class of bisphosphonates, which are used to treat osteonecrosis of the jaw, especially in women diagnosed with cancer. Trimethoprim-sulfamethoxazole (Bactrim), ciprofloxacin (Cipro), and amoxicillin (Amoxil) may be used to manage symptoms associated with urinary tract infections, not osteoporosis.

17. a

Macrolides are least likely to contribute to erectile dysfunction. H2 receptor blockers, antihypertensives, and diuretics are all strongly associated with erectile dysfunction, as well as other drugs such as antidepressants, NSAIDs, and anti-epileptics.

18. a

Terazosin, an alpha-blocker, serves to provide immediate symptom relief in cases of benign prostatic hyperplasia (BPH) by relaxing the muscles of the bladder and prostate. Dutasteride and other 5-alpha-reductase inhibitors may also see use in shrinking enlarged prostates; however, these drugs are primarily effective in patients with larger prostates or in patients who cannot tolerate alpha-blockers. Saw palmetto, an herb, has seen use in treatment of BPH in the past, but studies are inconclusive on the full efficacy. Phosphodiesterase-5 inhibitors, such as avanafil, may be useful in treating concomitant erectile dysfunction and BPH, but evidence regarding efficacy in the treatment of BPH is limited at this time.

19. c

A dipstick urinalysis detecting esterase would confirm a lower urinary tract infection in a patient presenting with descriptions of dysuria, nocturia, and increased urinary frequency. A dipstick urinalysis detecting esterase yields evidence of infection and is considered to be very sensitive but not specific. Visual examination of the urine's appearance is neither highly sensitive nor specific, as the patient's urine sample may have an unusual appearance due to medication or other factors. A urinalysis detecting nitrates yields highly specific, but not sensitive, test results for bacteriuria. A blood test is usually not required unless it is to confirm suspicion of other disorders (e.g., kidney damage, blood disorders).

20. b

Calcium supplementation is not as necessary in a 56-year-old menopausal patient on hormone therapy (HT) because of the increased levels of estrogen from HT. Potassium, phosphorus, and iron are not significantly affected by HT and therefore do not need to be decreased.

21. a

Calcium supplementation is a mainstay of treatment for osteoporosis, as indicated by the patient's reduced stature, altered balance, and dowager hump; as such, dietary recommendations should include yogurt and green leafy vegetables. Although salmon is also rich in calcium, legumes are not particularly high in calcium. Fruits and raw vegetables would be better suited to treating a vitamin C deficiency than osteoporosis. Red meats and iron-fortified breads are a good source of iron, but not calcium.

22. c

Menopause, which often presents with breast size reduction, sleep disturbances, and stress incontinence, may result in an increase, not decrease, in melanin synthesis. Melanin synthesis becomes less regulated by the lack of estrogen, resulting in brown spots. Other common signs of menopause include thinning of the vagina, dry skin, and decreased skin elasticity.

23. b

A history of infertility is not a contraindication for menopausal or postmenopausal women seeking hormone therapy. A history of breast cancer, uterine cancer, or myocardial infarction—or any combination of these—are contraindications for hormone therapy in menopausal and postmenopausal women.

24. c

Three-fourths of all bone loss in individuals with osteoporosis is due to hypoestrogenic states, rather than the aging process itself. Age is also a factor, but it is not responsible for all bone loss in osteoporosis cases.

25. c

A finding of CIN 2 under the Bethesda System (TBS) indicates moderate cervical dysplasia. TBS, a standardized measure of the degree of abnormal cells in Pap test results, ranges from the least amount of dysplasia to the highest (CIN 1 to CIN 3). Human papillomavirus and mild dysplasia, which cause low-grade dysplasia, are classified under CIN 1, and severe dysplasia and carcinoma in situ are under CIN 3. Atypical squamous cells of undetermined significance are classified as ASC-US.

26. c

Of the choices, nocturia is not a typical finding of pelvic inflammatory disease (PID); rather, it is a symptom of urinary tract infection. Symptoms of PID may include chills, dysuria, and dyspareunia, among others.

27. a

A dual-energy x-ray absorptiometry scan that returns with a T-score of -2.7 indicates fully-developed osteoporosis; as such, a regimen of alendronate, a bisphosphonate, is the best course of treatment at this time. Increases in calcium through diet and supplements are helpful measures in both prevention and treatment of osteoporosis; however, as the patient's condition is fully developed, pharmacological intervention is more important. Coumadin, an anticoagulant, is generally used in the treatment of thrombosis, not osteoporosis.

28. a

Tension is an emotional symptom of premenstrual syndrome (PMS), which may also be accompanied by irritability, confusion, and mood swings, among other symptoms. Headaches, breast tenderness, and poor coordination are somatic symptoms of PMS.

29. c

Scrotal edema is not a sign of acute bacterial prostatitis; rather, it is an indication of epididymitis. Findings of acute bacterial prostatitis include fever, chills, and low back pain, as well as dysuria, increased urgency or frequency of urination, and nocturia.

30. d

The projection of areola and nipple as a secondary mound indicates Tanner stage 4 of female breast development. Tanner stage 1 presents with preadolescent breasts, whereas Tanner stage 2 presents with breast buds with areolar enlargement. Lastly, Tanner stage 3 presents with breast enlargement without separate nipple contour.

31. b

Corticosteroids are not recommended for relief of symptoms associated with premenstrual syndrome (PMS) because the symptoms may actually worsen due to the possibility of causing emotional side effects, such as mood swings. Pharmacologic options for managing PMS may include selective serotonin reuptake inhibitors to help relieve physical and emotional symptoms; hormonal birth control, which may help to relieve severe PMS symptoms; and vitamins, such as vitamins E and B6.

32. d

A patient who is going through menopause may experience decreased, rather than increased, sebaceous gland activity. Furthermore, loss of skin elasticity and changes in pigmentation commonly occur during menopause. Breasts typically decrease in tone and size during this time as well.

33. d

Acute bacterial prostatitis, most often caused by *Escherichia coli*, is the most likely diagnosis because the patient's symptoms include low back pain, fever, nocturia, and dysuria, as well as findings of a boggy, tender prostate. The positive urine culture also indicates acute bacterial prostatitis. *Chlamydia trachomatis* is the most common causative agent of epididymitis in younger men but is also known to cause nonbacterial prostatitis. *Mycoplasma genitalium* and *Gardnerella vaginalis* may also produce nonbacterial prostatitis in men, but are not common causes of acute bacterial prostatitis.

34. d

As pelvic inflammatory disease (PID) most often stems from infection, a thyroid-stimulating hormone test would not likely be ordered to diagnose the condition. Diagnostics for PID include sexually transmitted disease screenings and erythrocyte sedimentation rate tests to rule out other conditions. Ultrasounds are used to see ovarian cysts and scarring in the reproductive organs.

35. b

Menopause causes the epithelium tissue to atrophy and become thinner, not thicker, which may result in decreased stimulation in the vagina. Other findings of menopause include thinning cervical mucus and increased pH levels in vaginal lactic acid, which may increase susceptibility to vaginitis and urinary tract infections.

36. d

Based on the patient's presentation of lower abdominal pain, vomiting, fever over 38 °C, positive cervical motion tenderness, and positive test for *Chlamydia trachomatis*, she is most likely experiencing pelvic inflammatory disease, which is commonly treated with a combination of ceftriaxone and doxycycline with or without metronidazole. Other regimens include ofloxacin or levofloxacin with or without metronidazole, or cefoxitin plus probenecid and doxycycline with or without metronidazole.

37. a

African American ethnicity, overweight status, and family history of uterine cancer are not predisposing factors for osteoporosis. Although Hispanics are not considered to be at increased risk of developing osteoporosis, a predominantly sedentary lifestyle may contribute to this disorder. Caucasian and Asian women are more likely to develop osteoporosis. Risk factors for osteoporosis include being underweight, using tobacco, and experiencing early onset menopause.

38. b

A suspected diagnosis of trichomoniasis, which is characterized by vaginal erythema, "strawberry patches" on the cervix or vagina, vaginal erythema, pruritus, and a malodorous, yellowish-green discharge, would be confirmed with a wet prep test that shows motile trichomonads. Clue cells would typically turn up on a wet prep test if bacterial vaginosis is the cause, and candidiasis would generally produce pseudo hyphae. White blood cells are not diagnostic criterion for trichomoniasis.

39. c

Chlorophyllin is not a phosphodiesterase inhibitor but an internal deodorant used to improve breath odor and improve odors from bodily fluids. Sildenafil, vardenafil, and tadalafil are phosphodiesterase inhibitors used to treat erectile dysfunction.

40. a

Although cultures for gonorrhea and chlamydia may be performed to confirm a diagnosis of pelvic inflammatory disease (PID), a Venereal Disease Research Laboratory test would not see use, as it is used to screen for syphilis. Elevated erythrocyte sedimentation rate and C-reactive protein would both improve diagnostic specificity for PID, and an ultrasound helps to isolate ovarian cysts.

DISCUSSION

Tanner Staging for Girls: Breast Development

Presentation

In Tanner staging for girls, breast development occurs in five stages. Tanner stage 1 begins with preadolescent breasts, which bud with areolar enlargement in Tanner stage 2. The breasts then enlarge without separate nipple contour in Tanner stage 3. In Tanner stage 4, the areolas and nipples project as secondary mounds on each breast. Finally, in Tanner stage 5, adult breasts develop, the areola recedes, and the nipple projects.[1]

As for Tanner staging in boys, the testes, scrotum, and penis are present in preadolescence in stage 1. In Tanner stage 2, the scrotum and testes enlarge; the scrotum also roughens and reddens. In Tanner stage 3, the penis elongates. Then, it enlarges in breadth during stage 4. Additionally, in this stage, the glans develops and rugae appear. The testes, scrotum, and penis reach the adult shape and appearance in Tanner stage 5.[2]

Amenorrhea

Overview

Amenorrhea is the absence of menstrual flow. Primary amenorrhea is indicated by the absence of menarche by 16 years of age. Important initial primary care screens include a vaginal exam and a determination of a negative human chorionic gonadotropin (hCG) test. Teenagers with this type of amenorrhea are often referred to specialists for evaluation for underlying conditions, such as chromosomal defects, anatomic anomalies, hormonal imbalances, tumors, and trauma. Secondary amenorrhea, on the other hand, is the cessation of menses after a normal menstrual cycle has been established. Pregnancy is the most common cause of secondary amenorrhea and should also be ruled out in a diagnosis of primary amenorrhea.[3]

Presentation

Primary amenorrhea often presents with abnormal growth and development, as well as an absence of menarche and secondary sexual characteristics. Secondary amenorrhea, on the other hand, is indicated by an absence of expected menses and the loss of a history of regular cycles, which would warrant a review of the patient's overall health.[3] The most common cause of secondary amenorrhea is pregnancy.

Workup

Patients with amenorrhea should receive an hCG test, which is the first recommended step in evaluating secondary amenorrhea.[4] In addition to this pregnancy test, patients with amenorrhea should undergo a complete physical evaluation to identify etiology; specifically, the pelvic exam aids in identifying any anatomical defects. Additionally, patients with primary amenorrhea should be referred to a gynecologist or endocrinologist, whereas secondary amenorrhea patients should be referred for other studies, such as blood tests to check the patient's hormone levels.[5]

Treatment

Treatment of amenorrhea is directed at the underlying cause.[6] If possible, treatment should aim to help patients achieve fertility, if desired, and prevent complications of the disease process.[4] Moreover, amenorrhea patients may also respond to weight control and a change in exercise routine in cases that are caused by obesity, weight loss, or vigorous exercise.[5]

Cervical Cytology Test: Abnormal Results

Overview

A cervical cytology test is used to detect the presence of abnormal and precancerous cells within the cervix. As a screening test, the cervical cytology test has lowered the cervical cancer rate by more than 50%.[7] However, because one-third of all cervical cytology tests may have false-negative results, it is necessary to screen the patient as recommended. Cervical cancer stands as one of the most common gynecologic cancers in the United States. Additional risk factors for abnormal cervical cytology test results include cigarette smoking and the presence of human papillomavirus (HPV). Finally, abnormal cervical cytology test results may occur in patients who have had multiple sexual partners early in life, or those who have a male partner with a history of multiple sexual partners.[8]

Workup

The interpretations of cervical cytology test results are classified by the categories of the Bethesda Classification System. Normal cervical cytology test results are often indicated by the absence of atypia and malignancy. Abnormal test results, on the other hand, may include infections and reactive or reparative changes.[8] Low-grade squamous intraepithelial lesions (SIL) are categorized as cervical intraepithelial neoplasia (CIN) 1. HPV and mild dysplasia are classified as CIN1. High-grade SIL are categorized as CIN2, CIN3, and carcinoma in situ. Moderate and severe dysplasia are classified as CIN2 and CIN3, respectively.[7]

Treatment

When a cervical cytology test shows abnormal changes, further testing is needed, depending on the test results. Follow-up testing may include a colposcopy-directed biopsy and an HPV test, which assesses for HPV types that most likely cause cancer.[9] Patients with a Bethesda classification of CIN2 or higher should be referred for treatment.

Cervical Cancer Screening Guidelines for Average-Risk Women (see table 8.1)

Vulvovaginitis

Overview

Vulvovaginitis is an inflammation or infection rooted in the vulva and vagina that often produces from bacteria, protozoa, and fungi. Common causative sources of vulvovaginitis include trichomoniasis, bacterial vaginosis, and candidiasis. Of these causes, only trichomoniasis, which is often asymptomatic in men, is classified as a sexually transmitted infection (STI).[10,11]

Presentation

In cases of trichomoniasis, patients often present with a malodorous, frothy, and yellowish-green discharge. Additional findings of trichomoniasis may include pruritus and "strawberry patches" on the cervix and vagina. Moreover, patients may also experience dyspareunia, dysuria, and vaginal erythema. Vulvovaginal erythema with pruritus is also a common finding of candidiasis, which presents with a thick, white, and curd-like discharge. Finally, bacterial vaginosis may also present with a discharge, but this discharge is watery, gray, and "fishy" smelling.[10,11,12]

Workup

In the microscopic wet-prep diagnostic tests for vulvovaginitis, normal saline mixture is used to test for trichomoniasis and bacterial vaginosis. Normal saline typically shows motile trichomonads in patients with trichomoniasis and clue cells in patients with bacterial vaginosis. In candidiasis, on the other hand, a potassium hydroxide mixture commonly shows pseudo-hyphae.[10,11,12]

Treatment

Trichomoniasis is commonly treated by metronidazole (Flagyl) in a single dose of 2 grams by mouth, or 500 mg administered orally twice a day for 7 days. Metronidazole is also a treatment for bacterial vaginosis and is given according to the following dosage guidelines: either 500 mg administered orally twice a day for 7 days, 2 grams by mouth in a single dose, or gel (0.75%) 5 grams intravaginally twice a day for 5 days. Clindamycin (Cleocin) vaginal cream (2%) is another possible treatment for bacterial vaginosis, administered in a single dose of 5 grams intravaginally at bedtime for 7 days, or 300 mg administered orally twice a day for 7 days. Candidiasis, on the other hand, is often treated by miconazole (Mono-stat) or clotrimazole (Gyne-Lotrimin) (1%), 5 grams intravaginally at bedtime for 7 days. A terconazole (Terazol) 80 mg suppository is also a viable treatment for candidiasis, with one suppository at bedtime for 3 days. Lastly, butoconazole cream (2%) may also be given to candidiasis patients, administered in a single dose of 5 grams intravaginally at bedtime for 3 days.[13]

Pelvic Inflammatory Disease (PID)

Overview

Pelvic inflammatory disease (PID) is a general term for inflammation and infection that affects the uterus, ovaries, fallopian tubes, and surrounding tissues. The most predominant sexually transmitted disease (STD) associated with PID is *Chlamydia trachomatis*.[14] *Neisseria gonorrhoeae*, which is also transmitted sexually, is another common cause of PID.[15] Other prevalent polymicrobial causative agents of PID include *Escherichia coli*, *Gardnerella vaginalis*, *Haemophilus influenzae*, and *Streptococcus agalactiae*.[16,17,18]

Presentation

PID typically presents with fever, vaginal discharge, and pain in the lower abdomen, as well as in the pelvis and lower back.[19] Chills, nausea, and vomiting are other common signs and symptoms of PID. Moreover, patients may experience dysuria, dyspareunia, and infertility.[16,17,18]

Workup

Physical examination findings of PID include positive cervical motion tenderness, a fever greater than 38 °C, and adnexal and abdominal tenderness. PID workup may also include STD testing and ultrasound documentation for a potential ovarian cyst. An elevated erythrocyte sedimentation rate (ESR) and an elevated C-reactive protein level are typical diagnostic findings of PID.[16,17,18]

Treatment

Empiric, broad-spectrum antibiotic coverage is recommended for patients with PID. Outpatient management of PID may include one of the regimens listed in table 8.2.

Dysmenorrhea

Overview

Dysmenorrhea is a disorder of cramping pain that occurs with menstruation. The two categories of dysmenorrhea are primary and secondary. Primary dysmenorrhea, which is more common, occurs after the onset of menses and when no pelvic pathology is identified.[20] Secondary dysmenorrhea, on the other hand, is commonly associated with variants of pelvic disease and also results from identifiable organic diseases.[21] Primary dysmenorrhea occurs in adolescent women, resulting from high levels of prostaglandin, whereas secondary dysmenorrhea occurs in women over 20 years of age.[22]

Table 8.1 Cervical Cancer Screening Guidelines for Average-Risk Women[a]

	American Cancer Society (ACS), American Society for Colposcopy and Cervical Pathology (ASCCP), and American Society for Clinical Pathology (ASCP)[b]	U.S Preventive Services Task Force (USPSTF)[c]	American College of Obstetricians and Gynecologists (ACOG)[d]
When to start screening[e]	Age 21. Women younger than 21 years should not be screened regardless of the age of sexual initiation or other risk factors. (Strong recommendation)	Age 21. (A recommendation) Recommend against screening women younger than 21 years. (D recommendation)	Age 21 regardless of the age of onset of sexual activity. Should be avoided in women younger than 21 years. (Level A evidence)
Statement about annual screening	Women of any age should not be screened annually by any screening method. (Strong recommendation)	Individuals and clinicians can use the annual cervical cytology screening visit as an opportunity to discuss other health problems and preventive measures. Individuals, clinicians, and health systems should seek effective ways to facilitate the receipt of recommended preventive services at intervals that are beneficial to the patient. Efforts also should be made to ensure that individuals are able to seek care for additional health concerns as they present.	Physicians should inform their patients that annual gynecologic examinations may be appropriate. (Level C evidence)[f]
Screening method and intervals[g]			
Cytology (conventional or liquid based)			
21–29 years of age	Every 3 years[h] (Strong recommendation)	Every 3 years (A recommendation)	Every 3 years (Level A evidence)
30–65 years of age	Every 3 years[h] (Strong recommendation)	Every 3 years (A recommendation)	May screen every 3 years with history of 3 negative cytology tests (Level A evidence)
HPV co-test (cytology + HPV test administered together)			
21–29 years of age	HPV co-testing should not be used for women younger than 30 years	Recommend against HPC co-testing women younger than 30 year (D recommendation)	Not recommended for women younger than 30 years
30–65 years of age	Every 5 years (Strong recommendation); this is the preferred method (Weak recommendation)	For women who want to extend their screening interval, HPV co-testing every 5 years is an option (A recommendation)	Every 5 years if cytology normal, HPV test negative (Level A evidence)

Table 8.1	Cervical Cancer Screening Guidelines for Average-Risk Women		
	American Cancer Society (ACS), American Society for Colposcopy and Cervical Pathology (ASCCP), and American Society for Clinical Pathology (ASCP)[b]	U.S Preventive Services Task Force (USPSTF)[c]	American College of Obstetricians and Gynecologists (ACOG)[d]
Primary HPV testing[i]			
	For women aged 30–65 years, screening by HPV testing alone is not recommended in most clinical settings (Weak recommendation)[j]	Recommends against screening for cervical cancer with HPV testing (alone or in combination with cytology) in women younger than 30 years (D recommendation)	Not addressed
When to stop screening	Women older than 65 years with adequate screening history should not be screened. Women younger than 65 years with a history of CIN2, CIN3, or AIS should continue screening for at least 20 years after spontaneous regression or appropriate management (Weak recommendation)	Women older than 65 years with adequate recent screening with normal cervical cytology tests, who are not otherwise at high risk for cervical cancer (D recommendation)[k]	Between 65–70 years of age with 3 consecutive normal cytology tests and no abnormal tests in the past 10 years (Level B evidence). An older woman who is sexually active and has multiple partners should continue to have routine screening.
Screening post-total hysterectomy	Women who have had a total hysterectomy (removal of the uterus and cervix) should stop screening, unless the hysterectomy was done as a treatment for cervical pre-cancer or cancer. Women who have had a hysterectomy without removal of the cervix (supra-cervical hysterectomy) should continue screening according to guidelines. (Strong recommendation)	Recommend against screening in women who have had a hysterectomy with removal of the cervix and who do not have a history of a high-grade precancerous lesion (CIN2 or CIN3) or cervical cancer (D recommendation)	If removal for benign disease and no history of high-grade CIN or worse, may discontinue screening. (Level A evidence). Women whom a negative history cannot be documented should continue to be screened. (Level B evidence)
The need for bimanual pelvic exam	Not addressed in 2012 guidelines but was addressed in 2002 ACS guidelines.[l]	Addressed in USPSTV ovarian cancer screening recommendations (draft).[m]	Physicians should inform their patients that annual gynecologic examinations may be appropriate. (Level C evidence)[f]
Screening among those immunized against HPV 16/18	Women at any age with a history of HPV vaccination should be screened according to the age-specific recommendations for the general population.	The possibility that vaccination might reduce the need for screening with cytology alone or in combination with HPV testing is not established. Given these uncertainties, women who have been vaccinated should continue to be screened.	Recommendations remain the same regardless of vaccination status. (Level C evidence)

Table 8.2	Treatment Options for Pelvic Inflammatory Disease
Parenteral treatments	Cefotetan, 2 grams IV every 12 hr *or* cefoxitin, 2 grams IV ever 6 hr *Plus* Doxycycline, 100 mg PO/IV every 12 hr
	Clindamycin, 900 mg IV every 8 hr *Plus* Gentamicin, loading dose IV/IM of 2 mg/kg followed by maintenance dose of 1.5 mg/kg every 8 hr
Oral treatments	Ceftriaxone, 250 mg IM single dose *Plus* Doxycycline, 100 mg PO twice a day for 14 days *With or without* Metronidazole, 500 mg PO twice a day for 14 days
	Cefoxitin, 2 grams IM single dose plus Probenecid, 1 gram PO, administered concurrently *Plus* Doxycycline, 100 mg PO twice a day for 14 days *With or without* Metronidazole, 500 mg PO twice a day for 14 days
	A parenteral third-generation cephalosporin, such as ceftizoxime or cefotaxime *Plus* Doxycycline, 100 mg PO twice a day for 14 days *With or without* Metronidazole, 500 mg PO twice a day for 14 days

Note. Pelvic Inflammatory Disease: Sexually Transmitted Diseases Treatment Guidelines, 2010. http://www.cdc.gov/std/treatment/2010/pid.htm. Published 2014. Accessed April 2015. Reproduced with permission.

Presentation

The cramping pain of dysmenorrhea is usually located in the lower abdomen above the pelvis.[23] In primary dysmenorrhea, the patient's cramping pain often radiates towards the upper thighs and back. Additional findings of primary dysmenorrhea include headaches, diarrhea, nausea, vomiting, and fatigue. Moreover, primary dysmenorrhea is self-limiting and may last up to 72 hours. Physical exam findings of secondary dysmenorrhea, on the other hand, are related to the etiology of the condition. Signs and symptoms occur due to pelvic abnormalities from such conditions as endometriosis.[20]

Workup

A diagnosis of dysmenorrhea is based on clinical findings.[21] Primary dysmenorrhea often presents with a normal pelvic exam; typically, the only exceptional finding is uterine tenderness during menses. Conversely, physical exam findings of secondary dysmenorrhea are closely related to etiology, and a pelvic examination focuses on detecting causes of secondary dysmenorrhea.[20] Further tests that may be used to diagnose dysmenorrhea include a complete blood count (CBC), laparoscopy, and ultrasound. Additionally, cultures may help to rule out STIs.[24]

Treatment

The treatment of primary dysmenorrhea is directed at relieving the patient's cramping pelvic pain.[21] Patients may be prescribed oral contraceptive pills or prostaglandin synthetase inhibitors such as naproxen (Naprosyn), indomethacin (Indocin), and Advil or other forms of ibuprofen. Recommended non-pharmacological treatments for primary dysmenorrhea include exercise, a high-fiber diet, and reduction of the patient's sugar, caffeine, and salt intake. Management of secondary dysmenorrhea, on the other hand, depends upon the etiology and involves correcting the underlying organic cause, which may involve specific measures, such as surgery, to treat pelvic pathologic conditions.[21]

Abnormal Uterine Bleeding

Overview

Abnormal uterine bleeding usually stems from endocrine dysfunction. Heavy bleeding episodes may also indicate an underlying condition such as polycystic ovarian disease, immature hypothalamic-pituitary-ovarian axis (most often seen during adolescence), resistant follicular stimulation (i.e., perimenopause), and other conditions.[25]

Presentation

Abnormal uterine bleeding can be extremely heavy and vary in frequency and duration. Patterns of abnormal bleeding include oligomenorrhea, which is infrequent and irregular with a frequency of more than 40 days. Polymenorrhea is also irregular, but has a frequency of less than 18 days. Menorrhagia occurs in regular frequency, but bleeding is excessive and prolonged. Another form of prolonged, frequent, and excessive bleeding is menometrorrhagia, which is indicated by irregular bleeding patterns. Metrorrhagia is a pattern of bleeding between cycles, whereas intermenstrual bleeding varies in quantity between cycles.[25]

Workup

The initial diagnostic test of abnormal uterine bleeding is a quantitative hCG test, which helps to rule out ectopic pregnancy and threatened or incomplete abortion.[26] A urinalysis is also done, and patients may also receive a CBC and hormone measurement tests, such as thyroid stimulating hormone and prolactin tests.[27,28] Furthermore, a pelvic examination should be performed to look for infections, in addition to an STD screening.

Treatment

It is recommended that patients receive a consultation and referral for treatment of abnormal uterine bleeding.[7] Other common treatments of abnormal uterine bleeding include oral contraceptives, estrogen, and progestins.[26] Oral contraceptives and progestins are often tried first in perimenopausal women, and progestins may be used alone when estrogen is contraindicated.[27]

Premenstrual Syndrome (PMS)/ Premenstrual Dysphoric Disorder (PDD)

Overview

Premenstrual syndrome (PMS) and premenstrual dysphoric disorder (PDD) consist of somatic and affective symptoms that typically occur 7–10 days prior to menstruation and end with the onset of menses. Although the precise etiology of PMS is unknown, the incidence slowly increases from adolescence and peaks during a patient's 30s. PMS then quickly decreases after 41 years of age. PDD is considered a severe form of PMS.[29]

Presentation

Usually, no physical findings are specifically helpful in establishing a diagnosis of PMS, which more often presents with somatic and emotional symptoms.[30] The most common somatic symptoms of PMS are fatigue and feelings of being bloated.[31] Other symptoms may include headaches, body aches, breast tenderness, poor coordination, and food cravings. Emotional symptoms of PMS often include mood swings as well as depressive symptoms, irritability, and fear of loss of control.[32] Hypersensitivity, anxiety, tension, and confusion are also emotional signs and symptoms of PMS.[29]

Workup

Diagnosis of PMS is often made by the patient's history, which may be recorded in a menstrual and PMS diary. Additionally, PMS can be diagnosed by a physical exam, which works to rule out other possible causes of the patient's complaints.[32] For patients suspected of having PDD, a diagnosis is made based on the criteria of the fifth edition of the Diagnostic and Statistical Manual of Mental Disorders, which includes a demonstration of five or more of the aforementioned somatic and emotional symptoms.[31]

Treatment

A number of strategies have been suggested for assisting in symptomatic management of PMS. For patients with mild symptoms, lifestyle changes including exercise and taking supplements such as vitamin E or vitamin B6 are recommended.[33] Other dietary guidelines may include salt and caffeine restriction; caffeine intake can escalate tension, depression, anxiety, and irritability, whereas salt intake may result in bloating and fluid retention.[32,33]

As for pharmacological treatments of PMS, selective serotonin reuptake inhibitors (SSRIs) are often implemented as first-line treatment and recommended for relief of emotional symptoms, such as anxiety and irritability.[27,32] Other medications—such as clomipramine (Anafranil)—may also inhibit the patient's serotonin reuptake, even though these drugs may not be classified as SSRIs.[31] Oral contraceptive pills and progesterone are options for hormone manipulation, which may be effective for some women.[27] Antianxiety medications that may be given to patients with PMS include buspirone (BuSpar), alprazolam (Xanax), and tricyclic antidepressants, such as nortriptyline (Pamelor).[30] Other medications used in the treatment of PMS include bromocriptine (Parlodel) and atenolol (Tenormin).[34]

Fibrocystic Breast Disease

Overview

Fibrocystic breast disease is a benign breast condition characterized by increased growth and development of fibrosis of the breast tissue. Fibrocystic changes are the most commonly reported breast symptoms, and approximately 50% of all women will present with such findings; however, these findings are generally not indicative of breast cancer.[35,36,37] The exact cause of fibrocystic breast disease is unknown, although estrogen may play a role.[38]

Presentation

In a presentation of fibrocystic breast disease, the patient's breasts may be tender. Breast tenderness is often related to the patient's cycle and found in the affected area. A physical examination may also reveal nodularity, as well as formation and enlargement of cysts in the patient's breasts. The number of cysts is variable, and the cysts themselves are mobile. Moreover, the cysts vary in location, size, shape, and consistency, and may be round or nodular as well as soft or firm. Lastly, the patient may present with breast discharge, but rarely nipple discharge; however, when nipple discharge is present, the fluid is typically clear.[35,39,40]

Workup

After an initial ultrasound, other diagnostics may include a mammography, fine needle aspiration cytology, and excisional biopsy.[41]

Treatment

Treatment of fibrocystic breast disease is aimed at the underlying cause of the patient's condition.[41] The patient may be treated with vitamin supplements, warm soaks three times a day, and a low-sodium diet. Additional treatments of fibrocystic breast disease include hormonal therapy and surgical intervention.[39,40]

Breast Cancer

Overview

Breast cancer is a type of cancer that presents with malignant breast tissue and most often involves glandular breast cells in the ducts or lobules.[42] Among women, breast cancer is the second most common type of diagnosed cancer and the second most common cause of cancer deaths.[43] Moreover, the lifetime risk for breast cancer in the United States is one in eight women. If breast cancer has presented in a first degree relative, the risk of breast cancer typically increases two-fold to four-fold.[44]

Presentation

Breast cancer is often asymptomatic within the early stages and presents with a mass with poorly defined borders, which may be detected during physical examination or mammography.[42,45] The mass is typically non-tender and painless, although pain may occur later.[46] Other signs and symptoms that may occur during the later stages of the condition include nipple retraction, ulceration, and skin changes such as dimpling and erythema.[45] These findings, along with lymphadenopathy, are often detected during a physical examination. Lastly, blood or other types of fluids may discharge from the nipple as the cancer metastasizes.[47]

Workup

An evaluation of breast cancer should begin with the patient's complaints and clinical history.[45] A referral for diagnostic tests is subsequently required to differentiate benign lesions from cancerous lesions. The diagnostics of breast cancer are similar to those of fibrocystic breast disease and include ultrasonography, mammography, fine needle aspiration cytology, and excisional biopsy.[48] As with fibrocystic breast disease, excisional biopsy is the most reliable diagnostic, as it allows for staging and is used to identify masses and calcifications.[49]

Treatment

Treatment for breast cancer is based on factors such as the type and stage of the cancer, in addition to the patient's sensitivity to certain hormones.[47] Surgery is considered the primary treatment for early stage breast cancer and may eradicate the cancer completely without the need for other treatments.[45] Radiation therapy is also usually used in the treatment of breast cancer, and patients may be treated with chemotherapy and hormonal therapy as well.[42]

Breast Cancer Screening

Breast cancer screening guidelines from the American Cancer Society (ACS), the United States Preventive Service Task Force (USPSTF), and the American Congress of Obstetricians and Gynecologists (ACOG) are listed in table 8.3.

Menopause

Overview

Menopause is a cessation of ovarian function that heralds the conclusion of reproductive potential in women. The average age of onset of menopause is 51 years, but may typically begin anywhere from 45 to 55 years of age.[50] Furthermore, menopause may be induced by biological aging, surgical removal, chemotherapy, or radiation.[50]

Table 8.3	Breast Cancer Screening Recommendations		
	ACS	USPSTF	ACOG
When to begin?	Begin at age 40; if there is a family history of breast cancer, perform an MRI in addition to a mammogram	For ages 40–49, no routine screening; individualized decisions before 50	Annually for ages 40–49
How often?	Annually for ages 40–74	Every 2 years for ages 50–74	Annually for ages 50–74
When to end?	No recommendation for age to stop; "continue as long as the woman is in good health"	For ages 75 and older, no specific recommendations	No recommendation
Clinical breast exam?	For ages 20–39, every 3 years; annually, starting at age 40	Not recommended	Every year beginning at age 19
Self breast exam?	Optional beginning at age 21; women should be informed of potential benefits and harms	Not recommended	Can be recommended despite lack of supporting evidence

Presentation

Menopause commonly presents with neuroendocrine changes, such as mood changes, depression, and sleep disturbances. Menopause patients may also experience vasomotor instability, which results in symptoms such as hot flashes and night sweats.[51] Skin changes such as dryness, loss of elasticity, and altered sebaceous gland activity are also indicative of menopause, along with changes in pigmentation of the patient's skin.[52] Additionally, the patient's breasts may decrease in tone and size.[53]

Vaginal and urinary problems may start or increase around the time of menopause.[54] Estrogen deficiencies lead to a thinning and atrophy of the patient's vaginal epithelium, which may result in vaginitis and cause symptoms such as pruritus, dyspareunia, and dryness.[55] Reduced vaginal stimulation may also occur. In addition to vaginal atrophy, patients may also experience atrophy of the vulva and urethra. Atrophy of the vulva commonly occurs along with other changes of the vulva, such as thinning of tissue and loss or thinning of pubic hair. Atrophy of the urethra, on the other hand, is one of the genitourinary changes indicative of menopause; other genitourinary changes include cystitis and stress incontinence.[56] The patient's uterus may also prolapse, decrease in tone, and reduce in size.[57]

Other conditions associated with menopause include coronary artery disease, which is the leading cause of morbidity and mortality in postmenopausal women.[58] Menopause patients may also experience other cardiovascular issues such as atherosclerosis. Moreover, menopause may cause osteoporosis, which is pervasive in older women.[58]

Workup

A diagnosis of menopause is based on a clinical evaluation.[52] Blood and urine tests can be used to evaluate changes in the patient's hormone levels.[59] Other tests that may be performed include estradiol, follicle-stimulating hormone, and luteinizing hormone tests.[52]

Treatment

Hormonal therapy, which includes estrogen and progestin, is the most effective treatment for symptoms of menopause.[52] Types of estrogen that may be used to treat menopause include estradiol (Estrace, Estraderm, Climara), conjugated estrogen (Premarin), and estrone sulfate.[60] Progestin treatment, on the other hand, may be cyclic or continuous, although it is typically unnecessary if the patient has undergone a hysterectomy.[61] If hormonal therapy is contraindicated or refused, the patient may be treated by lifestyle changes in dietary and exercise regimens.[59] Additionally, calcium supplementation is recommended in cases where estrogen therapy is and is not pursued.[62] Finally, the benefits and risks of menopause treatment should

rely primarily on whether the family history shows one or more of the three major possible concerns: breast cancer, uterine cancer, or myocardial infarction or coronary artery disease.[63]

Systemic Lupus Erythematosus (SLE)

Overview

Systemic lupus erythematosus (SLE) is a chronic inflammatory disease that can affect any organ in the body and follows a relapsing and remitting course.[64,65] More than 90% of all cases occur in women, and signs and symptoms usually start around childbearing age.[64]

Presentation

The classical triad of signs and symptoms of SLE is fever, joint pain, and a butterfly rash.[64,7] The presentation and course is variable, however.[64] Musculoskeletal symptoms may include arthralgia and myalgia, among others. The most common dermatologic findings are a malar rash and photosensitivity.[64] Fatigue and weight changes are also common.[1b] Patients may also present with renal, neuropsychiatric, pulmonary, gastrointestinal, cardiac, or hematologic manifestations.[64]

Workup

The diagnosis of SLE is done through the manner of presentation and exclusion of alternative diagnoses.[65] A thorough drug history should be taken because some drugs (e.g., procainamide, hydralazine, isoniazid) may cause lupus-like syndrome. The workup should include a CBC to screen for leukopenia, lymphopenia, anemia, and thrombocytopenia. Tests for antinuclear antibodies (ANA) and antiphospholipid antibodies should also be completed.[64] An ANA test is positive in nearly all patients at some time in the course of their disease.[65] Imaging tests are not routinely performed.[65]

Treatment

Patients should practice sun protection to limit photosensitive rashes and should exercise to combat fatigue. During mild flare-ups, bed rest is often all that is necessary. Pharmacologic therapy consists of antimalarial drugs (e.g., hydroxychloroquine, chloroquine), NSAIDs, and glucocorticoids.[66]

Osteoporosis

Overview

Osteoporosis is a progressive metabolic bone disease that causes deterioration of bone structure and decreased bone density.[67] These changes in bone structure occur due to a reduction not in composition, but in quantity.[7] An abnormally low bone mass puts patients at an increased risk of fractures. Both genders commonly experience bone loss with aging; however, three-fourths of bone loss typically produces as a result of hypoestrogenic states rather than the aging process itself.[68] In addition, osteoporosis may occur in menopausal women due to the loss of estrogen.[67]

Signs and symptoms are more pronounced in Caucasian and Asian women with small or petite body frames.[69] In addition, patients may be at risk for osteoporosis if they are underweight or have a family history of osteoporosis, particularly a parental history of hip fractures.[67] Furthermore, early menopause and estrogen deficiency contribute to osteoporosis.

Other contributing factors to osteoporosis include alcoholism and smoking. High consumption of substances such as caffeine, phosphates, protein, and sodium are risk factors as well. Conversely, a low intake of dietary calcium may contribute to bone loss, which may also result from sedentary lifestyles.[67,70]

Certain medications, such as thyroid hormones, corticosteroids, and anticonvulsants, are risk factors for osteoporosis. Certain diseases may contribute to osteoporosis, such as liver dysfunction, intestinal malabsorption, kidney disease, thyroid and parathyroid conditions, and chronic obstructive pulmonary disease.[67]

Presentation

In the early stages of osteoporosis, no signs or symptoms are typically present, and the patient's condition often does not become apparent unless a fracture has occurred.[69] Loss of height is also suggestive of osteoporosis, and a stooped posture or kyphosis may develop.[70]

Workup

Screening for osteoporosis involves assessing fracture-risk and measuring bone mass density.[71] A dual-energy x-ray absorptiometry (DEXA) measures the consistency of bone in the wrist, spine, hip, and ankle. DEXA test results are reported as T- and Z-scores; the T-score is the number of standard deviations between the patient's result and the mean bone density for the patient's gender and race, while the Z-score compares the patient's density against the population adjusted for race, age, and gender. Normal T-score test results are greater than -1.0 standard deviations. T-scores between -1.0 and -2.5, on the other hand, indicate osteopenia, which is now known as low bone mass. A T-score below -2.5 confirms osteoporosis.

Bone density testing is recommended for all women 65 years of age and older.[7] Additionally, all postmenopausal women younger than 65 years of age should be screened if they have one or more of the following risk factors: a family history of osteoporosis, smoking or alcohol use, excessive exercise, hyperthyroidism, or petite body frame. Moreover, bone density testing is recommended for postmenopausal women with fractures, women who

are undergoing extensive hormone replacement therapy, and patients making decisions about treatment for the condition.[72]

Younger women should be screened for the female athlete triad, which consists of eating disorders, amenorrhea, and bone loss. In this triad, eating disorders and excessive exercise may lead to amenorrhea. Subsequently, amenorrhea leads to decreased amounts of estrogen, which in turn may result in bone loss.[72]

Treatment

In treatment of osteoporosis, prevention is key.[7] Estrogen replacement therapy and avoiding known risk factors are the main components in preventing the onset of osteoporosis. To strengthen the bone, the patient should perform weight-bearing exercises. These exercises include 30 minutes of moderate exercise three to five times a week, such as walking, jogging, dancing, climbing stairs, aerobics, and strength training.[73,74]

Patients with osteoporosis should increase their calcium intake or supplementation based on the daily calcium recommendations for their age.[7] Dietary sources of calcium include dairy products, sardines, salmon with bones, green leafy vegetables, tofu, and calcium-fortified food, among others. Additionally, it is recommended that the patient take 800–1,000 IU a day of vitamin D. The most common supplement used in the treatment of osteoporosis is calcium carbonate, which has the greatest amount of elemental calcium (40%). Supplements, however, should not be taken alongside high fiber foods, and the patient should avoid aluminum-containing antacids, as Ca++ binds with aluminum.[75]

Drug therapies for osteoporosis treatment include estrogens and bisphosphonates. There are rare but serious reports of osteonecrosis of the jaw stemming from the use of biphosphonates, especially in women with cancer undergoing chemotherapy. The Food and Drug Administration, however, has not established a valid connection between the use of biphosphonates and the risk of atypical subtrochanteric femur fractures. Drugs should be administered orally, and the patient should take them with a full glass of water. The patient should also sit upright and avoid food and fluids for the next 30 minutes to 1 hour.[75]

Urinary Tract Infections (UTIs)

Overview

Urinary tract infections (UTIs) are a type of inflammation and infection of the urinary tract caused by microbes such as fungi, viruses, and bacteria.[76] E. coli bacteria are the most common causative organisms of UTIs in women, whereas organisms of the proteus species are the most common causes in men.[76] There are two types of UTIs, both of which affect different parts of the body: Upper UTIs involve the kidneys, whereas lower UTIs involve the bladder, urethra, or prostate.[74] Lower UTIs may be caused by conditions such as cystitis, urethritis, and dysuria frequency syndrome. Upper UTIs, on the other hand, are often caused by other conditions such as pyelonephritis and renal abscesses.[78]

Presentation

UTIs do not always present with signs and symptoms and may be overlooked or mistaken for other conditions in older patients.[79] Signs and symptoms often vary by age and gender.[76] Dysuria is the key symptom of lower UTIs, which may also present with frequency, nocturia, and urgency.[78] Additionally, hematuria occurs in 40%–60% of all UTI patients, particularly when cystitis presents.[80]

Workup

Diagnostic tests of UTIs include analyzing the patient's urine sample to check for bacteria and red or white blood cells (WBCs).[79] A urinalysis usually shows pyuria, which is indicated by a WBC count greater than 10 WBC/ml; the presence of nitrate by dipstick is very specific but not sensitive for bacteriuria.[81] Conversely, esterase detection by dipstick is very sensitive but not specific.[82] Additional diagnostics, such as imaging tests, may be needed for patients who have recurrent UTIs.[76]

Treatment

In the management of lower UTIs, 3-day therapy commonly maximizes benefits of treatment while also minimizing drawbacks. This type of therapy is less costly than a 7-day course, and typically results in fewer side effects.[7] Commonly used agents in treatment of UTIs include nitrofurantoin monohydrate/macrocrystals (Macrobid), trimethoprim-sulfamethoxazole (Bactrim), and fosfomycin trometamol (Monuril, Zambon). Patients who cannot tolerate antimicrobials should be prescribed fluoroquinolones.[83]

Acute Pyelonephritis

Overview

Acute pyelonephritis is a type of UTI that is caused by a viral or bacterial infection of the kidneys. These infections may be caused by many types of bacteria and viruses, with *E. coli* frequently being the cause.[76]

Presentation

Acute pyelonephritis typically presents with fever and chills, which indicates a likely upper UTI.[7,77] Additional common signs and symptoms include vomiting, as well as pain in the flank, lower back, and abdomen. Moreover, although UTIs are often known to be asymptomatic in the elderly, older patients may experience changes in mental status.[77,84]

Workup

The diagnosis of acute pyelonephritis should begin with an assessment of the clinical history as well as a physical examination.[85] A diagnosis is further supported by results of a urinalysis if WBC casts or bacteria are present.[73,84] Among other diagnostics, an elevated ESR is also indicative of acute pyelonephritis.[86]

Treatment

Acute pyelonephritis is best treated with antibiotics, and upper UTIs may be managed in a 14-day to 6-week course.[7] Commonly used agents include trimethoprim-sulfamethoxazole and aminoglycosides, such as gentamicin and tobramycin. Ciprofloxacin (Cipro), quinolones, and amoxicillin/clavulanate (Augmentin) are also common treatment agents.[84] Lastly, hospitalization is recommended in more severe illness.[84]

Urinary Incontinence

Overview

Urinary incontinence is an involuntary loss of bladder control, which occurs when patients are unable to keep urine from leaking out of the urethra.[87] Among other risk factors, urinary incontinence is associated with ever-present risks such as fractures and falls. The condition is common, affecting 25% of all reproductive age women and 40% of all postmenopausal women, but it is also widely underreported, as many patients do not report urinary incontinence to their physicians.[88,89] Moreover, the diagnosis of urinary incontinence is costly at a price exceeding $26 billion annually, which constitutes more than the cost of all cancer care for women.[7]

Urinary incontinence appears in various forms. Stress incontinence, also known as urethral incompetence, is most commonly caused by muscles impairing urethral support.[90] Stress incontinence may also be caused by activities that place increased physical pressure or stress on the abdominal cavity, which affects the bladder.[90] Additionally, intrinsic sphincter deficiencies stemming from pelvic surgery are a common cause of urethral incompetence.[91]

Urge incontinence, on the other hand, is an involuntary leakage that occurs along with an urgent need to void.[89] This type of incontinence is often related to detrusor hyperactivity, which consists of uninhibited bladder contractions.[92] Additional causes of urge incontinence include infections of the genitourinary tract, urinary tones, and neoplasms.[90]

Finally, stress and urge incontinence may appear together in a combined condition, known as mixed incontinence, in which involuntary leakage is associated with urgency and exertion.[90]

Workup

Evaluation of urinary incontinence often includes a physical examination, as well as the patient's history.[89] A urinalysis is needed for all patients, along with a urine culture if an infection is suspected.[92] In certain patients, additional tests, such as post-void residual volume and a positive cough stress test, may also be needed.[90]

Treatment

All patients should keep a diary of recent urinary activities, such as fluids, voids, and incontinence events.[93] Other treatments depend on the patient's particular type of incontinence. Stress incontinence is treated by timed voids to prevent a full bladder, as well as stress control techniques such as squeezing the vaginal muscles before sneezing, lifting, etc.[94] Other treatment options may include surgery, which provides the best chance of curing patients for whom noninvasive procedures are ineffective.[00] The insertion of a vaginal pessary is an alternative to surgery, and a pessary trial may be offered to all women regardless of the patient's characteristics.[95]

Treatment of urge incontinence, on the other hand, usually begins with bladder training.[96] Relaxation techniques may be used to suppress and distract the patient's urge to void.[89] The patient may also benefit from pelvic floor exercises.[90] These exercises, known as Kegel exercises, are quick pelvic contractions and consist of the patient squeezing and holding for 2 seconds, then relaxing for 2 seconds. The patient should then increase each of these steps by 1 second each week, with a final goal of 10 seconds.[97] In addition to these exercises, medications such as anticholinergics and tricyclic antidepressants may help relax the patient's bladder contractions and improve bladder function.[96]

Non-pharmacologic treatments of urinary incontinence include weight loss and dietary changes.[92] Weight loss helps improve urge incontinence, which in turn is an effective motivator for weight loss.[7] Patients' fluids should be managed so that they drink for thirst only and take lozenges for dry mouth. Moreover, urinary incontinence patients should avoid caffeine.[90]

Epididymitis

Overview

Epididymitis is an acute inflammation or infection of the scrotum caused by the spread of a bacterial infection from the urethra, prostate, or bladder.[98] Chlamydia is the most common causative agent of epididymitis in men under 35 years of age, whereas cases of epididymitis in men over 35 years of age are likely caused by a bacterial ascension from the bladder.[99]

Presentation

Epididymitis usually presents with malaise, fever, and chills, as well as dysuria, urgency, and frequency.[98,100] Furthermore, epididymitis causes pain, swelling, and redness of the scrotum, and patients may also experience low back and perineal pain.[101] A physical examination will commonly reveal an enlarged, tender epididymis and a positive Prehn's sign.[100] Additionally, epididymitis patients may present with urethral discharge.[102]

Workup

A diagnosis of epididymitis is confirmed by finding swelling and tenderness of the epididymis.[102] Patients should be referred for diagnostic tests, such as a urine culture, a scrotal ultrasound, and STD testing.[100]

Treatment

Patients with epididymitis should receive supportive treatment, such as support and elevation of the scrotum, bed rest, ice packs, and heat.[100] Supportive treatment may also include medications such as analgesics and NSAIDs. If septicemia is suspected or has presented, a consultation or referral is often necessary.[100]

Antibiotic medications used to treat epididymitis depend on the causative agent.[7] Epididymitis most likely caused by sexually-transmitted chlamydia or gonorrhea should be treated with ceftriaxone (Rocephin) in a single dose of 250 mg intramuscularly in conjunction with doxycycline (Vibramycin) at 100 mg twice a day for 10 days. Epididymitis most likely caused by sexually-transmitted chlamydia and gonorrhea and enteric organisms should be treated with ceftriaxone in a single dose of 250 mg intramuscularly either in conjunction with levofloxacin (Levaquin) 500 mg orally one time per day for 10 days or in conjunction with ofloxacin (Floxin) 300 mg orally twice per day for 10 days. Cases most likely caused by enteric organisms should either be treated with levofloxacin 500 mg orally once per day for 10 days or treated with ofloxacin 300 mg orally twice per day for 10 days.[103]

Prostatitis

Overview

Prostatitis is a disorder of the prostate gland characterized by an increase of inflammatory cells.[86] Prostatitis either may be bacterial or may be nonbacterial and manifests with a combination of urinary symptoms and perineal pain.[104] Acute bacterial prostatitis is usually caused by Gram-negative bacteria, especially *E. coli*.[7] Nonbacterial prostatitis, on the other hand, mostly occurs in young men and is likely caused by bacteria such as *Chlamydia*, *Mycoplasma*, and *Gardnerella*.[105]

Presentation

Prostatitis patients are typically acutely ill and present with fever, chills, and irritative urinary symptoms such as dysuria, urgency, frequency, and nocturia.[104] A physical examination may show an edematous prostate, which may be warm and tender or boggy to palpation.[104] Patients may also feel pain in the lower back, abdomen, or genitals.[106]

Workup

Patients who present with signs and symptoms of prostatitis should receive a digital rectal exam, and a diagnosis is usually confirmed by an edematous and tender prostate.[107] A urine culture will reveal the causative pathogen.[86,108]

Treatment

Prostatitis is treated by antibiotics, including trimethoprim-sulfamethoxazole (Bactrim), ciprofloxacin (Cipro), or other fluoroquinolones.[107] Prostatitis patients should receive a consultation and referral if septicemia or urinary retention is evident.

Benign Prostatic Hypertrophy (BPH)

Overview

Benign prostatic hypertrophy (BPH) is a progressive, benign hyperplasia of the prostate.[104] Although its etiology is unknown, BPH is the primary cause of bladder obstruction in men over 50 years of age, and approximately 50% of all men will exhibit signs of this condition by age 50. Moreover, 80% of all men will acquire BPH by 80 years of age.[109]

Presentation

Among other findings, BPH often presents with dribbling and retention, as well as lower urinary tract symptoms such as urgency, frequency, and nocturia.[110] Physical examination usually indicates a non-tender prostate with a smooth, rubbery consistency; other possible physical examination findings include nodules, bladder distention, and asymmetrical or symmetrical enlargement.[104]

Workup

A diagnosis of BPH is often made on the basis of the patient's medical history.[109] After the patient's history is evaluated, the nurse practitioner (NP) should perform a digital rectal exam to assess the patient's prostate.[111] Diagnostics indicative of BPH include prostate-specific antigen (PSA) levels above 4 ng/ml. A urinalysis should also be taken, as the absence of hematuria often rules out a UTI. Similarly, upper tract pathology is ruled out by an abdominal ultrasound.[112] Patients may also be assessed with serum creatinine and blood urea nitrogen tests; both of these values should be normal.[109] Finally, uroflowmetry may sometimes be used in assessment of BPH.[104]

Treatment

Patients with BPH should be observed and receive consultation and referral to a urologist as needed. Alpha-blockers such as terazosin (Hytrin), prazosin (Minipress), or tamsulosin (Flomax) to relax the muscles of the prostate and bladder. Furthermore, to shrink large prostates, patients may be ordered 5-alpha-reductase inhibitors such as finasteride (Proscar) or dutasteride (Avodart).[113] Lastly, saw palmetto may also be effective for some patients.[111]

Prostate Cancer

Overview

As a malignant neoplasm of the prostate gland, prostate cancer is the second most prevalent cancer in men in the United States and the second leading cause of cancer deaths in men.[114] The cause of prostate cancer is unknown, although high-fat diets may be a contributing factor.[115]

Presentation

The majority of prostate cancer patients are asymptomatic, and symptoms rarely appear until the advanced stages of the condition.[116,117] In early stages, however, prostate cancer patients may present with findings similar to BPH, such as frequency, nocturia, and dribbling.[118] Conversely, symptoms that may appear in advanced stages of prostate cancer include bone pain from metastasis and uremia secondary to obstruction.[118] Furthermore, advanced stages of prostate cancer may also present with physical examination findings such as adenopathy and bladder distention, among others.[116] Moreover, the prostate palpates harder than normal, with obscure boundaries and possible nodules.[7]

Workup

Prostate cancer is diagnosed by a digital rectal exam and PSA.[119] Specifically, PSA values above 4 ng/ml are abnormal, and age-specific ranges derive from previously having a PSA below 4 ng/ml. Thus, the higher the patient's PSA value, the greater the possibility of a positive diagnosis for cancer.[120] Approximately 40% of all patients with prostate cancer, however, present with normal PSA values.[7] The patient should be referred to urology for an ultrasound or biopsy. Grading of the patient's tumor is based on histologic findings, whereas staging is determined by computed tomography and bone scanning.[117]

Treatment

Treatment of prostate cancer is determined by screening results and the patient's overall health. Among other recommendations, radiation therapy, surgery, and hormonal therapy are possible treatment options.[121]

Erectile Dysfunction

Overview

Erectile dysfunction is defined as "the consistent or recurrent inability to acquire or sustain an erection of sufficient rigidity and duration for sexual intercourse."[122] Erectile dysfunction may be caused by psychological factors such as stress, anxiety, and psychosocial issues; these factors may worsen the patient's condition even when the main cause is physical.[123] Major organic causes of erectile dysfunction include conditions such as atherosclerosis and diabetes, which often result in other vascular and neurologic disorders.[124]

Erectile dysfunction is also a side effect of many commonly prescribed medications, including antihistamines, most antidepressants, and some antihypertensives.[122,124,125] Other medications that may cause erectile dysfunction as a side effect include H2 blockers, anti-anxiety agents, anti-epileptics, NSAIDs, muscle relaxants, and Parkinson's disease medications, among others.[126]

Finally, alcohol and recreational drug use is also a potential cause of erectile dysfunction. Drugs that may cause this condition include amphetamines, barbiturates, cocaine, marijuana, methadone, nicotine, and opiates, among others.[126]

Workup

When assessing a patient with erectile dysfunction, the NP should gather the patient's medical, sexual, psychological, and surgical histories, as well as medication use.[125] Laboratory tests may include a CBC and PSA test, among others.[127] Additionally, the NP should check the patient's testosterone level.[127]

Treatment

Phosphodiesterase-5 inhibitors are usually first-line treatment for erectile dysfunction and include medications such as sildenafil (Viagra), vardenafil (Levitra), tadalafil (Cialis), and avanafil (Stendra).[124] However, phosphodiesterase-5 inhibitors should not be used concurrently with nitrates because a sudden drop in blood pressure may lead to syncope.[128]

Notes for Table 8.1

HPV=human papillomavirus; CIN= cervical intraepithelial neoplasia

[a]These recommendations do not apply to women who have received a diagnosis of a high-grade precancerous cervical lesion (CIN 2 or 3) or cervical cancer, women with in utero exposure to diethylstilbestrol, or women who are immunocompromised, or are HIV positive.

[b]Saslow D, Solomon D, Lawson HW, et al. American Cancer Society, American Society for Colposcopy and Cervical Pathology, and American Society for Clinical Pathology screening guidelines for the prevention and early detection of cervical cancer. *CA Cancer J Clin.* 2012 Mar 14. Available at http://www.cancer.org/Cancer/CervicalCancer/DetailedGuide/cervical-cancer-prevention

[c]USPSTF. Screening for Cervical Cancer. 2012. Available at http://www.uspreventiveservicestaskforce.org/uspstf11/cervcancer/cervcancerrs.htm. These recommendations apply to women who have a cervix, regardless of sexual history.

[d]ACOG Practice Bulletin No. 109: Cervical cytology screening. ACOG Committee on Practice Bulletins-Gynecology. *Obstet Gynecol.* 2009 Dec; 114(6): 1409–1420.

[e]Since cervical cancer is believed to be caused by sexually transmissible human papillomavirus infections, women who have not had sexual exposures (e.g., virgins) are likely at low risk. Women aged > 21 years who have not engaged in sexual intercourse may not need a Pap test depending on circumstances. The decision should be made at the discretion of the woman and her physician. Women who have had sex with women are still at risk of cervical cancer. About 10%–15% of women aged 21–24 years in the United States report no vaginal intercourse.

[f]More specific guidance from 2003 states an annual pelvic examination is a routine part of preventive care for all women aged > 21 years even if they do not need cervical cytology screening. (*Level C evidence*)

[g]Conventional cytology and liquid-based cytology are equivalent regarding screening guidelines, and no distinction should be made by test when recommending next screening.

[h]Primary HPV testing (HPV testing alone) is defined as conducting the HPV test as the first screening test. It may be followed by other tests (like a Pap) for triage.

[i]There is insufficient evidence to support longer intervals in women aged 30-65 years, even with a screening history of consecutive negative cytology tests.

[j]No further explanation of which clinical setting HPV testing should be used to screen women aged 30-65 years as a standalone test.

[k]Current guidelines define adequate screening as three consecutive negative cytology results or two consecutive negative co-tests within 10 years before cessation of screening, with the most recent test performed within 5 years, and are the same for ACS and USPSTF.

[l]2002 guidelines statement: The ACS and others should educate women, particularly teens and young women, that a pelvic exam does not equate to a cytology test and that women who may not need a cytology test still need regular health care visits including gynecologic care. Women should discuss the need for pelvic exams with their providers. Saslow D, Runowicz CD, Solomon D, et al. American Cancer Society Guideline for the Early Detection of Cervical Neoplasia and Cancer. *CA Cancer J Clin* 2002;52:342–362.

[m]The bimanual pelvic examination is often conducted (usually annually) in part to screen for ovarian cancer, although its effectiveness and harms are not well known and were not a focus of this review. No randomized trial has assessed the role of the bimanual pelvic examination for cancer screening. In the PLCO Trial, bimanual examination was discontinued as a screening strategy in the intervention arm because no cases of ovarian cancer were detected solely by this method and a high proportion of women underwent bimanual examination with ovarian palpation in the usual care arm.

References

1. Rosenbloom AL, Rohrs HJ, Haller MJ, Malasanos TH. Tanner stage 4 breast development in adults: Forensic implications. *Pediatrics.* 2012; 130(4): e978–e981. doi: 10.1542/peds.2011-3122.

2. Draper R, Tidy C. Normal and abnormal puberty. Patient.co.uk web site. http://www.patient.co.uk/doctor/Puberty-Normal-and-Abnormal.htm. Last updated June 22, 2011. Accessed March 25, 2015.

3. Bielak KM, Harris GS. Amenorrhea. In: Lucidi RS, ed. Medscape. http://emedicine.medscape.com/article/252928-overview#aw2aab6b2b3. Updated September 29, 2014. Accessed March 25, 2015.

4. Welt CK, Barbieri RL. Etiology, diagnosis, and treatment of secondary amenorrhea. In: Basow DS, ed. *UpToDate.* Waltham, MA: UpToDate; 2015. http://www.uptodate.com/contents/etiology-diagnosis-and-treatment-of-secondary-amenorrhea. Last updated April 25, 2014. Accessed March 25, 2015.

5. Secondary amenorrhea. A.D.A.M. Medical Encyclopedia. http://www.nlm.nih.gov/medlineplus/ency/article/001219.htm. Updated June 11, 2014. Accessed March 25, 2015.

6. Pinkerton JV. Amenorrhea. In: Porter RS, Kaplan JL, eds. The Merck Manual Online. http://www.merckmanuals.com/professional/gynecology_and_obstetrics/menstrual_abnormalities/amenorrhea.html?qt=amenorrhea&alt=sh. Last revised August 2012. Accessed March 25, 2015.

7. Barkley TW Jr. Gynecologic concerns/issues in men's health. In: Barkley TW Jr, ed. *Adult-Gerontology Primary Care Nurse Practitioner Certification Review/Clinical Update Continuing Education Course.* West Hollywood, CA: Barkley and Associates; 2015: 77–99.

8. American College of Obstetricians and Gynecologists. Understanding abnormal Pap smear results. Contemporary Obstetrics and Gynecology, PC web site. http://www.contemporarydoctors.com/webdocuments/ACOG/Understanding-Abnormal-Pap-Test-Results.pdf. Published May 2011. Accessed March 25, 2015.

9. Pap smear. A.D.A.M. Medical Encyclopedia. http://www.nlm.nih.gov/medlineplus/ency/article/003911.htm. Updated March 11, 2014. Accessed March 25, 2015.

10. Guile MW, Keller J. Infections of the genital tract. In: Hurt KJ, Guile MW, Bienstock JL, Fox HE, Wallach EE, eds. *The Johns Hopkins Manual of Gynecology and Obstetrics.* 4th ed. Philadelphia, PA: Wolters Kluwer Health/Lippincott Williams & Wilkins; 2011: 322–339.

11. Merritt DF. Vulvovaginitis. In: Kliegman RM, Behrman RE, Jenson HB, Stanton BF, eds. *Nelson Textbook of Pediatrics.* 19th ed. Philadelphia, PA: Elsevier Saunders; 2011: 1865–1868.

12. Trichomonas vaginalis. In: Bennett JE, Dolin R, Blaser MJ, eds. *Mandell, Douglas, & Bennett's Principles and Practice of Infectious Diseases.* 8th ed. Philadelphia, PA: Elsevier Saunders; 2014: Ch. 281.

13. United States Department of Health and Human Services, Centers for Disease Control and Prevention. Trichomoniasis - CDC Fact Sheet. http://www.cdc.gov/std/trichomonas/stdfact-trichomoniasis.htm. Last reviewed November 30, 2011. Last updated August 3, 2012. Accessed March 25, 2015.

14. Shepherd SM. Pelvic inflammatory disease. In: Revlin ME, ed. Medscape. http://emedicine.medscape.com/article/256448-overview. Updated March 27, 2014. Accessed March 25, 2015.

15. Soper DE. Pelvic inflammatory disease (PID). In: Porter RS, Kaplan JL, eds. The Merck Manual Online. http://www.merckmanuals.com/professional/gynecology_and_obstetrics/vaginitis_cervicitis_and_pelvic_inflammatory_disease_pid/pelvic_inflammatory_disease_pid.html?qt=pelvic%20inflammatory%20disease&alt=sh. Last reviewed March 2013. Accessed March 25, 2015.

16. Birnbaumer DM. Sexually transmitted diseases. In: Marx JA, Hockberger RS, Walls RM, et al., eds. *Rosen's Emergency Medicine: Concepts and Clinical Practice.* 8th ed. Philadelphia, PA: Elsevier Saunders; 2014: 1312–1325.

17. Pelvic inflammatory disease (PID). Penn Medicine web site. http://www.pennmedicine.org/encyclopedia/em_PrintArticle.aspx?gcid=000888&ptid=1. Reviewed July 28, 2014. Accessed March 26, 2015.

18. Workowski KA, Berman S. Sexually transmitted diseases treatment guidelines, 2010. *MMWR Morb Mortal Wkly Rep.* 2010; 59(RR-12): 1–110.

19. Pelvic inflammatory disease (PID). A.D.A.M. Medical Encyclopedia. http://www.nlm.nih.gov/medlineplus/ency/article/000888.htm. Updated August 5, 2013. Accessed March 26, 2015.

20. Pinkerton JV. Dysmenorrhea. In: Porter RS, Kaplan JL, eds. The Merck Manual Online. http://www.merckmanuals.com/professional/gynecology_and_obstetrics/menstrual_abnormalities/dysmenorrhea.html?qt=primary%20dysmenorrhea&alt=sh. Last reviewed August 2012. Accessed March 26, 2015.

21. Calis KA, Popat V, Dang DK, Kalantaridou SN, Erogul M. Dysmenorrhea. In: Rivlin ME, ed. Medscape. http://emedicine.medscape.com/article/253812-overview. Updated December 1, 2014. Accessed March 26, 2015.

22. American College of Obstetricians and Gynecologists. Gynecologic problems: Dysmenorrhea. American College of Obstetricians and Gynecologists web site. http://www.acog.org/-/media/For-Patients/faq046.pdf?dmc=1&ts=20150107T1405028500. Published January 2015. Accessed March 26, 2015.

23. Smith RP, Kaunitz AM. Patient information: Painful menstrual periods (dysmenorrhea) (Beyond the Basics). In: Basow DS, ed. UpToDate. Waltham, MA: UpToDate; 2015. http://www.uptodate.com/contents/painful-menstrual-periods-dysmenorrhea-beyond-the-basics. Last updated May 29, 2013. Accessed March 26, 2015.

24. Painful menstrual periods. A.D.A.M. Medical Encyclopedia. http://www.nlm.nih.gov/medlineplus/ency/article/003150.htm. Updated July 23, 2012. Accessed March 26, 2015.

25. American College of Obstetricians and Gynecologists. Abnormal uterine bleeding. American College of Obstetricians and Gynecologists web site. http://www.acog.org/~/media/For-Patients/faq095.pdf?dmc=1&ts=20131216T1606515476. Published December 2012. Accessed March 26, 2015.

26. Behera MA, Price TM. Dysfunctional uterine bleeding. In: Lucidi RS, ed. Medscape. http://emedicine.medscape.com/article/257007-overview. Updated September 29, 2014. Accessed March 26, 2015.

27. Pinkerton JV. Dysfunctional uterine bleeding (DUB). In: Porter RS, Kaplan JL, eds. The Merck Manual Online. Retrieved from http://www.merckmanuals.com/professional/gynecology_and_obstetrics/menstrual_abnormalities/dysfunctional_uterine_bleeding_dub.html. Last reviewed August 2012. Accessed March 26, 2015.

28. Vaginal bleeding – hormonal. A.D.A.M. Medical Encyclopedia. http://www.nlm.nih.gov/medlineplus/ency/article/000903.htm. Updated July 25, 2011. Accessed March 26, 2015.

29. Willacy H. Premenstrual syndrome. Patient.co.uk web site. http://www.patient.co.uk/doctor/The-Premenstrual-Syndrome.htm. Last updated April 19, 2012. Accessed March 26, 2015.

30. Moreno MA, Giesel AE, Rogers CB, Clark LR. Premenstrual syndrome. In: Zuckerman AL, ed. http://emedicine.medscape.com/article/953696-overview. Updated March 21, 2012. Accessed March 26, 2015.

31. Yonkers KA, Casper RF. Clinical manifestations and diagnosis of premenstrual syndrome and premenstrual dysphoric disorder. In: Basow DS, ed. UpToDate. Waltham, MA: UpToDate; 2015. http://www.uptodate.com/contents/clinical-manifestations-and-diagnosis-of-premenstrual-syndrome-and-premenstrual-dysphoric-disorder. Last updated November 14, 2015. Accessed March 26, 2015.

32. Premenstrual syndrome. A.D.A.M. Medical Encyclopedia. http://www.ncbi.nlm.nih.gov/pubmedhealth/PMH0002474. Accessed March 26, 2015.

33. American College of Obstetricians and Gynecologists. Premenstrual syndrome. American College of Obstetricians and Gynecologists web site. https://www.acog.org/-/media/For-Patients/faq057.pdf?dmc=1&ts=20150107T1409481943. Published May 2011. Accessed March 26, 2015.

34. Healthwise, Inc. Tricyclic antidepressants for premenstrual syndrome (PMS). Dartmouth-Hitchcock Norris Cotton Cancer Center web site. http://cancer.dartmouth.edu/pf/health_encyclopedia/hw138348. Last revised June 8, 2012. Accessed March 26, 2015.

35. Kosir MA. Breast masses (Breast lumps). In: Porter RS, Kaplan JL, eds. The Merck Manual Online. http://www.merckmanuals.com/professional/gynecology_and_obstetrics/breast_disorders/breast_masses_breast_lumps.html. Last reviewed September 2013. Accessed March 26, 2015.

36. Hosseini M, Tizmaghz A, Otaghvar HA, Shams M. The prevalence of fibrocystic changes of breast tissue of patients who underwent reduction mammoplasty in Rasool-Akram, Firuzgar, and Sadr hospitals during 2007–2012. Adv Surg Sci. 2014; 2(1): 5–8. doi: 10.11648/j.ass.20140201.12

37. Sabel MS. Overview of benign breast disease. In: Basow DS, ed. UpToDate. Waltham, MA: UpToDate; 2015. http://www.uptodate.com/contents/overview-of-benign-breast-disease. Last updated March 8, 2015. Accessed March 26, 2015.

38. Schindler AE. Dydrogesterone and other progestins in benign breast disease: An overview. Arch Gynecol Obstet. 2011; 283: 369–371. doi: 10.1007/s00404-010-1456-7.

39. Katz VL, Dotters D. Breast diseases: Diagnosis and treatment of benign and malignant disease. In: Lentz GM, Lobo RA, Gershenson DM, Katz VL, eds. Comprehensive Gynecology. 6th ed. Philadelphia, PA: Elsevier Mosby; 2012: 301–334.

40. Onstad M, Stuckey A. Benign breast disorders. Obstet Gynecol Clin North Am. 2013; 40(3): 459–473. doi: 10.1016/j.ogc.2013.05.004.

41. Kosir MA. Breast cancer. In: Porter RS, Kaplan JL, eds. The Merck Manual Online. http://www.merckmanuals.com/professional/gynecology_and_obstetrics/breast_disorders/breast_cancer.html. Last reviewed September 2013. Accessed March 26, 2015.

42. Breast cancer: What is cancer? American Cancer Society website. http://www.cancer.org/acs/groups/cid/documents/webcontent/003090-pdf.pdf. Last revised February 26, 2015. Accessed March 26, 2015.

43. United States Department of Health and Human Services, National Institutes of Health (NIH), National Cancer Institute (NCI). Genetics of breast and ovarian cancer (PDQ®). http://www.cancer.gov/cancertopics/pdq/genetics/breast-and-ovarian/Health-Professional. Updated February 6, 2015. Accessed March 26, 2015.

44. How many women get breast cancer? American Cancer Society web site. http://www.cancer.org/cancer/breastcancer/overviewguide/breast-cancer-overview-key-statistics. Last revised February 4, 2015. Accessed March 26, 2015.

45. Stopeck AT, Chalasani P, Thompson PA. Breast cancer. In: Harris JE, ed. Medscape. http://emedicine.medscape.com/article/1947145-overview#showall. Updated March 21, 2015. Accessed March 26, 2015.

46. Breast cancer symptoms: What you need to know. American Cancer Society web site. http://www.cancer.org/cancer/news/breast-cancer-symptoms-what-you-need-to-know. Published September 23, 2013. Accessed March 26, 2015.

47. Breast cancer. A.D.A.M. Medical Encyclopedia. http://www.nlm.nih.gov/medlineplus/ency/article/000913.htm. Updated October 30, 2013. Accessed April 2, 2015.

48. Breast cancer: How is breast cancer diagnosed? American Cancer Society web site. http://www.cancer.org/cancer/breastcancer/detailedguide/breast-cancer-diagnosis. Last revised February 26, 2015. Accessed March 26, 2015.

49. Harvey JA, Mahoney MC, Newell MS, et al. ACR Appropriateness Criteria® palpable breast masses. American College of Radiology web site. http://www.acr.org/~/media/ACR/Documents/AppCriteria/Diagnostic/PalpableBreastMasses.pdf. Last reviewed 2012. Accessed March 26, 2015.

50. American College of Obstetricians and Gynecologists. Menopause. American College of Obstetricians and Gynecologists web site. http://www.acog.org/~/media/For-Patients/faq047.pdf?dmc=1&ts=20131216T1821227692. Published February 2013. Accessed March 26, 2015.

51. Gass M. Menopause. In: Porter RS, Kaplan JL, eds. The Merck Manual Online. http://www.merckmanuals.com/professional/gynecology_and_obstetrics/menopause/menopause.html?qt=Menopause&alt=sh. Last reviewed May 2013. Accessed March 26, 2015.

52. Howard D. How does menopause affect the skin? International Dermal Institute web site. http://dermalinstitute.com/us/library/12_article_How_Does_Menopause_Affect_the_Skin_.html. Accessed March 26, 2015.

53. United States Department of Health and Human Services, NIH, National Institute of Aging. Menopause. http://www.nia.nih.gov/health/publication/menopause. Published December 2013. Last updated January 22, 2015. Accessed March 26, 2015.

54. Focus on . . . Urogenital concerns. Women's Health Concern web site. http://www.womens-health-concern.org/help/focuson/focus_urogenitalprobs.html. Accessed March 26, 2015.

55. Casper RF. Clinical manifestations and diagnosis of menopause. In: Basow DS, ed. *UpToDate*. Waltham, MA: UpToDate; 2015. http://www.uptodate.com/contents/clinical-manifestations-and-diagnosis-of-menopause. Last updated February 4, 2014. Accessed March 26, 2015.

56. Deen M, Ijaiya A, Raji HO. Treatment of pelvic organ prolapse. *Urogynaecologia*. 2012; 26(1): 8–11. doi: 10.4081/uij.2012.e3

57. Young SB. Vaginal surgery for pelvic organ prolapse. *Obstet Gynecol Clin North Am*. 2009; 36(3): 565–584. doi: 10.1016/j.ogc.2009.08.013.

58. Coney P. Menopause. In: Lucidi RS, ed. Medscape. http://emedicine.medscape.com/article/264088-overview#showall. Updated October 6, 2014. Accessed March 26, 2015.

59. Menopause. A.D.A.M. Medical Encyclopedia. http://www.ncbi.nlm.nih.gov/pubmedhealth/PMH0001896. Last updated August 29, 2013. Accessed March 26, 2015.

60. Brucker MC, Likis FE. Steroid hormones. In: King TL, Brucker MC, eds. *Pharmacology for Women's Health*. Sudbury, MA: Jones & Bartlett Publishers; 2010: 362–380.

61. North American Menopause Society. Estrogen and progestogen use in postmenopausal women: 2010 position statement of the North American Menopause Society. *Menopause*. 2010; 17(2): 242–255. doi: 10.1097/gme.0b013e3181d0f6b9.

62. United States Preventive Services Task Force. Vitamin D and calcium to prevent fractures: Preventative medication. U.S. Preventive Services Task Force webn site. http://www.uspreventiveservicestaskforce.org/uspstf12/vitamind/vitdfact.pdf. Published February 2013. Accessed March 26, 2015.

63. United States Preventive Services Task Force. Menopausal hormone therapy: Preventive medication. http://www.uspreventiveservicestaskforce.org/Page/Topic/recommendation-summary/menopausal-hormone-therapy-preventive-medication. Published October 2012. Accessed March 26, 2015.

64. Bartels CM, Muller D. Systemic lupus erythematosus (SLE). In: Diamond HS, ed. Medscape. http://emedicine.medscape.com/article/332244-overview. Last reviewed February 19, 2014. Accessed June 30, 2015.

65. Wallace DJ. Diagnosis and differential diagnosis of systemic lupus erythematosus in adults. In: Basow DS, ed. *UpToDate*. Waltham, MA: UpTo-Date; 2015. http://www.uptodate.com/contents/diagnosis-and-differential-diagnosis-of-systemic-lupus-erythematosus-in-adults?source=search_result&search=diagnosis+and+differential+diagnosis+of+sle&selectedTitle=1~150. Updated May 4, 2015. Accessed June 30, 2015.

66. Wallace DJ. Overview of the management and prognosis of systemic lupus erythematosus in adults. In: Basow DS, ed. *UpToDate*. Waltham, MA: Up-ToDate; 2015. http://www.uptodate.com/contents/overview-of-the-management-and-prognosis-of-systemic-lupus-erythematosus-in-adults?source=search_result&search=overview+of+the+management+and+prognosis+of+systemic+lupus+erythematosus&selectedTitle=1~150. Updated October 3, 2014. Accessed June 30, 2015.

67. Bolster MB. Osteoporosis. In Porter RS, Kaplan JL, eds. The Merck Manual Online. http://www.merckmanuals.com/professional/musculoskeletal_and_connective_tissue_disorders/osteoporosis/osteoporosis.html?qt=osteoporosis&alt=sh. Last revised December 2012. Accessed March 26, 2015.

68. Simon H. Osteoporosis. University of Maryland Medical Center web site. http://umm.edu/health/medical/reports/articles/osteoporosis. Last updated September 18, 2013. Accessed March 26, 2015.

69. Bethel M, Machua W, Carbone LD, Lohr KM. Osteoporosis. In: Diamond HS, ed. Medscape. http://emedicine.medscape.com/article/330598-overview#showall. Updated February 26, 2015. Accessed March 26, 2015.

70. Osteoporosis – overview. A.D.A.M. Medical Encyclopedia. http://www.ncbi.nlm.nih.gov/pubmedhealth/PMH0001400. Last updated April 9, 2014. Accessed March 26, 2015.

71. Kleerekoper M. Screening for osteoporosis. In: Basow DS, ed. *UpToDate*. Waltham, MA: UpToDate; 2015. http://www.uptodate.com/contents/screening-for-osteoporosis. Last updated October 17, 2013. Accessed March 26, 2015.

72. Milos G, Häuselmann HJ, Krieg MA, Rüegsegger P, Gallo LM. Are patterns of bone loss in anorexic and postmenopausal women similar? Preliminary results using high resolution peripheral computed tomography. *Bone*. 2012; 58: 146–150. doi: 10.1016/j.bone.2013.09.016.

73. Mayo Clinic Staff. Osteoporosis prevention. Mayo Clinic web site. http://www.mayoclinic.org/diseases-conditions/osteoporosis/basics/prevention/con-20019924. Reviewed December 13, 2014. Accessed March 31, 2015.

74. Exercise examples. National Osteoporosis Foundation web site. http://nof.org/articles/543. Accessed March 31, 2015.

75. *Dietary reference intakes for calcium and vitamin D*. Washington, DC: Institute of Medicine; 2011.

76. United States Department of Health and Human Services, NIH, National Institute of Diabetes and Digestive and Kidney Diseases (NIDDK), National Kidney and Urologic Diseases Information Clearinghouse (NKUDIC). Pyelonephritis: Kidney infection. http://kidney.niddk.nih.gov/KUDiseases/pubs/ pyelonephritis/index.aspx. Published April 2012. Last updated June 11, 2012. Accessed March 31, 2015.

77. Imam TH. Introduction to urinary tract infections. In: Porter RS, Kaplan JL, eds. The Merck Manual Online. http://www.merckmanuals.com/professional/genitourinary_disorders/urinary_tract_infections_uti/introduction_to_urinary_tract_infections.html. Last updated November 2013. Accessed March 31, 2015.

78. Urinary tract infection. Clinical Key web site. https://www.clinicalkey.com/topics/emergency-medicine/urinary-tract-infection.html. Accessed March 31, 2015.

79. Mayo Clinic Staff. Urinary tract infection. Mayo Clinic web site. http://www.mayoclinic.org/diseases-conditions/urinary-tract-infection/basics/definition/con-20037892. Reviewed August 29, 2012. Accessed March 31, 2015.

80. Walters MD, Karram MM. *Urogynecology and Reconstructive Pelvic Surgery*. 4th ed. Philadelphia, PA: Elsevier Saunders; 2015.

81. Urinary tract infections. UCLA Health Antimicrobial Stewardship Program web site. http://www.asp.mednet.ucla.edu/files/view/guidebook/UrinaryTractInfections.pdf. Accessed April 2, 2015.

82. Simati B, Kriegsman W. FPIN's clinical inquiries: Dipstick analysis for the diagnosis of acute UTI. *Am Fam Physician*. 2013; 87(10). http://www.aafp.org/afp/2013/0515/od2.html.

83. Gupta K, Hooton TM, Naber KG, Wullt B, et al. International clinical practice guidelines for the treatment of acute uncomplicated cystitis and pyelonephritis in women: A 2010 update by the Infectious Diseases Society of America and the European Society for Microbiology and Infectious Diseases. *Clin Infect Dis*. 2011; 52: e103–e120.

84. Fulop T. Acute pyelonephritis clinical presentation. In: Batuman V, ed. Medscape. http://emedicine.medscape.com/article/245559-clinical#showall. Updated April 18, 2014. Accessed March 31, 2015.

85. Hooton TM. Acute complicated cystitis and pyelonephritis. In: Basow DS, ed. *UpToDate*. Waltham, MA: UpToDate; 2015. http://www.uptodate.com/contents/acute-complicated-cystitis-and-pyelonephritis. Last updated May 30, 2014. Accessed March 31, 2015.

86. Deem SG, Rhee JJ, Piesman M, Costabile RA. Acute bacterial prostatitis. In: Kim ED, ed. Medscape. http://emedicine.medscape.com/article/2002872-overview. Updated November 12, 2014. Accessed March 31, 2015.

87. Urinary incontinence. Penn State Hershey web site. http://pennstatehershey.adam.com/content.aspx?productId=10&pid=10&gid=000050. Reviewed September 24, 2014. Accessed March 31, 2015.

88. American College of Obstetricians and Gynecologists. 2011 Women's health stats & facts. American College of Obstetricians and Gynecologists web site. http://www.acog.org/~/media/NewsRoom/MediaKit.pdf. Published 2011. Accessed March 31, 2015.

89. Shenot PJ. Urinary incontinence in adults. In: Porter RS, Kaplan JL, eds. The Merck Manual Online. http://www.merckmanuals.com/professional/genitourinary_disorders/voiding_disorders/urinary_incontinence_in_adults.html. Last reviewed August 2014. Accessed March 31, 2015.

90. Vasavada SP, Carmel ME, Rackley RR. Urinary incontinence. In: Kim ED, ed. Medscape. http://emedicine.medscape.com/article/452289-overview#aw2aab6b-2b1aa. Updated July 21, 2014. Accessed March 31, 2015.

91. Lovatsis D, Easton W, Wilkie D. Guidelines for the evaluation and treatment of recurrent urinary incontinence following pelvic floor surgery. J Obstet Gynaecol Can. 2010; 32(9): 893–904. http://sogc.org/wp-content/uploads/2013/01/gui248CPG1009E_000.pdf

92. Clemens JQ. Urinary incontinence in men. In: Basow DS, ed. UpToDate. Waltham, MA: UpToDate; 2015. http://www.uptodate.com/contents/urinary-incontinence-in-men. Last updated March 16, 2015. Accessed March 31, 2015.

93. Story CM. How a bladder diary can help you control bladder symptoms. Healthline web site. http://www.healthline.com/health-slideshow/bladder-diary#1. Reviewed February 27, 2014. Accessed March 31, 2015.

94. Stress incontinence. A.D.A.M. Encyclopedia. http://www.nlm.nih.gov/medlineplus/ency/article/000891.htm. Updated March 12, 2014. Accessed March 31, 2015.

95. Clemons JL. Vaginal pessary treatment of prolapse and incontinence. In: Basow, DS, ed. UpToDate. Waltham, MA: UpToDate; 2015. http://www.uptodate.com/contents/vaginal-pessary-treatment-of-prolapse-and-incontinence. Last updated March 10, 2014. Accessed March 31, 2015.

96. Urge incontinence. A.D.A.M. Medical Encyclopedia. http://www.nlm.nih.gov/medlineplus/ency/article/001270.htm. Updated October 2, 2013. Accessed March 31, 2015.

97. Kegel exercises—self-care. A.D.A.M. Encyclopedia. http://www.nlm.nih.gov/medlineplus/ency/patientinstructions/000141.htm. Updated December 12, 2012. Accessed March 31, 2015.

98. Epididymitis. A.D.A.M. Medical Encyclopedia. http://www.nlm.nih.gov/medlineplus/ency/article/001279.htm. Updated September 29, 2014. Accessed March 31, 2015.

99. United States Department of Health and Human Services, Centers for Disease Control and Prevention. Epididymitis. http://www.cdc.gov/std/treatment/2010/epididymitis.htm. Last reviewed January 28, 2011. Last updated August 14, 2014. Accessed March 31, 2015.

100. Ching CB, Sabanegh ES. Epididymitis. In: Kim ED, ed. Medscape. http://emedicine.medscape.com/article/436154-clinical. Updated December 15, 2014. Accessed March 31, 2015.

101. Patient information: Epididymitis (the basics). In: Basow DS, ed. UpToDate. Waltham, MA: UpToDate; 2015. Accessed March 31, 2015.

102. Shenot PJ. Epididymitis. In: Porter RS, Kaplan JL, eds. The Merck Manual Online. http://www.merckmanuals.com/professional/genitourinary_disorders/penile_and_scrotal_disorders/epididymitis.html?qt=epididymitis&alt=sh. Last reviewed December 2012. Accessed March 31, 2015.

103. Centers for Disease Control and Prevention (CDC). Sexually transmitted diseases treatment guidelines, 2015. MMWR Morb Mortal Wkly Rep. 2015; 64(3): 84.

104. Andriole GL. Prostatitis. In: Porter RS, Kaplan JL, eds. The Merck Manual Online. Retrieved from http://www.merckmanuals.com/professional/genitourinary_disorders/benign_prostate_disease/prostatitis.html?qt=prostatitis&alt=sh. Last reviewed March 2014. Accessed March 31, 2015.

105. Burns KA, Feeley NK. Renal and urinary disorders. In: Nettina SM, ed. Lippincott Manual of Nursing Practice. 10th ed. Philadelphia, PA: Wolters Kluwer Health/Lippincott Williams & Wilkins; 2013: 769–831.

106. Prostatitis - bacterial. A.D.A.M. Medical Encyclopedia. http://www.nlm.nih.gov/medlineplus/ency/article/000519.htm. Updated October 2, 2013. Accessed April 1, 2015.

107. Meyrier A, Fekete T. Acute bacterial prostatitis. In: Basow DS, ed. UpToDate. Waltham, MA: UpToDate; 2015. http://www.uptodate.com/contents/acute-bacterial-prostatitis. Last updated March 6, 2014. Accessed April 1, 2015.

108. Sharp VJ, Takacs EB, Powell CR. Prostatitis: Diagnosis and treatment. Am Fam Physician. 2010; 82(4): 397–406. http://www.aafp.org/afp/2010/0815/p397.html

109. Deters LA, Costabile RA, Leveillee RJ, Moore CR, Patel VR. Benign prostatic hypertrophy. In: Kim ED, ed. Medscape. http://emedicine.medscape.com/article/437359-overview. Updated March 28, 2014. Accessed April 2, 2015.

110. Cunningham GR, Kadmon D. Clinical manifestations and diagnostic evaluation of benign prostatic hyperplasia. In: Basow DS, ed. *UpToDate*. Waltham, MA: UpToDate; 2015. http://www.uptodate.com/contents/clinical-manifestations-and-diagnostic-evaluation-of-benign-prostatic-hyperplasia. Last updated March 18, 2013. Accessed April 2, 2015.

111. Enlarged prostate. A.D.A.M. Medical Encyclopedia. http://www.nlm.nih.gov/medlineplus/ency/article/000381.htm. Updated October 2, 2013. Accessed April 2, 2015.

112. Moodley P, Zareba P, Shayegan B. BPH and lower urinary tract symptoms in primary care. *The Canadian Journal of CME*. 2010; 22(5): 33–36. http://www.sta-communications.com/journals/cme/2010/5-May-2010/May%20Workshop.pdf

113. Kumar R, Malla P, Kumar M. Advances in the design and discovery of drugs for the treatment of prostatic hyperplasia. *Expert Opin Drug Discov*. 2013; 8(8) 1013–1027. doi: 10.1517/17460441.2013.797960

114. What are the key statistics about prostate cancer? American Cancer Society web site. http://www.cancer.org/cancer/prostatecancer/detailedguide/prostate-cancer-key-statistics. Last revised March 12, 2015. Accessed April 2, 2015.

115. United States Department of Health and Human Services, NIH, NCI. Prostate cancer prevention (PDQ): Risk factors for prostate cancer development. http://www.cancer.gov/cancertopics/pdq/prevention/prostate/healthprofessional/page3#_33_toc. Updated February 6, 2015. Accessed April 2, 2015.

116. Chodak GW, Krupski TL. Prostate cancer. In: Kim ED, ed. Medscape. http://emedicine.medscape.com/article/1967731-overview. Updated December 2, 2014. Accessed April 2, 2015.

117. Master VA. Prostate cancer. In: Porter RS, Kaplan JL, eds. The Merck Manual Online. http://www.merckmanuals.com/professional/genitourinary_disorders/genitourinary_cancer/prostate_cancer.html?qt=prostate%20cancer&alt=sh. Last reviewed November 2013. Accessed April 2, 2015.

118. Cooney MM, MacLennan G, Okuku F. Genitourinary cancers. In: Miller KD, Simon M, eds. *Global Perspectives on Cancer: Incidence, Care, and Experience*. Santa Barbara, CA: Praeger/ABC-CLIO; 2015: 205–218.

119. Kantoff PW, Taplin M, Smith JA. Clinical presentation and diagnosis of prostate cancer. In: Basow DS, ed. *UpToDate*. Waltham, MA: UpToDate; 2015. http://www.uptodate.com/contents/clinical-presentation-and-diagnosis-of-prostate-cancer. Last updated January 15, 2015. Accessed April 2, 2015.

120. How is prostate cancer staged? American Cancer Society web site. http://www.cancer.org/cancer/prostate-cancer/detailedguide/prostate-cancer-staging. Last reviewed March 12, 2015. Accessed April 2, 2015.

121. Prostate cancer. A.D.A.M. Medical Encyclopedia. http://www.ncbi.nlm.nih.gov/pubmedhealth/PMH0032722. Last updated September 12, 2014. Accessed April 2, 2015.

122. Cunningham GR, Rosen RC. Overview of male sexual dysfunction. In: Basow DS, ed. *UpToDate*. Waltham, MA: UpToDate; 2015. http://www.uptodate.com/contents/overview-of-male-sexual-dysfunction. Last updated November 10, 2014. Accessed April 2, 2015.

123. United States Department of Health and Human Services, NIH, NIDDK, NKUDIC. Erectile dysfunction. http://kidney.niddk.nih.gov/kudiseases/pubs/ED/#cause. Published June 2009. Last updated March 28, 2012. Accessed April 2, 2015.

124. Hirsch IH. Erectile dysfunction. In: Porter RS, Kaplan JL, eds. The Merck Manual Online. http://www.merckmanuals.com/professional/genitourinary_disorders/male_sexual_dysfunction/erectile_dysfunction.html?qt=erectile%20dysfunction&alt=sh. Last reviewed February 2013. Accessed April 2, 2015.

125. Kim ED, Brosman SA. Erectile dysfunction. In: Kim ED, ed. Medscape. http://emedicine.medscape.com/article/444220-overview#aw2aab6b2b4. Updated August 21, 2014. Accessed April 2, 2015.

126. Drugs that cause impotence. A.D.A.M. Encyclopedia. http://www.nlm.nih.gov/medlineplus/ency/article/004024.htm. Updated October 22, 2012. Accessed April 2, 2015.

127. Erection problems. A.D.A.M. Medical Encyclopedia. http://www.nlm.nih.gov/medlineplus/ency/article/003164.htm. Updated September 19, 2011. Accessed April 2, 2015.

128. Whelan PS, Nehra A. Basic principles of the Princeton recommendations. In: Viigimaa M, Vlachopoulos C, Doumas M, eds. *Erectile Dysfunction in Hypertension and Cardiovascular Disease: A Guide for Clinicians*. Heidelberg, Germany: Springer; 2015: 213–230.

Chapter 9
Hematologic and Oncologic Disorders

1. Iron deficiency anemia results in a decrease in the amount of iron available for which process?

    a. Hemoglobin production

    b. Red blood cell formation

    c. Transportation of oxygen in the body

    d. Absorption of vitamin B12

2. A 45-year-old patient presents to the clinic complaining of weak arms, pins and needles, and fingers that can't keep a pen steady. A blood panel shows that his hemoglobin, hematocrit, and red blood cell count are decreased, whereas his mean corpuscular volume is increased. Which follow-up diagnostic would be least helpful in confirming the most likely condition?

    a. Citrate agar gel electrophoresis

    b. Anti-intrinsic factor test

    c. Schilling test

    d. Antiparietal cell antibody test

3. The TNM classification for a patient reads as follows: T2, N1, M0. All of the following inferences are supported by the patient's TNM classification except:

    a. The patient's bladder tumor has spread to the muscle of the bladder wall.

    b. The patient's breast tumor has spread to axillary lymph nodes.

    c. The patient's colon tumor has spread to nearby lymph nodes.

    d. The patient's brain tumor has not spread to distant tissue.

4. A patient comes to the clinic with complaints of weakness, fatigue, and difficulty breathing during mild exercise. His lab results indicate a low serum iron level, a low total iron binding capacity level, and a low hemoglobin level. However, his mean corpuscular hemoglobin count and mean corpuscular volume are both normal. What condition would the patient's symptoms and lab results most strongly indicate?

    a. Anemia of chronic disease

    b. Iron deficiency anemia

    c. Sickle cell anemia

    d. Pernicious anemia

5. Immunosenescence refers to:

    a. The gradual decline of overall immune system function due to chronic disease

    b. The decline in innate immune system function

    c. The gradual decline of overall immune system function due to age

    d. The waning of vaccine-induced antibody response

6. Identify the finding that best indicates pernicious anemia.

    a. Increased red blood cells

    b. Presence of antiparietal cell antibodies

    c. Decreased mean corpuscular volume

    d. Presence of intrinsic factor

7. A 47-year-old male patient has signs of leukemia. Which of the following diagnostic tests would best distinguish acute leukemia from chronic leukemia?

    a. Erythrocyte sedimentation rate

    b. Complete blood count

    c. Peripheral blood smear

    d. Ultrasonography scan

8. Which of these anemias is properly paired with a dietary staple well-suited for treating the condition?

    a. Iron deficiency anemia; milk

    b. Folic acid deficiency; peanut butter

    c. Pernicious anemia; raisins

    d. Thalassemia; red meat

9. A patient's lab results show a mean corpuscular volume of 120 fL. Which of the following anemias would be most strongly indicated by this finding?

    a. Iron deficiency anemia

    b. Sickle cell anemia

    c. Folic acid deficiency

    d. Thalassemia

10. Non-Hodgkin's lymphoma is more likely than Hodgkin's disease to present with which characteristic?

    a. Unpredictable pattern of spread

    b. Reed-Sternberg cells

    c. An unknown etiology

    d. Cervical adenopathy

11. A 37-year-old male presents with recurring headaches, fatigue, and a decreased desire to eat. An examination and lab panel reveals that the patient has a resting heartbeat of 122 bpm and a normal mean corpuscular hemoglobin concentration. Which condition is the patient most likely experiencing?

    a. Iron deficiency anemia

    b. Folic acid deficiency

    c. Anemia of chronic disease

    d. Thalassemia

12. Sarah, a 35-year-old female, presents to your practice with anorexia, glossitis, and dizziness. She tests positive for both the Romberg and Babinski tests. Which of these is the most likely condition?

    a. Pernicious anemia

    b. Folic acid deficiency

    c. Sickle cell anemia

    d. Iron deficiency anemia

13. Which of these values is within the normal range for mean corpuscular volume?

    a. 77 fL

    b. 92 fL

    c. 101 fL

    d. 113 fL

14. A patient presents to the clinic with complaints of a constant headache, fatigue, and a "racing heart." A blood panel reveals elevated mean corpuscular volume, normal mean corpuscular hemoglobin concentration, and a red blood cell folate of 83 ng/mL. Which of the following supplements would be best for the patient?

    a. Vitamin B12

    b. Iron

    c. Vitamin C

    d. Folate

15. You suspect that your patient, Susana, has chronic, normocytic, hemolytic anemia. Select the best diagnostic procedure that would best confirm the most likely condition.

    a. Peripheral blood smear

    b. Erythrocyte sedimentation rate

    c. Electrophoresis on citrate agar gel

    d. Antiparietal cell antibody test

16. Benjamin, a 55-year-old male, presents with complaints of fatigue, a heartbeat that "races" even when sitting down, and difficulty breathing when lifting heavy objects. What finding would most strongly indicate a vitamin B12 deficiency rather than a folic acid deficiency?

    a. Decreased serum folate

    b. Decreased red blood cells

    c. Lack of intrinsic factor

    d. Increased mean corpuscular volume

17. Joshua, a 45-year-old male, comes to your practice with complaints of fatigue, weakness, and weight loss. After further investigation, you discover that he has generalized lymphadenopathy. You order a complete blood count, which reveals subnormal red blood cells and neutrophils. Given the most likely diagnosis, you might recommend any of the following methods of management except:

    a. Symptomatic control

    b. Oral ferrous sulfate

    c. Bone marrow transplantation

    d. Chemotherapy

18. The practitioner knows that conditions associated with an MCV = 124 u^3 include all of the following except:

    a. Alcoholism

    b. B12 deficiency anemia

    c. Folate deficiency anemia

    d. Thalassemia

19. Franklin, a 66-year-old male, presents to the clinic with fatigue, weakness, weight loss, and generalized lymphadenopathy. His lab results reveal a subnormal red blood cell count and neutrophils, as well as an elevated erythrocyte sedimentation rate. Which of the following laboratory tests would best confirm the most likely diagnosis?

    a. Peripheral blood smear

    b. Citrate agar gel electrophoresis

    c. Bone marrow aspiration

    d. Complete blood count

20. A patient in your care comes to the clinic with complaints of headache, weakness, and a constant craving for ice. A blood panel shows that the patient has microcytic, hypochromic anemia and is experiencing a low hematocrit. You decide to take a closer look at the patient's diet for purposes of confirming diagnosis and establishing a treatment plan. Given the most likely condition, which of the following staples should the patient be cautioned to avoid?

    a. Orange juice

    b. Steak

    c. Tea

    d. Lettuce

21. Which of the following lab findings is most likely to be indicative of iron deficiency anemia?

    a. Low mean corpuscular volume

    b. High mean corpuscular hemoglobin concentration

    c. Low red cell distribution width

    d. High serum ferritin

22. Jake, a 27-year-old male, presents to the clinic with fatigue and anorexia. A blood panel shows that he has a normocytic and normochromic anemia, but has low total iron binding capacity and a serum ferritin level of 120 ng/mL. Given the most likely diagnosis, which of these drugs would be best suited for resolving the condition?

    a. Isoniazid

    b. Red blood cell transfusions

    c. Cyanocobalamin

    d. Fluid administration

23. The Union for International Cancer Control uses all of the following parameters to classify tumor development except:

    a. Size or extent of the primary tumor

    b. Type of tissue in which the cancer originates

    c. Amount of spread to regional lymph nodes

    d. Presence of metastasis

24. Julie, a 44-year-old female of Middle Eastern descent, comes in for routine bloodwork. You note that she has a low hemoglobin level and a mean corpuscular volume of 75 fL/red cell. Her mean corpuscular hemoglobin concentration is 30%. She denies experiencing any changes in general well-being and assures you that she has been feeling normal. Which condition does Julie most likely have?

    a. Anemia of chronic disease

    b. Thalassemia

    c. Pernicious anemia

    d. Folic acid deficiency

25. The Schilling test is most closely associated with screening for which of the following conditions?

    a. Thalassemia

    b. Folic acid deficiency

    c. Iron deficiency anemia

    d. Pernicious anemia

26. The results of a patient's chromosome analysis show the presence of the Philadelphia chromosome. What type of leukemia does this finding most often indicate?

    a. Acute nonlymphocytic leukemia

    b. Acute lymphocytic leukemia

    c. Chronic lymphocytic leukemia

    d. Chronic myelogenous leukemia

27. Which of the following patients has the least normal hemoglobin count?

    a. Daisy, a 29-year-old mother with 15 grams/100 ml

    b. George, a 42-year-old father with 13 grams/100 ml

    c. Linda, a 50-year-old grandmother with 12 grams/100 ml

    d. Dan, a 21-year-old student with 18 grams/100 ml

28. All of these treatments may be necessary for a patient with severe thalassemia except:

    a. Red blood cell transfusion

    b. Chelation therapy

    c. Iron supplements

    d. Splenectomy

29. You would like to recommend oral ferrous sulfate to your 36-year-old patient with iron deficiency anemia, but you want to make sure the treatment is effective and that nothing inhibits the absorption of the medicine. Which of the following should you most strongly recommend the patient avoid for optimal absorption of the oral ferrous sulfate?

    a. Antacids

    b. Vitamin C

    c. Folate

    d. Analgesics

30. When using the TNM Classification of Malignant Tumors staging system to classify the spread to regional lymph nodes, all of the following grades would be appropriate <u>except</u>:

   a. A grade of "4"

   b. A grade of "0"

   c. A grade of "X"

   d. A grade of "3"

31. Which of these statements regarding folic acid deficiency and pernicious anemia is true?

   a. Folic acid deficiency is a normochromic anemia and pernicious anemia is a hypochromic anemia.

   b. Neither folic acid deficiency or pernicious anemia are normochromic anemias.

   c. Lack of folic acid and lack of intrinsic factor lead to malabsorption of vitamin B12.

   d. Both folic acid deficiency and pernicious anemia are macrocytic anemias.

32. After your patient undergoes diagnostic studies for lymphocytic malignancy, you determine that there are two lymph node groups involved on both sides of the patient's diaphragm, in addition to bone marrow involvement. Which stage of lymphocytic malignancy is best illustrated in the patient?

   a. Stage I

   b. Stage II

   c. Stage III

   d. Stage IV

33. All of the following statements regarding leukemia in adult patients are true <u>except</u>:

   a. Leukemia more frequently occurs in males.

   b. Acute myelogenous leukemia constitutes 80% of leukemia in adults.

   c. Acute lymphocytic leukemia is more difficult to cure in adults than in children.

   d. The median survival for chronic myelogenous leukemia is 4–7 years.

34. Which of the following values best represents a normal red blood cell concentration in a 50-year-old male patient?

   a. 32%

   b. 39%

   c. 48%

   d. 55%

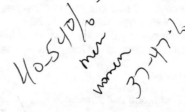

35. A 35-year-old male is presenting with complaints of fatigue and fever. No sign of infection is present. Diagnostic tests show decreased red and white blood cells, as well as the presence of circulating blast cells. Which of the following is the most likely type of cancer based on these findings?

   a. Acute myelogenous leukemia

   b. Acute lymphocytic leukemia

   c. Chronic lymphocytic leukemia

   d. Chronic myelogenous leukemia

36. Your female sickle cell patient reveals to you that she plans to go on vacation in the next few months. Which of the following environments should you most strongly advise the patient against visiting?

   a. Densely populated cities

   b. Beachy areas

   c. Valleys

   d. The mountains

37. Which of the following is the most appropriate choice of management for moderate thalassemia?

   a. Red blood cell transfusion or splenectomy

   b. Chelation therapy

   c. Oral ferrous sulfate

   d. No treatment

38. Your patient has just returned from competing in a soccer tournament in Denver. He complains of pain in his legs, nausea, tiredness, having trouble concentrating in school, and generally feeling unwell. The patient's history is positive for sickle cell trait. You order baseline studies to assess the patient. Which finding would you most expect to see in your patient?

    a. Elevated erythrocyte sedimentation rate

    b. Anorexia

    c. Glossitis

    d. Acidosis

39. Which of the following factors most strongly contributes to the development of anemia of chronic disease?

    a. Decreased erythrocyte life span

    b. Periodic malformation of red blood cells

    c. Deficiency of intrinsic factor

    d. Impaired absorption of iron

40. Your 62-year old patient has just been diagnosed with chronic lymphocytic leukemia. Which of these statements would you make to your patient regarding his condition?

    a. "Your condition is related to a shortening of chromosome 22."

    b. "Your condition stems from abnormalities in the myeloid cells."

    c. "Your condition is the most common leukemia in adults."

    d. "Pancytopenia with circular blasts were observed in your blood smear."

RATIONALES

1. b

Iron deficiency anemia results from a decrease in the amount of iron available for red blood cell formation. Thalassemia affects the production of hemoglobin and, thus, the transportation of oxygen in the body. Pernicious anemia results in the deficiency of intrinsic factor protein, thus affecting the absorption of vitamin B12.

2. a

The loss of motor control in addition to an increased mean corpuscular volume most strongly indicates pernicious anemia, which is not evaluated by citrate agar gel electrophoresis. Rather, electrophoresis with cellulose acetate and citrate agar gel is used to confirm hemoglobin genotype in a patient suspected of having sickle cell anemia. Anti-intrinsic factor and antiparietal cell antibody tests are used to affirm vitamin B12 deficiency, whereas a Schilling test may be helpful early in the diagnosis process to determine if the body is correctly absorbing vitamin B12.

3. d

Brain tumors do not have TNM classifications for several reasons: the size of the tumor in the brain is not as relevant as the histology and location, there are no lymphatics within the brain, and metastatic spread is not as observable because patients may not live long enough for the tumor to spread. The 'T' parameter of the TNM classification refers to the size or direct extent of the primary tumor. A 'T' parameter of T2 indicates that there has been some growth, such as a bladder tumor that has spread to the muscle of the bladder wall. The 'N' parameter of the TNM classification refers to the spread to regional lymph nodes. A classification of N1 indicates that there has been minimal spreading to regional lymph nodes. The 'M' parameter refers to the distant metastasis, the spread of cancer to other parts of the body.

4. a

Symptoms of weakness, fatigue, and labored breathing may suggest multiple hematological conditions; however, lab results indicating low serum iron, total iron binding capacity levels, and hemoglobin levels while also indicating normal mean corpuscular hemoglobin concentration (MCHC) and mean corpuscular volume (MCV) would likely suggest anemia of chronic disease. A patient with iron deficiency anemia would have low MCV and low MCHC, and sickle cell anemia would present with sickle-shaped red blood cells and elevated MCHC. In pernicious anemia, the Hgb and hematocrit counts typically decrease, whereas the MCV count increases.

5. c

Immunosenescence refers to the gradual decline in overall immune system function due to age. Because both the innate and adaptive immune systems are affected, the immune system's ability to respond to infection is reduced. Consequently, chronic disease may be exacerbated, and elderly patients may require new administration of prior vaccines because of waning vaccine-induced antibody response.

6. b

The presence of antiparietal cell antibodies affirms a deficiency of intrinsic factor, a major contribution to the development of pernicious anemia. The lack of intrinsic factor leads to malabsorption of vitamin B12, producing the anemia. Pernicious anemia is also characterized by decreased, not increased, red blood cells, as well as increased, not decreased, mean corpuscular volume.

7. c

A peripheral blood smear would best distinguish acute leukemia from chronic leukemia. The smear will typically show blasts in acute leukemias and mature cells in chronic leukemias. Erythrocyte sedimentation rates (ESR) are typically elevated in patients with leukemia; however, an ESR test would not differentiate between acute and chronic leukemia. Although a complete blood count is used to assess leukemia, it would likely reveal a subnormal red blood cell and neutrophil count for both acute and chronic cases of leukemia. An ultrasonography scan is not typically used to diagnose leukemia.

8. b

It is recommended that folic acid deficiency patients eat peanut butter, bananas, fish, green leafy vegetables, and other foods high in folic acid. Milk does not aid in treating iron deficiency anemia and may interfere with the body's ability to absorb iron. Pernicious anemia is treated through administration of vitamin B12, which is not found in raisins. Patients with thalassemia should monitor their intake of red meat and other foods rich in iron, as iron overload is a potential complication of severe thalassemia.

9. c

Folic acid deficiency would be the most strongly indicated anemia because it is characterized by a mean corpuscular volume (MCV) of greater than 100 fL. Iron deficiency anemia and thalassemia, on the other hand, are microcytic anemias and typically present with an MCV of less than 80 fL. Sickle cell anemia is a normocytic anemia that typically presents with an MCV in the normal range of 80–100 fL.

10. a

Non-Hodgkin's lymphoma typically has a less predictable pattern of spread than Hodgkin's disease, which often spreads in a predictable manner across lymph node groups. In both conditions, the cause is unknown. Lastly, Hodgkin's disease, rather than non-Hodgkin's lymphoma, presents with Reed-Sternberg cells and cervical adenopathy.

11. b

The patient's findings suggest that he may have folic acid deficiency. Headaches, fatigue, and tachycardia are also signs of iron deficiency anemia, but this anemia tends to present with pica, not anorexia, as indicated by the patient's lack of desire to eat. Furthermore, patients with iron deficiency anemia are likely to have a low mean corpuscular hemoglobin concentration, not a normal percentage. Patients with anemia of chronic disease may also exhibit fatigue and anorexia, but tachycardia is not a hallmark of the condition. Lastly, thalassemia major is usually diagnosed in childhood, and thalassemia minor does not present with remarkable findings, making the diagnosis of thalassemia less likely than that of folic acid deficiency.

12. a

Anorexia, glossitis, and dizziness, in addition to positive Romberg and Babinski tests, are signs of pernicious anemia. Glossitis and anorexia may be present in folic acid deficiency, and although neurological signs may also be present, it would not produce positive Romberg and Babinski tests. Anorexia and glossitis are not typical findings of sickle cell anemia. Although glossitis may be rarely seen in individuals with iron deficiency anemia, positive Romberg and Babinski tests would not be expected.

13. b

The normal range of mean corpuscular volume (MCV) is 80–100 fL; therefore, a value of 92 fL would be considered a normal MCV. An MCV of less than 80 fL may be indicative of microcytic conditions, such as iron deficiency anemia or thalassemia. An MCV of greater than 100 fL would be indicative of macrocytic conditions, such as folic acid deficiency or pernicious anemia.

14. d

The patient's symptoms and laboratory results most strongly indicate folic acid deficiency, which is best treated with folate supplements. Symptoms of folic acid deficiency include headache, fatigue, tachycardia, and anorexia. An elevated mean corpuscular volume (MCV), a normal mean corpuscular hemoglobin concentration (MCHC), and a red blood cell folate below 100 ng/mL further confirm the diagnosis of folic acid deficiency. Vitamin B12 injections are used to treat pernicious anemia, which presents with neurological signs and a low serum B12 level. Iron is a method of management for patients with iron deficiency anemia, which usually presents with unusual cravings, a low MCV, and a low MCHC. Iron should be taken with vitamin C to increase absorption.

15. c

In diagnosing sickle cell anemia, a chronic, normocytic, hemolytic anemia, the confirmation of the requisite hemoglobin genotype is often done through electrophoresis, using citrate agar gel or cellulose acetate. Although a peripheral smear is used to show the distorted sickle-shaped red blood cells, it does not confirm the condition. The erythrocyte sedimentation rate would be low in a patient with sickle cell anemia, but this test would be more useful in diagnosing a patient suspected of having leukemia. An antiparietal cell antibody test would more likely be used in diagnosing a patient suspected of having pernicious anemia.

16. c

Pernicious anemia is due to a deficiency of intrinsic factor, which results in the malabsorption of vitamin B12. An anti-intrinsic factor test can confirm this deficiency. Folic acid deficiency does not usually present with vitamin B12 deficiency. Folic acid deficiency and pernicious anemia both present with decreased serum folate, decreased red blood cells, and increased mean corpuscular volume.

17. b

Leukemia is not likely to be treated by oral ferrous sulfate. Oral ferrous sulfate is more likely to be a method of management in a patient with iron deficiency anemia. Chemotherapy, bone marrow transplantation, and control of symptoms with NSAIDs or opioids such as hydromorphone are all methods of management for patients with leukemia.

18. d

Thalassemia is the least likely condition because it is a microcytic anemia and would have a mean corpuscular volume (MCV) of less than 80 fL. Macrocytic anemias have MCVs above 100 fL. Macrocytic anemias are caused by folate deficiency, alcoholism, liver failure, drug effects, or vitamin B12 deficiency, the latter causing pernicious anemia.

19. c

Leukemia, indicated by the patient's fatigue, weakness, weight loss, generalized lymphadenopathy, and presence of neutrophils, can be confirmed through a bone marrow aspiration. A peripheral blood smear is also used when determining a diagnosis of leukemia, but is more likely implemented to distinguish acute leukemia from chronic leukemia. Citrate agar gel electrophoresis is a typical part of the workup for sickle cell anemia. A complete blood count is used to detect abnormalities indicating leukemia but will not confirm a diagnosis.

20. c

Tea should be avoided in patients with iron deficiency anemia—which is indicated by the patient's findings—because it blocks iron absorption and may stand in the way of treatment. Red meat, leafy greens, and citrus products, as well as raisins and iron-fortified bread and cereals, are all strongly recommended for dietary management of iron deficiency anemia.

21. a

Of the choices, iron deficiency anemia is most likely to be indicated by low mean corpuscular volume. Iron deficiency anemia also typically presents with a low mean corpuscular hemoglobin concentration, a high red cell distribution width, and low serum ferritin levels.

22. a

Anemia of chronic disease, a normocytic, normochromic anemia that presents with low serum ferritin and total iron binding capacity, is best treated through management of the underlying infectious, inflammatory, or malignant condition that produces the anemia; as tuberculosis has been closely linked to anemia of chronic disease, isoniazid would aid in resolving the anemia. Red blood cell transfusions may be warranted in severe cases of thalassemia. Cyanocobalamin, or vitamin B12, is more essential in the treatment of pernicious anemia; although pernicious anemia may present with weakness and anorexia, it is a macrocytic, not normocytic, anemia. Fluid administration is more often used to treat dehydration.

23. b

The type of tissue in which the cancer originates is not one of the three categories within the TNM classification of malignant tumors. The Union for International Cancer Control TNM classification system classifies tumors by the size or extent of the primary tumor, amount of spread to regional lymph nodes, and presence of metastasis.

24. b

General physical findings associated with thalassemia are typically unremarkable, except in severe forms. However, this condition, found mainly in Mediterranean, African, Middle Eastern, Indian, and Asian populations, may present with decreased hemoglobin and microcytic, hypochromic anemia. Anemia of chronic disease is normocytic and normochromic and typically results in fatigue, weakness, and dyspnea on exertion. Pernicious anemia presents with many signs and symptoms, including weakness, palpitations, and anorexia. Folic acid deficiency presents with fatigue, tachycardia, and anorexia, among other signs and symptoms.

25. d

The Schilling test may help diagnose pernicious anemia by determining if the body is absorbing vitamin B12 normally. However, the Schilling test is not typically used in diagnosing thalassemia, folic acid deficiency, or iron deficiency anemia, as vitamin B12 is not implicated in the etiologies of these conditions.

26. d

The Philadelphia chromosome is a specific characteristic of chronic myelogenous leukemia cells and is not typically found in other types of leukemia cells. Acute lymphocytic leukemia is most closely associated with the presence of pancytopenia with circulating blasts. Chronic lymphocytic leukemia is characterized by lymphocytosis. Acute nonlymphocytic leukemia may be associated with translocations on certain chromosomes; however, there is not a specific hallmark finding from chromosomal analysis that would distinguish acute nonlymphocytic leukemia.

27. b

George has the least normal hemoglobin count of the four patients. A normal hemoglobin count in males would range from 14 to 18 grams/100 ml. A normal hemoglobin count in females ranges from 12–16 grams/100 ml. Therefore, Daisy, Linda, and Dan all have normal hemoglobin counts for their respective genders.

28. c

Iron supplements are contraindicated in patients with severe thalassemia, as they may result in iron overload and increase the risk of organ damage. Red blood cell transfusion may be necessary for managing anemia in patients with severe thalassemia; as regular transfusion can result in iron build-up, chelation therapy may also be necessary. If the necessity for transfusion increases by more than half over a 1-year period, splenectomy may be considered to reduce demand.

29. a

Patients prescribed iron to treat iron deficiency anemia should be advised to avoid antacids, as these drugs may interfere with the absorption of iron. Iron should be taken in conjunction with vitamin C in order to facilitate absorption. Folic acid tablets are used to treat folic acid deficiency; although regular intake of folic acid is beneficial to all diets, it plays little role in facilitating or inhibiting iron absorption. Analgesics are a recommended method of pain management in patients with sickle cell anemia and do not interfere with oral ferrous sulfate.

30. a

The TNM Classification of Malignant Tumors staging system uses 0–3 or "X" when classifying the spread of the tumor to regional lymph nodes; therefore, a rating of 4 is not valid for measuring spread. The range of the size or extent of the primary tumor can be classified by "a," "is," or 1–4. Presence of distant metastasis can be designated by 0 or 1. In all of the above parameters, an "X" can be used instead of a number or letter to denote that the parameter was not assessed in the patient.

31. d

Folic acid deficiency and pernicious anemia are both macrocytic, normochromic anemias. Folic acid deficiency is caused by a lack or malabsorption of folic acid. Pernicious anemia is attributed to a deficiency of the intrinsic factor protein, which inhibits absorption of vitamin B12.

32. d

Stage IV of lymphocytic malignancy implies the involvement of liver or bone marrow. Stage I, on the other hand, refers to localized malignancy that affects a single lymph node or group. In stage II, the disease is in more than one lymph node or group, but is confined to one side of the diaphragm. Lastly, stage III refers to lymph node or splenic involvement on both sides of the diaphragm but does not involve the bone marrow.

33. b

Acute myelogenous leukemia constitutes 80% of acute leukemia in adults, but not all leukemia; chronic lymphocytic leukemia is the most common leukemia in adults. It is true that leukemia is more common in males, that acute lymphocytic leukemia is more difficult to cure in adults than in children, and that the median survival for chronic myelogenous leukemia is 4–7 years.

34. c

The normal percentage of red blood cell (RBC) concentration in a 50-year-old male patient would be best represented by a value of 48%. Normal RBC concentration values for a male patient range from 40–54%. Normal RBC concentration values for a female patient range from 37–47%.

35. b

Acute lymphocytic leukemia is most often characterized by indications of pancytopenia (i.e., reduced levels of white and red blood cells) and circulating blasts. In the early stages of leukemia, patients are typically asymptomatic. However, signs of anemia may present with all types of leukemia and may include complaints of fatigue and fever.

36. d

Sickle cell patients should be advised against visiting high-altitude regions, which can precipitate sickling in the blood due to the reduction of oxygen in these types of environments. Beaches and valleys do not offer significant additional risk to patients with sickle cell disease because these environments are at sea level. Densely populated cities generally do not pose a general risk to sickle cell patients, but can if they are in high-elevation areas.

37. d

No treatment is required for mild or moderate forms of thalassemia. A red blood cell transfusion or splenectomy, however, may be used in severe thalassemia. Chelation therapy is also administered to patients with severe thalassemia who experience iron overload from frequent blood transfusions. Oral ferrous sulfate recommended for treatment of iron deficiency anemia, not for thalassemia.

38. d

Cellular hypoxia causes acidosis and tissue ischemia in patients with either sickle cell anemia or, in rare instances, sickle cell trait. Sickle cell anemia is most likely to present with a reduced, not elevated, erythrocyte sedimentation rate. Anorexia and glossitis are more likely to occur with folic acid deficiency or pernicious anemia, rather than sickle cell trait.

39. a

Although the etiology is unclear, a decreased erythrocyte life span often contributes to the development of anemia of chronic disease. Sickle cell anemia, on the other hand, stems from a genetic marker that produces sickle-shaped red blood cells (RBCs), resulting in vessel obstruction. Pernicious anemia is a result of deficiency of intrinsic factor, which results in vitamin B12 malabsorption and macrocytosis of the erythrocytes. Impaired absorption of iron leads to iron deficiency anemia, which is not a chronic condition.

40. c

Chronic lymphocytic leukemia (CLL), which is distinguished by lymphocytosis and may present with fatigue, dyspnea, and abdominal fullness, is the most common leukemia in adults, most frequently presenting in middle-aged and elderly patients. A shortening of chromosome 22, also known as the Philadelphia chromosome, is linked to chronic myelogenous leukemia. Myelogenous leukemias stem from abnormalities in the myeloid cells, whereas lymphocytic leukemias stem from abnormalities in the lymphocytes. Pancytopenia with circulating blasts is more common in acute lymphocytic leukemia and rarely presents in cases of CLL.

DISCUSSION

General Concepts/Key Terms

Table 9.1	Hematologic Terms
Hgb: main component of red blood cells (RBCs) and the essential protein that combines with and transports O_2 to the body	Normal: 14–18 grams/100 ml (males) 12–16 grams/100 ml (females)
Hct: measures the % of a given volume of whole blood that is occupied by erythrocytes; the amount of plasma to total RBC mass (RBC concentration)	Normal: 40%–54% (males) 37%–47% (females)
TIBC: total iron binding capacity	Normal: 250–450 µg/dl
Serum Iron	Normal: 50–150 µg/dl
Mean Corpuscular Volume (MCV): expression of the average volume and size of individual erythrocytes	Normal: 80–100 u³
Microcytic = < 80; Normocytic = 80–100; Macrocytic = > 100)	
Mean Corpuscular Hemoglobin (MCH): expression of the average amount and weight of Hgb contained in a single erythrocyte	Normal: 26–34 pg
Mean Corpuscular Hemoglobin Concentration (MCHC): expression of the average Hgb concentration or proportion of each RBC occupied by Hgb as a percentage; more accurate measure than MCH	Normal: 32%–36%
Hypochromic < 32%, Normochromic 32%–36%, Hyperchromic* > 36% (*Most texts deny the existence of this state, in that it is impossible for an RBC to be too red)	

**The differential diagnosis of each category is well defined:

Low MCV:	Iron deficiency anemia and thalassemia
High MCV:	B12 or folate deficiency, alcoholism, liver failure, and drug effects
Normocytic:	Anemia of chronic disease, sickle cell disease, renal failure, blood loss, and hemolysis

Iron Deficiency Anemia

Overview

Iron deficiency anemia is a microcytic, hypochromic anemia that stems from an overall deficiency of iron.[1] This condition is considered to be the leading cause of anemia worldwide.

The principal cause of iron deficiency anemia is iron loss exceeding intake so that storage is depleted, causing a decrease in iron available for red blood cell (RBC) formation. Iron deficiency anemia typically stems from blood loss, but may also be caused by inadequate iron intake or impaired absorption of iron.[1]

Presentation

Signs and symptoms of iron deficiency anemia tend to be slow in onset. Patients with iron deficiency anemia present with low Hct levels. If Hct falls, pica may occur, characterized by unusual food cravings such as ice or clay. Exercise may also trigger dyspnea and mild fatigue. Other findings include headaches, palpitations, weakness, tachycardia, postural hypotension, and pallor.[2]

Workup

A complete blood count (CBC) is the first step in confirming a diagnosis for iron deficiency anemia. Results reveal a low Hgb, low Hct, low RBC count, and high red cell distribution width. A CBC will also demonstrate low MCV and MCHC. Blood tests for serum iron and ferritin will show low serum iron, low serum ferritin, and a high total iron binding capacity (TIBC).[3]

Treatment

Oral ferrous sulfate at 300–325 mg taken 1–2 hours after meals is a standard treatment for iron deficiency anemia. Antacids should not be taken with iron, as these drugs impair absorption. Taking iron with liquids rich in vitamin C, such as orange juice, aids in absorption. Foods high in iron are also recommended for treating iron deficiency anemia.[4] These foods include raisins, citrus products, green leafy vegetables, red meats, and iron fortified breads and cereals.

Thalassemia

Overview

Thalassemia is a genetically inherited disorder that generates abnormal Hgb production and results in microcytic, hypochromic anemia.[5] The condition results in abnormal production of the alpha or beta Hgb chains, and is regularly classified as alpha or beta thalassemia. Thalassemia is found mainly in African, Middle Eastern, Indian, Mediterranean, and Asian populations.[6]

Presentation

General physical findings for both alpha and beta thalassemia are noncontributory in mild to moderate cases; at worst, patients may experience signs and symptoms of mild anemia. In severe cases, however, signs and symptoms can begin anywhere from birth to the first 6 months of life. Findings of severe thalassemia may include hepatosplenomegaly, arrhythmias, osteopenia, and chronic pain.

Workup

A CBC will isolate findings that distinguish thalassemia from other anemias, such as decreased Hgb, low MCV, low MCHC, normal TIBC, and normal ferritin. Hgb electrophoresis can detect decreased alpha or beta Hgb chains; in some cases, however, gene mapping is necessary to differentiate between alpha and beta thalassemia.[6]

Treatment

Treatments are not necessary for mild to moderate forms of thalassemia. RBC transfusion and splenectomy are treatment options for more severe forms of thalassemia, but are rarely needed. Iron regimens are contraindicated in patients with severe cases, as iron overload can occur, increasing the risk of organ damage.[5]

Folic Acid Deficiency

Overview

Folic acid deficiency is a macrocytic, normochromic anemia that occurs due to a deficiency of folic acid, a synthetic form of vitamin B9. The cause of this anemia is usually inadequate intake of folic acid, which is generally needed for RBC production.[7]

Presentation

Findings of folic acid deficiency include fatigue, dyspnea on exertion, pallor, headache, tachycardia, anorexia, and glossitis.[7] Neurological signs and symptoms may be associated with folic acid deficiency but the Babinski and Romberg tests should be performed to rule out pernicious anemia.

Workup

In a CBC, findings consistent with folic acid deficiency include elevated MCV and normal MCHC. Decreased serum folate levels will aid in confirming the diagnosis, as will RBC folate levels below 100 ng/mL.[6]

Treatment

Treatment for folic acid deficiency focuses on foods high in folic acid, such as bananas, peanut butter, fish, iron fortified breads and cereals, and green, leafy vegetables.[8,9]

Pernicious Anemia

Overview

Pernicious anemia is a macrocytic, normochromic anemia that occurs due to a shortfall of intrinsic factor, resulting in impaired absorption of vitamin B12.[10]

Presentation

The classic findings that suggest pernicious anemia consist of mental sluggishness, glossitis, and shuffling gait; although this grouping is less common these days, these findings can still indicate vitamin B12 deficiency.[11] Weakness and fatigue are common, along with palpitations, anorexia, nausea, vomiting, or weight loss.[10] Positive neurological findings are classically associated with pernicious anemia, and may include dizziness, paresthesia, loss of vibratory sense, and loss of fine motor control.

Certain signs further indicate neurologic effects of pernicious anemia. Romberg's test is performed by having the patient stand straight up and close his or her eyes. If the patient begins to sway or otherwise lose balance, the test is considered positive. Likewise, a patient with pernicious anemia may test positive for Babinski sign, which is found when the big toe elevates upon stimulation of the sole of the foot.

Workup

Expected findings on a CBC in a patient with pernicious anemia include decreased Hgb, Hct, and RBCs, as well as increased MCV. Serum levels of vitamin B12 will be decreased, usually reading under 0.1 µg/mL, and tests for antiparietal cell and anti-intrinsic factor antibodies will also be positive. A Schilling test, used to measure absorption of vitamin B12, can help to determine whether the anemia stems from a lack of intrinsic factor or another possible cause of vitamin B12 deficiency.[10]

Treatment

The standard course of treatment for pernicious anemia is administration of vitamin B12 (cyanocobalamin).[10] The vitamin should be given intramuscularly at 100 µg daily for 1 week. Patients with pernicious anemia will require continuous lifelong monthly maintenance treatment for their condition.

Anemia of Chronic Disease

Overview

Anemia of chronic disease is a chronic anemia that is normocytic and normochromic in nature, and is linked to infection, chronic inflammation, renal failure, and malignancy, among others. Causes of this condition are unclear, but this anemia is closely associated with a decreased erythrocyte life span.

Anemia of chronic disease is the second most common cause of anemia, and is the most common cause of anemia in the elderly and in the hospital setting.[6,12]

Presentation

Findings of anemia of chronic disease often include fatigue, weakness, dyspnea on exertion, and anorexia.[6]

Workup

Expected findings on a CBC in a patient with anemia of chronic disease include low Hgb and Hct, normal MCV, and normal MCHC, whereas tests for serum iron reveal low serum iron and TIBC. High serum ferritin levels differentiate anemia of chronic disease from iron deficiency anemia.[12]

Treatment

Standard treatment for anemia of chronic disease includes ensuring good nutritional support and treating associated diseases that contribute to this condition. Recombinant erythropoietin (EPO) serves as a treatment option, but can require high doses and regular administration due to both reduced production of and marrow resistance to EPO.[12]

Sickle Cell Anemia

Overview

Sickle cell anemia is a chronic hemolytic anemia transmitted via genetics that results in sickle-shaped RBCs. The condition is characterized by episodes of acute, periodic exacerbation wherein RBCs become sickle-shaped. This sickling can be precipitated by factors such as infections, hypoxia, dehydration, high altitudes, physical and emotional stress, surgery, blood loss, and acidosis.[13] Such sickling can produce episodes of vessel obstruction; these episodes frequently cause cellular hypoxia, resulting in acidosis and tissue ischemia. Additionally, pain results from blood hyperviscosity and tissue ischemia.

Presentation

Signs of sickle cell anemia tend to develop in infancy or childhood. The condition can delay growth and development, thus increasing susceptibility to infections. In crisis, patients experience a sudden onset of severe pain in locations such as the extremities, back, chest, and abdomen; aching joint pain, weakness, and dyspnea may also occur during such crises.[13]

Workup

A peripheral smear demonstrates the distorted sickle-shaped RBCs classically associated with the condition, and electrophoresis with cellulose acetate and citrate agar gel confirms Hgb genotype.[13]

Treatment

Both acute and chronic complications must be treated when dealing with sickle cell anemia. Acute complications require fluids for dehydration, analgesics for pain, and oxygen for hypoxemia.[13]

Leukemias

Overview

Leukemia is a cancer of the body's blood-forming tissues, including the bone marrow and lymphatic system.[14] Leukemia has a higher incidence in males and rarely has a direct cause that can be reliably isolated.[6]

There are four major subtypes of leukemia. One is acute nonlymphocytic leukemia (ANL) or acute myelogenous leukemia (AML). Acute leukemias are characterized by immature abnormal cells, such as blast cells, and myelogenous leukemias stem from myeloid cells, which are responsible for the production of RBCs, WBCs, and megakaryocytes.[15] This classification of leukemia constitutes 80% of all cases of acute leukemia in adults. Remission rates for AML range from 50%–85%, with a long term survival rate of approximately 40%.[16]

Another classification is acute lymphocytic leukemia (ALL). Lymphocytic leukemias stem from abnormalities in the immune system cells known as lymphocytes.[15] This condition is generally more difficult to treat in adults than children. Although both populations experience similar initial remission rates (at least 95% in children, 70%–90% in adults), children tend to have a greater than 75% chance of continuous disease-free survival for 5 years, whereas adults have a 30%–40% chance of experiencing the same state.[17] Pancytopenia with circulating blasts usually occurs and is considered a hallmark of the disease.[18]

Chronic lymphocytic leukemia (CLL) is the most common leukemia in adults. Chronic leukemias are characterized by more mature abnormal cells and tend to appear as abnormal leukocytosis with or without reduced blood cell production.[14] Incidence of CLL increases with age, and the condition most frequently presents in middle-aged and elderly patients.[19] The median survival rate for CLL patients is 7–10 years.[14] Lymphocytosis is considered the hallmark finding of CLL.[19]

Lastly, chronic myelogenous leukemia (CML) tends to present in persons 40 years of age and older. Median survival is 4–7 years for CML patients. The classic finding for CML is the presence of the Philadelphia chromosome.[20]

Presentation

Leukemia is often asymptomatic until generalized lymphadenopathy and weight loss occur. For acute leukemia, findings may include fatigue, pallor, fever, malaise, and tachycardia, among others.[17] As for chronic leukemia, findings can include fatigue, anorexia, dyspnea on exertion, and a sense of abdominal fullness, among others.[19,20]

Workup

Expected laboratory findings of leukemia include a complete blood count (CBC) with subnormal RBCs and neutrophils. Elevated ESR will also suggest leukemia. A peripheral blood smear aids in distinguishing between acute and chronic leukemia; however, proper confirmation of the diagnosis requires bone marrow aspiration.[14]

Treatment

The three major treatment measures for leukemia are chemotherapy, bone marrow transplantation, and symptomatic management.[18] Potential control measures for acute leukemias include transfusions, hydration, and psychological support.[18] Treatment for chronic leukemias is focused on extending survival. In recent years, stem cell therapy has shown some curative value in patients with CML.[20]

Lymphomas: Lymphocytic Malignancy

Overview

Lymphoma is a type of blood cancer that develops in lymphatic cells. The condition begins in the lymphocytes, with the malignancy occurring when the lymphocytes are in a state of uncontrolled cell growth and multiplication.[21]

There are two types of lymphomas: non-Hodgkin's lymphoma and Hodgkin's disease. As these lymphomas may exhibit overlapping signs and symptoms, they are best distinguished at a microscopic level. Non-Hodgkin's lymphoma affects both B-cell and T-cell lymphocytes, whereas Hodgkin's disease tends to manifest through abnormal B-cell lymphocytes called Reed-Sternberg cells.[21]

Non-Hodgkin's lymphoma does not have a known cause, but it may have a viral etiology. The condition traditionally presents with lymphadenopathy and is the predominant neoplasm in patients between 20 and 40 years of age. Non-Hodgkin's lymphoma has a less predictable pattern of metastasis than Hodgkin's disease.[22]

Hodgkin's disease also has no known cause, but patients with a history of Epstein-Barr virus infection/infectious mononucleosis have an increased risk of developing the condition.[21] Hodgkin's is more likely to occur in males than in females and reaches peak incidence in patients either between the ages of 15 and 40 or over the age of 55.[23] The condition classically presents with cervical lymphadenopathy and expands through lymph node groups in a predictable fashion. Reed-Sternberg cells differentiate Hodgkin's disease from non-Hodgkin's lymphoma. With this type of lymphoma, cells in the lymphatic system grow abnormally and can spread beyond the lymphatic system. As the condition progresses, Hodgkin's lymphoma compromises the body's ability to fight infection.[23]

Presentation

Lymphomas present in various stages. In stage I, the disease is isolated to a single lymph node or group; by stage II, the disease has progressed to more than one lymph node group but is limited to one side of the diaphragm. In stage III, the condition involves nodes on both sides of the diaphragm, and may spread to the spleen or areas adjacent to the lymph nodes. By stage IV, the lymphoma has spread to the liver, bone marrow, or other organs distant from the affected node.[21] Other findings of lymphomas include heavy night sweats, fever, sudden weight loss, itching, abdominal pain, loss of appetite, and fatigue.[21]

Workup

Diagnostics for lymphomas may include the use of computed tomography, x-rays, ultrasonography, and magnetic resonance imaging, which aid in isolating and staging the disease.[21] Biopsy and histopathologic examination are used to confirm a diagnosis.

Treatment

Treatments for lymphomas include radiation, chemotherapy, and bone marrow transplantation.[21]

TNM Classification of Malignant Tumors (TNM)

Overview

Classification of malignant tumors (TNM) is a system for staging cancers created and regulated by the Union for International Cancer Control.[24] However, not all tumors fall within the TNM classification system (e.g., brain tumors).

There are three mandatory parameters of 'T', 'N', and 'M'. T, the first value, measures the size of the primary tumor and the degree to which it has involved nearby tissue. T is measured in values of 0–4, with a value of "Tis" indicating carcinoma in situ.[25] N, the second value, is graded from 0 to 3 and indicates the spread to regional lymph nodes. M, the third value, is rated as 0 or 1 and indicates the distant metastasis. If a parameter is assigned an "X" rating rather than a number or other suffix, that means the parameter in question could not be assessed.

References

1. Rote NS, McCance KL. Alterations of erythrocyte function. In: McCance KL, Huether SE, Brashers VL, Rote NS, eds. *Pathophysiology: The Biologic Basis for Disease in Adults and Children.* 7th ed. St. Louis, MO: Elsevier Mosby; 2014: 982–1007.

2. Harper JL, Conrad ME. Iron deficiency anemia. In: Besa EC, ed. *Medscape.* http://emedicine.medscape.com/article/202333-overview. Updated October 10, 2014. Accessed March 25, 2015.

3. Harper JL, Conrad ME. Iron deficiency anemia workup. In: Besa EC, ed. *Medscape.* http://emedicine.medscape.com/article/202333-workup. Updated October 10, 2014.

4. Harper JL, Conrad ME. Iron deficiency anemia treatment & management. In: Besa EC, ed. *Medscape.* http://emedicine.medscape.com/article/202333-treatment. Updated October 10, 2014. Accessed Marc h 25, 2015.

5. Benz EJ Jr. Clinical manifestations and diagnosis of the thalassemias. In: Basow DS, ed. *UpToDate.* Waltham, MA: UpToDate; 2015. http://www.uptodate.com/contents/clinical-manifestations-and-diagnosis-of-the-thalassemias. Updated December 17, 2014. Accessed March 25, 2015.

6. Barkley TW Jr. Hematologic and oncologic disorders. In: Barkley TW Jr, ed. *Adult-Gerontology Primary Care Nurse Practitioner.* West Hollywood, CA: Barkley & Associates; 2015: 100–106.

7. Folate deficiency. MedlinePlus Web site. http://www.nlm.nih.gov/medlineplus/ency/article/000354.htm. Updated September 20, 2013. Accessed March 25, 2015.

8. Mayo Clinic Staff. Folic acid (Oral route, injection route). Mayo Clinic Web site. http://www.mayoclinic.org/drugs-supplements/folic-acid-oral-route-injection-route/proper-use/drg-20063897. Updated December 1, 2014. Accessed March 25, 2015.

9. Folate-deficiency anemia. MedlinePlus Web site. http://www.nlm.nih.gov/medlineplus/ency/article/000551.htm. Updated February 24, 2014. Accessed March 25, 2015.

10. Pernicious anemia. PubMed Health Web site. http://www.ncbi.nlm.nih.gov/pubmedhealth/PMH0001595/. Accessed March 25, 2015.

11. Schrier SL. Etiology and clinical manifestations of vitamin B12 and folate deficiency. In: Basow DS, ed. *UpToDate.* Waltham, MA: UpToDate; 2015. http://www.uptodate.com/contents/etiology-and-clinical-manifestations-of-vitamin-b12-and-folate-deficiency. Last updated October 8, 2014. Accessed March 25, 2015.

12. Lichtin AE. Anemia of chronic disease. In: Porter RS, Kaplan JL, eds. *The Merck Manual Online.* http://www.merckmanuals.com/professional/hematology_and_oncology/anemias_caused_by_deficient_erythropoiesis/anemia_of_chronic_disease.html. Updated November 2013. Accessed March 25, 2015.

13. United States Department of Health and Human Services, National Institutes of Health, National Heart, Lung and Blood Institute. What is sickle cell anemia? http://www.nhlbi.nih.gov/health/health-topics/topics/sca/. Updated September 28, 2012. Accessed March 25, 2015.

14. Rytting ME. Overview of leukemia. In: Porter RS, Kaplan JL, eds. *The Merck Manual Online.* http://www.merckmanuals.com/professional/hematology_and_oncology/leukemias/overview_of_leukemia.html. Updated October 2014. Accessed March 25, 2015.

15. What is acute lymphocytic leukemia? American Cancer Society Web site. http://www.cancer.org/cancer/leukemia-acutelymphocyticallinadults/detailedguide/leukemia-acute-lymphocytic-what-is-all. Updated January 12, 2015. Accessed March 25, 2015.

16. Rytting ME. Acute myelogenous leukemia (AML). In: Porter RS, Kaplan JL, eds. *The Merck Manual Online.* http://www.merckmanuals.com/professional/hematology_and_oncology/leukemias/acute_myelogenous_leukemia_aml.html. Updated October 2014. Accessed March 25, 2015.

17. Rytting ME. Acute lymphocytic leukemia (ALL). In: Porter RS, Kaplan JL, eds. *The Merck Manual Online.* http://www.merckmanuals.com/professional/hematology_and_oncology/leukemias/acute_lymphocytic_leukemia_all.html. Updated October 2014. Accessed March 25, 2015.

18. Rytting ME. Acute leukemia overview. In: Porter RS, Kaplan JL, eds. *The Merck Manual Online.* http://www.merckmanuals.com/professional/hematology_and_oncology/leukemias/acute_leukemia_overview.html. Updated October 2014. Accessed March 25, 2015.

19. Rytting ME. Chronic lymphocytic leukemia (CLL). In: Porter RS, Kaplan JL, eds. *The Merck Manual Online.* http://www.merckmanuals.com/professional/hematology_and_oncology/leukemias/chronic_lymphocytic_leukemia_cll.html. Updated October 2014. Accessed March 25, 2015.

20. Rytting ME. Chronic myelogenous leukemia (CML). In: Porter RS, Kaplan JL, eds. *The Merck Manual Online.* http://www.merckmanuals.com/professional/hematology_and_oncology/leukemias/chronic_myelogenous_leukemia_cml.html. Updated October 2014. Accessed March 25, 2015.

21. MacGill M. Lymphoma causes, symptoms and treatments. Medical News Today Web site. http://www.medicalnewstoday.com/articles/146136.php. Updated February 10, 2015. Accessed March 25, 2015.

22. Mayo Clinic Staff. Non-Hodgkin's lymphoma. Mayo Clinic Web site. http://www.mayoclinic.org/diseases-conditions/non-hodgkins-lymphoma/basics/definition/con-20027792. Updated January 23, 2015. Accessed March 25, 2015.

23. What are the key statistics about Hodgkin disease? American Cancer Society Web site. http://www.cancer.org/cancer/hodgkindisease/detailedguide/hodgkin-disease-key-statistics#top. Revised March 4, 2015. Accessed March 25, 2015.

24. Buzaid AC, Gershenwald JE. Tumor node metastasis (TNM) staging system and other prognostic factors in cutaneous melanoma. In: Basow DS, ed. *UpToDate.* Waltham, MA: UpToDate; 2015. http://www.uptodate.com/contents/tumor-node-metastasis-tnm-staging-system-and-other-prognostic-factors-in-cutaneous-melanoma. Updated February 26, 2015. Accessed March 25, 2015.

25. United States Department of Health and Human Services, National Institutes of Health, National Cancer Institute. Cancer staging. http://www.cancer.gov/cancertopics/factsheet/detection/staging. Updated January 6, 2015. Accessed March 25, 2015.

26. Azar A, Ballas ZK. Immune function in older adults. In: Porter RS, Kaplan JL, eds. *UpToDate.* Waltham, MA: UpToDate; 2015. http://www.uptodate.com/contents/immune-function-in-older-adults. Updated January 5, 2015. Accessed March 25, 2015.

Chapter 10
Psychosocial Issues

1. Susan, age 67, has been experiencing difficulty planning and organizing her weekly errands. She frequently has trouble articulating her thoughts and putting sentences together, and struggles with remembering how to cook her favorite meals. Which of the following medications would be <u>least</u> helpful in treating Susan?

    a. Tacrine hydrochloride

    b. Clonazepam

    c. Donepezil

    d. Galantamine

2. Which of the following tasks is most pertinent in assessing a patient's attention in a mini-mental status exam?

    a. Repeating three objects

    b. Counting backwards from 100 in serial 7s

    c. Recalling three objects 5 minutes later

    d. Copying a design

3. A patient complains of insomnia, indecisiveness, and fatigue. His physical examination indicates that he has lost a considerable amount of weight since his last visit 2 months prior. When asked if anything is wrong, the patient explains that he is about to graduate college soon, and he has no job lined up or other future prospects. Which of the following signs or symptoms would best support depression in his case?

    a. Thoughts of suicide

    b. Psychomotor agitation

    c. Hypersomnia

    d. Anhedonia

4. Margaret, a 29-year-old, complains of feeling nervous, moody, and anxious. In addition, she experiences excessive tension and a "rapid heartbeat." To narrow your differential diagnosis, which of the following tests should be ordered first?

    a. VDRL

    b. Electroencephalography

    c. Cortisol test

    d. TSH

5. A 32-year-old Asian female is in the emergency department after being assaulted by her husband. Her history shows that she has been seen two times within the past 6 weeks for bruises and facial abrasions. Which of the following statements best demonstrates the nurse practitioner's ethical responsibility to this patient before discharge?

    a. "I will need to send a report to the health department social worker who can follow up with you at home."

    b. "I would like for you to see a counselor or therapist to really be honest and talk through some things going on with you at home. I can give you several referral names before you leave today."

    c. "I will need to call the police and file a small report. The policewoman will be glad to assist you."

    d. "I want you to know that this is not a normal relationship, and I would like for you to talk with someone here today about your family situation."

6. Which of the following drugs is an opiate antagonist used to help opiate-dependent patients with withdrawal?

 a. Buprenorphine

 b. Tramadol

 c. Clonidine

 d. Buspirone

7. You have diagnosed Jennifer, age 19, with depression. Her parents want you to prescribe her the safest antidepressant to help manage her symptoms, so you prescribe a SSRI. Which of the following is least pertinent in determining why SSRIs are the most commonly prescribed antidepressants?

 a. Fast symptom response

 b. Low overdose danger

 c. No withdrawal symptoms

 d. Low risk of postural hypotension

8. You are seeing Joshua, age 34, who is experiencing feelings of sadness and has trouble concentrating. When asked about why he is sad, Joshua explains that he "screws up all the time" with work and with his relationships. Which of the following explanatory styles is best illustrated by Joshua?

 a. Global thinking

 b. Stable causality

 c. Internal versus external causes

 d. Loss and deprivation

9. Which method is most commonly used in completed suicides?

 a. Hanging

 b. Overdose

 c. Cutting

 d. Firearms

10. Although tricyclics and monoamine oxidase inhibitors are less efficacious for generalized anxiety, these medications are most likely to be useful in treating which of the following issues associated with anxiety?

 a. Tachycardia

 b. Palpitations

 c. Panic attacks

 d. Breathlessness

11. Raphael, a 69-year-old retired professor, has gradually shown less and less interest in reading or interacting with others in the last few years. His wife and his kids both state that he will frequently say things that don't seem to make sense. They also complain that his memory has gradually and steadily worsened, that he can't remember certain daily or weekly activities, and sometimes can't remember most of what he taught in his 35 years of teaching. Considering the most common permanent cause of his issues, which of the following is attributable to Raphael's mental decline?

 a. Poor nutrition

 b. Electrolyte imbalances

 c. Trauma

 d. Cortical atrophy

12. Which of these would a practitioner use as a test to assess a patient's cerebellar function?

 a. Flexion posture

 b. Memory impairment

 c. Gait disturbances

 d. Balance and coordination

13. You want to assess cerebral function in a patient experiencing memory loss. All of the following are main components of the examination that specifically assess cerebral function except:

 a. Thought processes

 b. Cognition

 c. Coordination

 d. Appearance

14. Which of the following anxiety disorders is most commonly tied to the development of agoraphobia?

    a. Panic disorder

    b. Generalized anxiety disorder

    c. Post-traumatic stress disorder

    d. Obsessive compulsive disorder

15. Ingrid, your 26-year-old schizophrenic patient, has attempted suicide multiple times. You want to prescribe her an antipsychotic; however, extreme caution should be exerted when specifically prescribing which of the following medications for psychosis?

    a. Buspirone

    b. Lithium

    c. Donezepil

    d. Memantine

16. Your 63-year-old patient, Sal, suffers from emphysema from lifelong smoking in response to having chronic anxiety throughout most of his life. Although you routinely go through relaxation techniques with him on his visits, he is also interested in pharmacotherapy to deal with his anxiety. Which of the following medications would be the best choice for Sal?

    a. Buspirone

    b. Tranylcypromine

    c. Lorazepam

    d. Hydroxyzine

17. You have just prescribed your 42-year-old bipolar male patient risperidone. The patient may experience which of the following?

    a. Anorexia

    b. Suicidal ideation

    c. Weight gain

    d. Cataracts

18. You have visited a high school to teach young adults about the dangers of drug and alcohol abuse. A student asks what factors could place people at higher risk of developing alcoholism. You would discuss all of the following factors except:

    a. Lower level of psychosocial development

    b. Abnormal protein in the brain

    c. An alcoholic grandparent

    d. Low self-esteem

19. Which of these patients is most at risk of developing dementia?

    a. A 59-year-old who recently underwent a traumatic experience

    b. A 62-year-old with ventricular dilation

    c. A 65-year-old with poor nutrition

    d. A 56-year-old undergoing anesthesia

20. You are examining Patrick, age 65, to assess his cerebellar function. You want to examine his perception of his body in comparison to his surroundings, as well as his ability to sense his own motion and equilibrium. Which test would be least beneficial in making these assessments?

    a. Finger-to-nose test

    b. Romberg test

    c. Rovsing's test

    d. Heel-to-shin test

21. A patient with anxiety complains of heart palpitations and frequent shortness of breath. Her blood pressure is 155/100. Which of the following drugs would be the best choice for her condition at this time?

    a. Amitriptyline

    b. Buspirone

    c. Metoprolol

    d. Diazepam

22. Which of these patients represents a demographic for which suicide is the second leading cause of death?

    a. A 50-year-old Caucasian male

    b. A 77-year-old African-American female

    c. A 17-year-old African-American male

    d. A 22-year-old Caucasian female

23. Which of the following is least likely to present as a differential diagnosis in the assessment of dementia?

    a. Drug reactions and interactions

    b. Nutritional problems

    c. Emotional disorders

    d. Insomnia

24. In the context of depression management, which of the following statements from patients would least strongly indicate the need for referral?

    a. "I just screw everything in my life up; I always have and I probably always will."

    b. "At times, I kind of feel like everyone would just be better off without me."

    c. "I feel horrible that people died in the recent earthquake; I need to be held accountable."

    d. "I don't sleep much anymore because my wife just sneaks out to cheat whenever I do."

25. You have just diagnosed Harold, age 19, with depression. His concerned parents want to know what fast-acting, safe medications are available for his condition. Which of the following is the best first-line pharmacotherapeutic choice for Harold in this case?

    a. Diazepam

    b. Amitriptyline

    c. Phenelzine

    d. Fluoxetine

26. All of the following are standard components in assessing cerebellar function except:

    a. The patient stands with eyes closed, feet together, and arms at the side.

    b. The patient runs the heel of one foot along the shin of the opposite leg.

    c. The patient fully extends arms to the front, raising one while lowering the other, and alternating.

    d. The patient alternately points from his/her nose to the examiner's finger.

27. Susan, age 35, experiences excessive worry about life, which keeps her on edge and makes her always dread the future. She is interested in taking medication to ease her condition, but is very clear about her desire to not take a "tranquilizer." Which of the following medications would be the best choice for Susan?

    a. Lorazepam

    b. Buspirone

    c. Imipramine

    d. Selegiline

28. Going by the standard CAGE mnemonic, which of the following questions is least helpful in the diagnosis for alcohol abuse?

    a. "Have you ever felt the need to cut down on your drinking?"

    b. "Have you ever justified having a drink for any reason?"

    c. "Have you ever felt guilty about your drinking?"

    d. "Have people annoyed you by criticizing your drinking?"

29. All of the following statements regarding suicide are true except:

    a. Men are more likely to complete suicide.

    b. Adolescents and white males over 45 years of age have a higher incidence of suicide.

    c. Women are more likely to attempt suicide.

    d. Jumping is the second most common method of completed suicide.

30. Your colleague is worried that her patient is at risk of committing suicide. She states that he has other underlying psychosocial conditions that also increase this risk. Which of the following conditions accounts for the highest number of suicides?

    a. Alcoholism

    b. Drug abuse

    c. Terminal diseases

    d. Mental disorders

31. Jorge, age 74, learned how to play bingo last year. Since then, he has played twice a week at the community center. However, while playing during the last few weeks, he has constantly had to be reminded what the marking circles were next to his scorecard, though he still remembers how to play the game. Which of the following most accurately describes Jorge's condition?

    a. Apraxia

    b. Aphasia

    c. Agnosia

    d. Delirium

32. Of the following, which statement is most accurate regarding suicide?

    a. Overdose is present in the majority of completed suicides.

    b. Suicide is the leading cause of death among adolescents.

    c. Most people who state intent to commit suicide actually follow through.

    d. In the United States, men attempt suicide more often than women.

33. Rachel, age 33, comes to the clinic with complaints of frequent distraction, lack of focus, and disorientation. While in your office, Rachel's face goes blank and she forgets where she is, although she remembers a few minutes later. Which of the following is the most likely diagnosis?

    a. Panic disorder

    b. Alzheimer's disease

    c. Dementia

    d. Delirium

34. A patient complains of feeling anxious for no reason. He states he does not think he has panic attacks, but there will be moments of excessive worry about minute things seemingly triggered by nothing. He complains of not being able to breathe at moments and has a "tight feeling" in his chest. After these brief moments, the patient states that he feels fatigued. Which of the following should be your lowest priority to order?

    a. Complete blood count

    b. Electrocardiogram

    c. Glucose levels

    d. Thyroid stimulating hormone levels

35. Which of the following plays a role in 70% of all substance overdoses in the U.S.?

    a. Prescription narcotics

    b. Alcohol

    c. Heroin

    d. Cocaine

36. All of these statements regarding depression are true except:

    a. More women are affected by depression than men.

    b. Approximately 30% of depressed patients attempt suicide.

    c. It is estimated that at least 9 million Americans are affected.

    d. It is the most common psychiatric disorder.

37. Dave, a 72-year-old patient, receives a score of 22 on a mini-mental status exam. What does his score indicate?

    a. No cognitive impairment

    b. Mild cognitive impairment

    c. Moderate cognitive impairment

    d. Severe cognitive impairment

38. Which of the following is least likely to be used to treat patients with depression due to its side effects and high overdose potential?

a. Alprazolam

b. Memantine

c. Citalopram

d. Phenelzine

39. In general, depression must be present for at least how long to qualify for a dysthymia diagnosis?

a. One year

b. Two years

c. Three years

d. Four years

40. Megan, a 68-year-old patient, is brought to the clinic by her distressed daughter, Carol. Carol claims that her mom had missed their weekly lunch meetings the last two weeks, and she recently found out that Megan missed both an appointment with her optometrist and a DMV appointment in the last week. She also says that when she went to pick Megan up from her house, Megan almost fell because she didn't see the step from her kitchen to the living room. During the examination, Megan has trouble keeping her attention focused and articulating her thoughts in a coherent manner. Which condition is Megan most likely experiencing?

a. Delirium

b. Anxiety

c. Dysthymia

d. Alzheimer's disease

RATIONALES

1. b

Clonazepam is a benzodiazepine, a class of drugs most often used in treating anxiety, seizures, insomnia, and other conditions, but not used in the treatment of Alzheimer's. Tacrine hydrochloride is a parasympathomimetic agent, and donepezil and galantamine are acetylcholinesterase inhibitors; these drugs increase the availability of acetylcholine, and are thus used in the treatment of Alzheimer's patients.

2. b

In a mini-mental status exam, patients may be assessed for attention by counting backwards from 100 in serial 7s. The other answer choices represent tasks used to assess other aspects of a patient's mental status. The nurse practitioner can assess for recognition by asking the patient to repeat three objects, and can assess for recall by asking the patient to recall the same three objects 5 minutes later. Copying a design would demonstrate a patient's ability to copy and draw rather than his or her ability to pay attention.

3. d

The patient fulfills four diagnostic criteria of depression according to the Diagnostic and Statistical Manual of Mental Disorders-5 (DSM-5); but, for a diagnosis of depression, the patient would also need to present with either a consistently depressed mood for the majority of almost every day, or anhedonia, a markedly diminished interest in almost all activity. Suicidal ideation, psychomotor agitation, and hypersomnia are symptoms of depression, but are not required for a diagnosis of depression.

4. d

A nurse practitioner should order a TSH assay first to rule out the possibility of hyperthyroidism in patients experiencing symptoms similar to those of anxiety, like the patient in the question. Similar to anxiety, hyperthyroidism frequently presents with excessive tension, rapid heartbeat, and feelings of nervousness, moodiness, and anxiety. An electroencephalogram would be used to rule out seizure disorders, cortisol levels would be checked to rule out Cushing's syndrome, and a Venereal Disease Research Laboratory test would be ordered to rule out syphilis.

5. d

Informing the patient that abuse should not be tolerated and guiding her to immediate help most accurately demonstrates fulfilling the nurse practitioner's ethical responsibility. Sending a report to a social worker, giving referrals to therapists, and filing a report with the police are all methods of action that do not provide as immediate assistance, and do less to reassure the patient that help is immediately available.

6. a

Buprenorphine is an opiate antagonist used to help ease withdrawal in opiate-dependent patients. Tramadol is not an opiate antagonist, but a narcotic analgesic. Clonidine or buspirone may also be utilized to help opiate-dependent patients in withdrawal, but these drugs are not opiate antagonists.

7. c

Although SSRIs are not considered addictive, dosing should be gradually decreased when stopping treatment to reduce withdrawal-like symptoms. SSRIs are given to patients with depression because these medications present low overdose danger and fast symptom response. Moreover, SSRIs do not increase the risk of postural hypotension.

8. c

The internal versus external style is best illustrated by the patient because the patient assumes accountability and fault for all of the bad things in his life. The global thinking theory of depression, on the other hand, would explain a patient who thinks that everything is ruined. The stable causality theory would be best demonstrated by someone who feels that the causes of all negativity are absolute, and that nothing can be done to change them. Lastly, reactions to loss and deprivation are a psychodynamic cause of depression rather than a cognitive cause.

9. d

Approximately 60% percent of all completed suicides are accomplished with the aid of firearms. Hanging is the second most common method of completed suicide. Overdose is present in more than 70% of attempted suicides, but it does not account for the majority of completed suicides. Lastly, although cutting is one of the best-known suicide methods, it is not as common as the use of firearms.

10. c

Tricyclics and monoamine oxidase inhibitors (MAOIs) may be useful for treating panic attacks in patients with anxiety. Tachycardia, palpitations, and breathlessness are treated by beta blockers, not MAOIs or tricyclics.

11. d

Cortical atrophy is a possible cause of dementia, of which the patient has displayed key signs, such as the gradual and steady decline in memory and intellectual functioning. Poor nutrition, electrolyte imbalances, and trauma are not likely causes of dementia, but they are possible causes of delirium.

12. d

The cerebellum is primarily responsible for balance and coordination. Therefore, assessment techniques, such as the Romberg test and heel-to-shin test, primarily test for balance and coordination. Although flexion posture and gait disturbances may be impacted by the cerebellum, a standard test of cerebellum function does not assess posture and gait. Recent memory impairments indicate Alzheimer's disease, but memory impairments are not specifically tested for when evaluating cerebellar function.

13. c

Coordination is not one of the four main components of a mental status examination; rather, a patient's balance and coordination are examined in a series of assessment techniques for cerebellar function. The four main components of a mental status examination are appearance, behavior, cognition, and thought processes.

14. a

Panic disorder, the morbid dread of seemingly harmless objects or situations, may lead to agoraphobia. For some patients, generalized anxiety disorder or post-traumatic stress disorder can lead to agoraphobia, but panic disorder is more closely associated with agoraphobia. Agoraphobia is not typically associated with obsessive compulsive disorder.

15. b

Low therapeutic index medications, such as lithium, should be prescribed with extreme caution when used to manage the risk of suicide, due to the high risk of poisoning. Donezepil, memantine, and buspirone all have a higher therapeutic index than lithium, but are not typically used to manage suicide risk. Donezepil and memantine are prescribed for Alzheimer's disease; buspirone, on the other hand, is an antianxiety medication but is not typically prescribed to manage suicide risk.

16. d

Hydroxyzine would be the best choice for the patient, as it is an antihistamine used for the treatment of anxiety; antihistamines are especially warranted in anxiety patients with chronic obstructive pulmonary disorder—like the patient's emphysema—or a potential for abuse. Although buspirone, lorazepam, and tranylcypromine are appropriate treatments for anxiety, hydroxyzine is the best choice in this case because of the patient's emphysema.

17. c

Significant weight gain is an expected side effect of atypical antipsychotics, such as risperidone. Anorexia is not a typical side effect of antipsychotics. Suicidal ideation more often presents as a side effect in antidepressants, and does not typically present as a side effect in antipsychotics. There is a small risk of developing cataracts after using atypical antipsychotics, but developing cataracts would not be an expected side effect.

18. b

Abnormal protein in the brain may lead to Alzheimer's disease, but is not traditionally linked to alcoholism. Genetics, such as a parent, grandparent, or aunt or uncle with alcoholism, may increase one's risk for developing alcoholism. Psychosocial factors, such as poor impulse control, low psychosocial development, and low self-esteem, may also increase the risk of alcoholism.

19. b

A patient who is over 60 years old with ventricular dilation would typically be at high risk for dementia. Although the 65-year-old with poor nutrition is also over 60 years old, poor nutrition is more likely to lead to delirium than dementia. The 59-year-old and 56-year-old patients would be at lower risk for developing dementia as dementia typically occurs in patients over the age of 60. Additionally, trauma and anesthesia are more likely to lead to delirium than dementia.

20. c

Rovsing's test does not measure cerebellar function; rather, it is used to assess for appendicitis. The Romberg test, which consists of asking the patient to stand with feet together, eyes closed, and arms at his or her side, assesses a patient's proprioception, as well as cerebellar function. The finger-to-nose test and heel-to-shin test also evaluate a patient's balance and coordination and can be used to test proprioception.

21. c

Beta blockers, such as metoprolol, help reduce tachycardia, palpitations, and breathlessness in patients with anxiety. Amitriptyline is a tricyclic, which is more likely to be beneficial in treating panic attacks. The patient's symptoms would not be treated with buspirone, an antianxiety medication not classified as a tranquilizer. Benzodiazepines, such as diazepam, are the most commonly used antianxiety medication, but these are not specified to treat tachycardia, palpitations, or breathlessness.

22. c

Suicide is the second leading cause of death in adolescents; thus, an African-American male who is 17 years old would fit in that demographic. White males above 45 years of age, and persons of all ethnicities above 65 years of age have a higher suicide rate, but it is usually due to the sudden loss of a spouse or partner. Women are more likely than men to attempt suicide, but more men successfully complete suicide than women.

23. d

Of these choices, insomnia is least likely to present as a differential diagnosis in evaluating for dementia. Drug reactions, nutritional problems, and emotional disorders are all conditions that could present with signs and symptoms indicative of dementia. Other possible differential diagnoses include infection, metabolic disorders, eye and ear disorders, tumors, and arteriosclerosis.

24. a

The first patient would least strongly indicate a referral; although his statement demonstrates depressed behavior via stable causality and an internal versus external conflict, referrals for depressed patients are warranted by the occurrence of more serious issues, such as hallucinations, delusions, loss of reality contact, or suicidal ideation. The second patient indicates suicidal ideation in stating that everyone would probably be better off without him/her, and would thus warrant a referral. Both of the last two patients demonstrate delusional behavior; the third patient feels that he/she is responsible and to blame for a natural disaster, and the fourth patient refuses to sleep because he/she is convinced that his/her wife leaves and cheats every time the patient sleeps.

25. d

Fluoxetine and other selective serotonin reuptake inhibitors (SSRIs) would be the best choice of first line pharmacotherapy for the patient, as these antidepressants are most commonly prescribed due to their low overdose danger, fast symptom response, and lack of yielding postural hypotension. Diazepam is a benzodiazepine and would not typically be used to treat depression. Amitriptyline is a tricyclic antidepressant, whereas phenelzine is a monoamine oxidase inhibitor; although both these drugs can be used to treat depression, they are used less often than SSRIs due to their increased side effects and high overdose potential.

26. c

Fully extending the arms out, raising one while lowering the other, and alternating these movements is not a standard component in assessing for cerebellar function. The patient standing with eyes closed, feet together, and arms at the side is performing the Romberg test. The patient running the heel of one foot along the shin of the opposite leg is performing the heel-to-shin test. The patient alternately pointing from his/her nose to the examiner's finger is performing the finger-to-nose test. The Romberg, heel-to-shin, and finger-to-nose tests are all assessment techniques for cerebellar function.

27. b

Buspirone is the only antianxiety medication not classified as a "tranquilizer." It treats the anxiety-stimulating factors rather than the somatic response that anxiety causes. Lorazepam is a benzodiazepine; benzodiazepines are commonly used in cases of anxiety and are considered to be tranquilizers because they treat the somatic symptoms of anxiety, which include muscle tension and hyper-awareness. Imipramine is a tricyclic and selegiline is a monoamine oxidase inhibitor; both are tranquilizers.

28. b

The question, "Have you ever justified having a drink for any reason?" is not part of the CAGE mnemonic screening for alcohol abuse. The other questions are part of the CAGE mnemonic screening. The components of the CAGE mnemonic include questions regarding feeling the need to cut down drinking, feeling annoyed by criticism, feeling guilty about drinking, and needing a morning eye-opener.

29. d

Hanging, rather than jumping, is the second most common method of completed suicides. Women are more likely to attempt suicide, whereas men are more likely to complete suicide. Adolescents and white males over 45 years of age have a higher suicide rate.

30. d

Mental illness accounts for at least 90% of all suicides. Alcohol and drug use increases the risk of committing suicide. People with terminal illness make up a smaller percentage of suicides.

31. c

Agnosia would best describe Jorge's condition. Agnosia is the inability to recognize an object, and though it does not necessarily indicate memory loss or defective sensorium, it may increase with memory loss. Aphasia is characterized by difficulty with speech, which is not illustrated by Jorge in this context. Apraxia refers to the inability to perform a previously learned task; this would be more applicable if Jorge had forgotten how to play bingo altogether. Delirium is characterized by confusion and decreased awareness of one's environment.

32. c

Approximately 80% of all individuals who state their intentions to commit suicide actually follow through on their plans. Although overdose is present in the majority of attempted suicides, it is not the most common method used in completed suicides. The majority of completed suicides involve the use of a firearm, whereas hanging constitutes the second most common method of completed suicide. Furthermore, suicide is the second leading cause of death among adolescents, not the leading cause. Lastly, in the United States, women attempt suicide more often than men, whereas men are three times more likely to succeed in completing suicides.

33. d

Delirium is the most likely diagnosis, as the distraction, lack of focus, and the patient's age would all strongly indicate the condition. Though dementia may sometimes have a similar presentation, it is not likely to be seen in someone under the age of 60; furthermore, despite the loss of decreased intellectual functioning, people with dementia are typically more alert and not as distracted as people with delirium. The patient's quick lapse of disorientation in the office more closely demonstrates the transience of clouded sensorium associated with delirium rather than the permanent memory and cognitive impairment associated with Alzheimer's. Additionally, like dementia, Alzheimer's is not likely to be seen in a 33-year-old patient. Lastly, panic disorder is an anxiety disorder causing morbid dread of seemingly harmless objects or situations, and does not typically produce with clouded sensorium.

34. a

A nurse practitioner would typically perform all of the tests listed to rule out anxiety except a complete blood count (CBC), though such information is interesting as a baseline. CBCs are more commonly used to rule out anemia, infection, or other disorders in likely Alzheimer's patients. The electrocardiogram may be conducted to examine underlying causes of the patient's chest pain. Glucose levels may be checked to examine for causes of the patient's fatigue. Thyroid stimulating hormone levels may be assessed to look for hyperthyroidism, which can cause many symptoms similar to anxiety.

35. b

Alcohol plays a role in 70% of drug overdoses in the U.S. Approximately 10% of the population is alcoholic. Other potential causes for drug abuse include genetics, alterations in opiate receptors, neurotransmitter alterations, and psychosocial factors such as poor impulse control or low self-esteem.

36. b

Approximately 15% of depressed patients commit suicide, not 30%. It is true that women are more often diagnosed with depression compared to men, possibly because women are more likely to report it. Depression is the most common psychiatric disorder and an estimated 9–16 million Americans are affected by it.

37. b

The patient with a mini-mental status assessment score of 22 experiences mild cognitive impairment, which ranges from 18–23; furthermore, this score suggests that the patient is experiencing either delirium or dementia. Severe cognitive impairment is typically indicated by a score range of 0–7. Moderate cognitive impairment is not a category used in the mental status examination. Lastly, the absence of cognitive impairment is usually indicated by a score range of 24–30, with a score of 27 being the average.

38. d

Monoamine oxidase inhibitors, such as phenelzine, are not used as often as SSRIs because of the increase in side effects and potential for overdose. Alprazolam and memantine would most likely not be used for treatment of depression; alprazolam is a benzodiazepine that would be more pertinent in treating anxiety, and memantine is an NMDA receptor antagonist that is most often used to treat Alzheimer's disease or dementia. Citalopram is a SSRI and would most likely be used to treat patients with depression.

39. b

Dysthymia is a chronic form of depression that typically lasts at least 2 years. Dysthymia often occurs for a much longer period of time but depression only needs to last 2 years to qualify as dysthymia. Conversely, depression lasting only 1 year would not qualify as dysthymia.

40. d

Short-term memory loss is typically an early sign of Alzheimer's disease, which eventually impairs the ability to learn new information and recall previously learned information. Difficulty with speech and depth perception, as well as the inability to recognize objects, would further support the diagnosis of Alzheimer's disease. Delirium involves a sudden, transient onset of clouded sensorium, leading to an acute confusional state in the patient. Dysthymia is classified as chronic depression lasting for at least 2 years. Lastly, anxiety is typically distinguished by an unpleasant feeling of dread, apprehension, or tension.

DISCUSSION

Depression

Overview

Depression is a highly prevalent mood disorder interferes with daily life, characterized by fatigue, feelings of sadness, decreased interest in normal activities, and impaired concentration that occurs nearly every day. Dysthymia is a mild, chronic form of depression lasting for 2 years or longer.

Approximately 9–16 million Americans are affected by depression. Worldwide, twice as many women than men are diagnosed with depression. In many cases, depression is believed to be undertreated or not reported at all.[1]

Psychodynamic causes of depression include anger that is directed internally instead of being expressed directly, inordinate reactions to loss and deprivation, or a decrease in or loss of self-esteem resulting from a sense of not having lived up to certain expectations.

Cognitive causes include negative belief systems, dysfunctional thinking, stable causality (e.g., "It will always be this way"), global thinking (e.g., "Everything is ruined"), and internal versus external causes (e.g., "It's my fault").

Biochemical theories suggest that depression is caused by a neurotransmitter imbalance (e.g., dopamine, serotonin, epinephrine, norepinephrine), thyroid dysfunction, or medicinal side effects, among others.[2,3]

Presentation

The criteria to diagnose depression are outlined in the DSM-5. Patients must experience either a depressed mood for most or part of the day nearly every day, anhedonia (i.e., a clear decrease in pleasure or interest in almost all activities), or both.[4] In addition, a patient must demonstrate at least five of the following within the same 2-week period and represent a change in previous functioning: either weight loss or weight gain, resulting in a change of more than 5% in body weight; insomnia or hypersomnia; psychomotor agitation or retardation; fatigue or loss of energy; lack of concentration or indecisiveness nearly every day; excessive guilt or feelings of worthlessness; or recurrent thoughts of death or suicidal ideation without plan or attempt.[3]

"In Sad Cages" is a mnemonic device used to help memorize the symptoms of depression.[5] This mnemonic stands for INterest (loss of pleasure), Sleep disturbances, Appetite changes, Depressed mood, Concentration difficulty, Activity (agitation or retardation), Guilt feelings or low self-esteem, Energy loss, and Suicidal ideation.

Workup

The diagnosis relies primarily on the patient's clinical history. The patient's feelings should also be assessed in accordance with one of the following categories: mad, sad, glad, afraid, or ashamed. Initial laboratory tests include a thyroid-stimulating hormone (TSH) assay, basic metabolic panel (BMP), complete blood count (CBC), liver function tests, urinalysis, B12, and a Venereal Disease Research Laboratory (VDRL) test to exclude other potential conditions.[7]

Treatment (see table 10.1)

Patients who experience delusions, hallucinations, loss of contact with reality, or suicidal thoughts must receive immediate care by a mental health specialist.

For mild depression, weekly appointments are recommended. Contact by phone should also be provided to check on the patient's status. Therapeutic communication should focus on expression of feelings, fears, losses that have occurred, and cognitive errors in thinking.

Depressed patients require support during the five stages of grief, according to Kübler-Ross, which include denial, anger, bargaining, depression, and acceptance (DABDA).[8] One crucial aspect of therapeutic communication involves avoiding making judgments or blaming. The NP should also encourage interaction with others, alternative coping methods, planned or regular activities, and relaxation techniques.

Antidepressants may be considered in certain cases. Selective serotonin reuptake inhibitors (SSRIs) are the most commonly prescribed antidepressants due to their fast symptom response, low overdose danger, and no postural hypotension.[9] Tricyclics and monoamine oxidase inhibitors (MAOIs) are gaining popularity again, yet are known to produce side effects associated with anti-cholinergic activity, such as dry mouth and constipation. MAOIs have the potential to cause a hypertensive crisis when consumed with food products containing high amounts of tyramine, dopamine, or tryptophan.

Psychotherapy is another option to consider when managing depression. The use of electroconvulsive therapy, on the other hand, is controversial.

Anxiety

Overview

Anxiety disorders cause patients to experience physical symptoms that can interfere with a person's ability to lead a normal life. Anxiety develops from an emotionally learned reaction to stress and manifests as a symptom in many disorders. Anxiety produces an unpleasant sensation of tension, apprehension, or dread stemming from an unexpected threat to one's sense of self or well-being.

Table 10.1	Pharmacologic Agents for Depression		
Agent	**Initial Dosage**	**Adverse Effects**	**Comments**
Selective Serotonin Reuptake Inhibitors (SSRIs)			
citalopram (Celexa)	20 mg PO daily Max: 40 mg/day	nausea, dry mouth, insomnia, somnolence, headache, anxiety, GI disturbances, dizziness, anorexia, fatigue, sexual dysfunction, suicidal ideation, serotonin syndrome, SJS	Generally considered as first line therapy Many applications: OCD, anxiety, PTSD, others Well tolerated, but many drug-drug interactions **Black Box Warning**: increased risk of suicidal thinking/behavior[a] Onset of effect: 4–6 weeks
escitalopram (Lexapro)	10 mg PO daily Max: 20 mg/day		
fluoxetine (Prozac)	20 mg PO daily Max: 80 mg/day		
fluvoxamine (Luvox)	50 mg PO daily Max: 300 mg/day		
paroxetine (Paxil)	20 mg PO daily Max: 50 mg/day		
sertraline (Zoloft)	50 mg PO daily Max: 200 mg/day		
vilazodone (Viibryd)	10 mg PO daily Max: 40 mg/day		
Serotonin-norepinephrine Reuptake Inhibitors (SNRIs)			
duloxetine (Cymbalta)	20 mg PO BID Max: 120 mg/day	insomnia, nausea, dry mouth, constipation, hypertension, dizziness, somnolence, sweating, agitation, blurred vision, headache, tremor, vomiting, drowsiness, increased appetite, orthostatic hypotension, sexual dysfunction, suicidal ideation, serotonin syndrome	Other applications: pain disorders, fibromyalgia Several drug-drug interactions **Black Box Warning**: suicidal thinking/behavior[a] Withdrawal syndrome if stopped abruptly Onset of effect: 4–6 weeks
desvenlafaxine (Pristiq)	50 mg PO daily Max: 50 mg/day		
venlafaxine (Effexor, Effexor XR)	37.5 mg PO BID 37.5 mg PO daily Max: 225 mg/day		
Serotonin Antagonists			
nefazodone (Serzone)	100 mg PO BID Max: 600 mg/day	insomnia, nausea, dry mouth, constipation, dizziness, somnolence, sweating, agitation, blurred vision, headache, tremor, vomiting, drowsiness, increased appetite, orthostatic hypotension, sexual dysfunction, suicidal ideation, serotonin syndrome, QTc prolongation	Several drug-drug interactions **Black Box Warning**: suicidal thinking/behavior[a] Withdrawal syndrome if stopped abruptly Other applications: insomnia (trazodone) Onset of effect: 4–6 weeks
trazodone (Desyrel)	50 mg PO TID Max: 400 mg/day		

Table 10.1	Pharmacologic Agents for Depression		
Agent	**Initial Dosage**	**Adverse Effects**	**Comments**
Atypical Antidepressants			
bupropion (Wellbutrin, Wellbutrin SR, Wellbutrin XL)	100 mg PO TID 150 mg PO BID 150 mg PO daily Max: 450 mg/day	insomnia, nausea, dry mouth, dizziness, somnolence, sweating, agitation, blurred vision, headache, tremor, vomiting, drowsiness, weight gain, orthostatic hypotension, sexual dysfunction, suicidal ideation, serotonin syndrome, seizures	Several drug-drug interactions **Black Box Warning**: suicidal thinking/behavior[a] Withdrawal syndrome if stopped abruptly Bupropion lowers the seizure threshold Onset of effect: 4–6 weeks
mirtazapine (Remeron)	15 mg PO daily Max: 45 mg/day		
Monoamine Oxidase Inhibitors (MAOIs)			
isocarboxazid (Marplan)	10 mg PO BID Max: 40 mg/day	dry mouth, constipation, urinary retention, blurred vision, sedation, confusion, arrhythmias, insomnia, nausea, anorexia, drowsiness, orthostatic hypotension, sexual dysfunction, serotonin syndrome, suicidal ideation	Reserved for depression unresponsive to other agents Many drug-drug and drug-food (tyramine: HTN crisis) interactions **Black Box Warning**: suicidal thinking/behavior[a] Onset of effect: 4–6 weeks
phenelzine (Nardil)	15 mg PO TID Max: 90 mg/day		
tranylcypromine (Parnate)	10 mg PO TID Max: 60 mg/day		
Tricyclic Antidepressants (TCAs)			
amitriptyline (Elavil)	25 mg PO TID Max: 300 mg/day	dry mouth, constipation, urinary retention, blurred vision, sedation, confusion, arrhythmias, insomnia, nausea, dizziness, somnolence, sweating, agitation, headache, tremor, vomiting, drowsiness, weight gain, orthostatic hypotension, sexual dysfunction, suicidal ideation	Several drug-drug interactions Other applications: pain disorders, fibromyalgia **Black Box Warning**: suicidal thinking/behavior[a] Onset of effect: 4–6 weeks
amoxapine (Asendin)	50 mg PO BID Max: 300 mg/day		
desipramine (Norpramin)	50 mg PO BID Max: 300 mg/day		
doxepin (Sinequan)	25 mg PO daily Max: 300 mg/day		
imipramine (Tofranil)	25 mg PO TID Max: 300 mg/day		
nortriptyline (Aventyl, Pamelor)	25 mg PO TID Max: 150 mg/day		

Note. [a]Although injectable haloperidol is approved by the FDA only for intramuscular injection, there is considerable evidence from the medical literature that intravenous administration of haloperidol is a relatively common "off-label" clinical practice, primarily for treatment of severe agitation. Higher doses and intravenous administration of haloperidol appear to be associated with a higher risk of QT prolongation and Torsades de pointes (TdP). Because of this risk of TdP and QT prolongation, ECG monitoring is recommended if haloperidol is given intravenously. Used with permission from Vuckovich PK. Psychosocial Problems in Acute Care. In: Barkley TW Jr, Myers CM, eds. *Practice Considerations for the Adult-Gerontology Acute Care Nurse Practitioner.* West Hollywood, CA: Barkley and Associates; 2015: 417–419.

The majority of Americans experience symptoms of anxiety or an anxiety disorder at least once in their lifetime. Various theories attribute causes for the condition to psychodynamics, genetics, neuropsychological factors, and family dynamics.[10]

Presentation

Anxiety disorders are the most common group of emotional disorders, ranging from mild to severe. Two of the most serious forms of anxiety disorders are generalized anxiety disorder and panic disorder.

Generalized anxiety disorder involves excessive worry about life circumstances. Agoraphobia is a type of anxiety disorder that is characterized by a morbid sense of dread or terror of a seemingly harmless object or situation that may cause the patient to panic.[11]

Obsessive compulsive disorder (OCD) is characterized by uncontrollable obsessive, repetitive thoughts that escape the patient's control, which are called obsessions. To control these thoughts, the patient feels an overwhelming urge to perform acts that can only be resisted or avoided with great difficulty or effort (i.e., compulsion).

Post-traumatic stress disorder (PTSD) involves anxiety that lasts for at least 6 months after the patient experiences severe trauma or an event that he or she perceived as a threat to his or her integrity or safety. PTSD patients are prone to flashbacks, nightmares, and intrusive thoughts.

Workup

A physical examination helps to determine if the anxiety is secondary to a physical illness. A standard diagnostic workup may include a TSH, serum chemistries, serum glucose analysis, and electrocardiogram (ECG).[12]

Treatment (see table 10.2)

Treatment options depend on the category of anxiety. Treatment may involve psychotherapy, prescription medication, or both. Therapeutic communication identifies emotional and physical feelings while keeping the focus of responsibility on the patient. Relaxation techniques provide the patient with a means of managing the physiological component of anxiety.[13]

Pharmacological options include antianxiety medications such as benzodiazepines (e.g., lorazepam [Ativan]).[14] Buspirone (Buspar), which takes 3–4 weeks to reach a full therapeutic effect, is the only antianxiety medication not defined as a tranquilizer by pharmacological standards. Antihistamines are prescribed to anxiety patients with chronic obstructive pulmonary disease or with the potential for substance abuse. Beta blockers are used to reduce tachycardia, palpitations, and breathlessness. Tricyclic antidepressants and MAOIs help to manage panic attacks but are less efficacious for generalized anxiety.

Table 10.2	Pharmacologic Agents for Anxiety		
Agent	**Initial Dosage**	**Adverse Effects**	**Comments**
Benzodiazepines			
alprazolam (Xanax)	0.25 mg PO TID Max: 4 mg/day	drowsiness, sedation, lethargy, ataxia, confusion	Alprazolam, lorazepam, diazepam effective for situational anxiety
clonazepam (Klonopin)	1 mg PO daily Max: 4 mg/day		Preferred agent for insomnia caused by anxiety
lorazepam (Ativan)	0.5 mg PO BID Max: 10 mg/day		Many other applications: seizures, EtOH withdrawal, adjunct to anesthesia, nausea
diazepam (Valium)	2 mg PO QID Max: 40 mg/day		Adjust dose for liver/renal dysfunction Some agents have active metabolites
oxazepam (Serax)	10 mg PO TID Max: 120 mg/day		Antidote: flumazenil (Romazicon)
Serotonin Receptor Agonist			
buspirone (Buspar)	7.5 mg PO BID Max: 60 mg/day	nausea, dizziness, nervousness, headache, somnolence, tachycardia, heart failure, MI, CVA	Many drug-drug interactions Slow onset of action (14 days) Adjust dose for liver or renal impairment Not a controlled substance

Table 10.2	Pharmacologic Agents for Anxiety		
Agent	Initial Dosage	Adverse Effects	Comments
Antidepressant agents			
duloxetine (Cymbalta)	30 mg PO daily Max: 120 mg/day	nausea, dry mouth, insomnia, somnolence, headache, anxiety, GI disturbances, dizziness, anorexia, fatigue, sexual dysfunction, suicidal ideation, serotonin syndrome, SJS	Effective for: General anxiety disorder Panic disorder Social Anxiety disorder Post Traumatic Stress Disorder Obsessive-compulsive disorder
escitalopram (Lexapro)	10 mg PO daily Max: 20 mg/day		
paroxetine (Paxil)	20 mg PO daily Max: 50 mg/day		
sertraline (Zoloft)	50 mg PO daily Max: 200 mg/day		
venlafaxine (Effexor, Effexor XR)	37.5 mg PO BID 37.5 mg PO daily Max: 225 mg/day	insomnia, nausea, dry mouth, constipation, hypertension, dizziness, somnolence, sweating, agitation, blurred vision, headache, tremor, vomiting, drowsiness, increased appetite, sexual dysfunction, suicidal ideation, serotonin syndrome	

Used with permission from Vuckovich PK. Psychosocial Problems in Acute Care. In: Barkley TW Jr, Myers CM, eds. *Practice Considerations for the Adult-Gerontology Acute Care Nurse Practitioner.* West Hollywood, CA: Barkley and Associates; 2015: 725.

Suicide

Overview

Suicidal ideation is an attempt to intentionally kill oneself and is due to various factors that often lead the patient to feelings of despair.

Several risk factors may contribute to an individual's decision to commit suicide, including sudden loss or crisis, poor previous coping mechanisms, few or no significant others, past suicide attempts, and a family history of suicide. Some comorbid conditions (e.g., depression, anxiety, alcohol abuse) greatly increase the risk of suicide. Among the elderly, the major reasons for suicide are loneliness and medical disability. Substance abuse and mental disorders contribute to more than 90% of all suicides.

Suicide is a major preventable health concern because of its prevalence in the United States. Approximately 15% of patients suffering from depression commit suicide. Among those who state their intent to commit suicide, 80% actually commit the act.[1]

Suicide is the second leading cause of death among adolescents, and incidence increases among adults 24 years of age and older, particularly in white males older than age 45.[15] Although men are three times more likely to complete suicide, women attempt suicide more often than men. Drug overdose is involved in more than 70% of all attempted suicides; firearms are used in approximately 60% of all completed suicides. Hanging is the second leading cause of suicide deaths.[16]

Presentation

Major warning signs of suicide include contemplating or seeking ways to commit suicide, having no reason to live, and feeling like a burden to others or being trapped, and chronic pain. Other potential warning signs of suicide include sleep disturbances, substance abuse or reckless behavior, isolation and withdrawal from activities, and giving away one's possessions.[17]

Workup

The mnemonic **SUICIDAL** is useful in assessing a patient for risk factors of suicide: **S**ex; **U**nsuccessful previous attempts at suicide; **I**dentified family members with suicide attempt history; **C**hronic **I**llness history; **D**epression, drug abuse, drinking; **A**ge of patient; and **L**ethal method available.[18]

Treatment

Patients who are at a high risk for suicide may require hospitalization and psychotherapy. Substance abuse treatment may be referred if warranted.

Antidepressants are known to significantly reduce suicide rates. Antipsychotics such as lithium (Eskalith, Lithobid) should be prescribed with caution because they have a low therapeutic index and could lead to toxicity.[19] Significant weight gain is a common side effect of atypical antipsychotics.

Drug Abuse/Alcoholism

Overview

Alcohol is the most commonly abused substance in the United States, with alcohol-related fatalities being the third leading preventable cause of death. Severe alcohol abuse can lead to alcohol use disorder (AUD). According to the National Institute on Alcohol Abuse and Alcoholism, approximately 9.4% of men and 5.8% of women older than 18 years of age had an AUD in 2013.[20]

Drug abuse is also highly prevalent in the United States. According to a study by the National Survey on Drug Use and Health, approximately 20 million Americans older than 12 years of age used an illegal drug within the past 30 days. The most commonly abused drugs are marijuana, amphetamines, barbiturates, and cocaine. Drug abuse is closely associated with the spread of infectious diseases, death, adverse effects on unborn children, crime, and homelessness.[21]

Risk factors for alcohol and drug abuse include genetics, alterations in opiate receptors, neurotransmitter alterations, and psychosocial factors (e.g., poor impulse control, a low level of psychosocial development, low self-esteem).[22]

Presentation

Drug abuse and AUD can alter an individual's physical, behavioral, and psychological health. The physical warning signs of substance abuse include bloodshot eyes, seizures without a history of epilepsy, and deterioration of physical appearance (e.g., changes in weight). Some patients may also present with uncontrollable shaking, incoherent speech, and unstable coordination.

The effects of a drug or alcohol addiction can affect the patient's performance at work or school, and can lead to suspicious behavior and sudden changes in relationships. Mood changes, lack of motivation, or unexplained fear or paranoia may also suggest a drug or alcohol addiction.[21]

Workup

The **CAGE** mnemonic is useful when screening a patient for AUD. These assessment questions consist of the following: **C**: "Have you ever felt the need to **C**ut down on your drinking?"; **A**: "Have people **A**nnoyed you by criticizing your drinking?"; **G**: "Have you ever felt **G**uilty about your drinking?"; and **E**: "Have you **E**ver had a drink first thing in the morning to steady your nerves or get rid of a hangover?"[1]

If substance abuse is suspected, the patient can be assessed for dehydration and poor nutrition with a referral for electrolyte, glucose, blood urea nitrogen, and creatinine tests. A CBC may be ordered if there is suspicion of gastrointestinal bleeding, anemia, bone marrow complications, or infection. Patients with cocaine intoxication may be referred for an ECG or computed tomography (CT) scan.[23]

Treatment

Patients presenting with severe alcohol or drug intoxication may require immediate inpatient treatment. Patients with AUD should be referred to a substance abuse program or support group, such as Alcoholics Anonymous. The NP should be direct in communicating the diagnosis to the patient while letting the patient know that the disorder is treatable. Other appropriate referrals include behavioral approaches, psychodrama, and rational emotive psychotherapy.[1]

Cerebral Function (Mental Status Assessment)

Overview

The mental status assessment is a structured analysis that combines objective observations from the health professional and subjective descriptions from the patient in order to provide a comprehensive assessment of a patient's mental health.[24] The assessment can determine a diagnosis and exclude other potential causes of the patient's signs or symptoms. The principal components of the mental status examination are appearance, behavior, cognition, and thought processes.

Presentation

Prior to initiating the interview portion of the mental status assessment, the NP should observe the patient's appearance (e.g., personal grooming, clothing, etc.) and general behavior traits (e.g., how he or she interacts with others, pacing in the waiting area, talking to oneself). All observations should be recorded. The interview should begin once the NP determines if the patient seems wary and has established rapport with the patient.[25]

Workup

The Mini-Mental Status Exam (MMSE) aids in the assessment of the patient's cognitive and intellectual functions.[26] The MMSE is a 30-point questionnaire that incorporates the following 11 components: **O**rientation to time and place; **R**ecognition (ask the patient to repeat three objects); **A**: Attention (serial sevens, counting backwards from 100); **R**ecall (ask to recall three objects 5 minutes later); **L**anguage; Identify names of **two** objects; Follow a **three**-step command; **R**eading ("read this statement to yourself, do exactly what it says, but do not say it out loud"); **W**riting (ask the patient to write a sentence); **D**rawing.[1]

The maximum possible MMSE score is 30 points; the average score is 27. No cognitive impairment is indicated in patients who score between 24 and 30 points. A score less than 24 is indicative of delirium or dementia, or both. A score that is between 18 and 23 indicates mild impairment. A score between 0 and 7 indicates severe mental impairment.[27]

Delirium

Overview

Delirium is a clinical syndrome characterized by a disturbance in cognitive function that results in mental confusion and decreased awareness of one's environment. Onset of the condition is usually sudden and can occur at any age. This onset is associated with a physical stressor and has been associated with toxins, alcohol and drug abuse, trauma, infections, poor nutrition, electrolyte imbalances, anesthesia, and impactions in the elderly.[28,29]

Presentation

Delirium is characterized by a sudden, transient onset of clouded sensorium and cognitive changes. Typical findings include memory impairment, disorientation, and language disturbance. Some patients may exhibit changes in psychomotor behavior that involve agitation, slowing, or a mixture of features. Emotional disturbances associated with delirium include anxiety, fear, irritability, anger,

Table 10.3	Mini-Mental Status Exam Components
Orientation in place and time	-being able to identify dates and locations
Recognition	-being able to repeat three objects
Attention	-using serial 7s to count backward from 100
Recall	-recalling three objects 5 minutes later
Language	-identifying the names of two objects -following a three step command -reading statement to silently, doing what it says without saying it aloud -writing a sentence -copying a design

Adapted from Barkley TW Jr. *Adult-Gerontology Primary Care Nurse Practitioner.* West Hollywood, CA: Barkley & Associates; 2015.

depression, and euphoria. The condition may also alter the patient's sleep cycle.[30]

Workup

The diagnosis of delirium relies on exclusion of other possible causes. A mental status assessment is performed to ascertain a baseline. Blood and urine tests or brain imaging studies may be ordered if a diagnosis is unclear.[31]

Treatment

Management focuses on treating the underlying cause of delirium.[31] For example, opioid overdose is reversed through naloxone, whereas benzodiazepine overdose is reversed through flumazenil. Supportive care should focus on balanced fluid intake and may need to occur in an acute care facility, depending on cause.[32]

Dementia

Overview

Dementia is a broad category of symptoms characterized by gradual memory loss and decreased intellectual functioning. Dementia is primarily associated with older age because of its prevalence in adults older than age 60. The etiology of the disease is not clearly known, but associated causes include atherosclerosis, neurotransmitter deficits, cortical atrophy, ventricular dilation, loss of brain cells, viruses, and Alzheimer's disease (AD), among others.[33]

Presentation

A full dementia evaluation should be performed if cognitive impairment is suspected. Patients diagnosed with dementia must exhibit problems with at least two brain functions (e.g., memory loss, impaired judgment or language) and the incapacity to perform basic daily activities.[34]

Workup

Taking the patient's history should include questions that focus on determining the onset of signs or symptoms, the patient's emotional state, and overall medical condition. The physical examination helps to assess for treatable and preventable causes of dementia and other contributing factors, such as medications or overlapping illness.

A helpful mnemonic to help rule out the possibility of other diseases is **DEMENTIA**: **D**rug reactions/interactions, **E**motional disorders, **M**etabolic/endocrine disorders, **E**ye and ear disorders, **N**utritional problems, **T**umors, **I**nfection, and **A**rteriosclerosis.[35]

Treatment

Pharmacological agents are used to improve mental function, mood, or behavior. The most widely prescribed agents for dementia are acetylcholinesterase inhibitors (e.g., donepezil, galantamine, and rivastigmine). In addition, antidepressants and antipsychotics may be used as warranted. Dementia patients should also receive support and counseling to help the patient function independently.[36]

Alzheimer's Disease

Overview

Alzheimer's disease (AD) is the most common cause of dementia, characterized by multiple cognitive defects. AD is a progressive, neurodegenerative disorder that is primarily seen in elderly patients, linked to memory impairment and the gradual loss of physical and mental functions.[37,38]

AD affects millions of people in the United States.[39] Although the cause is not well understood, AD has been linked to genetic predisposition, age, gender, and vascular conditions (e.g., diabetes, uncontrolled hypertension). Acetylcholine deficiency, in particular, is postulated as a major cause in the development of AD.[38]

Presentation

Patients with AD exhibit memory impairment and at least one of the following findings: difficulty with speech (aphasia), inability to perform a previously learned task (apraxia), inability to recognize an object (agnosia), or inability to plan, organize, sequence, and make abstract differences. Many patients in the early stages of AD demonstrate the ability to function independently and may not show any indications for several years.

Other cognitive findings include changes in mood or personality, disorientation, and impaired judgment.[39] Additional physical findings may include

Table 10.4	Comparison of Delirium with Dementia	
	Delirium	**Dementia**
Onset	Sudden; days or weeks. Associated with a physical stressor	Gradual; months or years
Essential Features	Clouded sensorium, irritability and anxiety, misperception of sensory stimuli, possible hallucinations, lucid periods, alternating with confusion, suspiciousness, agitation	Memory loss, decreased intellectual functioning (confabulation and circumstantiality), loss of executive function
Causes	Toxins, alcohol/drug abuse, CNS or cardiac infarction, hypoxia, head trauma, adverse effects of medications, infections, electrolyte imbalance, poor nutrition, anesthesia, tumors, endocrine problems, impactions in the elderly	Neurotransmitter deficit, cortical atrophy, ventricular dilatation, cerebrovascular accident (multi-infarct dementia), Lewy bodies, Alzheimer's disease, Parkinson's disease, Huntington's chorea
Age	Any age	Usually older than 60 years

Note: CNS = central nervous system. Used with permission from Psychosocial Problems in Acute Care. In: Barkley TW Jr, Myers CM, eds. *Practice Considerations for the Adult-Gerontology Acute Care Nurse Practitioner.* West Hollywood, CA: Barkley and Associates; 2015: 731.

limb rigidity, flexion posture, and gait disturbances, among others.

A potentially dangerous symptom of AD is "sundowning"—a patient will experience changes in their sleep schedule and become restless at night.

Workup

A diagnosis based on a detailed clinical assessment should include a history of insidious onset and the progressive course of development, documentation of cognitive impairments, and exclusion of other conditions. The MMSE may be used to assess the patient for dementia.[37]

Additional diagnostic studies to rule out other diseases may include a CBC, BMP, liver function tests, vitamin B12 levels, VDRL tests, urinalysis, and thyroid function studies. A CT scan or MRI is also used.[40]

Treatment

Alzheimer's disease patients should be referred for a neurological consultation. Because there is no cure that can stop the death or malfunction of neurons, symptomatic treatment is aimed at slowing down the degenerative process. Acetylcholinesterase inhibitors can increase the availability of acetylcholine; therapeutic options include donepezil (Aricept), rivastigmine (Exelon), and galantamine (Razadyne). These agents are often prescribed in conjunction with NMDA receptor antagonists such as memantine (Namenda) to improve thinking and aid in activities of daily living. Others agents may be necessary to manage secondary symptoms such as depression, aggression, delusions, and sleep disorders.[41]

Structured routines for meals, medication administration, and daily activities and exercise can help to decrease stressors and reduce agitation. The patient and family should be referred for counseling as appropriate.[41]

Cerebellar Function

Overview

The cerebellum is a region of the brain that primarily helps with motor functions and may also play a role in some cognitive functions. This region of the brain helps to compensate for shifts in body position to maintain balance, coordinate the timing of certain muscle groups, and facilitate motor learning.[42] Damage to the cerebellum can result in balance and movement deterioration, intention tremors, and motor learning deficits.[43]

Workup

The assessment of cerebellar dysfunction involves testing and observation of the patient's gait pattern and coordination.

The Romberg test assesses cerebellar function and coordination by evaluating proprioception, vision, and vestibular sense. This test requires the patient to stand with his or her eyes closed, feet together, and arms at the side; the test is considered positive if the patient experiences a loss of balance during the assessment.[44]

The finger-to-nose test begins with the patient resting his or her hand on the thigh. The patient is then given a command to extend the arm and touch his or her nose with the index finger. This is followed by having the patient use his or her index finger to touch the examiner's finger.[1]

The heel-to-shin test requires the patient to run the heel of one foot along the shin of the opposite leg.[45]

References

1. Barkley TW Jr. *Adult-Gerontology Primary Care Nurse Practitioner*. West Hollywood, CA: Barkley & Associates; 2015.

2. Mayo Clinic Staff. Dysthymia definition. Mayo Clinic Web site. http://www.mayoclinic.org/diseases-conditions/dysthymia/basics/definition/con-20033879. Updated December 20, 2012. Accessed April 1, 2015.

3. Andrews LW. *Encyclopedia of Depression*. Santa Barbara, CA: ABC-CLIO; 2010.

4. Highlights of changes from DSM-IV-TR to DSM-5. American Psychiatric Association Web site. http://www.dsm5.org/Documents/changes%20from%20dsm-iv-tr%20to%20dsm-5.pdf. Published 2013. Accessed April 1, 2015.

5. Beebe R., Myers J. *Professional Paramedic, Vol. 1: Foundations of Paramedic Care*. Clifton Park, NY: Delmar; 2010.

6. Lyness JM. Unipolar depression in adults: Assessment and diagnosis. In: Basow DS, ed. *UpToDate*. Waltham, MA: UpToDate; 2015. http://www.uptodate.com/contents/clinical-manifestations-and-diagnosis-of-depression?detectedLanguage=en&source=search_result&search=depression&selectedTitle=2~150&provider=noProvider#H7. Updated January 29, 2015. Accessed March 25, 2015.

7. Meloche C, Mancell M. Psychiatric lab workup. Sharing in Health website. http://www.sharinginhealth.ca/labs/other/psychiatric_workup.html. Last reviewed January 2011. Accessed April 1, 2015.

8. Rana D, Upton, D. *Psychology for Nurses*. New York, NY: Routledge; 2013.

9. Darby-Stewart A, Dachs R, Graber MA. Antidepressants for initial treatment of depression. *Am Fam Physician*. 2010; 81(10): 1205–1212. http://www.aafp.org/afp/2010/0515/p1205.html

10. Nussbaumer B, Morgan LC, Reichenpfader U, et al. Comparative efficacy and risk of harms of immediate- versus extended-release second-generation antidepressants: A systematic review with network meta-analysis. *CNS Drugs*. 2014; 28(8); 699–712. doi: 10.1007/s40263-0169-z

11. Panic disorder & agoraphobia. Anxiety and Depression Association of America Web site. http://www.adaa.org/understanding-anxiety/panic-disorder-agoraphobia. Accessed April 1, 2015.

12. Higgins ES, George MS. *Neuroscience of Clinical Psychiatry: The Pathophysiology of Behavior and Mental Illness.* 2nd ed. Philadelphia, PA: Lippincott Williams & Wilkins; 2013.

13. Yates WR. Anxiety disorders treatment & management. In: Bienenfield D, ed. *Medscape.* http://emedicine.medscape.com/article/286227-treatment#showall. Updated April 21, 2014. Accessed April 1, 2015.

14. Bandelow B, Sher L, Bunevicius R, et al. Guidelines for the pharmacological treatment of anxiety disorders, obsessive-compulsive disorder and posttraumatic stress disorder in primary care. *Int J Psychiatry Clin Pract.* 2012; 16(2): 77–84. doi: 10.3109/13651501.2012.667114

15. United States Department of Health and Human Services, Centers for Disease Control and Prevention. National suicide statistics at a glance: Trends in suicide rates among both sexes, by age group, United States, 1991–2009. http://www.cdc.gov/violenceprevention/suicide/statistics/trends02.html. Updated December 16, 2014.

16. Brendel RW, Wei M, Lagomasino IT, Perlis RH, Stern TA. Care of the suicidal patient. In: Stern TA, Fricchione GL, Cassem NH, Jellinek M, Rosenbaum JF, eds. *Massachusetts General Hospital Handbook of General Hospital Psychiatry.* 6th ed. Philadelphia, PA: Saunders; 2010: 541–554.

17. Suicide warning signs. American Foundation for Suicide Prevention Web site. https://www.afsp.org/preventing-suicide/suicide-warning-signs. Accessed April 2, 2015.

18. Bryan CJ, ed. *Cognitive Behavioral Therapy for Preventing Suicide Attempts: A Guide to Brief Treatments Across Clinical Settings.* New York, NY: Routledge; 2015.

19. Moini J. *The Pharmacy Technician: A Comprehensive Approach.* 3rd ed. Boston, MA: Cengage Learning; 2015.

20. Unites States Department of Health and Human Services, National Institutes of Health, National Institute on Alcohol Abuse and Alcoholism. Alcohol facts and statistics. http://www.niaaa.nih.gov/alcohol-health/overview-alcohol-consumption/alcohol-facts-and-statistics. Updated March 2015. Accessed April 2, 2015.

21. Understanding drugs and drug dependence. National Council on Alcoholism and Drug Dependence Web site. https://ncadd.org/learn-about-drugs. Accessed April 2, 2015.

22. Czachowski CL, McBride WJ, Rodd ZA. Brain sites and neurotransmitter systems mediating the reinforcing effects of alcohol. In: Miller PM, ed. *Biological Research on Addiction: Comprehensive Addictive Behaviors and Disorders, Vol. 2.* San Diego, CA: Academic Press; 2013: 199–208.

23. Cohagan A, Worthington R, Krause RS. Alcohol and substance abuse evaluation. In: Brenner BE, ed. *Medscape.* http://emedicine.medscape.com/article/805084-overview#a7. Updated July 3, 2013. Accessed April 2, 2015.

24. Combs H. *Mental Status Exam.* [PowerPoint]. http://depts.washington.edu/psyclerk/secure/mentalstatusexam.pdf. Accessed April 2, 2015.

25. Brannon GE. History and mental status examination. In: Bienenfield D, ed. *Medscape.* http://emedicine.medscape.com/article/293402-overview. Updated March 15, 2013. Accessed April 2, 2015.

26. The Mini Mental State Examination. Alzheimer's Association Web site. http://www.alzheimers.org.uk/site/scripts/documents_info.php?documentID=121. Updated January 2012. Accessed April 2, 2015.

27. McGee, S. R. *Evidence-Based Physical Diagnosis.* 3rd ed. Philadelphia, PA: Elsevier Saunders; 2012.

28. Trzepacz PT, Meagher DJ. Neuropsychiatric aspects of delirium. In: Yodofsky SC, Hales RE, eds. *Essentials of Neuropsychiatry and Behavioral Neurosciences.* 2nd ed. Arlington, VA: American Psychiatric Publishing; 2010: 149–222.

29. Keltner NL, Steele D. *Psychiatric Nursing.* 7th ed. St. Louis, MO: Elsevier Mosby; 2014.

30. Fields C, Lyketsos C. Psychiatry. In: Durso SC, Bowker LK, Price JD, Smith SC, eds. *Oxford American Handbook of Geriatric Medicine.* New York, NY: Oxford University Press; 2010: 195–252.

31. Alagiakrishnan K. Delirium. In: Ahmed I, ed. *Medscape.* http://emedicine.medscape.com/article/288890-overview. Updated April 28, 2014. Accessed April 2, 2015.

32. Alagiakrishnan K. Delirium treatment & management. In: Ahmed I, ed. *Medscape.* http://emedicine.medscape.com/article/288890-treatment. Updated April 28, 2014. Accessed April 2, 2015.

33. Sheehan R, Sinai A, Bass N, et al. Dementia diagnostic criteria in Down syndrome. *Int J of Geriatr Psychiatry.* 2014. doi:10.1002/gps.4228

34. Mayo Clinic Staff. Dementia definition. Mayo Clinic Web site. http://www.mayoclinic.org/diseases-conditions/seo/basics/definition/con-20034399. Updated November 22, 2014. Accessed April 2, 2015.

35. Markovchick VJ, Pons PT, Bakes KA. *Emergency Medicine Secrets.* 5th ed. St. Louis, MO: Elsevier; 2011.

36. Healthwise Staff. Dementia treatment overview. WebMD Web site. http://www.webmd.com/alzheimers/tc/dementia-treatment-overview. Updated January 27, 2014. Accessed April 2, 2015.

37. Grabowski, TJ. Clinical features and diagnosis of Alzheimer disease. In: Basow DS, ed. *UpToDate*. Waltham, MA: UpToDate; 2015. http://www.uptodate.com/contents/clinical-features-and-diagnosis-of-alzheimer-disease?source=search_result&search=alzheimer+dementia&selectedTitle=1~150

38. Grossberg G, Kamat S. *Alzheimer's: The Latest Assessment & Treatment Strategies*. Burlington, MA: Jones and Bartlett Learning; 2011.

39. Alzheimer's Association. 2013 Alzheimer's disease facts and figures. *Alzheimers Dement*. March 2013; 9(2): 208–245. doi:10.1016/j.jalz2013.02.003.

40. Soucy JP, Bartha R, Bocti C, et al. Clinical applications of neuroimaging in patients with Alzheimer's disease: A review from the Fourth Canadian Consensus Conference on the Diagnosis and Treatment of Dementia 2012. *Alzheimers Res Ther*. July 2013; 5(Suppl 1): S3. doi: 101186/alzrt199. http://www.biomedcentral.com/content/pdf/alzrt199.pdf. Accessed January 7, 2015.

41. Anderson, HS. Alzheimer disease. In: Hoffman M, ed. *Medscape*. http://emedicine.medscape.com/article/1134817-treatment. Updated January 7, 2015. Accessed April 2, 2015.

42. Knierim, J. Cerebellum. In: Byrne JH, ed. *Neuroscience Online: An Electronic Textbook for the Neurosciences*. Houston, TX: University of Texas Medical School. http://neuroscience.uth.tmc.edu/s3/chapter05.html. Accessed April 2, 2015.

43. Reese NB. *Muscle and Sensory Testing*. 3rd ed. St. Louis, MO: Elsevier Saunders; 2012.

44. Schniepp R, Wühr M, Huth S, Pradhan C, Brandt T, Jahn K. Gait characteristics of patients with phobic postural vertigo: Effects of fear of falling, attention, and visual input. *J Neurol*. 2014; 261(4): 739–746. doi: 10.1004/s00415-014-7259-1

45. Arslan OE. *Neuroanatomical Basis of Clinical Neurology*. 2nd ed. Boca Raton, FL: CRC Press; 2015.

Chapter 11
Neurologic Disorders

1. A patient experiences tremors, impaired swallowing, and drooling, in addition to testing positive for Myerson's sign. Based on the above symptoms and lab results, you conclude that the patient is exhibiting the initial onset of Parkinson's disease. Which of the following would least likely describe the patient?

   a. A 50-year-old African American male

   b. A 55-year-old Caucasian female

   c. A 65-year-old Hispanic male

   d. A 70-year-old Asian female

2. A patient has just been diagnosed with multiple sclerosis. Your colleague is informing her about the different forms of management and mentions beta interferons, anticoagulants, immunosuppressives, and plasmapheresis as viable methods. You realize that your colleague misinformed the patient about one of the treatments. Which of the following is not a method of managing this disorder?

   a. Beta interferons

   b. Anticoagulants

   c. Immunosuppressives

   d. Plasmapheresis

3. Jessica, a 34-year-old female, presents with episodic, throbbing headaches that last for multiple hours at a time. She tells you that these headaches are usually accompanied by nausea and vomiting. Given the type of headache the patient is most likely experiencing, all of the following visual disturbances are usually expected except:

   a. Seeing stars

   b. Zigzag of lights

   c. Faded colors

   d. Luminous hallucinations

4. An adult comes to your practice with complaints of occasional weakness, numbness, and double vision but no reported breathing difficulties. You order lab tests and the results indicate lymphocytosis, an elevated protein level in the cerebrospinal fluid, and an elevated igG index level in the cerebrospinal fluid. Which of the following would be most appropriate for managing the patient's most likely condition at this time?

   a. Prescribe antiseizure drugs

   b. Order an MRI

   c. Prescribe anticholinesterase drugs

   d. Refer the patient to neurology

5. Doug, a 58-year-old male, has recently been diagnosed with cluster headaches. He had previously assumed that he was experiencing migraines and wants to know what the two types of headaches have in common. You tell him that cluster headaches and migraines may share which precipitating factor?

   a. Nitrate containing foods

   b. Changes in weather

   c. Genetic predisposition

   d. Alcohol ingestion

6. Sarah, a 26-year-old female, experiences recurring episodes of headaches that are characterized by unilateral and lateralized throbbing. She says that changes in weather and emotional stress tend to increase the incidence. Which of the following diagnostic tests would you <u>least</u> likely order, based on the patient's suspected condition?

   a. Erythrocyte sedimentation rate

   b. Computed tomography scan

   c. Electroencephalography

   d. Venereal Disease Research Laboratory test

7. The nurse practitioner witnesses a patient with a seizure disorder as he suddenly stops talking, sits down, and stares straight ahead. During the seizure, which lasts approximately two minutes, he makes chewing movements and repeatedly pulls at his shirt. After the seizure, the patient cannot recall the onset of the seizure or describe what happened to him. What type of seizure should the practitioner document?

   a. Simple partial

   b. Absence

   c. Complex partial

   d. Simple partial seizure with motor symptoms

8. Georgiana, age 69, who has a history of Parkinson's disease, explains that she's had trouble writing because her hand starts shaking. You ask her to move from the chair to the exam table, and you notice that she moves very slowly and has trouble navigating herself towards the table. The practitioner knows that which of the following drugs should be increased to help alleviate Georgiana's tremors?

   a. Selegiline

   b. Carbidopa-levodopa

   c. Tolcapone

   d. Benztropine

9. You are treating four patients who experience recurring headaches. Which of the following patients is most likely to be experiencing cluster headaches?

   a. A 70-year-old man whose headache lasts for several hours and is most intense at the back of the neck.

   b. A 30-year-old woman whose headache lasts for several hours and often comes after she skips breakfast.

   c. A 45-year-old man whose headache lasts for 1 hour and usually returns a month later.

   d. A 22-year-old woman whose headache lasts for a couple hours and coincides with her menstrual cycle.

10. Of the following, which method is commonly considered in addition to a computerized tomography scan in detecting ischemic infarcts?

    a. Electroencephalography

    b. Cerebral angiogram

    c. Carotid Doppler

    d. Magnetic resonance imaging

11. Yolanda, a 52-year-old female, states that her face seems "pulled to one side." However, no other neurological deficits are noted. Given the most likely diagnosis, what is most likely to be the underlying etiology of Yolanda's condition?

    a. Seizures

    b. Myasthenia gravis

    c. Herpes simplex

    d. Trigeminal neuralgia

12. Hannah, a 23-year-old female, comes to the clinic after having multiple episodes of headaches. She complains that the headaches throb and usually manifest on one side of her head, build "to a slow crescendo," and last for several hours. She also experiences visual disturbances and nausea. Which of the following foods would most likely be contributing to her complaints?

    a. Smoked salmon

    b. Cane sugar

    c. Chocolate

    d. Bananas

13. Which of the following patients would you expect to have the highest risk of developing multiple sclerosis?

    a. A 16-year-old African American male

    b. A 22-year-old Asian female

    c. A 35-year-old Irish female

    d. A 55-year-old Hispanic female

14. Mr. Thomas is a 74-year-old who was diagnosed with Parkinson's disease at the age of 57. During one visit, he states, "I'm really having trouble getting up from my recliner, and sometimes I can't even pull the chair up to the dinner table." Considering common drug regimens for Parkinson's patients, you realize that Mr. Thomas should be referred to his neurologist for an increase in which drug?

    a. Trihexyphenidyl (Artane)

    b. Benztropine (Cogentin)

    c. Primidone (Mysoline)

    d. Pramipexole (Mirapex)

15. Your patient is admitted to the hospital with slurred speech and tingling in his right arm and leg. An hour later, he appears to have fully recovered. However, he is alarmed to learn that about one-third of patients who have such attacks will experience which of the following within the next 5 years?

    a. Brain tumor

    b. Intraventricular hemorrhage

    c. Increased intracranial pressure

    d. Cerebral infarction

16. Harriet, age 54, is waiting in the clinic when her muscles become tense. She loses consciousness and develops consistent contractions. The episode lasts for about three minutes, and you notice that she loses control of her bladder during the event. How should the nurse practitioner document these findings?

    a. Status epilepticus

    b. Complex partial seizure

    c. Petit mal seizure

    d. Grand mal seizure

17. A patient complains of "this feeling like my head's in a vise" and "this tight aching sensation in my neck," symptoms that have never presented before. Suspecting a tension headache, you would inspect the patient's neck to rule out which condition?

    a. Transient ischemic attack

    b. Brain tumor

    c. Meningitis

    d. Bell's palsy

18. Damage to cranial nerve IX would most likely result in impairment of:

    a. Sensation of the face

    b. Equilibrium

    c. The gag reflex

    d. Swallowing

19. Which of these headaches occurs as a result of vasodilation and excessive pulsation of the external carotid artery branches but does not typically present with an aura?

    a. Classic migraine

    b. Cluster headaches

    c. Common migraine

    d. Tension headache

20. Anthony, age 62, presents to your practice with a droopy eye and difficulty swallowing. He comments that he usually swims laps every morning, but he's had to stop because he tires out after only a couple of laps. He also experiences shortness of breath and fatigue. He denies experiencing limb numbness and urinary difficulties. Which of the following lab results would be most helpful in establishing a diagnosis based on your suspicion?

    a. Elevated IgG in cerebrospinal fluid

    b. Elevated protein in cerebrospinal fluid

    c. Acetylcholine receptor antibodies in serum

    d. Mild lymphocytosis

21. Adam, age 26, has a seizure that initially originates in his arms before spreading to the entire left side of his body. He remains conscious through the entire seizure. Based on this type of seizure, which of the following would you most expect Adam to also experience?

    a. Akathisia

    b. Hand gestures

    c. Lip smacking

    d. Flashing lights

22. A patient comes to you with complaints of a "bad headache." He is not able to clearly articulate any other signs or symptoms. Which of the following features is most important for you to assess to determine the type of headache?

    a. Location

    b. Duration

    c. Chronology

    d. Quality

23. A 62-year-old male presents to urgent care saying that he has been experiencing trouble maintaining balance and coordinating his movement since early this morning. As he puts it, "every once in a while, I feel lightheaded and dizzy." Suddenly, he appears to lose his balance and states that "it feels as though the room is spinning." You notify the ER physician that you are transferring the patient based on which most likely diagnosis?

    a. Vertebrobasilar transient ischemic attack

    b. Trigeminal neuralgia

    c. Partial seizure

    d. Carotid transient ischemic attack

24. Which of these patient statements would most warrant a diagnosis of tension headaches?

    a. "I've been experiencing throbbing in my temples that is consistently dull."

    b. "The pain only occurs on one side of my head."

    c. "I feel pressure around my eyes."

    d. "It feels like something is squeezing my head."

25. Regarding the incidence of myasthenia gravis, which of the following is most accurate?

    a. Most common in the Caucasian population

    b. Age of onset is later in females

    c. More common in temperate climates

    d. More common in women

26. Nolan, a 22-year-old, has lost the ability to control lateral eye movement. Which cranial nerve (CN) has most likely been affected?

    a. CN II

    b. CN III

    c. CN IV

    d. CN VI

27. You are examining a new patient, Stacy, who has a history of focal seizures that do not cause loss of consciousness. Given this information, you know that if she were to have a seizure, it would likely include all of the following except:

    a. Tingling

    b. Vocalizations

    c. Flashing lights

    d. Impaired swallowing

28. A female patient presents to your office for a regular check-up and inquires about the incidence of myasthenia gravis for females. She tells you that her grandmother had the condition, and she is worried that she will develop it as well. The nurse practitioner should tell her that female incidence of myasthenia gravis peaks approximately:

    a. In the third decade of age

    b. In the fourth decade of age

    c. In the fifth decade of age

    d. In the sixth decade of age

29. You are treating a patient who is unable to move the right side of her face. As a nurse practitioner, you know that while this condition may resolve without treatment, some patients may benefit from treatment. Which of the following treatment options is <u>least</u> likely to be beneficial?

    a. Prednisone

    b. Artificial tears

    c. Pyridostigmine

    d. Acyclovir

30. Josephine, age 63, experiences severe pain in her face, claiming that it feels like "an electric shock." In discussing her history, she mentions that her gait has become stiff and unpredictable as of late, and reports experiencing blurred vision. Which of the following is the most likely diagnosis?

    a. Parkinson's disease

    b. Trigeminal neuralgia

    c. Bell's palsy

    d. Myasthenia gravis

31. Sandra, a 44-year-old, experiences a unilateral, lateralized throbbing headache with accompanying visual disturbances at least three times a month. She says that these headaches are usually preceded by auras. Of the following medications, which would be the best option to order for prophylactic therapy for the most likely type of headache?

    a. Acetaminophen

    b. Sumatriptan

    c. Propranolol

    d. Oxycodone

32. Your patient starts to have difficulty moving his extremities. He is coughing, wheezing, and having difficulty breathing. You look at his fingers and notice they are starting to turn blue. Which of the following tests would you order to distinguish between the two most likely causes of your patient's condition?

    a. Cerebral angiography

    b. Edrophonium test

    c. Cerebral spinal fluid analysis

    d. Acetylcholine receptor antibody test

33. Which of these patients would be most likely to be affected by a cluster headache?

    a. A 17-year-old male

    b. A 23-year-old female

    c. A 55-year-old male

    d. A 60-year-old female

34. You are testing a patient who you suspect has Parkinson's disease. You repeatedly tap the bridge of her nose. Which of the following responses or results would indicate a neurological disorder?

    a. Flared nostrils

    b. Impaired swallowing

    c. Sustained blinking

    d. Wooden facies

35. John, age 46, comes to your office with a history of headaches. He states that the headaches last for several hours and feel like a vise is gripping his head, yet he experiences no changes in movement or sensation. Given the most likely type of headache, where would you expect the headaches to be the most intense?

    a. Crown of the head

    b. Eyes

    c. Neck

    d. Jaw

36. A patient presents with an inability to move the left side of his face. The nurse practitioner identifies the cause as an inflammatory reaction involving the facial nerve. Which of the following medications would be best suited for treating the condition most evidenced by the patient's findings and the known cause?

    a. Sumatriptan

    b. Chlordiazepoxide

    c. Oxazepam

    d. Prednisone

37. Susana, age 60, exhibits slow tremors that are exacerbated when she experiences high levels of stress. She also complains of difficulty swallowing and increased muscle rigidity that has developed over the last 5 years. Upon tapping over the bridge of the patient's nose, you note repeated blinking of the eyes, which you recognize as Myerson's sign. Based on the most likely diagnosis, which of the following deficiencies does Susana most likely have?

    a. Dopamine

    b. Amino acids

    c. Acetylcholine

    d. Serotonin

38. Sally, a 27-year-old female, reports to your clinic with complaints of recurring headaches. When you ask her to describe the nature of the pain, she says: "I don't know, it just hurts." You decide to ask her about signs and symptoms that accompany the headaches. All of these statements would suggest Sally is experiencing cluster headaches except:

    a. "It feels like my nostrils just close up."

    b. "I keep crying and I don't know why."

    c. "My nose just starts running like a waterfall."

    d. "I feel like the light starts stabbing at my eyes."

39. You have just transferred a patient showing classical findings of a transient ischemic attack to emergency care. You know that, in the course of imaging the condition, your patient will likely first undergo a computed tomography scan. Why would this diagnostic be performed?

    a. To identify the need for urgent surgical intervention

    b. To determine whether antihypertensive therapy is warranted

    c. To evaluate for a cardioembolic source

    d. To rule out the possibility of hemorrhage

40. Sonia, a 23-year-old female, has lost the ability to move her eyes downward. Which cranial nerve has been affected?

    a. Trigeminal

    b. Trochlear

    c. Optic

    d. Vagus

RATIONALES

1. d

As the onset of Parkinson's disease occurs typically from 45–65 years of age with increased incidence among male and Caucasian patients, a 70-year-old Asian woman would be least likely to experience the onset of symptoms. All of the other answer choices contain at least one incidence-related factor and are henceforth incorrect.

2. b

Anticoagulants are commonly used in managing transient ischemic attack. Although the role of anticoagulant medications has been studied in the management of multiple sclerosis, findings do not indicate that anticoagulants assist in managing the condition. Beta interferons may reduce relapses in patients with relapsing-remitting multiple sclerosis. The immune system's attack on myelin in patients with multiple sclerosis is typically reduced by implementing immunosuppressants into the treatment regimen. Plasmapheresis is usually used in the treatment of multiple sclerosis by replacing the patient's blood plasma.

3. c

The patient's findings of a consistent throbbing headache, which is accompanied by nausea and vomiting, would most likely be attributed to a migraine headache, which does not typically present with the perception of faded colors. On the contrary, seeing faded colors is usually attributed to macular degeneration. Migraine headaches are linked to a variety of visual disturbances and often cause blind spots or defects in the patient's field of vision. Halos and luminous hallucinations, such as seeing stars or sparks and zigzagged lights, are also commonly attributed to migraine headaches.

4. d

A patient suspected of having multiple sclerosis is typically immediately referred to neurology. Although an MRI of the brain is a common diagnostic procedure in this case, it usually does not precede referring the patient to neurology. Although patients with multiple sclerosis may experience seizures, anti-seizure drugs are not typically incorporated into a regular regimen; since the patient in this scenario is not undergoing a seizure, this treatment would not take precedence over referral to neurology. Anticholinesterase drugs are more commonly used to manage myasthenia gravis; these drugs may also be used to treat patients with multiple sclerosis who experience breathing difficulties, which are not factors in this case.

5. d

Alcohol ingestion is a possible precipitating factor for cluster headaches and migraine headaches. Nitrate-containing foods, changes in weather, and genetic predisposition are considered precipitating factors for migraine headaches, but not cluster headaches.

6. c

Electroencephalography would most likely be performed on a patient with seizures, rather than one exhibiting symptoms of a migraine headache. Common laboratory tests to further evaluate migraines and to rule out other conditions include erythrocyte sedimentation rate, computed tomography scan, and Venereal Disease Research Laboratory test.

7. c

Complex partial seizures are usually accompanied by an aura and impaired level of consciousness, during which the patient stares blankly and loses awareness. In addition, this type of seizure is frequently characterized by automatisms such as repeated chewing movements or pulling at clothes. Patients affected by complex partial seizures often have trouble remembering the events that took place during these seizures. In cases of simple partial seizure, however, patients retain awareness and can remember what happens to them. While absence seizures also involve lapses of awareness, staring, and automatisms such as chewing or hand gestures, they are brief and last only a few seconds. Simple partial seizures affect muscle activity, typically causing jerking movements; they will not, however, cause impaired levels of consciousness.

8. d

Benztropine is an anticholinergic, a class of drugs typically prescribed to Parkinson's patients to alleviate tremors and rigidity. Selegiline is a controversial medication in the treatment of Parkinson's disease; it may be used to conserve dopamine levels, not to directly alleviate tremors or rigidity. Carbidopa-levodopa and tolcapone may also be prescribed to Parkinson's disease patients, but these medications are typically used to increase levels of available dopamine and not to alleviate tremors or rigidity.

9. c

Cluster headaches, which usually last less than 2 hours, are most common in middle-aged men. Patients can go several weeks or months between episodes. Tension headaches, on the other hand, can last for several hours. Tension headaches are more intense at the neck or back of the head. Migraine headaches are more common in women and can be triggered by stress, missed meals, and specific foods, among other factors. Menstrual cycles can also trigger migraine headaches.

10. d

Magnetic resonance imaging (MRI) can be used, in addition to a computerized tomography scan, in detecting ischemic infarcts. An electroencephalography, on the other hand, is an important test in determining seizure classification rather than ischemic infarcts. Although cerebral angiograms are used to diagnose transient ischemic attacks, this test is not usually superior to a computerized tomography scan in identifying ischemic infarcts. Lastly, a carotid doppler is used to assess the amount of plaque inside carotid arteries.

11. c

Herpes simplex activation is commonly considered to be a possible cause of Bell's palsy, which is indicated by the abrupt onset of unilateral facial paresis. Seizures and myasthenia gravis are usually not suggested as likely causes of Bell's palsy. Although family history may show an incidence of trigeminal neuralgia, Bell's palsy does not typically present as a direct result of this condition.

12. a

Foods containing nitrates, such as smoked, cured, or processed meats or fish, may serve as a trigger in patients predisposed to migraines, as indicated by a recurring unilateral headache that results in visual disturbances and nausea. High amounts of nitrate are also present in vegetables such as beets, lettuce, and spinach, as well as meat and dairy products. Although artificial sweeteners such as aspartame or saccharin are typically advised against, cane sugar is not artificial and thus is not considered a common trigger for migraine headaches. Chocolate has been previously thought to cause the onset of migraines; however, recent studies show that there is actually no correlation between chocolate and migraines. Citrus fruits are usually advised against as well; however, bananas are considered a safe food to eat for patients prone to migraines.

13. c

The greatest incidence of multiple sclerosis is between the ages of 20 and 50 and is more common in people of Western European descent who live in temperate regions; therefore, a 35-year-old Irish woman would be most likely to develop the condition. Even though the ages of 16 and 22 are within the range of greatest incidence, African Americans and Asians are not at a heightened risk of developing the disease. Lastly, a 55-year-old Hispanic woman is older than the typical age of onset for multiple sclerosis.

14. d

Pramipexole (Mirapex) is a dopamine agonist commonly used in the treatment of Parkinson's disease. By increasing available dopamine, the drug effectively treats stiffness, slowed movements, and other symptoms associated with Parkinson's disease. Dopamine agonists are particularly recommended when the patient's muscle feel "frozen," thereby inhibiting him or her to rise from a chair or perform other daily activities. Trihexyphenidyl (Artane) and benztropine (Cogentin) are anticholinergics that may be used to alleviate tremor and rigidity in cases of Parkinson's disease; they are not, however, specifically used to manage such symptoms as "stuck" or "frozen" muscles that inhibit movement. Lastly, primidone (Mysoline) is a long-acting anticonvulsant that is commonly prescribed for seizure prevention.

15. d

One-third of patients with transient ischemic attacks (TIAs) will experience a cerebral infarction within 5 years. Brain tumors, intraventricular hemorrhages, and increased intracranial pressure are less likely to follow TIAs within 5 years.

16. d

The initiation of tonic contractions, followed by clonic contractions that last for 2–5 minutes, is indicative of a grand mal seizure. This type of seizure may result in an aura or incontinence, and may end with a postictal period. Status epilepticus, the most life-threatening form of seizures, is commonly characterized by a series of grand mal seizures that last for more than 10 minutes. The patient usually remains unconscious throughout the duration of status epilepticus. Complex partial seizures tend to last for less than a minute and include loss of muscle control, flashing lights, hallucinations, and vocalizations. The sudden inability to move, paired with a blank stare, is characteristic of a petit mal seizure, which begins and ends suddenly.

17. c

Patients with new onset tension headache that present with neck pain should be assessed for nuchal rigidity, a classical finding of meningitis. Headache may occur at onset of transient ischemic attack, and brain tumor may present with pain similar to tension headache; however, assessing the neck would not serve to differentiate either condition from a tension headache. Bell's palsy does not typically present with neck pain or "vise-like" pressure on the head.

18. c

The glossopharyngeal nerve, also known as cranial nerve (CN) IX, is responsible for the gag reflex, phonation, reflex swallowing, and taste. The trigeminal nerve, or CN V, innervates the mastication muscles and provides sensation for parts of the face. The acoustic nerve, or CN VIII, provides hearing and equilibrium. Lastly, the CN X, or vagus nerve, is responsible for talking, swallowing, and maintaining the carotid reflex.

19. c

Though common migraines and classic migraines are closely related to dilation and excessive pulsation of branches of the external carotid artery, common migraines do not typically present with an aura, whereas classic migraines often do. Although the cause of cluster headaches is not fully understood, such headaches do not normally involve the external carotid artery as common migraines do. Lastly, tension headaches are not commonly associated with the focal neurological symptoms, such as changes in sensation and movement, that appear in classic and common migraines.

20. c

Approximately 85% of patients with myasthenia gravis, as indicated by ptosis, dysphagia, and extremity weakness, present with antibodies to acetylcholine receptors in serum. Mild lymphocytosis and elevated protein and IgG in cerebrospinal fluid are common diagnostic findings for multiple sclerosis, not myasthenia gravis. Multiple sclerosis would likely present with numbness in the limbs and urinary difficulties, which the patient is not experiencing.

21. d

Simple partial seizures typically originate in a single muscle group before spreading to an entire side of the body and may cause a patient to experience visual disturbances, such as seeing flashing lights. Tonic-clonic seizures usually begin with tonic contractions and loss of consciousness before progressing to clonic contractions during which muscles begin to spasm and jerking movements can be observed. Akathisia is the inability to control motor restlessness, which does not commonly occur in simple partial seizures. Petit mal seizures typically begin and end suddenly, with patients frequently having a blank stare during an episode. Complex partial seizures are simple partial seizures followed by an impaired level of consciousness. Automatisms, such as lip smacking, are common during complex partial seizures.

22. c

Each type of headache is characterized by a distinct chronology or timeline. Thus, a careful consideration of a pattern by which the patient's headache evolves would usually allow for a classification of the headache. In addition, consideration of a timeline would typically enable the patient to determine the duration of pain during an attack. Location of the headache can also be used for classification of headaches; however, this method is less precise since location of attacks may be the same for more than one headache type. Duration of headache attacks is typically considered in analysis of headache timeline; while it forms an important part of chronology, in itself, it is insufficient for a precise classification of headaches. Quality of pain should also be considered in diagnosis of headaches; in this particular case, however, it would not be helpful in determining the type of headache since the patient cannot clearly articulate his symptoms.

23. a

Ataxia, bouts of mild dizziness, and vertigo are indicative of a vertebrobasilar transient ischemic attack (TIA), which typically precipitates an impending stroke. The patient is not likely experiencing a carotid TIA, which, among other findings, is commonly characterized by aphasia and dysarthria. The patient also is not likely experiencing trigeminal neuralgia, which usually presents with painful, sharp spasms localized on one side of the face. Lastly, the patient is not experiencing a partial seizure because vertigo and mild dizziness are not typically symptoms of an impending seizure.

24. d

Tension headaches are characterized by a vise-like grip near the neck or back of the head. Dull throbbing is more commonly associated with migraines, whereas unilateral and periorbital pain can be attributed to cluster headaches.

25. d

Myasthenia gravis more commonly occurs in women than in men at about a reported 3:2 ratio. The incidence of the condition does not reveal a demographic inclination towards any particular ethnicity. The condition often peaks in incidence in the fifth and sixth decades for males and in the third decade for females. Because temperature fluctuations adversely affect individuals with myasthenia gravis, it is best for individuals diagnosed with this condition to live in temperate climates.

26. d

Cranial nerve (CN) VI controls lateral eye movement. CN II, on the other hand, controls vision, but not eye movement. CN III controls the extraocular muscles and the ability to open the eyelids, but not lateral eye movement. Finally, CN IV controls downward and inward eye movement.

27. d

A patient with simple partial seizures is not expected to experience dysphagia. Simple partial seizures are more likely to cause paresthesia, flashing lights, vocalizations, and hallucinations.

28. a

Although myasthenia gravis predominantly presents between the ages of 20 and 40 years in females, peak incidence usually occurs in the third decade. In males, on the other hand, incidence of myasthenia gravis commonly peaks in the fifth and sixth decades.

29. c

Pyridostigmine is an anticholinesterase commonly used in the management of myasthenia gravis, not Bell's palsy. Steroids, such as prednisone, are often used at the beginning of treatment of Bell's palsy. An antiviral, such as acyclovir, may also be used when facial weakness is severe. When patients cannot close their eyes, lubricating eye drops are typically recommended.

30. b

Trigeminal neuralgia may occur as a symptom of multiple sclerosis, which is a likely diagnosis, based on the patient's presentation of limb numbness, spastic paraparesis, and optic atrophy. Trigeminal neuralgia typically presents as an episodic, severe, jabbing pain that may feel like an electric shock. Parkinson's disease, myasthenia gravis, and Bell's palsy, on the other hand, do not commonly occur in patients with multiple sclerosis. Moreover, patients with Parkinson's disease and myasthenia gravis do not typically present with lacerating pain in the face. While Bell's palsy often involves pain about the eye and ear, it is not characterized by an episodic, lacerating, or jabbing quality of pain.

31. c

Patients who experience migraine headaches, which can present with throbbing and be accompanied by visual disturbances, more frequently than two or three times per month should receive prophylactic daily therapy, which may see use of propranolol and other beta blockers. Sumatriptan, acetaminophen, and oxycodone are not typically indicated for daily prophylactic therapy in migraine patients, but may be used to treat acute episodes.

32. b

The edrophonium test may be used to differentiate a myasthenic crisis from a cholinergic crisis. A cerebral angiography, on the other hand, is employed to assess transient ischemic attack. A cerebral spinal fluid analysis is used to detect slightly elevated protein levels in cases of multiple sclerosis, among others. Finally, while an acetylcholine receptor antibody test is a common diagnostic procedure for patients experiencing myasthenia gravis, this test is not used to differentiate a myasthenic crisis from a cholinergic crisis.

33. c

Cluster headaches are most common in middle-aged male patients. Females are more likely to be affected by migraine headaches than males. Furthermore, tension headaches, not cluster headaches, usually present in adolescence and early adulthood.

34. c

A positive Myerson's sign in patients with Parkinson's disease is usually elicited by repeatedly tapping over the bridge of the nose, causing continuous blinking. Wooden facies and impaired swallowing are other signs and symptoms of Parkinson's disease that are not commonly elicited by tapping on the bridge of the nose. Flared nostrils are not a sign of Parkinson's disease.

35. c

Tension headaches, as characterized by a vise-like quality, are likely to be most intense about the neck or back of the head. The forehead, scalp, and shoulder muscles may also experience pressure or tenderness. The eyes, jaw, and crown of the head, however, are not particularly affected by tension headaches.

36. d

The condition most strongly evidenced by the patient's facial paralysis and the doctor's listed cause of the signs is Bell's palsy, which can be treated with prednisone and other corticosteroids. Neither sumatriptan nor benzodiazepines, such as oxazepam and chlordiazepoxide, would help to reduce the inflammation of the facial nerve; therefore, these treatments would not likely be prescribed.

37. a

Parkinson's disease is a degenerative disorder that commonly occurs as a result of insufficient amounts of dopamine in the body that subsequently results in slow tremors. On the other hand, Parkinson's disease does not typically occur due to insufficient amounts of serotonin, acetylcholine, and amino acids.

38. d

Photophobia is a common finding of migraine headaches, not cluster headaches. Cluster headaches may present with nasal congestion, lacrimation, and rhinorrhea, all occurring on the same side of the head as the headache.

39. d

A computed tomography (CT) scan serves to distinguish between transient ischemic attack (TIA) and hemorrhage. A Carotid Doppler ultrasonography is used to identify patients in need of urgent surgery. Antihypertensive therapy would be deemed necessary based on the patient's blood pressure. A transthoracic or transesophageal echocardiography would be used to assess for a cardioembolic source of TIA.

40. b

The major function of the trochlear nerve is to control downward and inward movement of the eyes, which are motor functions. The trigeminal nerve, which controls mastication muscles and facial sensation, as well as vagus nerve, which is responsible for talking, swallowing, and the carotid reflex, serve as both sensory and motor function nerves. Lastly, the optic nerve is a sensory nerve, not a motor function nerve, and is responsible for vision rather than the movement of the eye.

DISCUSSION

Cranial Nerves (see figure 11.1 and table 11.1)

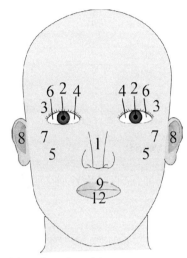

Figure 11.1. Location of cranial nerves.

Headache

Overview (see table 11.2)

Headaches are painful disorders with several types and etiologies. The causes of each type of headache can overlap, with many differences in the onset and progression of each. Some of the most common types of headaches are migraine, tension, and cluster. For a nurse practitioner (NP) to effectively assess the type of headache, a careful examination of the patient and a discussion of the patient's complaints are necessary.[1,2]

Workup

A standard headache evaluation is composed of several parts. Because the evaluation relies primarily on a patient's description of the headache, the most important component of the headache evaluation is the chronology of findings. Therefore, NPs must have a thorough discussion with the patient about his or her complaints, which seeks to identify any associated triggers, activities, or other health issues that have preceded or been present during each episode. The NP should identify the location of the headache, its duration, and its quality. In females, menstrual cycles can also relate to the history of the headache, especially migraines.[3,4]

Table 11.1	Cranial Nerves		
Number	**Name**	**Major Functions**	**Type**
CN I:	Olfactory	Smell	S = Some
CN II:	Optic	Vision	S = Say
CN III:	Oculomotor	Most EOMs, opening eyelids, papillary constriction	M = Marry
CN IV:	Trochlear	Down and inward eye movement	M = Money
CN V:	Trigeminal	Muscles of mastication, sensation of face, scalp, cornea, mucus membranes and nose	B = But
CN VI:	Abducens	Lateral eye movement	M = My
CN VII:	Facial	Move face, close mouth and eyes, taste (anterior 2/3), saliva and tear secretion	B = Brother
CN VIII:	Acoustic	Hearing and equilibrium	S = Says
CN IX:	Glossopharyngeal	Phonation, (one-third), gag reflex, carotid reflex swallowing, taste (posterior)	B = Big
CN X:	Vagus	Talking, swallowing, general sensation from the carotid body, carotid reflex	B = Bras
CN XI:	Spinal accessory	Movement of trapezius and sternomastoid muscles (shrug shoulders)	M = Matter
CN XII:	Hypoglossal	Moves the tongue	M = Most

Used with permission from Barkley TW Jr. Neurologic disorders. In *Adult-Gerontology Primary Care Nurse Practitioner: Certification Review/Clinical Update Continuing Education Course*. West Hollywood, CA: Barkley & Associates; 2015: 114-123.

Tension Headaches

Overview

Tension headaches are the predominant variety of headache, accounting for 90% of all cases.[4] Incidence may be episodic, which is associated with stress, or chronic, which usually involves tightening of muscles in the neck and scalp.[5]

Presentation

Patients with tension headaches tend to describe headache pain as tightness or pressure on each side of the head (i.e., a "vise-like" quality). The tension may be strongest in the neck or the back of the head. The pain traditionally follows a bilateral distribution in the frontal or temporal areas of the head, but can occur in the occipital or parietal regions as well. The headache can also be accompanied by generalized pain, but is not accompanied by focal neurological symptoms. Tension headaches can last anywhere from 30 minutes up to several hours and may even occur on a daily basis in some patients.[6]

Workup

The diagnosis of a tension headache is based on symptomatic presentation. A physical examination may reveal tenderness in the scalp, neck, or upper cervical muscles. Pain with flexion of the neck should be distinguished from nuchal rigidity to exclude meningeal irritation.[7]

Treatment

Tension headaches that are not chronic are controlled with over-the-counter analgesics.[2,8] For preventive treatment, a combination of sleep regulation, exercise, and dietary management can be recommended, as well as relaxation and biofeedback methods.[9]

Migraine Headaches

Overview

Migraine headache is one of the most frequently seen headache disorders. This disorder is characterized by recurrent headaches that are usually unilateral, are either pulsing or throbbing in nature, and may be preceded by an aura.[10] The classification of a migraine headache is further divided into two subtypes: classic migraines (i.e., migraines with an aura) and common migraines (i.e., migraines without an aura).[11,12]

The etiology of migraine headaches is unknown.[13] Many cases include a family history of migraine headaches, which strongly suggests a genetic component.[14] Patients with a history of cardiovascular or cerebrovascular disease are more susceptible to the disorder, and women are more frequently affected than males.

The traditional onset of migraine headaches is during adolescence or early adulthood. These headaches can be precipitated by a variety of "triggers" that include emotional or physical stress, excessive or insufficient sleep, changes in the weather, missed meals, specific foods (e.g., caffeine, nitrate-containing foods), and alcoholic beverages. In females, menstruation and the use of oral contraceptives are also known "triggers" (see table 11.3).[13]

Presentation

The characteristic feature of a migraine headache is a unilateral, lateralized headache that occurs episodically. Patients may describe the headache as "dull" or "throbbing." The headache tends to build gradually as pain develops in the back of the head prior to becoming diffuse, potentially lasting between 30 minutes and 72 hours.[14,15]

Migraines traditionally exhibit a gradual build in intensity and subsequently diminish within an hour.[16] Patients with classic migraines may report an aura (i.e., perceptual disturbance) preceding a migraine. Classic migraines may also be preceded or accompanied by focal neurologic disturbances, which may manifest as visual, sensory, motor, and/or verbal disturbances. Disturbances associated with classic migraines include vision loss, luminous visual hallucinations (e.g., stars, sparks, zigzagging lights, or other geometric patterns), photophobia, phonophobia, altered speech (i.e., aphasia), numbness, tingling, clumsiness, and weakness, among others.[17] These disturbances may lead to nausea and vomiting in some patients.[16,17]

Workup

A clinical diagnosis of migraine headache usually does not require additional investigation. Patients with migraine often appear ill and may exhibit neurological deficits. In some cases, such as with a new onset "migraine-like" headache, a careful neurological exam may be required to search for focal deficits or findings supportive of a brain tumor.[17]

Table 11.2	Characteristics of Primary Headaches		
	Migraine	**Cluster headache**	**Tension headache**
Pain location	Unilateral (60%)	Unilateral	Bilateral
	Bilateral (40%)	Behind the right or left eye	"Headband" configuration
Pain quality	Throbbing	Throbbing Sometimes piercing	Non-throbbing
Pain severity	Moderate to severe	Severe	Mild to moderate
Duration	4 hr to 3 days	15 min to 2 hr[a]	30 min to 7 days[b]
Impact of activity	Worsens pain	None	None
Associated symptoms	Nausea, vomiting, photophobia, phonophobia	Conjunctival redness, lacrimation, nasal congestion, rhinorrhea, ptosis, miosis—all on the same side as the headache	Uncommon
Usual time of onset	Early morning	Nighttime	Daytime
Preceded by aura	Yes, in 30%	No	No
Triggers	Many	Usually unidentified	Tension, anxiety
Gender prevalence	More common in females (3:1)	More common in males (5:1)	Slightly (10%) more common in females
Family history	Likely	Unlikely	Unlikely
Impact on daily life	Often substantial	Usually substantial	Minimal

Note. [a]Headaches occur in clusters that typically consist of one or more headaches, lasting 15 minutes to 2 hr each day for 2–3 months, with a headache-free interval between each cluster. [b]Chronic tension headaches occur at least 15 days out of the month for 6 months or longer. Used with permission from Gullette DL, Barkley TW Jr, Myers CM. Headache. In: Barkley TW Jr, Myers CM, eds. *Practice Considerations for the Adult-Gerontology Acute Care Nurse Practitioner.* West Hollywood, CA: Barkley and Associates; 2015: 669.

Table 11.3	Triggers for Migraine Headaches
Emotions	Anticipation
	Anxiety
	Depression
	Excitement
	Frustration
	Stress
Food Ingredients	Aspartame (e.g., diet sodas and artificial sweeteners)
	Monosodium glutamate (e.g., Chinese food and canned soups)
	Nitrates (e.g., cured meats)
	Phenylethylamine (e.g., chocolate)
	Tyramine (e.g., aged cheeses and Chianti wine)
	Yellow food coloring
Drugs	Alcohol
	Analgesics (excessive use or withdrawal)
	Caffeine (excessive use or withdrawal)
	Cimetidine
	Cocaine
	Estrogen (e.g., oral contraceptives)
	Nitroglycerin
Other Factors	Carbon monoxide
	Hormonal changes in women
	Flickering lights, glare
	Loud noises
	Hypoglycemia
	Change in altitude or barometric pressure
	Altered sleep pattern (excessive sleep or sleep deprivation)

Note. Adapted with permission from Lehne RA. *Pharmacology for Nursing Care.* 5th ed. St. Louis: Elsevier Saunders; 2004.

Laboratory and other diagnostic studies for migraine headaches may include a urinalysis, hCG, blood chemistries including a basic metabolic panel (BMP) and complete blood count (CBC), a VDRL, and ESR. A CT scan or MRI may also be ordered by a neurology specialist.[18]

Treatment

Non-pharmacologic therapy for migraine headaches can include biofeedback methods, relaxation techniques, avoidance of triggers, and stress management techniques. Prophylactic daily therapy may be considered if the patient's attacks occur more than two to three times per month. Examples of possible drugs for prophylactic therapy include amitriptyline (Elavil), divalproex (Depakote), propranolol (Inderal), imipramine (Tofranil), clonidine (Catapres), verapamil (Calan), topiramate (Topamax), gabapentin (Neurontin), methysergide (Sansert), and magnesium, among others.[19]

During a migraine headache acute attack, the patient should rest in a dark, quiet room. A simple analgesic, such as acetylsalicylic acid, acetaminophen, ibuprofen, or naproxen, may provide relief if taken immediately.[20] Sumatriptan (Imitrex), 6 mg subcutaneously may be prescribed at the onset of headache; further administrations are given hourly but are limited to a total of three times a day. Oral sumatriptan, 25 mg is also another option for patients.[21,22]

Cluster Headaches

Overview

A cluster headache (CH) is a very painful primary headache disorder characterized by attacks of severe, unilateral, periorbital pain that may occur daily for several weeks. The exact etiology and pathophysiology are not completely understood. Patients who experience CH often have no family history of headaches or migraines, but the condition is known to mostly affect middle-aged men. These headaches can be precipitated by triggers, which may include alcohol ingestion, stress, and hot weather, among others.[23]

Presentation

Cluster headaches predominantly occur at night, causing the patient to wake from sleep; such headaches rarely last longer than 2 hours. A patient can be pain-free for months or weeks between attacks.[23]

Many patients with CH report feeling agitated or restless during each attack. In addition to pain, the headache may also be accompanied by findings that include ipsilateral nasal congestion, nasal stuffiness or rhinorrhea, and eye redness, among others.[24]

Workup

The diagnosis of CH is based on clinical findings.[25] The NP should assess the history of the patient's headaches and any accompanying complaints that manifest during an attack, including the headache's character, location, distribution, onset, duration, frequency, periodicity, and remission.[24]

Treatment

Rapid, effective control of CH pain focuses on the administration of 100% oxygen via inhalation and/or the use of sumatriptan (Imitrex), 6 mg subcutaneously.[11,25] Prevention measures for future attacks may include avoiding the use of alcohol or tobacco products, dietary modifications, and a headache diary to identify triggers.[25,26]

Transient Ischemic Attack (TIA)

Overview

A transient ischemic attack (TIA) is a period of cerebral insufficiency that lasts for less than 24 hours without causing any residual deficits. A TIA does not cause permanent brain tissue death but can serve as a warning of an impending stroke. Approximately one-third of all patients who have experienced a TIA will have a cerebrovascular accident (CVA)/stroke within 5 years, with more than 10% of those patients at an increased risk of experiencing a stroke within 3 months.[27,28]

Patients with hypertension are at the highest risk of experiencing a TIA. Consequently, other conditions that can lead to a TIA include atherosclerosis, thrombus, arterial occlusion, and an embolus. Cardio-embolic events (e.g., atrial fibrillation, acute myocardial infarction [MI], endocarditis, or valve disease) can also lead to a TIA.[27,29]

Presentation

Signs and symptoms of a TIA are similar to those of a CVA, and patients should be immediately evaluated. Findings may include sensory deficits or changes in hearing, vision, taste, and touch. Changes in vision associated with a TIA include nystagmus, altered vision (e.g., hemianopsia), and ipsilateral monocular blindness (i.e., amaurosis fugax). Additionally, transient aphasia, motor impairment (i.e., paresthesias of contralateral arm, leg, or face), cognitive and behavioral abnormalities, dysphagia (i.e., difficulty swallowing), vertigo, and changes in alertness (e.g., sleepiness, unconsciousness) may also occur.[11,27]

TIAs are classified as either vertebrobasilar or carotid. Vertebrobasilar TIA results from insufficient blood flow from vertebral arteries and presents with vertigo, ataxia, dizziness, visual field deficits, weakness, or confusion. A carotid TIA, on the other hand, is due to carotid stenosis and classically produces an altered level of consciousness, dysarthria, weakness, numbness, or other "traditional" symptoms of stroke.[27,29]

Workup

A "FAST" exam (i.e., face, arm, speech test) should be performed on any patient suspected of having a stroke, especially if the onset of symptoms was rapid.[30] Upon recognition by an NP, patients who experience a TIA should be transported to the emergency department immediately for further evaluation. A physical exam and additional diagnostic studies will be performed, including an urgent CT scan, which is the best method to distinguish between ischemia and hemorrhage. A diagnosis relies on the patient's constellation of signs and symptoms, including onset and duration.[27,29]

Additional tests may include an MRI, echocardiogram, and a carotid Doppler ultrasound.[29]

Treatment

The emergency department management of acute TIA involves evaluation of the patient's CT scan and other findings. For those presenting with hypertension, the American Heart Association (AHA) does not recommend initial treatment of this complication unless the BP is higher than 220/120. Once hemorrhagic stroke is ruled out, treatment generally involves one of two TIA management pathways: noncardioembolic and cardioembolic.[30]

According to the AHA and the American Stroke Association (ASA) guidelines for the prevention of stroke in patients with stroke or TIA, recommendations include the following.[31] For patients experiencing a noncardioembolic TIA, antiplatelet agents, instead of oral anticoagulants, are recommended as initial therapy. Class 1 recommendations from the AHA/ASA guidelines support that aspirin, 50–325 mg/day, a combination of aspirin and extended-release dipyridamole, and clopidogrel are all reasonable first-line choices.[32] The AHA/ASA guidelines do not recommend clopidogrel plus aspirin for patients with a hemorrhagic contraindication to warfarin because this combination carries a risk of bleeding similar to that of warfarin.[32]

For those with a cardioembolic TIA secondary to atrial fibrillation, anticoagulation with warfarin and aspirin, 325 mg/day is recommended.[32] Low-molecular-weight heparin subcutaneously may also be used. A neurologist, and frequently a cardiologist, will further devise the patient's plan of care in the acute care facility.

Seizures

Overview

Seizures, paroxysmal events stemming from abnormal electrical activity in the brain, are the most prevalent acute neurologic problem in the United States. Some seizures, such as absence seizures, predominantly present in children and adolescents; however, the likelihood of epileptic seizures increases with age.[33,34]

Presentation

The International Classification of Seizures categorizes seizures as two basic types: partial or generalized, in addition to status epilepticus. Subcategories of partial seizures include simple partial and complex partial. The two main subcategories of generalized seizures are absence and tonic-clonic.

Simple partial seizures

Simple partial seizures are associated with cerebral lesions and cause no alteration of memory. These seizures rarely last more than a minute and do not result in a loss of consciousness. These seizures may present with twitching; abnormal sensations; abnormal visions, sounds, or smells; and distortions of perception. Moreover, these motor signs and symptoms traditionally start in a single muscle group and extend to the entire side of the body. Paresthesias, flashing lights, vocalizations, and hallucinations are also common occurrences in cases of simple partial seizures.[35]

Complex partial seizures

Complex partial seizures are any simple partial seizure followed by an impaired level of consciousness. These seizures may present with an aura, staring, and automatisms (e.g., lip-smacking, picking at clothing).[35]

Absence (previously known as petit mal) seizures

Absence seizures often present with a sudden arrest of motor activity, such as a blank stare that is sometimes accompanied by eyelid fluttering or head-nodding. These seizures begin and end suddenly and frequently first appear in childhood or adolescence.

Tonic–clonic (previously known as grand mal) seizures

Tonic-clonic seizures often present with an aura. These seizures begin with tonic contractions (i.e., repetitive involuntary contractions of muscle) and loss of consciousness followed by clonic contractions (i.e., maintained involuntary contractions of muscles). During the seizure, the patient may experience incontinence. These seizures last about two to five minutes and are followed by a postictal period characterized by sluggishness, sleepiness, confusion, and unconsciousness.[35]

Status epilepticus seizures

Status epilepticus seizures are a series of grand mal seizures lasting longer than 10 minutes. Status epilepticus can occur when a patient is awake or asleep; in either case, patients generally do not regain consciousness between attacks. These seizures are rarer than others but are also the most life-threatening. Patients experiencing these seizures require immediate attention via EMS with transport to an emergency department.[35,36]

Workup

The NP must take a detailed medical history to assess the patient's seizure symptoms to classify which type of seizure the patient is experiencing. Because many patients are unable to recall what happened during a seizure, the best accounts are those taken from someone who witnessed the seizure, such as a caregiver or family member. Seizure assessment includes determining the presence of an aura, the onset and duration of the seizure, its spread, the type of movement it causes, and the body parts involved in movement. In addition, NPs should note pupil changes and reactivity, the patient's loss/level of consciousness, and if the patient became incontinent. The NP should also determine if behavioral and neurological changes occurred after seizure activity ended.

The most important test in classifying seizures is an electroencephalogram, which can assess for brain wave abnormalities. A CT scan of the head is indicated for any patient who experiences the onset of a new seizure. An MRI can help to detect abnormalities in brain function or structure, whereas positron emission tomography is useful in isolating seizure foci.[11,35]

Treatment

Seizures should be treated aggressively. Because the majority of seizures are self-limiting, initial management is supportive. The NP should focus on maintaining the patient's airway, then focus on other vital signs.[36,37]

If the seizure is not self-limiting, parenteral anticonvulsants are standard measures for stopping convulsive seizures, usually in an emergency department setting. Standard agents used to break seizures include benzodiazepines (e.g., diazepam or lorazepam). Following a neurologist consult, phenytoin (Dilantin) or fosphenytoin (Cerebyx) may be employed. If phenytoin is unresponsive, phenobarbital (Luminal) may see use. A barbiturate coma or general anesthesia with neuromuscular blockade may also be used to treat unrelenting seizures.[11,36]

Long-acting anticonvulsants may be used to prevent subsequent seizures. Some long-acting anticonvulsants include carbamazepine (Tegretol), phenytoin, phenobarbital, valproic acid (Depakene), primidone (Mysoline), and clonazepam (Klonopin), among others. Dosages are titrated and should never be abruptly withdrawn.[36,38]

Parkinson's Disease

Overview

Parkinson's disease (PD) is a degenerative disorder associated with insufficient amounts of dopamine in the body. The disorder occurs in all ethnic groups, with men diagnosed more often than women. The onset of this condition mainly occurs between 45 and 65 years of age, and the exact cause remains unknown.

Presentation

Although signs and symptoms of PD vary from patient to patient, cardinal features that all PD patients eventually experience include tremor, rigidity, and bradykinesia (i.e., slow movement).[39] Tremors of the hands, arms, legs, jaw, or face are most conspicuous at rest and may be enhanced by stress. Rigidity (e.g., "cogwheel" rigidity) or stiffness can involve the limbs and trunk. Bradykinesia is closely associated with an impaired ability to initiate voluntary movement.[40] Additional findings of PD include wooden facies, impaired swallowing, drooling, decreased blinking, and Myerson's sign—a repetitive tapping over the bridge of the nose that produces a sustained blink response.[11,41]

Workup

The primary workup available for PD is an assessment of a patient's symptoms, making diagnosis largely based on clinical findings. An array of laboratory tests are further used to support the diagnosis as a matter of exclusion. MRIs are initially noncontributory but are used for comparison as the disease progresses.[40,42,43]

Treatment

Although PD is incurable, dopamine agonists are the gold standard in the treatment of PD. Dopamine agonists include carbidopa-levodopa (Sinemet), amantadine (Symmetrel), apomorphine (Apokyn), pramipexole (Mirapex), ropinirole hydrochloride (Requip), and rotigotine (Neupro). Anticholinergics, such as benztropine (Cogentin) and trihexyphenidyl (Artane), may be helpful in alleviating tremors and, to some degree, rigidity in some patients. Other possible agents that may be employed in PD treatment include monoamine oxidase (MAO)-B inhibitors and catechol-O-methyl transferase (COMT) inhibitors.[44]

Myasthenia Gravis

Overview

Myasthenia gravis (MG) is a chronic autoimmune disorder that causes a reduction in acetylcholine receptor sites at the neuromuscular junction. The condition stems from a defect in the transmission of nerve impulses to the muscles, which produces symptoms that lead to varying degrees of muscle weakness in specific areas of the body. MG has a variable clinical course, during which patients experience periods of remission and exacerbations.[45]

The disorder affects a significant portion of the U.S. population; approximately 36,000–60,000 new cases are estimated to occur annually.[46] The predominant age of onset is between 20 and 40 years of age, but MG can occur at any age. The incidence peaks in the third decade for females and in the fifth and sixth decades for males.[11] The disorder occurs more frequently in women, although recent studies show that incidence is rising in men.[46,47]

Presentation

Patients with MG typically initially complain of specific muscle weakness. Symptoms can suddenly onset, are sometimes not immediately recognizable, and regularly fluctuate throughout the day. Patients may also report experiencing weakness that worsens after exercise but feels better after rest.[46]

Although MG can affect any voluntary muscle and symptoms vary from patient to patient, the most commonly affected muscles are those that control eye and eyelid movements. In many cases, the initial findings involve weakness of the eye muscles; these presentations may include ptosis (i.e., drooping eyelid) or diplopia (i.e., double vision). Ocular MG, a disorder in which symptoms are only limited to the extrinsic ocular muscles, occurs in a small number of cases.[45,48]

In traditional cases, MG signs and symptoms progress and become more generalized, often affecting the facial and oropharyngeal muscles; in some patients, dysphagia or dysarthria are the initial findings.[45] Progression of the disease can involve weakness in the extremities and fatigue. In severe cases, the muscles involved in breathing may be affected, resulting in respiratory difficulty. Sensory modalities and deep tendon reflexes (DTRs) tend to exhibit normal activity.[46]

Workup

Neurological and physical exams to assess eye movement impairment or muscle weakness are initially performed.[47] If MG is suspected, a variety of blood tests are conducted, including a test for antibodies to acetylcholine receptors (AChR-ab). To help confirm the diagnosis during a potential crisis, an edrophonium (Tensilon) test can be ordered to assess whether the patient experienced a myasthenic crisis or a cholinergic crisis.[47]

Treatment

As there is no specific protocol for treatment of MG, patients are referred to a neurologist for individualized treatment plans. Current treatments for the condition include the use of anticholinesterase agents such as pyridostigmine bromide (Prostigmin), which block the hydrolysis of acetylcholine to improve neuromuscular transmission. Corticosteroids may be used for their immunosuppressive properties; other immunosuppressive drugs may be used to interfere with the growth of T cells and B cells. Plasmapheresis and ventilator support may be used to treat severe exacerbations of MG.[48]

Multiple Sclerosis

Overview

Multiple sclerosis (MS) is an autoimmune disease that causes the body's immune system to attack myelin, a nerve insulator that assists in nerve signal transmission.[11,49] The condition is marked by numbness, weakness, loss of muscle coordination, and difficulties with vision, speech, and bladder control. Like myasthenia gravis, the progression of MS varies from patient to patient, as it has a variable clinical course with periods of exacerbation and remission. The incidence of symptomatic episodes can be separated by months or years.[50]

The incidence of MS is highest in young adults, predominantly occurring in individuals between the ages of 20 and 50; however, the condition can occur at any age. The disorder occurs more often in women than in men, and presents with particular frequency in patients of Western European descent who live in temperate zones.[50,51]

Presentation

A common finding in cases of MS is weakness, numbness, tingling, or unsteadiness in one limb that may progress to all limbs over time. Findings may also include spastic paraparesis, diplopia, disequilibrium, urinary urgency or hesitancy, optic atrophy, and nystagmus, among others. Although specific signs and symptoms vary in each patient, findings of MS are often compounded by extreme fatigue. A classic feature of MS is for symptoms to become worse as a result of an internal or external increase in body temperature. Some patients describe symptoms as being worse in the afternoon.[52]

Workup

A diagnosis of MS is based on clinical findings and supporting evidence from laboratory findings and other tests. The physical exam should include an expert neurological assessment, which is absolutely essential in assessing for MS.[53]

An MRI is the diagnostic of choice for confirming MS and can also be used to monitor progression of the disease.[50] An MRI of the brain can identify MS plaques or lesions in different parts of the central nervous system. Lab studies, on the other hand, will tend to show normal findings and should not serve as the sole diagnostic process for MS. In a patient with MS, a CBC may show mild lymphocytosis, and a lumbar puncture (LP) may show slightly elevated protein levels and elevated cerebrospinal fluid immunoglobulin G.[53]

Treatment

The progression of MS cannot be reversed, but symptoms can be managed. Patients with MS should be referred to a neurologist for further care. Recovery from acute relapses can be hastened by steroids, but these drugs do little to alter or reverse the progression of the disease. Other treatments for MS include antispasmodics, interferon therapy, immunosuppressive therapy, and plasmapheresis.[54]

Rehabilitation programs can help patients maintain function. Some standard rehabilitation programs include physical therapy, occupational therapy, therapy for speech and swallowing problems, cognitive rehabilitation, and vocational rehabilitation.[54]

Bell's Palsy

Overview

Bell's palsy is characterized by unilateral facial paresis that gradually resolves, usually without any residual effects. The condition stems from an inflammatory reaction affecting the facial nerve. Although the etiology is idiopathic, a relationship to herpes simplex reactivation has been strongly suggested.[55]

Presentation

Bell's palsy presents with an abrupt onset of ipsilateral facial paresis involving the forehead and lower aspect of the face. Some patients complain of pain around the area of the eye accompanied by weakness, and the face may feel stiff and pulled to one side. Patients with Bell's palsy are unable to move their forehead and may show ipsilateral restriction of eye closure, difficulty with eating and fine facial movements, and a possible disturbance of taste.[56]

Workup

No specific laboratory test can determine if a patient has Bell's palsy. Diagnosis is typically made after consideration of the clinical presentation and the patient's history.[57]

Treatment

In many cases, Bell's palsy will resolve without treatment. However, traditional management includes a tapered dose of prednisone 60 mg divided in four to five doses over 7–10 days. Treatment should be initiated within 72 hours of symptom onset for best outcomes. Acyclovir or valacyclovir may also see use.[58] If the patient is unable to close his or her eyes, lubricating eye drops and a patch at night are recommended. Patients who do not respond favorably to initial treatment should be referred to a neurologist for further intervention.

Trigeminal Neuralgia

Overview

Trigeminal neuralgia is a nerve disorder that causes a stabbing or electric shock-like sensation in the face. This condition is caused by pressure on the trigeminal nerve; this pressure commonly stems from inflammatory changes related to multiple sclerosis, but may also stem from idiopathic causes, a tumor, or a swollen blood vessel.[59]

Presentation

Patients with trigeminal neuralgia typically present with pain that is characteristically localized on one side of the face. The patient experiences very painful, sharp spasms that last anywhere from a few seconds up to a few minutes.[60]

Workup

Diagnostics for trigeminal neuralgia may include trigeminal nerve testing and MRI, among other studies.[61]

Treatment

Management methods for trigeminal neuralgia include anti-seizure medications, with carbamazepine considered the gold standard for treatment. Carbamazepine is often used in combination with muscle relaxants and tricyclic antidepressants.[62,63]

Figures

Figure 11.1. Cranial nerves. Barkley & Associates, Inc. Published 2015.

References

1. United States Department of Health and Human Services, National Institutes of Health (NIH), National Institute of Neurological Disorders and Stroke (NINDS). NINDS Headache Information page. http://www.ninds.nih.gov/disorders/headache/headache.htm. Updated February 23, 2015. Accessed April 2, 2015.

2. Bajwa ZH, Wootton RJ. Patient information: Headache causes and diagnosis in adults (Beyond the basics). In: Basow DS, ed. *UptoDate*. Waltham, MA: UpToDate; 2015. http://www.uptodate.com/contents/headache-causes-and-diagnosis-in-adults-beyond-the-basics. Updated November 21, 2014. Assessed April 2, 2015.

3. Taylor FR. ABC's of headache trigger management. American Headache Society Web site. http://www.achenet.org/resources/abcs_of_headache_trigger_management. Published 2011. Accessed April 2, 2015.

4. Headache. MedLinePlus web site. http://www.nlm.nih.gov/medlineplus/headache.html. Reviewed October 2, 2014. Accessed April 2, 2015.

5. Blanda M, Sergeant LK. Tension headache. In: Dyne PL, ed. Medscape. http://emedicine.medscape.com/article/792384-overview#showall. Updated October 1, 2014. Accessed April 2, 2015.

6. Singh MK. Muscle contraction tension headache. In: Crystal HA, ed. Medscape. http://emedicine.medscape.com/article/1142908-overview. Updated August 29, 2013. Accessed April 2, 2015.

7. Blanda M, Sergeant LK. Tension headache workup. In: Dyne PL, ed. Medscape. http://emedicine.medscape.com/article/792384-workup#showall. Updated October 1, 2014. Accessed April 2, 2015.

8. Garza I, Schwedt TJ. Medication overuse headache: Etiology, clinical features, and diagnosis. In: Basow DS, ed. *UpToDate*. Waltham, MA: UpToDate; 2015. http://www.uptodate.com/contents/medication-overuse-headache-etiology-clinical-features-and-diagnosis. Updated December 15, 2014. Accessed April 2, 2015.

9. Taylor FR. Tension-type headache in adults: Preventive treatment. In: Basow DS, ed. *UptoDate*. Waltham, MA: UpToDate; 2015. http://www.uptodate.com/contents/tension-type-headache-in-adults-preventive-treatment. Updated March 12, 2015. Accessed April 2, 2015.

10. Rothrock JF. Migraine aura. American Headache Society Web site. https://www.americanheadachesociety.org/assets/1/7/Migraine_Aura_July-August_2009.pdf. Published 2009. Accessed April 2, 2015.

11. Barkley TW Jr. Neurologic disorders. In *Adult-Gerontology Primary Care Nurse Practitioner: Certification Review/Clinical Update Continuing Education Course*. West Hollywood, CA: Barkley & Associates; 2015: 114–123.

12. Chawla J. Migraine headache clinical presentation. In: Lutsep HL, ed. Medscape. http://emedicine.medscape.com/article/1142556-clinical#showall. Updated September 15, 2014. Accessed April 2, 2015.

13. Cowan R, Sahai S. Causes and treatments of migraines and related headaches. In: Carcione J, Talavera F, Halsey JH, eds. Emedicinehealth Web site. http://www.emedicinehealth.com/causes_and_treatments_of_migraine_headaches/article_em.htm. Updated July 22, 2014. Accessed April 2, 2015.

14. Chawla J. Migraine headache. In: Lutsep HL, ed. Medscape. http://emedicine.medscape.com/article/1142556-overview#showall. Updated September 15, 2014. Accessed April 2, 2015.

15. Hutchinson S. What kind of headache do I have? In *The Woman's Guide to Managing Migraine: Understanding the Hormone Connection to Find Hope and Wellness*. New York, NY: Oxford University Press; 2013: 31–42.

16. Cutrer F, Bajwa ZH, Sabahat A. Pathophysiology, clinical manifestations, and diagnosis of migraine in adults. In: Basow DS, ed. *UptoDate*. Waltham, MA: UpToDate; 2015. http://www.uptodate.com/contents/pathophysiology-clinical-manifestations-and-diagnosis-of-migraine-in-adults. Updated April 21, 2014. Accessed April 2, 2015.

17. Headache Classification Subcommittee of the International Headache Society. The International Classification of Headache Disorders, 3rd edition. *Cephalalgia*. 2013; 33(9): 629–808. http://www.ihs-classification.org/_downloads/mixed/International-Headache-Classification-III-ICHD-III-2013-Beta.pdf.

18. Chawla J. Migraine headache workup. In: Lutsep HL, ed. Medscape. http://emedicine.medscape.com/article/1142556-workup#showall. Updated September 15, 2014. Accessed April 2, 2015.

19. Chawla J. Migraine headache treatment and management. In: Lutsep HL, ed. Medscape. http://emedicine.medscape.com/article/1142556-treatment#showall. Updated September 15, 2014. Accessed April 2, 2015.

20. Questions and answers for migraine patients. UCLA Headache Research and Treatment Program Web site. http://hartp.neurology.ucla.edu/QUESTIONS%20AND%20ANSWERS.html. Accessed April 2, 2015.

21. Bajwa ZH, Sabahat A. Acute treatment of migraine in adults. In: Basow DS, ed. *UptoDate*. Waltham, MA: UpToDate; 2015. http://www.uptodate.com/contents/acute-treatment-of-migraine-in-adults?detectedLanguage =en&source=search_result&search=Sumatriptan&selectedTitle=2~26&provider=noProvider. Updated March 17, 2015. Accessed April 2, 2015.

22. Gilmore B, Michael M. Treatment of acute migraine headache. *Am Fam Physician*. 2011; 83(3): 271–280. http://www.aafp.org/afp/2011/0201/p271.html.

23. Blanda M, Dafer RM. Cluster headache. In: Crystal HA, ed. Medscape. http://emedicine.medscape.com/article/1142459-overview#showall. Updated April 8, 2014. Accessed April 2, 2015.

24. Blanda M, Dafer RM. Cluster headache clinical presentation. In: Crystal HA, ed. Medscape. http://emedicine.medscape.com/article/1142459-clinical#showall. Updated April 8, 2014. Accessed April 2, 2015.

25. Cluster headache. A.D.A.M. Medical Encyclopedia. http://www.nlm.nih.gov/medlineplus/ency/article/000786.htm. Updated October 29, 2013. Accessed April 2, 2015.

26. Ashkenazi A, Schwedt T. Cluster headache-acute and prophylactic therapy. *Headache*. 2011; 51(2): 272–286. doi:10.1111/hed.2011.51.issue-2

27. Transient ischemic attack. A.D.A.M. Medical Encyclopedia. http://www.nlm.nih.gov/medlineplus/ency/article/000730.htm. Updated May 28, 2014. Accessed April 2, 2015.

28. United States Department of Health and Human Services, NIH, NINDS. NINDS transient ischemic attack information page. http://www.ninds.nih.gov/disorders/tia/tia.htm. Updated March 5, 2015. Accessed April 2, 2015.

29. Furie KL, Ay H. Etiology and clinical manifestations of transient ischemic attack. In: Basow DS, ed. *UptoDate*. Waltham, MA: UpToDate; 2015. http://www.uptodate.com/contents/etiology-and-clinical-manifestations-of-transient-ischemic-attack. Updated January 10, 2014. Accessed April 2, 2015.

30. Hayashi T, Seahara Y, Kato Y, et al. Clinical characters of cardioembolic transient ischemic attack: Comparison with noncardioembolic transient ischemic attack. *J Stroke Cerebrovasc Dis*. 2014; 23(8): 2169–2173. doi: 10.1016/j.jstrokecerebrovasdis.2014.04.005.

31. Morgenstern LB, Hemphill JC III, Anderson C, et al. Guidelines for the management of spontaneous intracerebral hemorrhage: A guideline for healthcare professionals from the American Heart Association/American Stroke Association. *Stroke*. 2010;41:2108–2129. doi: 10.1161/STR.0b013e3181ec611b

32. Nanda A, Singh NN. Transient ischemic attack treatment and management. In: O'Connor RE, ed. Medscape. http://emedicine.medscape.com/article/1910519-treatment#d10. Updated December 15, 2014. Accessed April 4, 2015.

33. Segan S. Absence seizures. In: Benbadis SR, ed. Medscape. http://reference.medscape.com/article/1183858-overview#aw2aab6b4. Updated March 28, 2013. Accessed April 4, 2015.

34. Epilepsy later in life. Epilepsy Society Web site. http://www.epilepsysociety.org.uk/epilepsy-later-life#.VK7S_CvF-So. Accessed April 4, 2015.

35. United States Department of Health and Human Services, NIH, NINDS. Seizures and epilepsy: Hope through research. http://www.ninds.nih.gov/disorders/epilepsy/detail_epilepsy.htm. Updated March 20, 2015. Accessed April 4, 2015.

36. Roth JL, Blum AS. Status epilepticus treatment & management. In: Berman SA, ed. Medscape. http://emedicine.medscape.com/article/1164462-treatment#showall. Updated April 28, 2014. Accessed April 4, 2015.

37. United States Department of Health and Human Services, Centers for Disease Control and Prevention. Epilepsy: First aid for seizures. http://www.cdc.gov/epilepsy/basics/first_aid.htm. Updated August 1, 2011. Accessed April 4, 2015.

38. Discontinuing anti-epileptic drugs. Epilepsy Foundation of Greater Chicago Web site. http://www.epilepsychicago.org/epilepsyfacts/treatment/discontinuing-antiepileptic-drugs. Accessed April 7, 2015.

39. Chou KL. Clinical manifestations of Parkinson disease. In: Basow DS, ed. *UptoDate*. Waltham, MA: UpToDate; 2015. http://www.uptodate.com/contents/clinical-manifestations-of-parkinson-disease. Updated March 31, 2015. Accessed April 7, 2015.

40. Gonzalez-Usigli HA, Espay A. Parkinson's disease. In: Porter RS, Kaplan JL, eds. The Merck Manual Online. http://www.merckmanuals.com/professional/neurologic_disorders/movement_and_cerebellar_disorders/parkinsons_disease.html. Updated January, 2013. Accessed April 7, 2015.

41. Progression. Parkinson's Disease Foundation Web site. http://www.pdf.org/en/progression_parkinsons. Accessed April 7, 2015.

42. Malthur S. Physical examination in diagnosing Parkinson's disease. Parkinsons.about.com website. http://parkinsons.about.com/od/diagnosingpd/fl/Physical-Examination-in-Diagnosing-Parkinsons-Disease.htm. Updated April 11, 2014. Accessed April 7, 2015.

43. Hauser RA, Lyons KE, McClain TA, Pahwa R. Parkinson disease clinical presentation. In: Benbadis SR, ed. Medscape. http://emedicine.medscape.com/article/1831191-clinical#a0256. Updated January 23, 2015. Accessed April 7, 2015.

44. Politynska B. *The Clinical Presentation of Parkinson's Disease and the Dyadic Relationship Between Patients and Carriers: A Neuropsychological Approach.* Newcastle upon Tyne, UK: Cambridge Scholars Publishing; 2013.

45. United States Department of Health and Human Services, NIH, NINDS. Myasthenia gravis fact sheet. http://www.ninds.nih.gov/disorders/myasthenia_gravis/detail_myasthenia_gravis.htm. Updated March 12, 2015. Accessed April 7, 2015.

46. Howard JF. Clinical overview of MG. Myasthenia Gravis Foundation of America Web site. http://www.myasthenia.org/healthprofessionals/clinicaloverviewofmg.aspx. Updated June, 2010. Accessed April 7, 2015.

47. Shah AK, Goldenberg WD. Myasthenia gravis. In: Lorenzo N, ed. Medscape. http://emedicine.medscape.com/article/1171206-overview#a0156. Updated May 2, 2014. Accessed April 7, 2015.

48. Luchanok V, Kaminski HJ. Natural history of myasthenia gravis. In: Engel AG, ed. *Myasthenia Gravis and Myasthenic Disorders.* 2nd ed. New York, NY: Oxford University Press; 2012: 90–107.

49. Definition of MS. National Multiple Sclerosis Society Web site. http://www.nationalmssociety.org/about-multiple-sclerosis/what-we-know-about-ms/what-is-ms/index.aspx. Accessed April 7, 2015.

50. Luzzio C, Dangond F. Multiple sclerosis. In: Keegan BM, ed. Medscape. http://emedicine.medscape.com/article/1146199-overview#a0156. Updated November 24, 2014. Accessed April 7, 2015.

51. Who gets MS? (Epidemiology). National Multiple Sclerosis Society Web site. http://www.nationalmssociety.org/What-is-MS/Who-Gets-MS. Accessed April 7, 2015.

52. What are the symptoms of MS? Multiple Sclerosis Association of America Web site. http://www.mymsaa.org/about-ms/symptoms/. Updated October 16, 2013. Accessed April 7, 2015.

53. Luzzio C, Dangond F. Multiple sclerosis workup. In: Keegan BM, ed., Medscape. http://emedicine.medscape.com/article/1146199-workup#showall. Updated November 24, 2014. Accessed April 7, 2015.

54. Luzzio C, Dangond F. Multiple sclerosis treatment & management. In: Keegan BM, ed. Medscape. http://emedicine.medscape.com/article/1146199-treatment#showall. Updated November 24, 2014. Accessed April 7, 2015.

55. Taylor DC, Zachariah SB. Bell palsy. In: Keegan BM, ed. Medscape. http://emedicine.medscape.com/article/1146903-overview. Updated September 11, 2014. Accessed April 7, 2015.

56. Taylor DC, Zachariah SB. Bell palsy clinical presentation. In: Keegan BM, ed. Medscape. http://emedicine.medscape.com/article/1146903-clinical#showall. Updated September 11, 2014. Accessed April 7, 2015.

57. Berkeley RP. Trigeminal neuralgia and Bell's palsy. In: Wolfson AB, Cloutier RL, Hendey GW, Ling LJ, Rosen CL, Schaider JJ, eds. *Harwood-Nuss' Clinical Practice of Emergency Medicine.* 6th ed. Philadelphia, PA: Wolters Kluwer Health/Lippincott Williams and Wilkins; 2015: 781–784.

58. Ramsay-Hunt syndrome. MedlinePlus Web site. http://www.nlm.nih.gov/medlineplus/ency/article/001647.htm. Updated May 28, 2014. Accessed April 7, 2015.

59. United States Department of Health and Human Services, NIH, NINDS. Trigeminal Neuralgia Fact Sheet. http://www.ninds.nih.gov/disorders/trigeminal_neuralgia/detail_trigeminal_neuralgia.htm. Updated February 23, 2015. Accessed April 7, 2015.

60. Trigeminal neuralgia. John Hopkins Medicine Web site. http://www.hopkinsmedicine.org/neurology_neurosurgery/specialty_areas/trigeminal_neuralgia/conditions/trigeminal_neuralgia.html. Accessed April 7, 2015.

61. Trigeminal diagnosis. Johns Hopkins Medicine Web site. http://www.hopkinsmedicine.org/neurology_neurosurgery/specialty_areas/trigeminal_neuralgia/conditions/trigeminal_diagnosis.html. Accessed April 7, 2015.

62. Fillmore EP, Seifert MF. Anatomy of the trigeminal nerve. In: Tubbs RS, Rizk E, Shoja MM, Loukas M, Barbaro N, Spinner RJ, eds. *Nerves and Nerve Injuries, Vol. 1: History, Embryology, Anatomy, Imaging, and Diagnostics*. San Diego, CA: Academic Press; 2015: 319–350.

63. Trigeminal neuralgia treatments. John Hopkins Medicine Web site. http://www.hopkinsmedicine.org/neurology_neurosurgery/specialty_areas/trigeminal_neuralgia/conditions/trigeminal_neuralgia_treatments.html. Accessed April 7, 2015.

Chapter 12

Gastrointestinal Disorders

1. Ms. Swanson, age 60, presents with complaints of constipation and "a painful cramp" in her lower left side. She tells you that she has also been "feeling nauseated and even threw up." During the practitioner's physical exam, it is noted that the patient has a low-grade fever, tenderness in the left lower quadrant, and slight abdominal distention. After referring the patient to the emergency room, the nurse practitioner knows that which test is a priority at this time?

    a. Barium enema

    b. Abdominal x-ray

    c. Colonoscopy

    d. Computed tomography scan

2. Jonathan, a 44-year-old male, is undergoing an evaluation for his complaints of severe heartburn. He tells you that the pain normally occurs after he eats large meals and is usually alleviated after vomiting. You note that there is tenderness in the right upper quadrant of the patient's abdomen, and that the patient reports pain upon inspiration as you press down under his right rib cage with your fingers. Based on these findings, which of the following tests would be most effective in confirming the patient's likely condition?

    a. White blood cell count

    b. Plain film radiography

    c. Ultrasound

    d. Serum bilirubin test

3. You are evaluating a 24-year-old patient who is being seen for severe abdominal pain and nausea. He says a mild pain originated around his belly button earlier today, and that it has "just gotten worse." For which condition should you assess the patient, and what finding would you most likely expect to see in this patient that would further indicate this condition?

    a. Bowel obstruction; pronounced abdominal distention

    b. Appendicitis; the patient reports pain with internal rotation of flexed right thigh

    c. Cholecystitis; the patient experiences deep pain when you place your fingers under his rib cage

    d. Diverticulitis; the patient reports pain in the right lower abdomen when you apply pressure to the left lower quadrant

4. Which variant of hepatitis is a bloodborne RNA virus that is most commonly associated with intravenous drug use?

    a. Hepatitis A

    b. Hepatitis B

    c. Hepatitis C

    d. Hepatitis D

5. Which of the following signs or symptoms would you <u>not</u> expect to see in a patient who is in the icteric phase of hepatitis C?

    a. Low-grade fever

    b. Dark urine

    c. Clay-colored stool

    (d.) Headaches

6. Phoebe, a 23-year-old female, has gastroenteritis. While reviewing her medical history and discussing management options, she inquires about treatment for her severe diarrhea. Which of the following findings would contraindicate an anti-motility agent regimen to help manage the patient's diarrhea?

    a. The patient has a history of alcohol abuse and is a regular tobacco user.

    b. The patient is prescribed antidepressants to treat an unrelated condition.

    c. The patient is obese and has a lifelong history of diabetes.

    d. The initial workup shows that the patient has a temperature of 38.5 °C.

7. You are examining the serologic test results of a patient's hepatitis workup. The practitioner knows that the appearance of _____ and the disappearance of _____ indicate recovery from the hepatitis B virus, non-infectivity, and protection from recurrent infection.

    (a.) Anti-HBs; HBsAg

    b. HBsAg; Anti-HBc and IgM

    c. Anti-HBs; Anti-HBsAg

    d. Anti-HBc; HBs and IgG

8. Irritable bowel syndrome is a clinical syndrome with uncertain etiology that affects what percentage of the general population?

    a. Approximately 5%–6%

    b. Approximately 10%–12%

    c. Approximately 20%–24%

    d. Approximately 30%–32%

9. With regard to hepatitis and prevention, the practitioner knows that all of the following are true <u>except</u>:

    a. Hepatitis A immunization requires three injections over a 6-month period of time.

    b. A low- or no-protein diet may be appropriate.

    c. Hepatitis B immune globulin provides passive immunity.

    d. The leading cause of fulminant liver failure is hepatitis B.

10. Which of these serologic markers would provide the first definitive evidence of a current hepatitis B viral infection?

    a. Anti-HBs

    b. HBcAb

    c. HBsAg

    d. HBeAg

11. Which of the following physiological changes is <u>least</u> likely a result of the effects of aging in older adults?

    a. Increased intestinal transit time

    b. Decreased liver size

    c. Constipation

    d. Impaired defecation signal

12. An 18-year-old college student presents to urgent care with complaints of severe periumbilical pain. While being evaluated, the patient is lying very still with his right thigh drawn to his chest. Upon extension of the right thigh, the patient complains of strong pain. Which of the following signs should you determine is positive?

    a. McMurray   — knee

    b. Obturator

    c. Psoas

    d. Rovsing

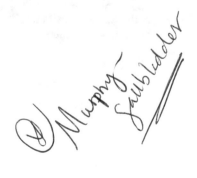
Murphy – gallbladder

13. You are seeing a 64-year-old female whose complaints include cramping in her lower abdomen that is only relieved by defecation. She says that the pain "tends to come and go" and that she often experiences heartburn and fatigue. She adds that her bowel habits sometime alternate between constipation and diarrhea. As you perform the examination, she tells you that she has been working long hours recently to meet an approaching deadline. Based on these findings, which of the following would you most likely suspect as a cause of the patient's most likely condition?

    a. Fecalith obstruction

    b. *Helicobacter pylori* infection

    c. High-fat diet

    d. Anxiety

14. A male patient presents with a noticeable yellow tint to his skin. In the workup, which of the following lab values would most likely be of priority to be assessed?

    a. Total bilirubin

    b. Prothrombin time

    c. Blood urea and nitrogen

    d. Serum creatinine

15. You are prescribing medication for *Helicobacter pylori* eradication to a 44-year-old female with NSAID-induced peptic ulcer disease. Considering the fact that the patient must still remain on a chronic, daily NSAID regimen, which of the following drugs should you strongly consider including as part of the patient's prophylactic therapy?

    a. Misoprostol *Cytotec*

    b. Amoxicillin

    c. Bismuth subsalicylate

    d. Omeprazole

16. You are ordering tests to confirm a diagnosis of bowel obstruction for a 36-year-old male who presents with complaints of vomiting, inability to pass stool, bloating, and severe abdominal pain around his "belly button." Which of the following indications would provide the earliest suggestion that the patient's condition may be due to colon cancer?

    a. Elevated white blood cell count

    b. Elevated serum bilirubin

    c. Sigmoidoscopy showing inflamed mucosa

    d. Positive guaiac test

17. Which of the following serology markers indicates a previous exposure to hepatitis A?

    a. Anti-HAV

    b. IgM

    c. IgG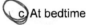

    d. HAV

18. You are prescribing a patient an initial trial of H2 receptor blockers for management of peptic ulcer disease. When should these be ordered?

    a. Every morning

    b. Four times daily with food

    c. At bedtime

    d. Three times each day with meals and once at bedtime

19. You are consulting Amber, a 41-year-old female who has gastroesophageal reflux disease. In discussing her diet, you should advise her to avoid consumption of all of the following food products <u>except</u>:

    a. Caffeine

    b. Spices

    c. Peanut butter

    d. Alcohol

20. You are evaluating a 45-year-old male who presented to your clinic with a low-grade fever, itching, and pain in the right upper area of his abdomen. He mentions during the evaluation that he has noticed his stool is "really pale, like, kind of grey." Based on the patient's signs and symptoms, which of the following lab results is least likely to help in confirming a diagnosis?

    a. Elevated aspartate aminotransferase

    b. Elevated alanine transaminase

    c. Elevated total bilirubin

    d. Elevated white blood cell count

21. Which agent is used specifically for the treatment of peptic ulcer disease and may also see use as an alternative drug for H2 receptor blockers to manage gastroesophageal reflux disease?

    a. Famotidine

    b. Senna

    c. Sucralfate

    d. Omeprazole

22. You notice on your patient's charts that he is dealing with a recurrent case of ulcerative colitis. Given your knowledge of ulcerative colitis, which of the following symptoms would you most expect your patient to report?

    a. Clay-colored stool

    b. Vomiting of blood

    c. Bloody diarrhea

    d. Thin stools

23. As a nurse practitioner, you know that a diagnosis of diverticulitis usually involves a physical exam, imaging studies, and which of the following lab findings?

    a. Elevated total serum bilirubin, elevated erythrocyte sedimentation rate (ESR)

    b. Normal white blood cell (WBC) count, elevated total serum bilirubin

    c. Elevated WBC count, elevated ESR

    d. Elevated total serum bilirubin, normal ESR

24. You are performing a health exam on James, a 54-year-old patient with a long history of alcohol addiction. You notice that his abdomen is swollen and his skin is a slight shade of yellow. When you ask him about his diet, he tells you that he does not normally have an appetite because he usually feels nauseous and his stomach "has been bothering [him] lately." Suspecting hepatitis resulting from his history of alcohol abuse, you know that all of the following options would be usually used in the patient's treatment plan except:

    a. Mesalamine

    b. Vitamin K

    c. Oxazepam

    d. Folic acid

25. You are discussing treatment options for a patient with severe case irritable bowel syndrome. What three medications would you most strongly consider to help manage this condition?

    a. Anticholinergic agents, antidiarrheal agents, and antidepressant agents

    b. Proton pump inhibitors, antidiarrheal agents, and antidepressant agents

    c. Histamine-2 blockers, antidiarrheal agents, and proton pump inhibitors

    d. Proton pump inhibitors, anticholinergic agents, and antidiarrheal agents

26. Which of the following patients has the lowest risk of developing colon cancer?

    a. A female whose aunt and grandmother both developed ovarian cancer

    b. A Hispanic male with a history of peptic ulcer disease

    c. A female with a high-fat diet that includes red meat and refined carbohydrates

    d. A male with a history of recurrent inflammatory bowel disease

27. A 56-year-old patient presents with complaints of nausea, vomiting, and watery diarrhea, all of which have lasted for 4 days. Upon examination, you note hyperactive bowel sounds, abdominal distension, and tachycardia. Based on these findings, which of the following lab tests would best help to diagnose the patient's condition?

    a. Colonoscopy

    b. Urea breath test

    c. Barium study

    d. Stool test

28. Which of the following indications would the nurse practitioner most likely expect to see during a physical exam that would suggest a diagnosis of cholecystitis?

    a. Mild tenderness but no peritoneal findings

    b. Pain upon inspiration while fingers are placed under the right rib cage

    c. Pronounced abdominal distention

    d. Pain with extension of the right thigh

29. Which test is used to differentiate prior exposure to the hepatitis C virus from a current infection?

    a. Enzyme immunoassay

    b. Recombinant immunoblot assay

    c. Polymerase chain reaction

    d. Prothrombin time

30. Which of these statements would most likely suggest that your female patient was predisposed to the hepatitis A virus?

    a. "I recently returned from a trip to Haiti doing hurricane relief work. Had some good oysters over there."

    b. "I am very sexually active with my partner, but I always insist on using condoms."

    c. "I've never had a blood transfusion, but I've recently donated blood while in Haiti."

    d. "I got a tattoo recently. The place was real professional, kept everything neat."

31. Owen, a 45-year-old male, presents to the clinic complaining of watery diarrhea, stomach cramps, and vomiting. He states that he has been under tremendous pressure at work and is so stressed out that he often feels nauseous. Based on these findings for the most likely diagnosis, which of the following indications would you least expect to find during a physical examination?

    a. Abdominal distention

    b. Hyperactive bowel sounds

    c. Fever

    d. Left lower quadrant pain

32. A 52-year-old male presents with complaints of heartburn and a persistent "stomach ache" that has increased in intensity over the past 2 weeks. He points to his upper abdomen to indicate the location of the pain, and he says that he usually "feels better" after he eats. These findings most strongly suggest:

    a. Pancreatitis

    b. Gastric ulcer

    c. Gastroesophageal reflux disease

    d. Duodenal ulcer

33. Casey, a 28-year-old male, is admitted to the emergency room after complaining of a sharp pain in his right side and of a fever. He says that he noticed he woke up feeling nauseous the day prior, and that the pain slowly started around his "belly button" and shifted to his right side slowly throughout the day. What complication is Casey most at risk of developing if the patient's condition were to be left untreated any longer?

    a. Volvulus

    b. Gangrene

    c. Bowel obstruction

    d. Biliary colic

34. Which of these statements is false in regard to ulcerative colitis and Crohn's disease?

    a. Ulcerative colitis and Crohn's disease may occur at any age in both males and females.

    b. Crohn's disease may affect the mouth.

    c. Ulcerative colitis can occur in any part of the gastrointestinal tract.

    d. Ulcerative colitis and Crohn's disease both have unknown etiologies.

35. Which of the following indications of bowel obstruction is properly paired with the source of obstruction?

    a. Minimal abdominal distension; proximal obstruction

    b. Vomiting within hours of pain; proximal obstruction

    c. Vomiting within minutes of pain; distal obstruction

    d. No abdominal distension; distal obstruction

36. What two gastrointestinal disorders are more common in women than in men?

    a. Peptic ulcer disease and diverticulitis

    b. Diverticulitis and irritable bowel syndrome

    c. Gastroesophageal reflux disease and gastroenteritis

    d. Gastroenteritis and irritable bowel syndrome

37. Following a regimen for *Helicobacter pylori* eradication therapy, a patient is continued on for antiulcer therapy to ensure symptomatic relief and promote ulcer healing. Which of the following regimens would be best suited for treating duodenal ulcers as a part of this therapy?

    a. Amoxicillin 1 gram twice a day with meals, omeprazole 20 mg twice a day before meals, and clarithromycin 500 mg twice a day with meals for 7 days

    b. Metronidazole 500 mg twice a day with meals, omeprazole 20 mg twice a day before meals, and clarithromycin 500 mg twice a day with meals for 7 days

    c. Bismuth subsalicylate 2 tabs four times daily, metronidazole 250 mg four times daily, and tetracycline 500 mg four times daily; all taken with food and at bedtime

    d. Omeprazole 40 mg daily or lansoprazole 30 mg daily for 7 weeks

38. You are seeing a 62-year-old female patient for a health assessment. Her medical history shows that she is a longtime smoker, and that she is currently taking NSAIDs for rheumatoid arthritis. Considering her age and history, you would know that these risk factors most likely further increase the risk of developing what condition?

    a. Decreased metabolism of drugs

    b. Gastric ulcers

    c. Colon cancer

    d. Duodenal ulcers

39. Considering a likely diagnosis of peptic ulcer disease, which of the following findings would be most indicative of a bleeding duodenal ulcer?

    a. Hematemesis

    b. Melena

    c. Coffee-ground emesis

    d. Maroon stools

40. You are considering medications to manage a patient's gastroenteritis. Which of the following agents should <u>not</u> be used if the patient's symptoms include bloody stools?

    a. Ciprofloxacin

    b. Loperamide

    c. Doxycycline

    d. Metronidazole

RATIONALES

1. b

When a patient is referred to the emergency room for presenting with indications of diverticulitis, the nurse practitioner knows that an abdominal x-ray is the priority test for an initial diagnostic. An abdominal x-ray is not only the least invasive test to order, but it can provide evidence of free air under the diaphragm, as well as initial indications of inflammation or perforation. A computerized tomography scan is effective in providing indications of an abscess or to detect if a rupture has occurred, but it would not be the initial test to order in an emergency room setting. Neither a barium enema x-ray nor a colonoscopy would be ordered as initial tests because these tests may worsen the condition if a rupture or perforation has occurred.

2. c

Recurrent, severe epigastric pain that is precipitated by large or fatty meals and usually relieved with vomiting most likely indicate cholecystitis. The most effective test to confirm the diagnosis is ultrasound, which is often the initial test for cholecystitis. Plain film radiography may help to show gallstones, but is not as effective as an abdominal ultrasound. Laboratory criteria are not always reliable in the diagnosis of cholecystitis; however, elevated white blood cells and elevated serum bilirubin may suggest common duct obstruction.

3. b

A complaint of nausea accompanied with pain in the lower right quadrant that originated as mild umbilical pain most likely indicates appendicitis. The obturator test assesses for appendicitis by checking for pain while the patient performs an internal rotation of the flexed right thigh. The patient does not present with signs of distal bowel obstruction, which presents with pronounced abdominal distention. Cholecystitis is assessed by checking for Murphy's sign, which is confirmed by the presence of pain upon inspiration while fingers are placed under the patient's right rib cage. Producing right lower quadrant pain by applying pressure to the patient's left lower quadrant also indicates appendicitis (i.e., positive Rovsing's sign), but this test is not used to assess for diverticulitis.

4. c

Hepatitis C is a bloodborne RNA virus that is most commonly associated with intravenous drug use. Hepatitis D is also a bloodborne RNA virus, but is least likely to be acquired via intravenous drug use, as it requires the presence of the hepatitis B virus to take root and reproduce. Hepatitis A is an enteral virus that is most commonly transmitted via the oral-fecal route and, rarely, parentally. Hepatitis B is a bloodborne DNA virus most commonly transmitted through serum, saliva, semen, and vaginal secretions.

5. d

Headaches are more likely to present during the pre-icteric phase of hepatitis C. During the icteric phase, dark urine and clay-colored stool are two common findings of the disorder. Some patients in the icteric phase may also present with a low-grade fever.

6. d

Anti-motility medicine should not be recommended to gastroenteritis patients who presented with fever or bloody stool. Alcohol abuse, tobacco use, antidepressant medications, pre-existing diabetes, and obesity are not known contraindications for anti-motility agents.

7. a

Serologic test results that show the presence of hepatitis B surface antibody (anti-HBs) and the absence of hepatitis B surface antigen (HBsAg) would indicate the patient has recovered from the hepatitis B virus (HBV), has entered into a non-infective stage, and is protected from recurrent infection. The other pairings do not work. The appearance of HBsAg would indicate the patient is experiencing either active or chronic HBV and has yet to enter recovery. Also, although the appearance of hepatitis B core antibodies (anti-HBc) and the disappearance of IgM or IgG may indicate recovery, there are no hepatitis B surface antigen antibodies (anti-HBsAg) or sickle hemoglobin (HBs) markers in serological exams for HBV.

8. b

Irritable bowel syndrome (IBS) currently affects approximately 10%–12% of the general population, with a higher incidence among women. Despite its prevalence, etiology for IBS is unknown but may be associated with a combination of physical and mental issues.

9. a

In children and adults, the hepatitis A vaccine requires two injections, not three, with a booster shot administered at least 6 months after the initial dose. A low- or no-protein diet is often appropriate for patients with hepatitis, as the disease may present with proteinuria. Hepatitis B immune globulin can provide passive immunity to hepatitis B, which is the leading cause of fulminant liver failure.

10. c

A hepatitis B blood panel that shows the hepatitis B surface antigen (HBsAg) is the first definitive evidence of a current hepatitis B viral infection, the results of which would remain positive in asymptomatic carriers and chronic hepatitis B patients. A hepatitis B blood panel would also test for hepatitis B surface antibodies, which would provide evidence of immunity or previous exposure to the virus, and for hepatitis B core antibodies (HBcAb), which also could provide evidence of a past or present infection but is less reliable because HBcAb may provide false-positive results. The hepatitis B e-antigen (HBeAG) is another serologic marker that can provide evidence of an active hepatitis B infection, but HBeAG would not provide initial evidence because HBeAG appears soon after HBsAG becomes detectable.

11. c

Constipation is least likely to be seen in older adults advancing in age because, although constipation may be common in older adults, it is not a normal physiological change that is directly caused by the effects of aging. Normal physiological changes commonly seen in the gerontologic population due to the effects of aging include increased intestinal transit time, decreased liver size, and an impaired defecation signal.

12. c

Pain upon extension of the right thigh is a positive marker for Psoas sign, which is often indicative of appendicitis. The obturator sign and Rovsing's sign are also markers for appendicitis; however, the obturator sign is indicated by pain with internal rotation of the flexed right thigh, and Rovsing's sign is indicated by right lower quadrant pain upon application of pressure to the left lower quadrant. McMurray's sign, an audible click upon rotation of the tibia on the femur, is a sign of injury to meniscal structures, not appendicitis.

13. d

Of the choices, anxiety is the most likely cause of the patient's most likely diagnosis of irritable bowel syndrome (IBS). The patient's symptoms of intermittent abdominal cramping relieved by defecation, heartburn (i.e., dyspepsia), fatigue, and alternating changes in bowel habits are likely indicative of IBS, which can be caused by stress, although the connection between stress and IBS is unknown. Fecalith obstruction is a known cause of acute diverticulitis and appendicitis, but is not a cause of IBS. *Helicobacter pylori* infection should be suspected in patients showing presentations of peptic ulcer disease, which would include gnawing epigastric pain as a hallmark symptom. A high-fat diet, on the other hand, is more likely to be associated with cholecystitis, which typically presents with vomiting and sudden onset of severe, steady pain in the epigastrium or right hypochondrium.

14. a

Total bilirubin values would most likely be initially assessed in patients presenting with skin that is noticeably yellow because elevated total bilirubin is associated with jaundice. Because jaundice is most often associated with viral hepatitis, serum creatinine levels, blood urea and nitrogen (BUN) levels, and prothrombin time would also be assessed. However, prolonged prothrombin time, which would indicate impaired synthetic function of the liver, is not always present in patients with viral hepatitis. Serum creatinine and BUN levels are assessed to find evidence of renal impairment after viral hepatitis is confirmed.

15. a

Prostaglandins, such as misoprostol, should be strongly considered as part of prophylactic therapy when treating patients with NSAID-induced peptic ulcer disease (PUD). Prostaglandins are effective at preventing NSAID-induced ulcers because they protect the stomach lining by stimulating mucous and bicarbonate production. Amoxicillin, bismuth subsalicylate, and omeprazole should all be considered when treating PUD, but these drugs are not effective at reducing the risk of NSAID-induced PUD or protecting the stomach lining from the effects of NSAIDs.

16. d

A positive guaiac test for fecal occult blood would warrant further diagnostic testing for colon cancer in patients presenting with indications of bowel obstruction. This finding may indicate a partial bowel obstruction due to a tumor in the upper intestine in advanced colon cancer cases. Sigmoidoscopy can aid in the diagnosis of colon cancer, but it would not be an initial test to order to confirm bowel obstruction. A complete blood count (CBC) also would be included in the diagnostic for colon cancer, but a CBC would not be ordered to confirm bowel obstruction because an elevated white blood cell count could also suggest cholecystitis. Elevated serum bilirubin is often an indication of problems involving the liver, such as hepatitis.

17. c

A serology test that shows the presence of IgG indicates previous exposure to the hepatitis A virus (HAV). Anti-HAV and IgM indicate antibodies to HAV and would be seen in a serology test during the first couple weeks of illness.

18. c

Patients should be ordered to take H2 receptor blockers (e.g., cimetidine) at bedtime, rather than the morning, for management of peptic ulcer disease (PUD). Misoprostol is a mucosal protective agent that is beneficial in the treatment of PUD, but the patient would be advised to take misoprostol four times daily with food. Combination regimens that pair a proton pump inhibitor with two antibiotics may require administration twice per day before meals. Bismuth regimens paired with antibiotics also may be administered four times per day—once before each meal and once at bedtime.

19. c

Gastroesophageal reflux disease (GERD) is not known to be exacerbated by eating peanut butter. Caffeine, spices, alcohol, and peppermint may increase the symptoms of GERD and should be recommended to be avoided.

20. d

Symptoms that include low-grade fever, pruritus, right upper quadrant pain, and clay-colored stools most likely indicate viral hepatitis. Thus, an elevated white blood cell (WBC) count would be least likely to be expected with this condition, as WBCs are typically normal or slightly lowered with hepatitis. Elevated levels of aspartate aminotransferase or total bilirubin would be expected in patients with viral hepatitis, as well as elevated levels of alanine transaminase.

21. d

Proton pump inhibitors (PPIs) such as omeprazole are mostly used in the treatment of peptic ulcer disease (PUD) but may also see use as an alternative in managing gastroesophageal reflux disease for cases in which H2 receptor blockers (e.g., famotidine) are found to be ineffective. Senna is a laxative, which would more likely see use in treating constipation, and sucralfate is a cytoprotective drug used in the treatment of active duodenal ulcers.

22. c

Bloody diarrhea is a hallmark symptom of ulcerative colitis, which is an idiopathic inflammatory condition characterized by diffuse mucosal inflammation of the colon and involvement of the rectum. Patients in the icteric phase of hepatitis are more likely to report passing clay-colored stool. Vomiting of blood (i.e., hematemesis), on the other hand, is more likely to be reported by a person with peptic ulcer disease. Thin stools may be a sign of colon cancer.

23. c

A diagnosis of diverticulitis involves a physical exam, imaging studies, and lab findings that may show elevated white blood cells and elevated erythrocyte sedimentation rate (ESR). Although findings of an elevated WBC and ESR indicate inflammation, these results are non-specific and not always present in diverticulitis patients. Elevated total serum bilirubin, on the other hand, is not a diagnostic of diverticulitis, as elevated values would be indicative of diseases affecting the liver, such as hepatitis or cholecystitis.

24. a

When developing a treatment plan to manage a patient's hepatitis associated with a long history of alcohol addiction, mesalamine would not be considered, as this drug is an anti-inflammatory agent typically used in the treatment of ulcerative colitis. The primary objective of management in this case should be the cessation of alcohol consumption. Oxazepam would be administered to manage alcohol withdrawal symptoms, and vitamin K would see use in treating coagulopathy. Folic acid is also helpful in treating individuals with alcoholic hepatitis, as these patients tend to be malnourished.

25. a

In severe cases of irritable bowel syndrome (IBS), patients may be prescribed a combination of anticholinergics, antidiarrheals, and antidepressants as warranted, depending on the patient's presentation. Proton pump inhibitors and histamine-2 receptor antagonists are mainly used for managing peptic ulcer disease and, in some cases, gastroesophageal reflux disease.

26. b

Of the choices, a Hispanic male with a history of peptic ulcer disease has the lowest risk of developing colon cancer, as the patient does not possess strong risk factors for the disease. Although colon cancer has an uncertain etiology, risk factors for the condition include a family history of adenocarcinomas, such as ovarian or endometrial cancer, a history of recurrent inflammatory bowel disease, and a diet high in fat or refined carbohydrates.

27. d

A diagnostic for gastroenteritis is indicated in cases involving symptoms that have persisted for more than 72 hours; in this case, the nurse practitioner should order a stool test to determine if an infection is present. A colonoscopy would more likely be indicated for a patient presenting with indications of colon cancer, rather than gastroenteritis. Although gastroenteritis may have a bacterial etiology, a urea breath test would more likely be ordered to test for *Helicobacter pylori* infection in patients presenting with indications of peptic ulcer disease. A barium study is a diagnostic for irritable bowel syndrome, not gastroenteritis.

28. b

Cholecystitis typically presents with Murphy's sign, which is indicated during a physical exam by deep pain upon inspiration while fingers are placed under the right rib cage. Physical exams often show that the right upper quadrant is tender to palpation, and the gallbladder may also be palpable. Patients presenting with mild tenderness but no peritoneal findings should be further examined for bowel obstruction. Pronounced abdominal distention is more indicative of distal bowel obstruction. The psoas sign, which is characterized by pain with extension of the right thigh, is a sign of appendicitis.

29. c

A polymerase chain reaction is used to differentiate prior exposure to the hepatitis C virus from a current infection because the serology marker for both acute and chronic hepatitis C is the same. An enzyme immunoassay detects the presence of hepatitis C antibodies (anti-HCV), but does not necessarily distinguish whether the antibodies are from a previous or current infection. Likewise, a recombinant immunoblot assay detects anti-HCV, which is present in both acute and chronic hepatitis C patients. Prothrombin time does not distinguish prior exposure from a current exposure of hepatitis C.

30. a

Hepatitis A is commonly transmitted through improperly prepared shellfish and contaminated food and water, with the latter more common in hurricane-stricken areas with poor sewage. Hence, a trip to Haiti to perform hurricane relief work and consumption of shellfish are more likely to predispose a patient to the hepatitis A virus. Vaginal intercourse is a common transmission route for hepatitis B, not hepatitis A, but the risk of transmission is lowered because the patient has one steady sex partner and practices safe sex. Blood transfusions and tattooing are potential transmission routes for hepatitis C, but modern standards and screening make contracting the disease through such means a rare occurrence.

31. d

Left lower quadrant pain is more likely a sign of diverticulitis. However, the patient is more likely experiencing gastroenteritis, based on the patient's emotional stress in addition to the presenting signs and symptoms. Hypotension is a common finding of gastroenteritis, and physical examination findings may include abdominal distention, fever, and hyperactive bowel sounds.

32. d

The patient's symptoms of gnawing epigastric aching pain that is relieved after eating most strongly indicate pain produced from duodenal ulcers, which is an indication of peptic ulcer disease (PUD). Gastric ulcers also produce from PUD, but the pain is worsened by eating. Gastroesophageal reflux disease may also be relieved by eating but typically presents with retrosternal burning, not aching pain, as well as belching and a bitter taste in the mouth. Pancreatitis may present with aching epigastric pain; however, this pain is typically not relieved by eating and may present alongside anorexia.

33. b

If left untreated, appendicitis may result in gangrene within 36 hours; thus, a patient who has been experiencing symptoms of appendicitis for more than 24 hours is at risk of developing gangrene. Bowel obstruction, volvulus of the colon, and biliary colic are not typical results of untreated appendicitis.

34. c

Ulcerative colitis is an inflammatory disorder that is not known to produce in any part of the gastrointestinal tract. Rather, ulcerative colitis is typically limited to the large intestine (i.e., the colon) but may also involve the rectum. Crohn's disease, however, can affect any part of the gastrointestinal tract from the mouth to the rectum. Both ulcerative colitis and Crohn's disease are inflammatory disorders that can occur at any age in both males and females, and both are known to have uncertain etiologies.

35. a

Proximal bowel obstruction typically presents with minimal abdominal distention. Vomiting also occurs within minutes of pain, not hours. Distal bowel obstruction usually presents with pronounced abdominal distention and vomiting within hours of pain.

36. b

Diverticulitis and irritable bowel syndrome are more commonly seen in women than in men. Peptic ulcer disease, on the other hand, is slightly more common in men, whereas gastroesophageal reflux disease is not known to be more common in one gender than the other. Some bacterial causes of gastroenteritis, such as *Campylobacter* bacteria, are more common in women, but the condition has equal incidence in men and women.

37. d

For treating duodenal ulcers during antiulcer therapy, which typically occurs following completion of the initial *Helicobacter pylori* therapy regimen, omeprazole 40 mg daily or lansoprazole 30 mg daily for 7 weeks is the recommended regimen to ensure symptomatic relief and ulcer healing. Prescribing amoxicillin with omeprazole and clarithromycin is a popular initial regimen utilizing antibiotics and a proton pump inhibitor for *H. pylori* therapy. Another popular regimen involving antibiotics and a proton pump inhibitor includes metronidazole, omeprazole, and clarithromycin. Bismuth subsalicylate with metronidazole and tetracycline is another combination therapy for *H. pylori* treatment, but is used as initial treatment and is not specifically administered for duodenal ulcers.

38. b

Gastric ulcers are more likely to be seen in older patients with peptic ulcer disease (PUD) who are between 55 and 65 years of age. The 62-year-old patient in this case is at an increased risk of developing NSAID-induced PUD, and her daily smoking habit further increase this risk. Duodenal ulcers are more likely to be seen in younger patients with PUD between 30 and 55 years of age. Decreased metabolism of drugs is an expected finding in gerontology patients because it is a normal effect of aging, not due to the patient's risk factors. Colon cancer, on the other hand, has an unknown etiology, but some gastrointestinal disorders, such as inflammatory bowel disease, are considered to increase the risk of producing the condition.

39. c

Of the various gastrointestinal (GI) bleeds that can occur from peptic ulcer disease (PUD), coffee-ground emesis would most strongly indicate the presence of a bleeding duodenal ulcer. Although melena and hematemesis indicate a GI bleed, hematemesis would most likely indicate bleeding from a gastric ulcer. Melena would signal that the location of the bleed is from a higher source of the lower part of the GI tract. Maroon stools, on the other hand, indicate a bleed lower in the GI tract.

40. b

Antimotility agents, such as loperamide, are contraindicated in patients with bloody stools or fever related to gastroenteritis. Ciprofloxacin and doxycycline, on the other hand, are antibiotics that would be administered in cases involving vibrio cholera infection. Metronidazole would be an antibiotic used to treat a *Clostridium difficile* infection.

DISCUSSION

Peptic Ulcer Disease

Overview

Peptic ulcer disease (PUD) is often caused by an infection with *Helicobacter pylori*.[1] *H. pylori* is present in more than 90% of all duodenal ulcers and more than 75% of all gastric ulcers.[2] Some medications, such as non-steroidal anti-inflammatory drugs (NSAIDs), acetylsalicylic acid (ASA), and glucocorticoids, increase the risk of developing PUD.[1] Smoking also increases the risk of developing ulcers.[3] The role of stress as a cause of these ulcers is uncertain; however, a higher incidence has been reported in individuals with type A personalities.[2] Duodenal ulcers are more common in those aged 30–55, and gastric ulcers are more common in adults aged 55–65.[2]

Presentation

Clinical findings differ for duodenal and gastric peptic ulcers. Both gastric and duodenal ulcers often present with gnawing epigastric pain. For duodenal ulcers, relief of pain usually occurs with eating. For gastric ulcers, on the contrary, eating as a rule, worsens the pain.[4]

Physical exam findings are often unremarkable but may include some mild epigastric tenderness. For patients with PUD, gastrointestinal (GI) bleeding may occur in 20% of all cases, and perforations occur in approximately 5%–10% of all cases.[5] Perforation with peritonitis presents with classic features of the "acute abdomen," including severe epigastric pain, rigidity, quiet bowel sounds, and a "board-like" abdomen.[2]

Workup

Laboratory tests are usually normal, but a complete blood count (CBC) may reveal anemia.[5]

Treatment

Acid-antisecretory agents are used to treat PUD. Two main types of acid-antisecretory agents are histamine-2 receptor antagonists and proton pump inhibitors (PPIs).[5]

Histamine-2 receptor antagonists used for PUD include cimetidine (Tagamet), ranitidine (Zantac), famotidine (Pepcid), and nizatidine (Axid).[2] These agents are initially ordered once a day at bedtime, then twice a day if warranted.[6]

With regard to peptic ulcer disease, a PPI is added to the regimen after twice daily H2-antagonists and should be ordered once a day, 30 minutes before a meal. PPIs include lansoprazole (Prevacid), rabeprazole (Aciphex), pantoprazole (Protonix), omeprazole (Prilosec), dexlansoprazole (Dexilant), and esomeprazole (Nexium).[2] Although more expensive, these drugs have been shown to be more effective than antacids or H2 blockers in treating ulcers.[7] However, health care professionals should be aware of the possible risk of osteoporotic fractures of the hip, wrist, and spine associated with the use of PPIs.[8]

Other mucosal protective agents may be used to treat PUD. These agents should be taken 2 hours apart from other medications.[2] One mucosal protective agent is bismuth subsalicylate (Pepto-Bismol), which frequently has direct antibacterial action against *H. pylori,* promotes prostaglandin production, and stimulates gastric bicarbonate. An unfavorable taste makes this agent less popular.[5] Antacids (e.g., Mylanta, Maalox, etc.) are also mucosal protective agents used to treat PUD, but these agents do not reduce the amount of gastric acidity.[2]

Another mucosal protective agent is misoprostol (Cytotec) which may be prescribed four times daily with food.[2] This agent may also be used as prophylaxis against NSAID-induced ulcers.[5] Misoprostol also works to stimulate mucus and bicarbonate production.[9] PPIs are often prescribed in patients who cannot discontinue NSAIDs.[2]

The two main options for *H. pylori* eradication therapy are triple therapy and quadruple therapy.[5] Triple therapy may consist of a PPI, amoxicillin, and clarithromycin, but metronidazole can be substituted for amoxicillin.[10] Quadruple therapy generally consists of a PPI, bismuth, metronidazole, and tetracycline; however, this regimen is not used as frequently because of the more frequent dosing requirements and unpleasant taste associated with bismuth.[5] Quadruple therapy is also appropriate for individuals who live in areas that have a high prevalence of clarithromycin resistance.[10]

Following a course of treatment with these agents, antiulcer therapy is usually recommended for 3–7 weeks to ensure continued ulcer healing and symptom relief. For duodenal ulcers, patients should continue to take PPIs for 7 additional weeks. H2 blockers may be administered for 6–8 weeks.[2]

Emergency department initial management for PUD includes baseline lab studies such as CBC, prothrombin time (PT), partial thromboplastin time, and basic metabolic panel. A gastrointestinal specialist may choose to perform an endoscopy, among other tests and treatments.[2,5]

Gastroesophageal Reflux Disease (GERD)

Overview

Gastroesophageal reflux disease (GERD) is a disorder in which acidic gastric contents of the stomach undergo back flow (reflux) into the esophagus.[2] The condition is believed to stem from an incompetent lower esophageal sphincter.[11]

Presentation

Findings of GERD may include retrosternal "burning," belching, hiccupping, difficulty swallowing, and excessive salivation. Patients may likewise complain of a bitter taste. GERD often occurs at night or while in the recumbent position and may be relieved by sitting up or ingesting antacids, cool water, or food.[2,11]

Workup

Physical exam findings for GERD are noncontributory in most cases.[2,12] Patients with troublesome findings, such as weight loss, iron deficiency anemia, or odynophagia, may be referred for to a gastrointestinal specialist for an esophagogastroduodenoscopy. Endoscopy should also be considered in all patients with long standing GERD to rule out Barrett's esophagus, a precursor to esophageal cancer.

Treatment

Non-pharmacologic measures are first used to treat mild cases of GERD. These include elevating the head of the bed, smoking cessation, losing weight if overweight, and avoiding alcohol, caffeine, spices, and peppermint.[11]

Although antacids can be used for rapid relief of occasional heartburn, the duration of action is generally short, and the overall amount of gastric acid is not appreciably reduced.[11] H2 blockers are often initially ordered, either in high nightly doses or divided twice daily doses; however, with these drugs, relief can take up to 30 minutes.[12] If twice-daily dosing with H2 blockers is ineffective, PPIs are employed.[11]

Gastroenteritis

Overview

Gastroenteritis is a nonspecific term used to describe a syndrome of acute nausea, vomiting, cramping, and diarrhea resulting from an acute inflammation or irritation of the gastric mucosa.[2] Common causes of gastroenteritis include viruses, bacteria, and parasites, with the most common being viruses.[13]

Presentation

Signs and symptoms of gastroenteritis include nausea, vomiting, watery diarrhea, anorexia, abdominal cramps, and a general "sick" feeling.[2,13] Physical exam findings may include hyperactive bowel sounds, abdominal distention, tachycardia, hypotension, and fever.[13]

Workup

Laboratory tests for gastroenteritis are not typically indicated in the adult patient unless symptoms are severe or persist for more than 72 hours.[13] At that point, diagnostic tests may include collecting a stool sample for culture, WBC count, and ova and parasites. A stool guaiac test may also be conducted to check for occult blood.[2,13]

Treatment

Treatment for gastroenteritis mainly includes supportive care and fluids for rehydration.[13] Antimotility drugs are not ordinarily recommended for adults with mild cases of the disease. Further, bloody stool and fever serve as contraindications for antimotility agents.[2] Antibiotics are only indicated when certain bacteria, such as those belonging to the *Campylobacter*, *Shigella*, and *Vibrio* genera, are the cause of diarrhea.[13] In many cases, traveler's diarrhea is most simply treated with bismuth subsalicylate (Pepto-Bismol).[14]

Hepatitis

Overview

Hepatitis is an inflammation of the liver that leads to dysfunction in the organ.[2] Most forms of hepatitis are caused by a virus, but heavy alcohol consumption, toxins, and certain medications may predispose a patient to the condition.[15]

Presentation

In the prodromal or preicteric phase of hepatitis, patients experience fatigue, anorexia, nausea, vomiting, and headaches. Some individuals may exhibit an aversion to alcohol and cigarette smoke.[2]

The icteric phase of hepatitis is characterized by weight loss, jaundice, pruritus, and right upper quadrant pain. In addition to presenting with GI findings such as clay-colored stools, some patients may note dark urine. Low-grade fever and hepatosplenomegaly may also be present in this phase.[2]

Workup

Patients diagnosed with hepatitis typically present with low to normal WBC count. A urinalysis may reveal increased protein, unconjugated bilirubin, and urinary urobilinogen levels.[16] Abnormal liver function tests often yield elevated aspartate transanimase (AST) and alanine transaminase (ALT) levels in the range of 500–2000 IU/L. Additional tests of the liver may reveal elevated bilirubin, alkaline phosphatase, and serum lactate dehydrogenase levels, as well as increased prothrombin time.[2,17]

Treatment

Management for hepatitis is generally supportive, focusing on rest during the active phase and increased fluid intake of 3,000–4,000 ml per day. Individuals with hepatitis should avoid alcohol and other drugs detoxified by the liver. A low- to no-protein diet is also advised.[2]

Hepatitis A

Overview

Hepatitis A is an enteral virus; the primary route of transmission for the virus is the oral-fecal route, but parenteral transmission may occur in rare circumstances.[2] Common sources of transmission include contaminated water or food such as shellfish. Additionally, hepatitis A may be transmitted by oral sexual activity.[18] Patients are contagious during the 2–6 week incubation period.[19,20] The disease has a very low incidence and mortality rate, and fulminant liver failure is rare.[18]

Presentation

The initial presentation of hepatitis A may be characterized by malaise, myalgia, or easy fatigability.[19] Nausea and vomiting often occur, and a low-grade fever is common.[18] Constant, mild abdominal pain is also typically present.[18,19] After 5–10 days, jaundice occurs.[19] Within 2–3 weeks, symptoms subside.[18]

Workup

Patients with a clinical suspicion of hepatitis A should receive a serology test to confirm the diagnosis.[20] Early in the course of the illness, detectable antibodies to the hepatitis A virus (anti-HAV) appear, such as immunoglobulin M (IgM anti-HAV) and immunoglobulin G (IgG anti-HAV).[19] IgM anti-HAV disappear within 3–6 months, whereas IgG anti-HAV persist for lifelong immunity against HAV.[2]

The presence of IgG anti-HAV without IgM anti-HAV indicates previous exposure to hepatitis A, non-infectivity, and immunity.[19,20]

Hepatitis B

Overview

Hepatitis B is a bloodborne DNA virus found in all body secretions: saliva, serum, semen, and vaginal secretions.[2] Thus, the virus is commonly transmitted via blood, blood products, and sexual activity.[21,22]

Workup

Serology tests are used in diagnosing hepatitis B.[23] The appearance of hepatitis B surface antigen (HBsAg) is the first evidence of a hepatitis B infection.[2,23] Hepatitis B e antigen (HBeAg) is only found in HBsAg-positive sera and indicates viral replication and infectivity. In addition, hepatitis B core antibody (anti-HBc) and IgM appear. When HBeAg disappears, antibodies to HBeAg (anti-HBe) appear, indicating a decrease in viral replication and infectivity.[19,23]

Acute hepatitis B is diagnosed based on the appearance of HBsAg, HBeAg, anti-HBc, and IgM. HBsAg that persists for more than 6 months, coupled with the appearance of anti-HBe, IgM, and

IgG, indicates chronic hepatitis B. Recovery from hepatitis B is heralded by the appearance of anti-HBc and antibodies to HBsAg (anti-HBsAg), both of which persist for life and confer immunity to hepatitis B.[19,23]

Hepatitis C

Overview

Hepatitis C is a blood-borne RNA virus with a typically uncertain source of infection.[2] However, the virus was traditionally associated with blood transfusions and is now most often associated with intravenous drug use.[19,24,25] Several newer agents offer the promise of recovery for hepatitis C in some patients.

Workup

Within days to weeks following exposure, hepatitis C RNA is usually detectable in serum by polymerase chain reaction testing.[26] About two months after exposure, hepatitis C antibodies will appear.[19]

On initial serology for hepatitis C, anti-HCV and HCV RNA are present in both acute and chronic hepatitis C patients.[19] Therefore, polymerase chain reaction testing is used to differentiate prior exposure to HCV from current viremia.[26,27]

Diverticulitis

Overview

Diverticulitis is an inflammation of diverticula that results in formation of an abscess.[12] If a diverticulum perforates, septic shock and death can ensue. This condition is more common in women than men and occurs more often in individuals with diets low in fiber.[2]

Presentation

Signs and symptoms of diverticulitis include mild to moderate abdominal pain characterized by aching in the left lower quadrant, constipation or loose stools, nausea, and vomiting.[12] Physical findings may include low grade fever, left lower quadrant tenderness to palpation, and a palpable mass.[12] Perforation is suggested by peritoneal signs.

Workup

A diagnosis of diverticulitis is supported by findings of leukocytosis, lower abdominal pain, and abdominal tenderness.[28] For patients with mild signs and symptoms, empiric therapy may be initiated without the need for further imaging.[12]

If patients do not improve within 2–4 days of empiric therapy, if not already conducted, an abdominal computed tomography (CT) scan should be conducted to look for evidence of diverticulitis, such as colonic diverticula, bowel wall thickening, and pericolic fat infiltration. CT scans can also be used to exclude other disorders.[12]

Treatment

Uncomplicated cases with diverticulitis can usually be treated with oral antibiotics and a clear liquid diet.[12,29] Bowel rest and a nothing-by-mouth diet may be required to treat severe episodes. Intravenous antibiotics and a clear liquid diet are often used to treat complicated cases, which typically require referral to the GI specialist.[30] Surgery is required in the event of peritonitis, large undrainable abscesses, or clinical deterioration.[2,12] Approximately 20%–30% of all patients diagnosed with diverticulitis will require surgical management.

Irritable Bowel Syndrome

Overview

Irritable bowel syndrome (IBS) is a clinical syndrome distinguished by lower abdominal pain with constipation, diarrhea, or alternating bouts of both.[2] Although IBS has no certain etiology, one theory posits a connection between this condition and anxiety. IBS affects approximately 10% of the population and is about twice as common in women as in men.[31,32]

Presentation

Patients with IBS may report chronic abdominal pain, altered bowel habits, and other GI signs and symptoms.[32] Abdominal pain is usually in the lower abdominal region, but the location can vary widely.[12,32] The pain is normally relieved with defecation.[2,12] Patients may also note gastroesophageal reflux, dysphagia, dyspepsia, nausea, or other GI signs and symptoms.[32]

Workup

Patients whose findings fulfill diagnostic criteria do not often require further diagnostic testing.[12] Patients with diarrhea-predominant IBS may warrant celiac disease screening or a colonoscopy, whereas those with constipation-predominant IBS can benefit from barium studies or a flexible sigmoidoscopy to rule out organic causes.[32]

Treatment

Patients with mild and intermittent symptoms of IBS should begin treatment by first making lifestyle and dietary modifications.[33] Dietary modifications may include exclusion of flatus-producing foods, avoidance of lactose, and incorporation of high-fiber foods into the patient's diet.[33,34] If symptoms are severe or not improved by dietary and lifestyle changes, anticholinergics or antidiarrheals may be prescribed as warranted.[34] IBS symptoms can be exacerbated by psychiatric conditions such as depression and anxiety. Some patients may require counseling, therapy, and antidepressant agents such as selective serotonin reuptake inhibitors.

Cholecystitis

Overview

Cholecystitis is an inflammation of the gallbladder usually associated with gallstones.[2]

Presentation

Symptoms of cholecystitis often occur after a large or fatty meal.[19] About one hour after the meal, steady, severe epigastric pain typically appears.[35] Vomiting often relieves this pain.[2]

Another physical exam finding characteristic of cholecystitis is tenderness to palpation on the right upper quadrant.[2] About 15% of all cases will present with a palpable gallbladder.[19] Patients frequently demonstrate muscle guarding upon physical examination.[35]

Workup

The preferred initial imaging modality in diagnosing cholecystitis is ultrasonography of the abdomen, which can effectively confirm the diagnosis if gallstones are shown.[19] Findings are often suggestive of cholecystitis if gallbladder wall thickening or pericholecystic fluid is shown.[19,35] Gallstones can also be observed on plain film radiography.

Expected lab findings for cholecystitis include an elevated WBC count, as well as elevated AST, ALT, and LDH.[19] Elevated alkaline phosphatase levels may indicate complicating conditions such as cholangitis or choledocholithiasis.[35] Total serum bilirubin values normally lie between 1 and 4 mg/dL.[19] Serum amylase may also be slightly elevated.[19]

Acute cholecystitis may also be indicated by a positive Murphy's sign, which manifests as right upper quadrant pain on inspiration while fingers are placed firmly beneath the right rib cage.[2]

Treatment

Acute cholecystitis is treated in an acute care facility by way of fasting nothing by mouth diet, antibiotics, and pain management.[36] A cholecystectomy may often be required.[37]

Bowel Obstruction

Overview

Bowel obstruction is a blockage of the intestinal lumen that results in decreased passage of bowel contents with increasing colonic pressure.[2] Causes of bowel obstruction include hernias, adhesions, volvulus, fecal impaction, ileus, and tumors.[38]

Presentation

Signs and symptoms of bowel obstruction include nausea, vomiting, cramping abdominal pain, and inability to pass gas or stool.[39] Vomiting within minutes of pain often indicates a proximal obstruction, and vomiting within hours of pain usually indicates a distal obstruction.[2]

Physical exam findings typically consist of manifestations of dehydration, such as tachycardia, orthostatic hypotension, and abdominal distention.[39] Patients with distal obstructions will frequently present with more pronounced abdominal distention, whereas patients with proximal obstructions will present with minimal abdominal distention but marked emesis.[38] Acute mechanical bowel obstruction regularly produces high-pitched "tinkling" sounds; then, as the bowel distends, the sounds become hypoactive.[39]

Workup

Laboratory tests for patients with suspected bowel obstruction include a CBC with differential and electrolytes, including blood urea nitrogen and creatinine.[39] These studies help to determine the presence and severity of hypovolemia, leukocytosis, and metabolic abnormalities.[39] A workup should also include either an abdominal x-ray or CT scan.[40] Air-fluid levels and horizontal dilated loops of bowel typically indicate a small bowel obstruction.[2,39] A frame pattern commonly indicates a large bowel obstruction.[2]

Treatment

Patients with a small bowel obstruction should be seen in the emergency department, where a gastroenterologist will be consulted. Initial management of a small bowel obstruction includes supportive care and fluid therapy, with electrolyte replacement if surgery is indicated.[41] Some patients may require placement of a nasogastric tube.[40,41]

Ulcerative Colitis

Overview

Ulcerative colitis is an idiopathic inflammatory condition that presents with diffuse inflammation of mucosa in the colon.[2] Crohn's disease and ulcerative colitis are both inflammatory ulcerative conditions of the colon; however, unlike Crohn's disease, which most commonly affects the small intestine, ulcerative colitis affects the rectum and extends upward.[42]

Presentation

The hallmark sign of ulcerative colitis is bloody diarrhea.[2] Patients with a mild form of the disease may present with infrequent diarrhea with occasional rectal bleeding and mucus, whereas those with a moderate form of the disease often have more severe diarrhea and frequent bleeding.[12] Patients with severe ulcerative colitis may present with severe anemia, hypovolemia, and impaired nutrition due to having more than six bloody bowel movements per day.[12]

Table 12.1	Assessment of Disease Activity in Ulcerative Colitis		
	Mild	Moderate	Severe
Albumin	Normal	3–3.5 grams/dl	Less than 3.0 grams/dl
Erythrocyte sedimentation rate	Less than 20 mm/hr or normal	20–30 mm/hr	More than 30 mm/hr
Heart rate (beats/minute)	Less than 90	90–100	Higher than 100
Hematocrit	Normal	30–40 mg/dl	Less than 30 mg/dl
Stool, #/day	Fewer than four	Four to six	More than six (bloody)
Temperature	Normal	99 °F to 100 °F	Above 100 °F
Weight loss	None	1% to 10%	Greater than 10%

Used with permission from Johnson LA, Myers CM. Inflammatory Gastrointestinal Disorders. In: Barkley TW Jr, Myers CM, eds. *Practice Considerations for the Adult-Gerontology Acute Care Nurse Practitioner.* West Hollywood, CA: Barkley and Associates; 2015: 361.

Workup (see table 12.1)

Laboratory findings suggestive of ulcerative colitis include low serum albumin levels, decreased hematocrit, and elevated erythrocyte sedimentation rate among other abnormalities that may appear on a BMP.[12,43] A sigmoidoscopy is often used to confirm a diagnosis of ulcerative colitis.

Treatment

Patients with mild to moderate ulcerative colitis are treated with corticosteroids (e.g., hydrocortisone) or aminosalicylates (e.g., mesalamine), usually in the form of suppositories or enemas.[12,44] Severe ulcerative colitis often requires hospitalization and corticosteroid therapy.[12]

Colon Cancer

Overview

The cause of colon cancer is unknown, but risk factors include diets rich in fat or refined carbohydrates, a family history of colon cancer or other adenocarcinomas (e.g., ovarian, endometrial), and inflammatory bowel disease.[45] Patients with such risk factors must be extremely aggressively screened.

Presentation

Adenocarcinomas usually grow slowly and may not present for several years.[45] Changes in bowel habits typically involve thin stools or constipation.[46] Patients may also present with abdominal pain and an abdominal mass.[45]

Workup

Colon cancer is diagnosed through a stool guaiac test, colonoscopy, and CBC.[44,45,47] Once colorectal cancer is confirmed, the patient is referred to an oncologist. A carcinoembryonic antigen (CEA) is measured and used as a prognostic indicator.[45]

Normal CEA levels in non-smokers are 2.5 ng/mL and below, whereas normal levels in smokers are 5 ng/mL and below.[2]

Treatment

Patients with colon cancer are managed by an oncologist, often in concert with a gastroenterologist initially. Treatments for the condition include surgical resection followed by chemotherapy.[48]

Appendicitis

Overview

Appendicitis is an inflammation of the appendix.[2] Appendicitis affects approximately 10% of the population, with the most common presentation among men 18–30 years of age. The condition often results from fecalith, foreign bodies, inflammation, or neoplasms.[49] If the condition goes without treatment, perforation and gangrene may develop within 36 hours.[12]

Presentation

Signs and symptoms of appendicitis frequently begin with vague, colicky umbilical pain.[2] After several hours, pain characteristically shifts to the right lower quadrant. Nausea with one or two episodes of vomiting may occur, but more vomiting often suggests another diagnosis.[12] Pain is typically worsened and localized with coughing.[50]

Guarding in the right lower quadrant with rebound tenderness, psoas sign (i.e., pain with right thigh extension), obturator sign (i.e., pain that presents upon internal rotation of flexed right thigh), positive Rovsing's sign (i.e., right lower quadrant pain that presents upon application of pressure to the left lower quadrant), and low grade fever are common findings of appendicitis.[12,51] High fever typically suggests perforation or a diagnosis other than appendicitis.

Workup

Diagnostics for appendicitis include a WBC count and either a CT scan or ultrasound.[52] WBC levels indicating leukocytosis (10,000–20,000 cells/μL) are common.[12] CT scans are more accurate than ultrasonography, but either imaging study can be used.[12]

Treatment

A patient presenting with appendicitis immediately receives surgical treatment and pain management.[12,49]

References

1. Ratini M. What is peptic ulcer disease? WebMD Web site. http://www.webmd.com/digestive-disorders/digestive-diseases-peptic-ulcer-disease?page=2. Reviewed December 16, 20 14. Accessed April 2, 2015.

2. Barkley TW Jr. Gastrointestinal disorders. In: Barkley TW Jr, ed. *Adult-Gerontology Primary Care Nurse Practitioner*. West Hollywood, CA: Barkley & Associates; 2015: 78–88.

3. Understanding peptic ulcer disease. American Gastroenterological Association Web site. http://www.gastro.org/info_for_patients/2013/6/6/understanding-peptic-ulcer-disease. Accessed April 2, 2015.

4. Healthwise Staff. Types of peptic ulcers. eMedicineHealth Web site. http://www.emedicinehealth.com/types_of_peptic_ulcers-health/article_em.htm. Updated January 4, 2012. Accessed April 2, 2015.

5. Anand BS. Peptic ulcer disease clinical presentation. In: Katz J, ed. *Medscape*. http://emedicine.medscape.com/article/181753-clinical#showall. Updated January 9, 2015. Accessed April 2, 2015.

6. Mayo Clinic Staff. Histamine H2 receptor antagonist (oral route, injection route, intravenous route). Mayo Clinic Web site. http://www.mayoclinic.org/drugs-supplements/histamine-h2-antagonist-oral-route-injection-route-intravenous-route/proper-use/drg-20068584. Updated July 1, 2015. Accessed July 1, 2015.

7. Thompson EG, Simon JB. Proton pump inhibitors (PPIs) for peptic ulcer disease. WebMD Web site. http://www.webmd.com/digestive-disorders/proton-pump-inhibitors-for-peptic-ulcer-disease. Updated November 13, 2015. Accessed April 2, 2015.

8. United States Department of Health and Human Services, Food and Drug Administration. FDA Drug Safety Communication: Possible increased risk of fractures of the hip, wrist, and spine with use of proton pump inhibitors. http://www.fda.gov/Drugs/DrugSafety/PostmarketDrugSafetyInformationforPatientsandProviders/ucm213206.htm. Updated March 28, 2011. Accessed April 2, 2015.

9. Feldman M, Das S. NSAIDs (including aspirin): Primary prevention of gastroduodenal toxicity. In: Basow DS, ed. *UpToDate*. Waltham, MA: UpToDate; 2015. http://www.uptodate.com/contents/nsaids-including-aspirin-primary-prevention-of-gastroduodenal-toxicity. Updated January 8, 2015. Accessed April 2, 2015.

10. Crowe SE. Treatment regimens for Helicobacter pylori. In: Basow DS, ed. *UpToDate*. Waltham, MA: UpToDate; 2015. http://www.uptodate.com/contents/treatment-regimens-for-helicobacter-pylori?source=see_link. Updated September 25, 2014. Accessed April 2, 2015.

11. Kahrilas PJ. Patient information: Acid reflux (gastroesophageal reflux disease) in adults (beyond the basics). In: Basow DS, ed. *UpToDate*. Waltham, MA: UpToDate; 2015. http://www.uptodate.com/contents/acid-reflux-gastroesophageal-reflux-disease-in-adults-beyond-the-basics?source=search_result&search=Patient+information%3A+Acid+reflux+%28gastroesophageal+reflux+disease%29+in+adults+%28Beyond+the+Basics%29&selectedTitle=1~150. Updated November 4, 2013. Accessed April 2, 2015.

12. McQuaid KR. Gastrointestinal disorders. In: Papadakis MA, McPhee SJ, Rabow MW, eds. *CURRENT Medical Diagnosis & Treatment 2014*. 53rd ed. New York, NY: McGraw Hill Professional; 2014: 547–640.

13. Boyce TG. Overview of gastroenteritis. In: Porter RS, Kaplan JL, eds. *The Merck Manual Online*. http://www.merckmanuals.com/home/digestive_disorders/gastroenteritis/overview_of_gastroenteritis.html. Updated December 2014. Accessed April 2, 2015.

14. United States Department of Health and Human Services, Centers for Disease Control and Prevention. Travelers' diarrhea. http://wwwnc.cdc.gov/travel/page/travelers-diarrhea. Updated April 26, 2013. Accessed April 2, 2015.

15. Davis CP. Hepatitis (Viral hepatitis, A, B, C, D, E, G). In: Marks JW, ed. *eMedicineHealth*. http://www.medicinenet.com/viral_hepatitis/article.htm. Updated October 1, 2014. Accessed April 2, 2015.

16. Hepatitis. In: Swearingen PL, ed. *All-in-One Care Planning Resource*. 3rd ed. St. Louis, MO: Elsevier Mosby; 2012: 426–429.

17. Rhee C. Ischemic hepatitis (DDX acute hepatitis). Stanford School of Medicine Web site. http://errolozdalga.com/medicine/pages/ischemichepatitis.cr.5.23.11.html. Updated May 23, 2011. Accessed April 2, 2015.

18. Mayo Clinic Staff. Hepatitis A. Mayo Clinic Web site. http://www.mayoclinic.com/health/hepatitis-a/DS00397. Updated September 9, 2014. Accessed April 2, 2015.

19. Friedman LS. Liver, biliary tract, & pancreas disorders. In: Papadakis MA, McPhee SJ, Rabow MW, eds. *CURRENT Medical Diagnosis & Treatment 2014*. 53rd ed. New York, NY: McGraw Hill Professional; 2014: 641–697.

20. Cheney CP. Overview of hepatitis A virus infection in adults. In: Basow DS, ed. *UpToDate*. http://www.uptodate.com/contents/overview-of-hepatitis-a-virus-infection-in-adults?source=search_result&search=hepatitis+a&selectedTitle=1~150. Updated February 19, 2015. Accessed April 2, 2015.

21. United States Department of Health and Human Services, National Institutes of Health, National Institute of Diabetes and Digestive and Kidney Disease. What I need to know about hepatitis B. http://digestive.niddk.nih.gov/ddiseases/pubs/hepb_ez/. Published December 2012. Accessed April 2, 2015.

22. Mayo Clinic Staff. Hepatitis B. Mayo Clinic Web site. Retrieved from http://www.mayoclinic.org/diseases-conditions/hepatitis-b/basics/symptoms/con-20022210. Updated August 29, 2014.

23. Lok ASF. Diagnosis of hepatitis B virus infection. In: Basow DS, ed. *UpToDate*. Waltham, MA: UpToDate; 2015. http://www.uptodatc.com/contents/diagnosis-of-hepatitis-b-virus-infection?source=search_result&search=hepatitis+b&selectedTitle=1~150. Updated February 5, 2015. Accessed April 2, 2015.

24. United States Department of Health and Human Services, National Institutes of Health, National Institute of Diabetes and Digestive and Kidney Disease. What I need to know about hepatitis C. http://digestive.niddk.nih.gov/ddiseases/pubs/hepc_ez/#symptoms. Published December 2012.

25. Mayo Clinic Staff. Hepatitis C. Mayo Clinic Web site. http://www.mayoclinic.org/diseases-conditions/hepatitis-c/basics/definition/con-20030618. Updated January 15, 2015. Accessed April 2, 2015.

26. Lorenz R, Endres S. Clinical manifestations, diagnosis, and treatment of acute hepatitis C in adults. In: Basow DS, ed. *UpToDate*. Waltham, MA: UpToDate; 2015. http://www.uptodate.com/contents/clinical-manifestations-diagnosis-and-treatment-of-acute-hepatitis-c-in-adults?source=see_link&anchor=H2#H2. Updated July 31, 2014. Accessed April 2, 2015.

27. Terrault NA, Chopra S. Diagnosis and evaluation of chronic hepatitis C virus infection. *UpToDate*. Waltham, MA: UpToDate; 2015. http://www.uptodate.com/contents/diagnosis-and-evaluation-of-chronic-hepatitis-c-virus-infection?source=search_result&search=hepatitis+c&selectedTitle=2~150. Updated March 19, 2015. Accessed April 2, 2015.

28. Pemberton JH, Young-Fadok T. Clinical manifestations and diagnosis of acute diverticulitis in adults. In: Basow DS, ed. *UpToDate*. Waltham, MA: UpToDate; 2015. http://www.uptodate.com/contents/clinical-manifestations-and-diagnosis-of-acute-diverticulitis-in-adults?source=search_result&search=diverticulitis&selectedTitle=3~18#H87395179. Updated April 14, 2014. Accessed April 2, 2015.

29. Young-Fadok T, Pemberton JH. Nonoperative management of acute uncomplicated diverticulitis. In: Basow DS, ed. *UpToDate*. Waltham, MA: UpToDate; 2015. http://www.uptodate.com/contents/nonoperative-management-of-acute-uncomplicated-diverticulitis?source=search_result&search=diverticulitis+treatment&selectedTitle=1~18. Updated July 10, 2014. Accessed April 2, 2015.

30. Young-Fadok T, Pemberton JH. Management of acute complicated diverticulitis. In: Basow DS, ed. *UpToDate*. http://www.uptodate.com/contents/management-of-acute-complicated-diverticulitis?source=search_result&search=diverticulitis+treatment&selectedTitle=2~18. Updated March 3, 2015. Accessed April 2, 2015.

31. Camilleri M. Peripheral mechanisms in irritable bowel syndrome. *N Engl J Med*. 2012; 367: 1626–1635. doi:10.1056/NEJMra1207068

32. Wald A. Clinical manifestations and diagnosis of irritable bowel syndrome in adults. In: Basow DS, ed. *UpToDate*. Waltham, MA: UpToDate; 2015. http://www.uptodate.com/contents/clinical-manifestations-and-diagnosis-of-irritable-bowel-syndrome-in-adults?source=search_result&search=irritable+bowel+syndrome&selectedTitle=2~150. Updated October 24, 2014. Accessed April 2, 2015.

33. Wald A. Treatment of irritable bowel syndrome in adults. In: Basow DS, ed. *UpToDate*. Waltham, MA: UpToDate; 2015. http://www.uptodate.com/contents/treatment-of-irritable-bowel-syndrome-in-adults?source=search_result&search=irritable+bowel+syndrome&selectedTitle=1~150#H2. Updated October 2, 2014. Accessed April 2, 2015.

34. Mayo Clinic Staff. Irritable bowel syndrome. Mayo Clinic Web site. http://www.mayoclinic.com/health/irritable-bowel-syndrome/DS00106/DSECTION=treatments-and-drugs. Updated July 31, 2014. Accessed April 2, 2015.

35. Zakko SF, Afdhal NH. Acute cholecystitis: Pathogenesis, clinical features, and diagnosis. In: Basow DS, ed. *UpToDate*. Waltham, MA: UpToDate; 2015. http://www.uptodate.com/contents/acute-cholecystitis-pathogenesis-clinical-features-and-diagnosis?source=search_result&search=cholecystitis&selectedTitle=1~150. Updated November 19, 2013. Accessed April 2, 2015.

36. Acute cholecystitis. MedlinePlus Web site. http://www.nlm.nih.gov/medlineplus/ency/article/000264.htm. Updated September 20, 2013. Accessed April 2, 2015.

37. Vollmer CM, Zakko SF, Afdhal NH. Treatment of acute calculous cholecystitis. In: Basow DS, ed. *UpToDate*. Waltham, MA: UpToDate; 2015. http://www.uptodate.com/contents/treatment-of-acute-calculous-cholecystitis?source=search_result&search=cholecystitis&selectedTitle=2~150. Updated February 3, 2015. Accessed April 2, 2015.

38. Jackson PG, Manish R. Evaluation and management of intestinal obstruction. *Am Fam Physician*. 2011; 83(2): 159–165. http://www.aafp.org/afp/2011/0115/p159.html. Accessed April 2, 2015.

39. Bordeianou L, Yeh DD. Epidemiology, clinical features, and diagnosis of mechanical small bowel obstruction in adults. In: Basow DS, ed. *UpToDate*. Waltham, MA: UpToDate; 2015. http://www.uptodate.com/contents/epidemiology-clinical-features-and-diagnosis-of-mechanical-small-bowel-obstruction-in-adults?source=search_result&search=bowel+obstruction&selectedTitle=1~150#H413451751. Updated March 4, 2014.

40. Mayo Clinic Staff. Intestinal obstruction. Mayo Clinic Web site. http://www.mayoclinic.org/diseases-conditions/intestinal-obstruction/basics/tests-diagnosis/con-20027567. Updated 18, 2012. Accessed April 2, 2015.

41. Bordeianou L, Yeh DD. Overview of management of mechanical small bowel obstruction in adults. In: Basow DS, ed. *UpToDate*. Waltham, MA: UpToDate; 2015. http://www.uptodate.com/contents/overview-of-management-of-mechanical-small-bowel-obstruction-in-adults?source=search_result&search=bowel+obstruction&selectedTitle=2~150. Updated May 27, 2014. Accessed April 2, 2015.

42. Bernstein CN, Fried M, Krabshuis JH, et al. World Gastroenterology Organization practice guidelines for the diagnosis and management of IBD in 2010. *Inflamm Bowel Dis*. 2010; 16(1): 112–124. doi:10.1002/ibd.21048

43. Peppercorn MA, Kane SV. Clinical manifestations, diagnosis, and prognosis of ulcerative colitis in adults. In: Basow DS, ed. *UpToDate*. http://www.uptodate.com/contents/clinical-manifestations-diagnosis-and-prognosis-of-ulcerative-colitis-in-adults?source=search_result&search=ulcerative+colitis&selectedTitle=1~150#H1844649662. Updated April 22, 2014. Accessed April 2, 2015.

44. MacDermott RP. Management of mild to moderate ulcerative colitis. In: Basow DS, ed. *UpToDate*. Waltham, MA: UpToDate; 2015. http://www.uptodate.com/contents/management-of-mild-to-moderate-ulcerative-colitis?source=search_result&search=ulcerative+colitis&selectedTitle=3~150#H432583317. Updated July 22, 2014. Accessed April 2, 2015.

45. Cornett PA, Dea TO. Cancer. In: Papadakis MA, McPhee SJ, eds. *CURRENT Medical Diagnosis & Treatment 2014*. 53rd ed. New York, NY: McGraw Hill Professional; 2014: 1539–1607.

46. Katoh H, Yamashita K, Wang G, Sato T, Nakamura T, Watanabe M. Prognostic significance of preoperative bowel obstruction in stage III colorectal cancer. *Ann Surg Oncol*. 2011; 18(9): 2432–2441. http://www.ncbi.nlm.nih.gov/pubmed/21369738. Accessed April 2, 2014.

47. United States Department of Health and Human Services, National Institutes of Health, National Cancer Institute. Tests to detect colorectal cancer and polyps. http://www.cancer.gov/cancertopics/factsheet/Detection/colorectal-screening. Reviewed November 12, 2014. Accessed April 2, 2015.

48. Rodriguez-Bigas MA, Grothey A. Overview of the management of primary colon cancer. In: Basow DS, ed. *UpToDate*. Waltham, MA: UpToDate; 2015. http://www.uptodate.com/contents/overview-of-the-management-of-primary-colon-cancer?source=search_result&search=Overview+of+the+management+of+primary+colon+cancer&selectedTitle=1~150. Updated January 19, 2015. Accessed April 2, 2015.

49. Ben-David K, Sarosi GA Jr. Appendicitis. In: Feldman M, Friedman LS, Brandt LJ, eds. *Sleisenger and Fordtran's Gastrointestinal and Liver Disease*. 9th ed. Philadelphia, PA: Saunders Elsevier; 2010: 2059–2072.

50. Appendicitis. MedlinePlus Web site. http://www.nlm.nih.gov/medlineplus/ency/article/000256.htm. Updated July 18, 2013. Accessed April 2, 2015.

51. Martin RF. Acute appendicitis in adults: Clinical manifestations and differential diagnosis. In: Basow DS, ed. *UpToDate*. Waltham, MA: UpToDate; 2015. http://www.uptodate.com/contents/acute-appendicitis-in-adults-clinical-manifestations-and-differential-diagnosis?source=search_result&search=appendicitis&selectedTitle=2~150. Updated July 9, 2014. Accessed April 2, 2015.

52. Krajewski S, Brown J, Phang PT, Raval M, Brown CJ. Impact of computed tomography of the abdomen on clinical outcomes in patients with acute right lower quadrant pain: A meta-analysis. *Can J Surg*. 2011; 54(1): 43–53. http://www.ncbi.nlm.nih.gov/pubmed/21251432. Accessed April 2, 2015.

Chapter 13
Respiratory Disorders

QUESTIONS

1. Lauren, a 29-year-old female, presents to the clinic with a sudden onset of productive cough that is accompanied by wheezing and a high-grade fever. During the physical exam, you find no evidence of lung consolidation, as the lungs are clear to auscultation and resonant to percussion. Given the most probable condition, which of the following pathogens would be the least likely cause?

   a. *Streptococcus pneumoniae*

   b. *Neisseria gonorrhoeae*

   c. *Mycoplasma pneumoniae*

   d. *Haemophilus influenzae*

2. Your patient has severe restrictive lung disease. The nurse practitioner would expect that all of the following pulmonary function test results should be significantly lower than normal except:

   a. Functional residual capacity

   b. Forced vital capacity

   c. Forced expiratory volume in one second

   d. Residual volume

3. A patient comes to you with the complaint that he cannot stop coughing. He has trouble speaking in sentences but manages to describe a tight feeling in his chest. A physical exam indicates his pulse is 115 bpm. The patient explains that he used his albuterol and inhaled budesonide today but is still having symptoms. Of the following, which would be the most appropriate treatment option?

   a. Add oral prednisone.

   b. Add an inhaled ipratropium bromide.

   c. Increase the dosage of albuterol.

   d. Add a regular dose of salmeterol.

4. An examination and series of lab panels for an elderly patient with pneumonia is most likely to show which finding?

   a. Low white blood cell count

   b. Increased hematocrit

   c. Decreased fremitus

   d. Rigid chest wall

5. Of the following choices, the practitioner recognizes which two as the most common pathogens responsible for sinusitis in the adult?

   a. *Haemophilus influenzae* and *Streptococcus pneumoniae*

   b. *Esherichia coli* and *Haemophilus influenzae*

   c. *Klebsiella pneumoniae* and *Moraxella catarrhalis*

   d. *Streptococcus pneumoniae* and *Staphylococcus aureus*

6. Which of the following is <u>not</u> an expected type of pleural effusion?

   a. Hyperemic

   b. Transudate

   c. Empyema

   d. Exudate

7. A thin patient with a slight build presents with constant difficulty breathing and clear mucus. A physical exam also indicates an increased chest anteroposterior diameter and hyperresonance on percussion. Given the most likely diagnosis, which class of medications is best suited for long-term treatment?

   a. Antibiotics

   b. Anticholinergics

   c. Antileukotrienes

   d. Short-acting beta-2 adrenergic agonists

8. Which of these manifestations is <u>least</u> likely to present with the onset of asthma?

   a. Plugging of airways by thick mucus

   b. Hypertrophy of the mucus glands

   c. Thinning of the epithelial basement membrane

   d. Hypertrophy of smooth muscle

9. Your patient was seen by a pulmonologist 2 months ago and diagnosed with asthma. The pulmonologist ordered a short acting beta-2 agonist for initial symptom relief. However, on today's visit to your office, the patient states, "I don't think this stuff is really working because I'm still short of breath." You refer the patient back to the pulmonologist. Which of the following would you anticipate to be the next step in the patient's management following the latest national guidelines?

   a. An antileukotriene

   b. A long-acting beta-2 adrenergic agonist

   c. A metered anticholinergic

   d. An inhaled corticosteroid

10. Jackie, a 25-year-old female, comes to the clinic experiencing respiratory distress and difficulty speaking. Her lungs are hyperresonant and show hyperinflation on the x-ray. Which result would most strongly indicate that Jackie should be admitted to a hospital?

    a. Forced expiratory volume is below 30%

    b. Respiratory rate is 25 breaths per minute

    c. Pulsus paradoxus of 8 mmHg

    d. Pulse is 112 bpm

11. Which of these is <u>not</u> a common indoor trigger for asthma?

    a. Cockroaches

    b. Dust mites

    c. Exercise

    d. Termites

12. Wilfred, a 45-year-old male, is diagnosed with tuberculosis. You order a common drug regimen for treating the infectious disease. You may suspect drug resistance if Wilfred's symptoms persist for approximately how long after initiating treatment?

    a. One month

    b. Three months

    c. Six months

    d. Nine months

13. Upon examination, you notice that Alex, an obese 63-year-old male, has moderate dyspnea and purulent sputum. His lungs are normal upon percussion. Laboratory results reveal an increased hematocrit level. Given the most likely diagnosis, which of the following drugs would you be <u>least</u> likely to prescribe for the patient's condition?

    a. Ipratropium bromide

    b. Albuterol

    c. Budesonide

    d. Montelukast

14. Nancy, a 62-year-old female, presents to the clinic with a dry cough and complaints of fatigue, weight loss, and night sweats. Upon looking at her medical history, you note that she has diabetes. You order a series of labs to confirm the most likely diagnosis. Which finding would provide the most definitive diagnosis for tuberculosis?

    a. Acid-fast bacilli on a sputum smear

    b. Positive purified protein derivative

    c. Homogenous infiltrates in the upper lobes on an x-ray

    d. Positive culture for tubercle bacilli

15. A patient presents with sudden onset of wheezing, coughing, and headache, but no fever. A physical exam reveals lungs with clear auscultation that are resonant to percussion. Given these findings, you conclude the patient has bronchitis. With these particular findings in mind, which of the following drugs would be least suited for treating the patient's condition?

    a. Ibuprofen

    b. Guaifenesin/dextromethorphan

    c. Albuterol

    d. Doxycycline

16. Which of the following medications is considered to be the mainstay of treatment for chronic obstructive pulmonary disease?

    a. Budesonide

    b. Ipratropium bromide

    c. Salmeterol

    d. Triamcinolone

17. A 52-year-old female patient comes to your practice with complaints of breathlessness and a cough accompanied by excessive phlegm. She produces a sputum sample, which appears clear upon inspection. You order a pulmonary function test; in reviewing the results, you find evidence indicating both an increased functional residual capacity and an increased total lung capacity. Which of the following respiratory diseases would be the most likely diagnosis?

    a. Acute bronchitis

    b. Emphysema

    c. Tuberculosis

    d. Pneumonia

18. A patient with tuberculosis is being treated with a regimen of isoniazid, rifampin, pyrazinamide, and ethambutol. The patient's condition is improving significantly and there is evidence indicating that the isolate being treated is fully susceptible to the current regimen. At this time, which change would be recommended to incorporate into the patient's regimen?

    a. Rifampin may be dropped.

    b. Isoniazid may be dropped.

    c. Pyrazinamide may be dropped.

    d. Ethambutol may be dropped.

19. Victor, a stocky 40-year-old male, presents to the clinic with complaints of difficulty breathing and "endless amounts of gunk whenever [he] cough[s]." During the visit, he coughs up a substantial amount of yellow phlegm. A blood test reveals an increased hematocrit level, and a physical examination detects lungs that are normal upon percussion. You order a pulmonary lab for the patient. Given the most likely condition, which of the following findings would you least expect?

    a. Increased forced expiratory volume in 1 second

    b. Increased total lung capacity

    c. Increased functional residual capacity

    d. Increased residual volume

20. An HIV-positive patient develops a low grade fever. During his visit, he complains of fatigue, a reduced desire to eat, and a dry cough. He coughs in front of you, producing sputum that is tinged red. You order a chest x-ray, which reveals a small homogeneous infiltrate in the upper lobes. Given the most likely condition, what combination of drugs would be most effective for treatment?

    a. Isoniazid, ipratropium bromide, pyrazinamide, ethambutol

    b. Isoniazid, rifampin, pyrazinamide, theophylline

    c. Isoniazid, rifampin, ethambutol, pyrazinamide

    d. Isoniazid, rifampin, albuterol, ethambutol

21. Which of the following findings would be least indicative of chronic obstructive pulmonary disease?

    a. Hyperinflated lungs

    b. Elevated diaphragm

    c. Reduced FEV_1

    d. Increased residual volume

22. A patient who has been using inhaled corticosteroids to manage his asthma has started to experience symptom breakthrough. Which of these steps should you take next?

    a. Add a short-acting beta-2 adrenergic agonist

    b. Increase the dose of the inhaled corticosteroid

    c. Add an inhaled anticholinergic

    d. Start an antileukotriene

23. A thin, 70-year-old patient with a wasted appearance comes to the clinic complaining of difficulty breathing and a cough. She states that she had to stop taking her senior water aerobics class because she couldn't make it through the 30 minutes without tiring out. Which of these characteristics would lead you to believe she has emphysema and not chronic bronchitis?

    a. Thin and wasted habitus

    b. Cough

    c. Exercise intolerance

    d. Dyspnea

24. In cases of asthma, the trachea and bronchi typically become more:

    a. Thickened

    b. Narrowed

    c. Responsive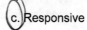

    d. Hyperemic

25. Winston, a 42-year-old male, is an HIV-positive patient whose tuberculosis (TB) skin test returns with an elevation of 5 mm. After confirming a diagnosis of TB, you prescribe a traditional drug regimen. For what minimum period of time is Winston expected to continue his regimen?

    a. Seven months

    b. Eight months

    c. Nine months

    d. Ten months

26. A patient presents to you with a productive cough and headache. The patient displays no other signs or symptoms and is afebrile. Upon physical examination, you note that his lungs are clear upon auscultation and resonant upon percussion. You suspect acute bronchitis; as the indications are far from definitive, however, you wish to rule out other conditions. Which of the following diagnostics would be least helpful in confirming or excluding probable conditions at this time?

    a. Sputum culture

    b. Chest x-ray

    c. Sputum sensitivity

    d. Pulmonary function test

27. Jordan, a 45-year-old male, comes to the clinic with a dry cough, weight loss, night sweats and fatigue. A chest x-ray reveals small, homogenous infiltrates in the upper lobe of the right lung. Given the most likely condition, which of the following tests are you most interested in ordering to confirm the most likely diagnosis?

    a. Complete blood count

    b. Acid-fast bacilli smear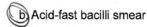

    c. Liver function

    d. Serum creatinine

28. A 29-year-old dental assistant returns to your practice to have her annual purified protein derivative test read. The nurse in your office documents an 8 mm induration that is reddened. Which of the following is your best plan of action?

    a. Order an acid-fast bacilli test.

    b. Send the patient for a chest x-ray.

    c. Order a complete blood count.

    d. Have her return for testing in 1 year.

29. Samuel, a 45-year-old male, presents to the clinic with a cough, headache, sore throat, and soreness in the chest. You take his temperature, which reveals that he has a fever, and notice that his shirt is drenched from sweating excessively. A chest x-ray reveals the presence of infiltrates. Given the most likely diagnosis, which of these would not be associated with an atypical pathogen that may have caused his condition?

    a. *Chlamydophila*

    b. *Streptococcus*

    c. *Legionella*

    d. *Mycoplasma*

30. Iris, a 32-year-old patient, presents with fever, shaking chills, and malaise. A physical examination reveals lung consolidation, purulent sputum, and an increased fremitus. Further diagnostic evaluation shows a low white blood cell count and infiltrates on the chest x-ray. Given the most likely diagnosis, which medication would be best suited for treating Iris's condition?

    a. Doxycycline

    b. Gemifloxacin

    c. Griseofulvin

    d. Moxifloxacin

31. All of the following would be consistent with a typical manifestation of severe asthma except:

    a. Respiratory rate of 35 bpm

    b. Pulse of 125 bpm

    c. Pulsus paradoxus of 15 mmHg

    d. White blood cell count of 1,800 eosinophils/mcl

32. Ethel, a 90-year-old female, presents to the clinic with fever, headache, excessive sweating, and soreness in the throat and chest. Results from a complete blood count reveal a low white blood cell count, and a chest x-ray shows infiltrates. Based on the most likely diagnosis, which antibiotic should Ethel be treated with?

    a. Doxycycline

    b. Azithromycin

    c. Clarithromycin

    d. Levofloxacin

33. In interpreting pulmonary function test results, which set of results below would most be expected in your patient who has idiopathic pulmonary fibrosis?

Patient	FVC[a]	FEV$_1$[a]	FEV$_1$[b]	TLC[a]	RV[a]
A	97	96	99	102	99
B	60	60	100	60	60
C	80	45	57	300	180
D	82	26	59	200	168

[a]percent predicted; [b]as a percent of the FVC

    a. Patient A

    b. Patient B

    c. Patient C

    d. Patient D

34. Zeke, a 37-year-old male, presents to the clinic with a cough, lack of hunger, weight loss, and a low-grade fever that is accompanied by night sweats. He states that his cough is not accompanied by phlegm. You order a regimen of antibiotics to treat his condition, which includes 15 mg/kg of ethambutol. With this medication as part of the regimen, Zeke should be tested for which of the following conditions?

    a. Drug resistance and diabetes

    b. Visual acuity and red-green color perception

    c. Red-green color perception and drug resistance

    d. Diabetes and visual acuity

35. An otherwise healthy 45-year-old patient with atypical pneumonia would best be treated with which medication?

a. Macrolide

b. Antileukotriene

c. Short-acting beta-2 adrenergic agonist

d. Fluoroquinolone

36. With regard to obstructive versus restrictive ventilatory defects, the practitioner knows that which of these is not a restrictive disorder?

a. Tuberculosis

b. Bronchiectasis

c. Heart failure

d. Kyphoscoliosis

37. Julia, a 19-year-old female, comes to the clinic with a cough, headache, sore throat, and excessive sweating. After ordering some diagnostic measures, you find an elevated white blood cell count and infiltrates in the lungs. Which condition is Julia most likely experiencing?

a. Typical pneumonia

b. Chronic bronchitis

c. Atypical pneumonia

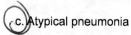

d. Acute bronchitis

38. Percy, a 38-year-old male, comes to your practice with fever, cough, headache, sore throat, and excessive sweating. After ordering a series of labs and diagnostics, you find that he has an elevated white blood cell count and chest infiltrates. Given the many ways the microorganism responsible for the most likely condition might gain access to the host, which route for infection is least likely?

a. Aspiration

b. Inhalation

c. Exogenous penetration

d. Hematogenous dissemination

39. The practitioner recognizes that all of these are expected pulmonary findings in the geriatric patient except:

a. Total lung capacity decreases

b. Residual volume increases

c. Vital capacity decreases

d. The number of mucus-producing cells increases.

40. Kyle, a 32-year-old male, is HIV-positive. When initiating a TB skin test, which result would show the minimal amount of elevation that would indicate he is positive for TB?

a. Approximately 5 mm

b. Approximately 10 mm

c. Approximately 15 mm

d. Approximately 20 mm

RATIONALES

1. b

A high-grade fever that is accompanied by a productive cough and wheezing usually indicates acute bronchitis with a bacterial etiology; *Neisseria gonorrhoeae* is more often a cause of pharyngitis than a cause of acute bronchitis. Common bacterial causes of acute bronchitis include *Mycoplasma pneumoniae*, *Streptococcus pneumoniae*, *Haemophilus influenzae*, and *Moraxella catarrhalis*.

2. c

Reduced forced expiratory volume in one second would be a measure of obstructive disease, not restrictive disease. Obstructive lung diseases reduce airflow rates while leaving volumes significantly unchanged, whereas restrictive disease reduces volumes but provides minor alterations to airflow rates.

3. d

The patient's symptoms of coughing, trouble speaking full sentences, chest tightness, and elevated pulse are most indicative of an acute asthma attack, which the patient already treats with a short-acting beta-2 adrenergic agonist (SABA) and an inhaled corticosteroid (ICS); if symptoms persist, treatment protocols may include increasing corticosteroid dosage, adding a long-acting beta-2 adrenergic agonist (LABA), such as salmeterol, or adding theophylline or antimediators. Adding oral corticosteroids, such as prednisone, would not be recommended at this stage, as oral corticosteroids are typically prescribed after treatment with ICS and LABA has failed to control symptoms. Adding ipratropium bromide or other anticholinergic agents would typically not be beneficial because these medications see more use in chronic bronchitis than asthma. Additionally, increasing the dosage of the SABA would not be recommended because overuse of the drug could reduce its future effectiveness.

4. a

Although pneumonia typically presents with an elevated white blood cell (WBC) count, a low WBC count may be expected in elderly or immunocompromised patients due to natural decreased immune function. Increased hematocrit is more often associated with pulmonary conditions such as chronic bronchitis and is not a specific finding in elderly or immunocompromised patients with pneumonia. Increased fremitus, rather than decreased fremitus, is common in patients with pneumonia. Although the development of a rigid chest wall commonly occurs during aging, it is not a specific result of developing pneumonia.

5. a

Haemophilus influenzae and *Streptococcus pneumoniae* are the two pathogens most commonly responsible for bacterial sinusitis in adults. *Moraxella catarrhalis* and *Klebsiella pneumoniae* are common pathogens in community-acquired and nosocomial bacterial sinusitis, respectively, but not as common as *H. influenzae* and *S. pneumoniae*. *Staphylococcus aureus* may likewise produce sinusitis, but is not a common pathogen. Finally, *Escherichia coli* is more likely to cause pneumonia than sinusitis.

6. a

Of the choices, hyperemic is not a type of pleural effusion. Hyperemia is an increase of blood flow to tissues in the body. Types of pleural effusions include transudates, exudates, empyema, and hemorrhagic pleural effusions.

7. b

Progressive and constant dyspnea, mild sputum, and an increased chest anteroposterior diameter are most indicative of emphysema; as such, core symptoms of the condition are best managed in the long term through inhaled anticholinergics, such as ipratropium bromide. Antibiotic treatment is usually aimed at preventing complications resulting from emphysema and does not treat the condition itself. Short-acting beta-2 adrenergic agonists may also be used to treat emphysema, but ipratropium bromide is often preferred due to greater efficacy and minimal cardiac stimulation effects. Antileukotrienes are not typically considered in management of emphysema.

8. c

Asthma produces as a result of increased responsiveness of the trachea and bronchi to stimuli, often leading to the thickening, not thinning, of the epithelial basement membrane. Other physical changes likely to produce from asthma include plugging of the airways by thick mucus and hypertrophy of both the mucus gland and smooth muscle.

9. d

By national guidelines for asthma management, a low-dose inhaled corticosteroid (ICS) is usually the first step for increased management after a short-acting beta-2 agonist (SABA) shows insufficient results in controlling symptoms. While an antileukotriene, such as montelukast, may serve as alternative treatment at this step, a low-dose ICS is considered to be the standard medication. Long-acting beta-2 agonists typically see use if treatment with a low-dose ICS fails to manage symptoms, whereas metered anticholinergics are usually paired with a SABA for short-term symptom relief, not long-term symptom control.

10. a

Hospitalization for asthma is typically recommended when the forced expiratory volume in one second (FEV1) is 30% below the predicted value. A respiratory rate of 25 breaths per minute is higher than the average breaths per minute for an adult, but does not indicate a need for hospitalization. Pulsus paradoxus of 8 mmHg and pulse of 112 bpm are not necessarily indicative of severe manifestations of asthma and would not indicate the need for hospitalization.

11. d

Although termites may trigger asthma, they are not commonly considered to be an indoor trigger for the condition. Dust mites, pets, cockroaches, indoor molds, exercise and cigarette smoke are all common indoor causes of asthma.

12. b

If symptoms of tuberculosis (TB) are still present or cultures for the disease are still positive after 3 months of therapy, drug resistance is typically indicated. A tuberculosis patient should have 6 weeks of weekly sputum smears after the initiation of therapy. After this time frame has passed and a negative culture has been confirmed, the sputum smear regimen may be reduced to once a month. Six months is the standard length of treatment for TB, with treatment for HIV-positive TB patients typically lasting 9 months.

13. d

A patient with dyspnea, purulent sputum, obesity, and an increased hematocrit level most likely has chronic bronchitis, which would not require the administration of montelukast. Mainstays of chronic bronchitis treatment include anticholinergics such as ipratropium bromide, as well as beta-2 adrenergic agonists, such as albuterol. Budesonide and other corticosteroids may likewise see use in improving lung function. Leukotriene receptor antagonists, such as montelukast, are not commonly used to treat chronic bronchitis, and would more likely see use in the management of asthma.

14. d

The patient's signs and symptoms of a dry cough, fatigue, weight loss, and night sweats most likely indicate tuberculosis (TB); the most definitive diagnosis for this condition is achieved by isolating *Mycobacterium tuberculosis* in a culture. The other tests may be used to rule out other conditions but do not provide a definitive diagnosis because of limited efficacy. Although acid-fast bacilli smears are rapid and cost-effective, the concentration needed to detect the bacteria does not always provide an accurate assessment. Infiltrates are not always present on x-rays of patients with TB, and this method does not effectively rule out other conditions that may cause scarring in the pulmonary lobes. The purified protein derivative test can help to determine whether a patient has been exposed to TB, but it is not commonly used to provide a definitive diagnosis as to whether or not a patient is actually infected.

15. d

Although the patient's findings of headache, wheezing, cough, and lungs with clear auscultation that are resonant to percussion all commonly present in acute bronchitis, the lack of fever most likely indicates a viral etiology rather than a bacterial one; as such, doxycycline, a macrolide antibiotic, would not be recommended for treatment. Treatment of acute bronchitis, regardless of etiology, often focuses on pain management and control of cough and wheezing. As such, ibuprofen, guaifenesin/dextromethorphan, and albuterol would likely be recommended for treatment.

16. b

Chronic obstructive pulmonary disease (COPD) is often best treated with anticholinergic agents, such as ipratropium bromide. Beta-agonists, such as salmeterol, and inhaled corticosteroids, such as budesonide and triamcinolone, may also see use in treatment of COPD, but anticholinergics often show better results in producing bronchodilation.

17. b

Emphysema is the most likely diagnosis, as it typically presents past the age of 50 and is characterized by productive cough, clear sputum, and breathlessness, as well as an increase in both functional residual capacity (FRC) and total lung capacity (TLC). Acute bronchitis may present with bronchospasm and bronchial hyperreactivity, but does not present with changes to FRC or TLC. Furthermore, tuberculosis does not result in an increased FRC or TLC; rather, decreased respiratory capacity often presents in patients with advanced tuberculosis. Pneumonia may produce a decrease, rather than increase, in FRC and TLC.

18. d

If a patient with tuberculosis shows susceptibility of the isolate while on a treatment regimen of isoniazid, rifampin, pyrazinamide, and ethambutol, then ethambutol may be dropped. Pyrazinamide should be continued for at least 2 more months, and isoniazid and rifampin should be continued as daily or intermittent therapy for 4 or more months.

19. a

The patient most likely has chronic bronchitis, which is indicated by excessive purulent sputum, mild to moderate dyspnea, a stocky body habitus, lungs that are normal on percussion, and an increased hematocrit level; chronic bronchitis commonly results in a decreased, rather than increased, forced expiratory volume in 1 second. Patients with chronic bronchitis also typically exhibit increases in total lung capacity, functional residual capacity, and residual volume alike.

20. c

Isoniazid, rifampin, ethambutol, and pyrazinamide make up the recommended combination of medications to treat tuberculosis, which may present with low-grade fever, anorexia, fatigue, and a dry cough that progresses to producing blood-tinged sputum. The diagnosis of tuberculosis would be confirmed by a chest x-ray, which shows the presence of a small homogeneous infiltrate in the upper lobes. Ipratropium bromide is an anticholinergic usually implemented in the treatment of chronic bronchitis, emphysema, or other respiratory conditions, but is not included in the typical regimen to treat tuberculosis. Theophylline is a methylxanthine, and albuterol is a beta-2 adrenergic agonist. Both medications are often used to treat asthma and other respiratory conditions, rather than tuberculosis.

21. b

A chest x-ray for a patient with chronic obstructive pulmonary disease (COPD), often broken up into the diagnoses of chronic bronchitis and emphysema, would commonly show a flattened, not elevated, diaphragm. Hyperinflation can also be detected on a chest x-ray and is a common finding for both chronic bronchitis and emphysema. In addition, increased residual volume and reduced FEV1 are diagnostic findings indicative of COPD.

22. a

A short-acting beta-2 adrenergic agonist, such as albuterol, may be added to an asthma patient's regimen for control of breakthrough symptoms. Although the dosage of inhaled corticosteroids may be increased to aid in management, this is meant to assist in daily maintenance, not in controlling breakthrough symptoms. Inhaled anticholinergics and antileukotrienes may likewise aid in daily maintenance.

23. a

Patients with emphysema often present with a thin and wasted body habitus, not a normal body habitus. On the other hand, a patient with chronic bronchitis would typically present with a stocky and obese body habitus. Both chronic bronchitis and emphysema typically present with dyspnea, cough, and exercise intolerance.

24. c

Asthma commonly results in the increased responsiveness of the trachea and bronchi to stimuli. Thickening of the epithelial basement membrane and mucosal edema and hyperemia typically result in narrowing of the respiratory airways.

25. c

HIV-positive patients who test positive for tuberculosis are expected to be treated for 9 months. In patients who are not immunocompromised and who test positive for tuberculosis, the regimen may be tapered before 9 months, with 6 months standing as the traditional cut-off point.

26. d

Pulmonary function testing measures the airflow and volume of air in the patient's lungs and is commonly used to diagnose such disorders as asthma, bronchitis, and emphysema; it does not, however, aid in differentiating acute bronchitis from other respiratory diseases. Sputum culture and sensitivity are usually performed to identify bacterial causes, as well as rule out other conditions that may present with similar symptoms. Additionally, chest x-rays may be normal in patients with acute bronchitis; however, they are useful in ruling out pneumonia and chronic bronchitis as differential diagnoses.

27. b

The patient most likely has tuberculosis (TB), as indicated by a dry cough, weight loss, night sweats, anorexia, and fatigue; as such, an acid-fast bacilli smear is most likely to be used as the baseline diagnostic, as it is quick and most useful in patients with pulmonary manifestations of TB. Complete blood count, liver function tests, and serum creatinine levels should be evaluated when beginning treatment, not when diagnosing TB.

28. d

A purified protein derivative (PPD) test is considered indicative for tuberculosis (TB) in health workers if it presents with an induration of 10 mm, not 8 mm; as such, the patient is not expected to undergo any management measures beyond an annual repeat of the test. As a positive PPD test indicates TB exposure but does not confirm infection, a chest x-ray may be ordered to confirm the condition; if the x-ray presents with negative results, it may be repeated 6 months later. An acid-fast bacilli test would likewise indicate exposure but not confirm infection, whereas a complete blood count is typically ordered after TB infection has been confirmed to evaluate potential side effects from isoniazid treatment.

29. b

The *Streptococcus* genus, specifically *Streptococcus pneumoniae*, is the most common cause of typical pneumonia, rather than atypical pneumonia, which is indicated by cough, headache, sore throat, soreness in the chest, excessive sweating, fever, and the presentation of infiltrates on a chest x-ray. Atypical pathogens for pneumonia include *Legionella pneumophila*, *Mycoplasma pneumoniae*, and *Chlamydophila pneumoniae*.

30. a

Doxycycline and other macrolides would be best suited for treatment of typical pneumonia, indicated by fever, chills, malaise, purulent sputum, and increased fremitus. A low white blood cell count and infiltrates on a chest x-ray would confirm this diagnosis. Fluoroquinolones, such as gemifloxacin and moxifloxacin, may also be used to treat pneumonia, but are typically used in patients who are over 60 years of age or who have existing health problems, such as diabetes or heart failure. Griseofulvin, an antifungal, would see more use in tinea infections.

31. c

A pulsus paradoxus of 15 mmHg does not strongly indicate severe asthma; rather, it would more strongly indicate moderate asthma, which typically presents with pulsus paradoxus of 10–20 mmHg. A respiratory rate that exceeds 28 bpm is a sign of asthma in older children. Furthermore, the patient's pulse of 125 bpm is consistent with the elevated pulse that typically occurs in severe cases of asthma. A white blood cell count that detects more than 1,500 eosinophils/mcl may also indicate severe asthma.

32. d

Elderly patients with atypical pneumonia, as indicated by fever, headache, excessive sweating, soreness in the throat and chest, low white blood cell count, and infiltrates on the chest x-ray, should be treated with fluoroquinolones, such as levofloxacin. Patients younger than 60 years old with no comorbidities and no recent antibiotic use should be treated with doxycycline or a macrolide, such as azithromycin or clarithromycin.

33. b

A patient presenting with forced vital capacity (FVC) and forced expiratory volume in 1 second (FEV1) below the normal ranges of 80%–120%, as well as total lung capacity (TLC) and residual volume (RV) below the normal ranges of 75%–120%, would most likely have a restrictive ventilatory disease such as idiopathic pulmonary fibrosis. A patient with values within the 75%–120% range is considered normal, whereas a patient who demonstrates reduced FEV1 but increased TLC and RV would likely have an obstructive ventilatory disease.

34. b

Patients taking ethambutol to treat tuberculosis (TB), as indicated by a dry cough, anorexia, weight loss, and a fever, should be tested for visual acuity and red-green color perception. Drug resistance is likely indicated if symptoms persist after 3 months of treatment; however, it does not need to be tested for when specifically initiating ethambutol. Diabetes may increase the risk of TB, but prescribing ethambutol does not normally indicate the need for testing for diabetes.

35. a

In patients under the age of 60 who are otherwise healthy, atypical pneumonia is best treated with macrolides, such as azithromycin. A fluoroquinolone, such as levofloxacin or gemifloxacin, would typically be used to treat a patient with pneumonia who is elderly, immunocompromised, or experiencing comorbidities. Short-acting beta-2 adrenergic agonists and antileukotrienes are medications that are often useful in treating asthma, but provide little benefit in treating pneumonia.

36. b

Bronchiectasis is an obstructive, not restrictive, respiratory disorder, as it affects exhalation through enlargement of parts of the airway and lungs. Tuberculosis, heart failure, and kyphoscoliosis are all restrictive disorders, as they prevent the full expansion of the lungs and thus affect inhalation.

37. c

Although typical and atypical pneumonia often both present with an elevated white blood cell (WBC) count and chest infiltrates, atypical pneumonia is more likely to present with a cough, headache, sore throat, and excessive sweating. Typical pneumonia, on the other hand, commonly presents with fever, chills, malaise, and an increased fremitus, among other findings. Although bronchitis may present with cough, headache, and sore throat, lung infiltrates would typically present only if pneumonia or influenza was the underlying cause. Furthermore, elevated hematocrit, not elevated WBCs, would be more likely to present in a patient with chronic bronchitis.

38. c

In order for a patient to contract atypical pneumonia, as indicated by fever, cough, headache, sore throat, and excessive sweating, the pathogen must invade the host; although the pathogen may invade via exogenous penetration, entering the lung directly after trauma or surgery, this is not a common route of invasion. More commonly, pathogens gain access to the host and cause inflammation of the lower respiratory tract via aspiration, inhalation, or hematogenous dissemination.

39. a

A geriatric patient is likely to experience an unchanged, not decreased, total lung capacity (TLC). Patients in the geriatric population commonly experience an increase in residual volume alongside a decrease in vital capacity, meaning that TLC typically remains constant. Geriatric patients are also likely to experience an increase in the number of mucus-producing cells.

40. a

In an HIV-positive patient, a skin test for tuberculosis (TB) would be considered positive if it is presented with an elevation of 5 mm. An elevation of 10 mm primarily indicates positive results in immigrants from high prevalence areas, those in high risk groups, or health care workers. A positive skin test is 15 mm for all others not in high prevalence groups. A skin test for TB is not expected to yield a result of 20 mm.

DISCUSSION

Pulmonary Function Tests (PFTs)

Overview

Pulmonary function tests (PFTs) assess how well the lungs take in and release air. PFTs also measure how well the lungs transfer gases such as oxygen from the atmosphere into a person's circulatory system.[1]

The types of PFTs and what these tests specifically measure are explained in table 13.1.[2,3]

Table 13.1	Pulmonary Function Tests (PFTs)
PFT	**Measurements**
FVC	Volume of gas forcefully expelled from lungs after maximal inspiration
FEV1	Volume of gas expelled in the first second of the FVC maneuver
FEV 25–75	Maximal mid-expiratory airflow rate
PEFR	Maximal airflow rate achieved in FVC maneuver
TLC	Volume of gas in lungs after maximal inspiration
FRC	Functional residual capacity
RV	Volume of gas remaining in lungs after maximal expiration

Adapted from Barkley TW Jr. Diagnosis and management of pulmonary disorders. In: Barkley TW Jr, ed. *Adult-Gerontology Acute Care Nurse Practitioner: Certification Review/Clinical Update Continuing Education Course*. West Hollywood, CA: Barkley & Associates; 2015: 136–142.

Acute Bronchitis

Overview

Acute bronchitis is characterized by acute inflammation of the upper airways that presents with persistent cough and sputum.[4] Mucous membranes typically become edematous and hyperemic while the condition manifests. Acute bronchitis may be either viral or bacterial in nature. Viral causes include the following: rhinovirus, coronavirus, and adenovirus. Bacterial causes include the following: *Mycoplasma pneumoniae, Streptococcus pneumoniae, Haemophilus influenzae,* and *Moraxella catarrhalis.*[4,5] The incidence of acute bronchitis is higher in smokers and is most common in patients younger than 50 years of age.[4]

Presentation

Acute bronchitis often presents with cough, wheezing, and complaints of headache. The cough may be productive, with sputum that is clear, yellow, green, or tinged with small amounts of blood. Other findings of acute bronchitis include sore throat, muscle aches, and runny or stuffy nose.[6]

Workup

A physical exam should be conducted to identify any evidence of lung consolidation. Clear auscultation strongly indicates no lung consolidation; moreover, the thorax will be resonant to percussion, and upper airway rhonchi are typically clear with coughing. If viral acute bronchitis is present, the patient either has no fever or has a low-grade temperature. If bacterial acute bronchitis is present, the patient will likely have a more pronounced temperature.[7,8,9]

Usually, no laboratory or additional diagnostic tests are needed; however, if the diagnosis is unclear, the nurse practitioner (NP) should order a chest X-ray (CXR).[7,8,9]

Treatment

Acute bronchitis is managed with supportive treatment, including humidifiers, an increased fluid intake, cough suppressants, analgesics for chest soreness or fever, and B2 adrenergic agonists, such as albuterol (Proventil), for wheezing.[10]

Antibiotics are indicated only for bacterial infections. The following antibiotics may commonly be used to treat bacterial acute bronchitis: macrolides, doxycycline, and trimethoprim-sulfamethoxazole.[11]

Asthma

Overview (see table 13.2)

Asthma occurs when the trachea and bronchi are hyperresponsive to stimuli. This response triggers acute inflammation and production of thick, viscid mucus, leading to airway constriction. The airways may likewise be narrowed by smooth muscle enlargement and remodeled through thickening of the epithelial basement membrane. Mucosal edema, hyperemia, and hypertrophy of the mucus glands may also occur.[12]

Asthma may be triggered by any or all of the following agents: dust mites, pets, cockroaches, indoor molds, exercise, or cigarette smoke.[13]

Presentation

Asthma patients may present with a variety of signs and symptoms, such as respiratory distress at rest, difficulty speaking in sentences, diaphoresis, and use of accessory muscles. Patients may also exhibit tachypnea or tachycardia. Asthma sufferers may experience pulsus paradoxus of more than 12 mmHg, hyperresonance, cough, and chest tightness.[14] Ominous signs of asthma include fatigue, absent breath sounds, paradoxical chest or abdominal movement, inability to maintain recumbency, and cyanosis.[14]

Workup

In patients with asthma, a complete blood count (CBC) may show a slight white blood cell (WBC) elevation with eosinophilia. PFTs reveal abnormalities typical of obstructive dysfunction. Hospitalization may be recommended if forced expiratory volume in 1 second (FEV1) is less than 30% predicted value or does not increase to at least 40% predicted value after 1 hour of vigorous therapy. Hospitalization may also be recommended if peak flow is less than 60 L per minute initially or does not improve to 50% predicted value after 1 hour of treatment.[15]

A bronchodilator may also be administered prior to conducting a spirometry; if used, a patient with asthma will most likely see a 15% improvement in forced vital capacity (FVC) or FEV1, as well as a 25% improvement in forced expiratory flow at 25%–75%. Initially upon treatment, respiratory alkalosis is expected as the primary acid/base imbalance. A CXR may show hyperinflation; however, it is often unnecessary unless the NP is attempting to rule out other conditions.[15]

Treatment

For asthma symptom relief or alleviation of exercise-induced reactions, a patient may use a short-acting B2 adrenergic agonist, such as albuterol (Proventil). For daily maintenance, a patient may be prescribed inhaled corticosteroids, such as budesonide (Pulmicort) and triamcinolone (Azmacort). Side effects of corticosteroids, such as candidal infection of the oropharynx, dry mouth, and sore throat, may be experienced.[16,17]

Asthma patients may also use short-acting B2 adrenergic agonists for symptom breakthrough.[18] If symptoms persist, the NP may increase the inhaled corticosteroids dose; add a long-acting B2 adrenergic agonist such as salmeterol (Serevent); or include the use of theophylline, antimediators, or inhaled anticholinergics such as ipratropium bromide (Atrovent). Antileukotrienes such as montelukast (Singulair) may be ordered to manage chronic asthma.[7,16]

Table 13.2 Assessing Asthma Control in Those ≥ 12 Years of Age

Components of Control		Well Controlled	Not Well Controlled	Very Poorly Controlled
Impairment	Symptoms	≤ 2 days/week	> 2 days/week	Throughout the day
	Nighttime awakenings	≤ 2x/month	1–3x/week	≥ 4x/week
	Interference with normal activity	None	Some limitation	Extremely limited
	SABA use for symptom control (not prevention of EIB)	≤ 2 days/week	> 2 days/week	Several times per day
	FEV_1 or peak flow	> 80% predicted/personal best	60%–80% predicted/personal best	< 60% predicted/personal best
	ATAQ	0	1–2	3–4
	ACQ	≤ 0.75[a]	≥ 1.5	n/a
	ACT	≥ 20	16–19	≤ 15
Risk	Exacerbations requiring oral corticosteroids	0–1/year	≥ 2/year[b]	
		Consider severity and interval since last exacerbation		
	Progressive loss of lung function	Evaluation requires long-term followup care		
	Treatment-related adverse effects	Medication side effects can vary in intensity from none to very troublesome and worrisome. The level of intensity does not correlate to specific levels of control but should be considered in the overall assessment of risk.		
Recommended Action for Treatment		Maintain current steps and regular follow-ups every 1–6 months to maintain control. Consider stepping down if well controlled for at least 3 months.	Step up 1 step and reevaluate in 2–6 weeks. For side effects consider alternative treatment options.	Consider short course of oral systemic corticosteroids. Step up 1–2 steps and reevaluate in 2 weeks. For side effects, consider alternative treatment options.

Note. SABA = short-acting beta$_2$ agonist; ACT = asthma control test; EIB = exercised-induced bronchospasm; FEV_1 = forced expiratory volume in 1 second; ATAQ = asthma therapy assessment questionnaire; ACQ = asthma control questionnaire. [a]ACQ values of 0.76–1.4 are indeterminate regarding well-controlled asthma. [b]The level of control is based on the most severe impairment or risk category. Assess impairment domain by patient's recall of previous 2–4 weeks and by spirometry/or peak flow measures. Symptom assessment for longer periods should reflect a global assessment, such as inquiring whether the patient's asthma is better or worse since the last visit. At present, there are inadequate data to correspond frequencies of exacerbations with different levels of asthma control. In general, more frequent and intense exacerbations (e.g., requiring urgent, unscheduled care, hospitalization, or ICU admission) indicate poorer disease control. For treatment purposes, patients who had ≥ 2 exacerbations requiring oral systemic corticosteroids in the past year may be considered the same as patients who have not-well-controlled asthma, even in the absence of impairment levels consistent with not-well-controlled asthma. Adapted from "Expert Panel Report 3: Guidelines for the Diagnosis and Management of Asthma" by the National Heart, Lung, and Blood Institute, 2007.

Chronic Obstructive Pulmonary Disease (COPD)

Overview

Chronic obstructive pulmonary disease (COPD) affects approximately 5% of the population and contributes to the third leading cause of death in the United States.[19,20] COPD is characterized by airflow obstruction and symptoms of chronic bronchitis and emphysema.[19,20] Chronic bronchitis is defined as excessive secretion of bronchial mucus and productive cough for three months or more in at least two consecutive years. Emphysema is defined as the abnormal, permanent enlargement of the alveoli.[7]

Presentation

The three cardinal symptoms of COPD are dyspnea, chronic cough, and sputum production.[19] Wheezing and chest tightness are less common findings.[19] Patients frequently present with characteristics of both chronic bronchitis and emphysema. Signs and symptoms of chronic bronchitis often present after age 35.[7] Patients have a frequent cough with purulent sputum production.[1,7] Patients may complain of mild to moderate dyspnea.[20] An examination may reveal use of accessory respiratory muscles and coarse rhonchi. Individuals with chronic bronchitis are likely to be obese.[20]

In contrast to chronic bronchitis, emphysema patients are likely to be very thin with a barrel chest.[20] Signs and symptoms of emphysema often manifest after age 50.[7] Patients with emphysema have little or no cough or expectoration. Like chronic bronchitis, emphysema patients may use accessory respiratory muscles. An examination may reveal a hyperresonant chest and distant heart sounds.[20] The disease is also marked by wheezing and severe dyspnea.[20,21]

Workup

Patients with suspected COPD are evaluated with PFTs. Spirometry should be performed pre- and post-bronchodilator administration to determine whether airflow limitation is reversible. Airflow limitation is indicated if the post-bronchodilator FEV1/FVC is reduced.[19]

If reduced FVC is detected in the post-bronchodilator spirometry, lung volume should be measured by a body plethysmography. Increased total lung capacity (TLC), functional residual capacity (FRC), and residual volume indicate hyperinflation. Increased FRC and normal TLC indicate air trapping without hyperinflation.[19]

A CXR is ordered to exclude alternative diagnoses. A low, flattened diaphragm is a common finding in COPD patients.[19]

Treatment

Inhaled anticholinergic agents (e.g., ipratropium bromide) and beta agonists are the mainstay of COPD therapy. These drugs help to diminish the number of acute exacerbations, slow the rate of decline in quality of life, and reduce the rate of decline in FEV1. Bronchodilators may be ordered to reduce dyspnea. Patients with emphysema are prescribed oral corticosteroids and antibiotics, if needed. Oral corticosteroids should not be used for long-term therapy, however.[21]

Non-pharmacological management should begin with smoking cessation. Additional management techniques include pulmonary rehabilitation, improved nutrition, and breathing techniques. Chest physical therapy includes deep breathing and postural drainage.[21]

Pneumonia

Overview

Pneumonia presents as inflammation stemming from microorganisms gaining access to the lower respiratory tract via aspiration, inhalation, or hematogenous dissemination.[22,23] Pneumonia accounts for approximately 10% of all admissions to medical services.[7]

The most common etiological agent of community-acquired pneumonia in adults is *S. pneumoniae*. Atypical pneumonia, however, may be caused by atypical pathogens such as *Legionella pneumophila*, *M. pneumoniae*, and *Chlamydophila pneumoniae*.[24]

Presentation

Typical pneumonia presents with fever, shaking chills, purulent sputum, malaise, and increased fremitus. A physical exam will often detect the presence of lung consolidation.[25] Atypical pneumonia usually manifests with cough, headache, sore throat, excessive sweating, fever, and soreness in the chest.[26]

Workup

A CBC is conducted to check for an elevated WBC count. In elderly patients or the immunocompromised, the WBC count may be lower. A CXR should be ordered to look for infiltrates. A Gram stain and a culture is the standard follow-up diagnostic. Blood cultures may also be ordered as needed.[27]

Treatment

According to the Infectious Diseases Society of America/American Thoracic Society, patients younger than 60 years of age with no comorbidities and no recent antibiotic use should be treated with doxycycline or a macrolide, such as azithromycin (Zithromax), clarithromycin (Biaxin), or erythromycin.[28] Older patients and patients with comorbidities—such as COPD, heart failure, or cancer—should be treated with fluoroquinolones, such as levofloxacin (Levaquin), gemifloxacin mesylate (Factive), or moxifloxacin (Avelox).[28]

Tuberculosis

Overview

Tuberculosis (TB) is a systemic disease caused by *Mycobacterium tuberculosis*. The most common site of TB is the lungs. Other sites of involvement include the lymphatic system, the genitourinary system, the bones, the meninges, the peritoneum, and the heart. Patients who are at increased risk include those residing in crowded living conditions, the institutionalized, and the immunosuppressed.[29,30]

Presentation

The majority of TB patients are asymptomatic. Some may experience the following: fatigue, anorexia, dry cough progressing to a productive cough, blood-tinged sputum, weight loss, low-grade fever, night sweats, and pleuritic chest pain.[31]

Workup

The most definitive diagnosis for TB involves taking at least three sputum cultures of *M. tuberculosis*. Acid-fast bacilli (AFB) smears can provide presumptive evidence of active TB. A CXR may likewise reveal if small homogeneous infiltrates are present in the upper lobes. A purified protein derivative (PPD) skin test may reveal exposure to TB; however, this test does not diagnose active disease.

Patients with TB must follow a medication regimen. However, before a patient begins this regimen, the doctor must conduct a baseline evaluation. Tests include liver function studies, CBC, and serum creatinine. Patients who are prescribed ethambutol should be assessed for visual acuity and red-green color perception, in addition to drug resistance.[32]

Treatment

A PPD test has different standards for positive results based on the patient's background and circumstances. A skin test result of 5 mm or greater is considered positive for HIV-infected persons, contacts of an individual with a known case of TB, or persons with a chest film typical for TB. A skin test result of 10 mm or greater is considered positive for immigrants from high prevalence areas, individuals in high-risk groups, or health care workers. In all other patients, a skin test result of 15 mm or greater is considered positive. In all patients with a positive PPD test, the patient should be given regular doses of isoniazid for 6 months.[33] If a PPD shows that a patient has been exposed to TB, a CXR is ordered. Patients with a positive PPD but a negative CXR

should receive 6 months of chemoprophylaxis with isoniazid.[34,35]

Patients with a positive PPD and a positive CXR should be prescribed the following regimen: isoniazid, 300 mg PO daily; rifampin, 600 mg PO each day; ethambutol, 15–25 mg/kg PO each day, and pyrazinamide, 15–30 mg/kg in three divided doses daily. If the patient proves fully susceptible to isoniazid and rifampin, then ethambutol may be discontinued. Isoniazid, rifampin, ethambutol, and pyrazinamide should be continued every day for 2 months, followed by a 4-month regimen of isoniazid and rifampin taken daily.[33] If the patient is HIV-positive or otherwise immunocompromised, the course of treatment should follow the same schedule, but run for 9 months total.

TB patients must be monitored during treatment. Patients with pulmonary TB should have sputum smears every week, in addition to cultures for the first 6 weeks after the initiation of therapy. Cultures should be continued every month until it is documented that the disease is no longer present. After 3 months, if cultures are still positive, the patient is likely to be resistant to the drugs used during treatment.[36]

Because TB is highly contagious, the local health department must be alerted of any cases. Patients who are diagnosed with TB must reduce exposure to susceptible individuals. However, hospitalization in a negative pressure room is required for those who are not compliant with this request.[37]

References

1. Hegewald MJ, Crapo RO. Pulmonary function testing. In: Mason RJ, Broaddus VC, Martin TR, et al., eds. *Murray and Nadel's Textbook of Respiratory Medicine.* 5th ed. Philadelphia, PA: Elsevier Saunders; 2010: 522–553.

2. Pulmonary function tests. Johns Hopkins University web site. http://www.hopkinsmedicine.org/healthlibrary/test_procedures/pulmonary/pulmonary_function_tests_92,P07759. Accessed April 2, 2015.

3. McCarthy K, Dweik RA. Pulmonary function testing. In: Byrd RP Jr, ed. Medscape. http://emedicine.medscape.com/article/303239-overview#showall. Updated February 18, 2015. Accessed April 2, 2015.

4. Fayyaz J, Olade RB, Lessnau K-D. Bronchitis. In: Mosenifar Z, ed. Medscape. http://emedicine.medscape.com/article/297108-overview#showall. Updated March 28, 2014. Accessed April 2, 2015.

5. Bronchitis – acute. A.D.A.M. Medical Encyclopedia. http://www.nlm.nih.gov/medlineplus/ency/article/001087.htm. Updated April 26, 2014. Accessed April 2, 2015.

6. Fayyaz J, Olade RB, Lessnau K-D. Bronchitis clinical presentation. In: Mosenifar Z, ed. Medscape. http://emedicine.medscape.com/article/297108-clinical. Updated March 28, 2014. Accessed April 2, 2015.

7. Barkley TW Jr. Lower respiratory disorders. In: Barkley TW Jr, ed. *Adult-Gerontology Primary Care Nurse Practitioner: Certification Review/Clinical Update Continuing Education Course.* West Hollywood, CA: Barkley & Associates; 2015: 136–142.

8. Fayyaz J, Olade RB, Lessnau K-D. Bronchitis workup. In: Mosenifar Z, ed. Medscape. http://emedicine.medscape.com/article/297108-workup. Updated March 28, 2014. Accessed April 2, 2015.

9. Tackett KL, Atkins A. Evidence-based acute bronchitis therapy. *J Pharm Pract.* 2012; 25(6): 586–590. doi: 10.1177/0897190012460826

10. Pacheco SM, Cook JL. Upper and lower respiratory tract infections. In: Mahon CR, Lehman DC, Manuselis G, eds. *Textbook of Diagnostic Microbiology.* 5th ed. 765–803). Maryland Heights, MO: Elsevier Saunders; 2015: 765–803.

11. Cropp AJ, Bigdeli G. Bronchitis, acute. In: Domino FJ, Baldor RA, Golding J, Grimes JA, eds. *The 5-Minute Clinical Consult 2014.* 22nd ed. Philadelphia, PA: Wolters Kluwer Health/Lippincott Williams & Wilkins; 2014: 182–183.

12. United States Department of Health and Human Services, National Institutes of Health (NIH), National Heart Lung and Blood Institute (NHLBI). What is asthma? http://www.nhlbi.nih.gov/health/health-topics/topics/asthma. Updated August 4, 2014. Accessed April 2, 2015.

13. United States Department of Health and Human Services, Centers for Disease Control and Prevention. Asthma. http://www.cdc.gov/asthma/faqs.htm, Last updated November 18, 2014. Accessed April 2, 2015.

14. Morris MJ. Asthma clinical presentation. In: Mosenifar Z, ed. Medscape. http://emedicine.medscape.com/article/296301-clinical#showall. Updated September 30, 2014. Accessed April 2, 2015.

15. Morris MJ. Asthma workup. In: Mosenifar Z, ed. Medscape. http://emedicine.medscape.com/article/296301-workup. Updated September 30, 2014. Accessed April 2, 2015.

16. Asthma: Treatment and management. American Academy of Allergy, Asthma, & Immunology web site. http://www.aaaai.org/conditions-and-treatments/asthma.aspx. Accessed April 2, 2015.

17. Godara N, Godara R, Khullar M. Impact of inhalation therapy on oral health. *Lung India.* 2011; 28(4), 272–275. doi: 10.4103/0970-2113.85689

18. Family medicine. In: Klostranec JM, Kolin DL, eds. *Essential Med Notes 2012: Comprehensive Medical Practice & Review for USMLE II & MCCQE I.* Toronto, ON: Toronto Notes; 2012: FM1–FM54.

19. Rennard SI. Chronic obstructive pulmonary disease: Definition, clinical manifestations, diagnosis, and staging. In: Basow DS, ed. *UpToDate.* Waltham, MA; 2015. http://www.uptodate.com/contents/chronic-obstructive-pulmonary-disease-definition-clinical-manifestations-diagnosis-and-staging?source=search_result&search=copd&selectedTitle=1~150. Updated May 7, 2015. Accessed June 30, 2015.

20. Mosenifar Z, Kamangar N. Chronic obstructive pulmonary disease. In: Byrd RP Jr, ed. Medscape. http://emedicine.medscape.com/article/297664-overview. Updated September 25, 2014. Accessed June 30, 2015.

21. Brashers VL, Huether SE. Alterations of pulmonary function. In: McCance KL, Huether SE, eds. *Pathophysiology.* 7th ed. St. Louis, MO: Elsevier Mosby; 2014: 1248–1289.

22. Kamangar N, Harrington A. Bacterial pneumonia. In: Byrd RP Jr, ed. Medscape. http://emedicine.medscape.com/article/300157-overview#showall. Updated October 8, 2014. Accessed April 2, 2015.

23. United States Department of Health and Human Services, NIH, NHLBI. What is pneumonia? http://www.nhlbi.nih.gov/health/health-topics/topics/pnu. Updated March 1, 2011. Accessed April 2, 2015.

24. United States Department of Health and Human Services, NIH, NHLBI. What causes pneumonia? http://www.nhlbi.nih.gov/health/health-topics/topics/pnu/causes. Updated March 1, 2011. Accessed April 2, 2015.

25. What are the symptoms of pneumonia? American Lung Association web site. http://www.lung.org/lung-disease/pneumonia/symptoms-diagnosis-and.html. Accessed April 2, 2015.

26. Limper AH. Overview of pneumonia. In: Goldman L, Schafer AI, eds. *Goldman's Cecil Medicine.* 24th ed. Philadelphia, PA: Elsevier Saunders; 2011: 587–595.

27. United States Department of Health and Human Services, NIH, NHLBI. How is pneumonia diagnosed? http://www.nhlbi.nih.gov/health/health-topics/topics/pnu/diagnosis. Updated March 1, 2011. Accessed April 2, 2015.

28. File TM Jr. Treatment of community-acquired pneumonia in adults who require hospitalization. In: Basow DS, ed. *UpToDate.* Waltham, MA: UpToDate; 2015. http://www.uptodate.com/contents/treatment-of-community-acquired-pneumonia-in-adults-who-require-hospitalization. Last updated April 1, 2015. Accessed April 2, 2015.

29. Tuberculosis: Fact sheets. Centers for Disease Control and Prevention web site. http://www.cdc.gov/TB/publications/factsheets/general/tb.htm. Last updated October 28, 2011. Accessed April 2, 2015.

30. Herchline TE, Amorosa JK. Tuberculosis. In: Bronze MS, ed. Medscape. http://emedicine.medscape.com/article/230802-overview#showall. Updated December 15, 2014. Accessed April 2, 2015.

31. Tuberculosis: Symptoms, diagnosis and treatment. American Lung Association web site. http://www.lung.org/lung-disease/tuberculosis/symptoms-diagnosis.html. Accessed April 2, 2015.

32. Herchline TE, Amorosa JK. Tuberculosis treatment & management. In: Bronze MS, ed. Medscape. http://emedicine.medscape.com/article/230802-treatment. Updated December 15, 2014. Accessed April 2, 2015.

33. Solanki RN, Borisagar GB, Sisodia JA. Prevention of tuberculosis. In: Jindal SK, Shankar PS, Raoof S, Gupta D, Aggarwal AN, Agarwal R, eds. *Textbook of Pulmonary and Critical Care Medicine, Vol. 1*. New Delhi, India: Jaypee Brothers Medical Publishers Ltd; 2011: 608–615.

34. Du Preez K, Hesseling AC, Mandalakas AM, Marais BJ, Schaaf HS. Opportunities for chemoprophylaxis in children with culture-confirmed tuberculosis. *Ann Trop Paediatr.* 2011; 31(4): 301–310. doi: 10.1179/1465328111Y.0000000035

35. Herchline TE, Amorosa JK. Tuberculosis workup. In: Bronze MS, ed. Medscape. http://emedicine.medscape.com/article/230802-workup. Updated December 15, 2014. Accessed April 2, 2015.

36. Hopewell PC, Fair EL, Pai M. International standards for tuberculosis care: Integrating tuberculosis care and control. In: Bronzino JD, Peterson DR, ed. *Medical Devices and Human Engineering*. 4th ed. Boca Raton, FL: CRC Press; 2014: 253–267.

37. Curry International Tuberculosis Center. Tuberculosis infection control: A practical manual for preventing TB. http://www.currytbcenter.ucsf.edu/sites/default/files/ic_book_2011.pdf. Published 2011. Accessed April 2, 2015.

Chapter 14

Cardiovascular Disorders

1. Your colleague's patient experiences a sudden onset of pain in her lower leg. The area where the patient identifies the pain is erythematous and warm to the touch but not swollen. The patient also has a consistent temperature. Your colleague suggests elevating the leg and applying warm compresses at night. He also prescribes a non-steroidal anti-inflammatory drug and suggests bed rest for at least a week to help the pain subside. Based on these findings, which of these measures is <u>not</u> a correct form of treatment for the patient's condition?

    a. Elevating the leg

    b. Applying warm compresses

    c. Prescribing non-steroidal anti-inflammatory drugs

    d. Ordering bed rest

2. Which of the following is <u>not</u> a common finding of acute left-sided heart failure?

    a. Coarse rales in all lung fields

    b. Hepatomegaly

    c. Wheezing, frothy cough

    d. An S3 gallop sound

3. With regard to S3 and S4 heart sounds, which statement is true?

    a. An S3 sounds like "Kentucky" and is expected during pregnancy but otherwise, it is not a normal finding in the adult.

    b. An S3 is an atrial gallop and sounds like "Tennessee."

    c. An S4 sounds like "Kentucky" and is expected during pregnancy but otherwise, it is not a normal finding in the adult.

    d. An S4 is a ventricular gallop and sounds like "Tennessee."

4. Which of the following statements is <u>not</u> typical of the heart murmur with which it is associated?

    a. A grade I/VI murmur is barely audible.

    b. A grade II/VI murmur is associated with a thrill.

    c. A grade III/VI murmur can easily be heard.

    d. A grade V/VI murmur can be heard off the chest wall with one corner of the stethoscope.

5. You hear a low-pitched diastolic rumble at the fifth intercostal space with the patient in the left lateral position. The murmur does not radiate. You refer the patient to cardiology to "rule out _____."

    a. Aortic stenosis

    b. Mitral regurgitation

    c. Mitral stenosis

    d. Aortic regurgitation

6. Which type of heart sound is caused by aortic and pulmonic valve closures?

   a. S1

   b. S2

   c. S3

   d. S4

7. Frank, age 56, has just been diagnosed with hypertension. After looking at his medical history, you decide that propranolol would be the most effective form of treatment, as it would treat his hypertension while also managing other conditions. Given the decided treatment, Frank most likely has which of the following co-occurring conditions?

   a. Migraines

   b. Diabetes mellitus

   c. Edema

   d. Chronic kidney disease

8. According to the Eighth Joint National Committee hypertension guidelines, which of the following is not used to estimate 10-year and lifetime atherosclerotic cardiovascular disease risks?

   a. High-density lipid cholesterol

   b. Race

   c. Diastolic blood pressure

   d. Diabetes status

9. Dependent rubor is a physical finding associated with which of these diseases or conditions?

   a. Chronic venous insufficiency

   b. Superficial thrombophlebitis

   c. Deep vein thrombosis

   d. Peripheral vascular disease

10. Sarah, age 24, comes to your practice complaining of sudden pain in her legs and a low-grade temperature. A physical exam reveals her right leg is hot to the touch and erythematous. Sarah has been bed-ridden for the past few weeks due to a minor surgical operation. Her medical history indicates that she is a smoker and uses an intrauterine device for contraception. Given the most likely condition, which of the following is least likely to be considered a risk factor?

   a. The patient is female.

   b. The patient is bed-ridden.

   c. The patient is a smoker.

   d. The patient has an intrauterine device.

11. According to the latest guidelines regarding statin therapy, which of these should you prescribe to specifically reduce low-density lipid cholesterol by approximately 30% to less than 50%?

   a. Atorvastatin, 40 mg

   b. Simvastatin, 10 mg

   c. Rosuvastatin, 20 mg

   d. Pravastatin, 40 mg

12. Which cardiovascular disorder is best defined as impaired venous return due to either destruction of valves, leg trauma, or sustained elevation of venous pressure?

   a. Superficial thrombophlebitis

   b. Chronic venous insufficiency

   c. Peripheral vascular disease

   d. Deep vein thrombosis

13. According to the New York Heart Association Functional Classification system, if a heart failure patient has marked limitations of physical activity but is comfortable at rest, which classification of the disease best applies to the patient?

   a. Class I

   b. Class II

   c. Class III

   d. Class IV

14. A 62-year-old patient has recently been diagnosed with heart failure. With respect to the standard of care, the best treatment regimen for this patient would include non-pharmacologic steps, such as sodium restriction and weight reduction, alongside pharmacologic measures, such as which of these drugs?

a. Prazosin

b. Captopril

c. Candesartan

d. Atenolol

15. Israel, age 55, presents with chest pain that is exacerbated by exercise but relieved by rest within several minutes. The patient expresses the pain he feels by clenching a fist to his chest. The nurse practitioner suspects angina. An electrocardiogram (ECG) returns normal findings. Which of the following is most true?

a. Approximately half of all patients with angina present with normal ECG findings, so an exercise test should be conducted for more definitive results.

b. Normal ECG findings indicate the patient does not have angina, but the patient's serum lipid levels should be evaluated to assess for heart disease.

c. Approximately half of all patients with angina present with normal ECG findings. If the patient also has normal angiogram findings, the nurse practitioner can rule out angina.

d. Normal ECG findings indicate the patient does not have angina and is not having a myocardial infarction.

16. A physical examination of a patient reveals a heart murmur near the second intercostal space (ICS). You suspect the patient may have aortic stenosis and you auscultate again for more details. Which details of the murmur would most likely confirm your diagnosis?

a. Low-pitched, mid-diastolic, builds to crescendo

b. Musical, blowing, radiates to left axilla

c. Blowing, rough, radiates to neck

d. Diastolic, blowing, at second left ICS

17. A patient with a history of heart failure presents to your practice complaining of classic symptoms of his disease. On examination, numerous murmurs are noted throughout the chest. In addition to a 12-lead electrocardiogram, what is the next diagnostic study to order that would be most helpful to identify the severity of the patient's problem?

a. Chest x-ray

b. Angiography

c. Echocardiogram

d. Complete blood count with differential and a urinalysis

18. You are conducting a physical exam on a patient with severe chest pain that occurred while he was at home watching television. He also complains of sudden sweating in a room temperature environment, weakness, difficulty breathing, and nausea. He comments that he had an uneasy feeling of impending doom during the event. When he experiences somewhat similar angina pain, he takes nitroglycerin, but this time, the nitroglycerin did not help with the pain. Based on the likely diagnosis, which of the following would you least expect to find?

a. S4 heart sound

b. Wheezing

c. Shiny, hairless skin

d. Pulmonary crackles

19. Adam, age 65, presents with intense chest pain that has persisted for the last 30 minutes, in addition to what he describes as "fading in and out." His wife elaborates that on the drive here, Adam passed out a couple times. Your examination reveals a low-grade fever, dysrhythmia, and an S4 heart sound. Which of the following cardiovascular conditions would most likely present with these signs and symptoms?

a. Hypertension

b. Angina

c. Heart failure

d. Myocardial infarction

20. Your 68-year-old patient has a blood pressure reading of 145/82 mmHg. As a nurse practitioner, you know that these readings can be caused by certain conditions and tests should be ordered to rule out other causes. Which of the following tests would you be <u>least</u> likely to order at this time?

    a. Renal angiogram

    b. Plasma aldosterone

    c. D-dimer

    d. Morning and evening cortisol levels

21. Susana, age 45, presents to urgent care with severe chest pain, accompanied by cold sweats and nausea. An examination reveals pulmonary crackles. You administer nitroglycerin; however, it proves ineffective. Which of the following lab results would be <u>least</u> consistent with the most likely diagnosis?

    a. Peaked T waves

    b. Elevated ST segment

    c. Leukopenia

    d. Development of Q waves

22. A cardiologist has prescribed a pharmacologic treatment for your 54-year-old Caucasian patient diagnosed with hypertension. When the patient comes back to your practice for a check-up, he says that the medication causes him to cough and sometimes have trouble breathing. Of the following, which medication was he most likely prescribed?

    a. Metolazone

    b. Amlodipine

    c. Lisinopril

    d. Olmesartan

23. ST-segment elevation in leads I and aVL indicates which type of infarction?

    a. Anterior wall

    b. Inferior wall

    c. Anteroseptal wall

    d. Lateral wall

24. Richard, age 55, presents with pain and tenderness in his left ankle while walking, as well as a low-grade temperature. A physical examination finds edema around Richard's ankle. Which of the following conditions should you most suspect?

    a. Superficial venous thrombosis

    b. Deep vein thrombosis

    c. Peripheral vascular disease

    d. Chronic venous insufficiency

25. Which of the following patients' lipid panels has two of the four values as abnormal, warranting attention by the nurse practitioner?

	Total Cholesterol	LDL	Fasting Triglycerides	HDL
a.	210	80	120	62
b.	180	96	160	45
c.	180	112	143	32
d.	190	72	135	25

26. A patient has a negative D-dimer test. Which of the following conditions would this lab result most strongly rule out?

    a. Hypertension

    b. Myocardial infarction

    c. Congestive heart failure

    d. Deep vein thrombosis

27. During a routine physical for Leonard, age 56, you note a diastolic murmur. The murmur presents with a blowing at the second left intercostal space. He most likely has which valvular disease?

    a. Mitral stenosis

    b. Mitral regurgitation

    c. Aortic stenosis

    d. Aortic regurgitation

28. Which of the following patient findings constitute the strongest indication for pharmacologic revascularization?

    a. Chest pain that has lasted for 1 hour, an ST segment elevation of 0.4 mV in the precordial lead, followed by an ST segment depression of 0.2 mV in lead I

    b. Chest pain that has lasted for 2 hours, an ST segment elevation of 0.1 mV in lead III, followed by an ST segment elevation of 0.3 mV in the precordial lead

    c. Chest pain that has lasted for 3 hours, an ST segment elevation of 0.3 mV in the precordial lead, followed by an ST segment elevation of 0.3 mV in lead I

    d. Chest pain that has lasted for 7 hours, an ST segment elevation of 0.6 mV in lead I, followed by an ST segment elevation of 0.2 mV in lead III

29. You are examining Victor, age 67, and identify a heart murmur. This murmur is fairly loud and can be heard with one corner of the stethoscope off the chest wall. You are most likely listening to which of the following murmurs?

    a. Grade II/VI

    b. Grade III/VI

    c. Grade IV/VI

    d. Grade V/VI

30. Which statement is false regarding hypertension?

    a. A classic presentation of hypertension includes a subparietal, "pulsating" headache, usually in the morning, which resolves throughout the day.

    b. Approximately 95% of all cases of hypertension are "primary" in nature.

    c. Hypertension related to contraceptive estrogen therapy would be classified as "secondary."

    d. Hypertension affects approximately 20%–30% of the African American population.

31. Benjamin, age 62, presents with wheezing, a frothy cough, and shortness of breath at rest. The cardiologist's report reveals that his condition derives from the inability of the heart to contract, which results in decreased cardiac output. Which of these is Benjamin most likely experiencing?

    a. Systolic acute

    b. Systolic chronic

    c. Diastolic acute

    d. Diastolic chronic

32. You are examining a chest x-ray of a patient with chronic right-sided heart failure. Which of the following would you least expect to find?

    a. Kerley B lines

    b. Enlarged aorta

    c. Pulmonary edema

    d. Pleural effusions

33. You are performing a fundoscopic exam on George, age 55, who presents with changes that include flame-shaped retinal hemorrhages, superficial white areas with feathered edges, and a swollen optic disc. Which of the following conditions is he most likely experiencing?

    a. Hypertensive urgency

    b. Malignant hypertension

    c. Macular degeneration

    d. Dissecting aortic aneurysm

34. As a nurse practitioner, you know that which two cardiac enzymes are entirely cardioselective and only elevate when myocardial damage is present?

    a. Myoglobin and CK-MB

    b. Troponin I and troponin T

    c. Troponin T and myoglobin

    d. CK-MB and troponin I

35. The practitioner is considering antihypertensive therapy for a patient. Which statement is most accurate?

 a. Angiotensin-converting enzyme (ACE) inhibitors may cause vasodilation, rash, taste disturbances, hyperkalemia, and renal impairment.

 b. Central alpha-2 agonists prevent vasoconstriction, slow the heart rate, and are primarily used as monotherapy agents.

 c. Angiotensin II-receptor blockers should be reserved for patients intolerant to ACE inhibitors and may cause hyperglycemia and hypokalemia.

 d. Calcium channel blockers may be used for angina, arrhythmias, and migraines and are associated with dry mouth, sedation, and nausea.

36. You hear a loud pansystolic murmur that is "blowing" at the apex of the heart. You refer the patient to a cardiology service to rule out which of these?

 a. Mitral regurgitation

 b. Aortic stenosis

 c. Mitral stenosis

 d. Aortic regurgitation

37. Your patient asks, "I really thought I was having a heart attack. How can you tell the difference between angina and having a myocardial infarction?" Which of the following responses would provide the patient the most accurate information?

 a. "Pain of angina can usually be relieved by resting or lying down."

 b. "Pain associated with a heart attack is much more severe."

 c. "Pain associated with a heart attack radiates into the jaw and down the left arm."

 d. "Pain of angina is generally easier to describe than that of a heart attack."

38. Sandra, age 65, presents to the clinic with chest discomfort. She describes her pain by clenching a fist to her chest. Upon examination you detect transient S4 sound. Which of the following would not be in the treatment plan for Sandra?

 a. Nitroglycerin

 b. Cholestyramine

 c. Atenolol

 d. Diltiazem

39. Peter, a 55-year-old Caucasian man, has a consistent blood pressure reading of 145/90 mmHg. His medical history reveals he was diagnosed with diabetes a few years prior. Which of the following would most likely be the drug class of choice for Peter at this time?

 a. Beta blockers

 b. Angiotensin-converting enzyme inhibitors

 c. Diuretics

 d. Adrenergic inhibitors

40. Your patient comes to the clinic with a blood pressure reading of 184/112 mmHg, but is otherwise asymptomatic. Your clinic does not have the appropriate medication to treat his condition, so you refer him to the local ER. Which medication would you most expect your patient to receive at the ER?

 a. Clonidine

 b. Nitroprusside

 c. Nitroglycerin

 d. Nicardipine

RATIONALES

1. d

Based on the sudden simultaneous presentation of pain, heat, and erythema in the affected leg, accompanied by lack of swelling, the patient is most likely experiencing superficial thrombosis, which is generally not treated with bed rest. Rather, mobility is encouraged in patients with superficial thrombosis, whereas bed rest would be a standard treatment for deep thrombosis. Elevating the leg, applying warm compresses, and taking non-steroidal anti-inflammatory drugs are all effective methods of managing superficial thrombosis.

2. b

Hepatomegaly is common in chronic right-sided heart failure but is much less common in acute heart failure. Coarse rales over all lung fields; a wheezing, frothy cough; and an S3 gallop are all common findings of acute, left-sided heart failure.

3. a

An S3 heart sound is a ventricular gallop that matches the cadence of the word "Kentucky" and typically presents as a result of increased fluid states; although it may be normal during pregnancy, presentation of the S3 heart sound at other times may indicate conditions such as chronic heart failure. An S4 heart sound, on the other hand, is an atrial gallop that matches the cadence of "Tennessee" and is often associated with conditions that result in a stiff ventricular wall, such as myocardial infarction and chronic hypertension.

4. b

A grade IV/VI heart murmur, not a grade II/VI murmur, is often accompanied by a palpable thrill. A grade I/VI murmur is barely audible, whereas a grade II/VI murmur is audible but faint. A grade III/VI murmur can easily be heard, and a V/VI murmur is loud enough to be heard with one corner of the stethoscope off the chest wall.

5. c

Mitral stenosis often presents at the fifth intercostal space (ICS) with a low-pitched diastolic rumble with minimal radiation. Mitral regurgitation likewise often presents at the fifth ICS, but with a systolic "blowing" murmur that may radiate to the base or left axilla. Aortic stenosis is systolic and often presents at the second right ICS, whereas aortic regurgitation is diastolic and typically presents at the second left ICS; both murmurs may be characterized by a "blowing" sound.

6. b

The S2 heart sound is caused by aortic and pulmonic valve closures. The S1 sound, on the other hand, is caused by mitral and tricuspid valve closures, whereas the S3 sound is typically caused by increased fluid states. Lastly, the S4 sound is usually caused by a stiff ventricular wall.

7. a

Beta blockers, such as propranolol, are particularly effective for treating hypertension as well as remedying migraines. Patients with hypertension and diabetes mellitus may benefit from calcium channel blockers or angiotensin-converting enzyme (ACE) inhibitors, but the potential side effects of those treatments include edema. Propranolol may also cause edema. If a patient has hypertension, chronic kidney disease is one of the conditions that must be considered when deciding course of treatment. Hypertension associated with chronic kidney disease is not usually treated with beta blockers, but more commonly with ACE inhibitors or angiotensin II receptor blockers.

8. c

By the hypertension recommendations of the Eighth Joint National Committee, systolic, not diastolic, blood pressure is used to estimate 10-year and lifetime atherosclerotic cardiovascular disease risks. Other such risks include high-density lipid cholesterol, race, and diabetes status, as well as sex, total cholesterol, and history of smoking.

9. d

Dependent rubor, or a dusky, red tint to the foot when it is placed on the floor, is a finding associated with peripheral vascular disease. Chronic venous insufficiency is more likely to present with stasis leg ulcers and edema of the lower extremities. Superficial thrombophlebitis is often characterized by localized heat and erythema, whereas a limb affected by deep vein thrombosis may be cool to the touch and manifest with edema distal to the occlusion.

10. d

The risk of superficial thrombosis is increased in patients who are taking estrogen-based oral contraceptives; thus, options such as intrauterine devices are the recommended form of birth control in patients with a history of coronary complications. Females, individuals bed-ridden due to surgery or sickness, and smokers are all at increased risk of developing superficial thrombosis.

11. d

By the latest standards for statin therapy, a daily dose of 40–80 mg of pravastatin is indicated for moderate-intensity statin therapy and expected to reduce low-density lipid cholesterol (LDL-C) by approximately 30% to less than 50%. Atorvastatin 40–80 mg and rosuvastatin 20–40 mg are both indicated for high-intensity statin therapy and expected to lower LDL-C by more than 50%, whereas simvastatin 10 mg is indicated for low-intensity statin therapy and expected to lower LDL-C by less than 30%.

12. b

Chronic venous insufficiency is characterized by impaired venous return most commonly due to either destruction of valves, changes due to deep thrombophlebitis, leg trauma, or sustained elevation of venous pressure. Superficial thrombophlebitis, on the other hand, is defined as obstructive inflammation of a vein just below the surface of the skin. Peripheral vascular disease is defined as an arteriosclerotic narrowing of the lumen of the arteries, resulting in decreased blood supply to the extremities. Lastly, deep vein thrombosis is defined as a partial or complete occlusion of a vein deep inside the body by a thrombus.

13. c

The New York Heart Association Functional Classification places heart failure presenting with marked limitations of physical activity but ease at rest as class III. A patient with class II heart failure would also be comfortable at rest but would present with slight, not marked, limitations of physical activity. There would be no physical limitations in a normal patient with class I heart failure. Conversely, a patient with class IV heart failure would be unable to carry out any physical activity and would experience symptoms even at rest.

14. b

Angiotensin-converting enzyme (ACE) inhibitors, such as captopril, are mainstays in the treatment of heart failure, as these drugs reduce aldosterone secretion, improve symptoms, and increase survival. Peripheral alpha-1 antagonists, such as prazosin, and beta-blocking agents, such as atenolol, may play a role in treating heart failure but would be better suited for treating hypertension. Candesartan and other angiotensin II-receptor blockers treat heart failure but are reserved for patients who cannot tolerate ACE inhibitors. Therefore, captopril would be the best treatment at this time.

15. a

An exercise stress test can be used to evaluate chest pain in patients suspected of having angina if an electrocardiogram returns normal results. Approximately 50% of all patients with angina will have normal electrocardiogram results so normal results do not rule out a diagnosis of angina. Many angina patients also return normal angiogram findings so these findings cannot be used to rule out a diagnosis of angina either. Serum lipid levels can be used to assess a patient for heart failure risk.

16. c

Aortic stenosis typically presents with a systolic, "blowing," rough- and harsh-sounding murmur that manifests at the second right intercostal space (ICS) and usually radiates to the neck. Mitral stenosis usually presents with a diastolic, low-pitched "crescendo" rumble. Mitral regurgitation can also present with a blowing sound, but it classically appears at the fifth ICS and may radiate to the base or left axilla. Aortic regurgitation normally presents with a blowing murmur at the second left ICS and is diastolic, not systolic.

17. c

Following an electrocardiogram, an echocardiogram would be most helpful in identifying the severity of heart failure, as well as tracing deviations or underlying problems such as dysrhythmia and myocardial infarction. A chest x-ray would be helpful in checking for edema and effusions; however, patients with a history of heart failure do not always show signs of pulmonary congestion on x-ray. An angiography would be useful in cases where symptoms of heart failure worsen with no clear cause; however, most patients will not require such an invasive procedure. A complete blood count with differential may help to assess complications of heart failure, such as anemia and renal insufficiency, but would not necessarily help in determining the severity of the disease.

18. c

Shiny, hairless skin is a physical finding of peripheral vascular disease, not myocardial infarction (MI), which is indicated by anginal pain during rest that is not relieved by nitroglycerin, cold sweats, weakness, dyspnea, nausea, and a sense of impending doom. The nurse practitioner (NP) should expect to find dysrhythmia, S4 heart sounds, and wheezing in the majority of MI patients. Additionally, in most patients, the NP should expect to find pulmonary crackles, tachycardia, and low-grade fever during the first 48 hours when diagnosing MI.

19. d

Myocardial infarction (MI) often presents with intense chest pain lasting 30–60 minutes and syncope, which is the partial or complete loss of consciousness. Physical exam findings may include dysrhythmia, S4 heart sounds, and a low-grade fever. Hypertension commonly presents with dizziness or lightheadedness; however, syncope and chest pain are not common findings. Although heart failure can cause syncope, syncope is more common in MI. Additionally, heart failure does not typically present with S4 heart sounds. Angina does not commonly present with syncope, low-grade fever, or dysrhythmia.

20. c

The D-dimer test is used in diagnosing individuals with blood-clotting problems, specifically deep vein thrombosis, pulmonary embolism, and disseminated intravascular coagulation, but is not typically used in diagnosing hypertension. Morning and evening cortisol levels are useful in ruling out Cushing's syndrome in hypertensive patients. Plasma aldosterone levels are useful in ruling out aldosteronism. Renal angiograms are useful in diagnosing renovascular disease, which can cause hypertension.

21. c

Myocardial infarctions (MIs), which present with chest pain that does not subside with nitroglycerin, cold sweats, and nausea, typically result in leukocytosis, rather than leukopenia. Furthermore, MIs also usually demonstrate peaked T waves and elevated ST segments on an electrocardiogram (ECG). Although not all infarctions result in these ECG changes, elevated ST segments help with the diagnosis of an MI and generally indicate an increased risk of damage to the heart, compared to MIs that may occur without elevated ST segments. Another change that MIs may cause is the development of Q waves, although this does not occur in all cases.

22. c

Although the drug of choice for Caucasian men younger than 65, angiotensin-converting enzyme inhibitors, such as lisinopril, are known to cause cough and bronchospasm as side effects in patients with hypertension. Although much less likely, olmesartan and other angiotensin II receptor blockers may also cause coughing as a side effect, but bronchospasms are not a known side effect. Diuretics, such as metolazone, are more often recommended for elderly patients with isolated systolic hypertension or patients with congestive heart failure, and are unlikely to produce cough and bronchospasm as side effects. Amlodipine and other calcium channel blockers are unlikely to produce cough and bronchospasm, and are more likely to produce headache, flushing, and bradycardia as side effects.

23. d

A lateral wall myocardial infarction would present with ST-segment elevation in leads I and aVL. An anterior wall infarction would present with ST-segment elevation in leads V1–V6, whereas an inferior wall infarction would show reciprocal ST-segment depression, not elevation, in leads I and aVL. An anteroseptal wall infarction would present with Q waves in leads V1–V4.

24. b

Deep vein thrombosis often presents with a low-grade temperature, unilateral edema distal to occlusion, and pain or tenderness that may be strongest when walking. Superficial thrombosis, on the other hand, usually involves a sudden onset of pain accompanied by localized heat and a low-grade temperature. Peripheral vascular disease typically presents with calf pain and numbness in the extremities, as well as pain at rest. Lastly, chronic venous insufficiency is often indicated by aching in the lower extremities that is relieved with elevation.

25. c

An optimal lipid panel would show total cholesterol at under 200 mg/dL, low-density lipids (LDLs) at under 100 mg/dL, triglycerides at under 150 mg/dL, and high-density lipids (HDLs) at over 40 mg/dL; therefore, a patient whose lipid panel returns with LDLs at 112 mg/dL and HDLs at 32 mg/dL would show abnormal results in two fields, warranting further attention. All the other returns show abnormal results in one field, be it total cholesterol at 210 mg/dL, triglycerides at 160 mg/dL, or HDLs at 25 mg/dL; these may warrant attention, but do not demonstrate the degree of risk that two abnormal results would.

26. d

A patient with deep vein thrombosis typically has a D-dimer level that is greater than 500 ng/mL; therefore, a patient with a negative D-dimer level would most likely be diagnosed with something other than deep vein thrombosis. D-dimer levels are especially useful in diagnosing individuals with blood-clotting problems, specifically deep vein thrombosis, pulmonary embolism, and disseminated intravascular coagulation; thus, this test would see little use in confirming or ruling out hypertension, myocardial infarction, or congestive heart failure.

27. d

Aortic regurgitation often presents with a diastolic "blowing" murmur at the second left intercostal space (ICS). Mitral stenosis, on the other hand, is typically indicated by a loud, low-pitched, and mid-diastolic S1 murmur with an apical "crescendo" rumble. A classic finding of mitral regurgitation is a third heart sound with a systolic murmur at the fifth ICS mid-clavicular line. Lastly, aortic stenosis typically presents with a systolic, "blowing," rough harsh murmur at the second right ICS, usually radiating to the neck.

28. c

Pharmacologic revascularization is generally indicated by the patient experiencing unrelieved chest pain for 30 minutes to 6 hours, accompanied by two or more elevated ST segments in either the left lateral ventricular wall, inferior chest, or precordial leads; therefore, chest pain that has lasted for 3 hours with ST segment elevations of 0.3 mV in the precordial lead and lead I would meet the general criteria for pharmacologic revascularization. Chest pain that has lasted for 1 hour would fall within the proper time frame; however, the presence of ST segment depression would not usually indicate pharmacologic revascularization. Chest pain that has lasted for 2 hours with ST segments of 0.1 mV and 0.3 mV would not fit the standard criteria, as the ST segment in lead III is normal. Chest pain that has lasted for 7 hours, with or without elevated ST segments, would fall outside the typical range that indicates pharmacologic revascularization.

29. d

Grade V/VI heart murmurs are often very loud and can be heard with one corner of the stethoscope off the chest wall, in contrast to grade IV/VI heart murmurs that are generally loud and associated with a thrill. Grade II/VI murmurs are typically audible but faint, whereas grade III/VI murmurs are usually classified as moderately loud but easily heard.

30. a

Although severe hypertension may present with a "pulsating" headache that appears in the morning and usually resolves over the course of the day, this headache is typically suboccipital, not subparietal, in nature. Approximately 95% of all cases of hypertension are "primary" in nature, with no identifiable cause; the remaining cases of "secondary" hypertension have a traceable etiology, such as contraceptive estrogen therapy, pregnancy, or renal disease. African American adults have the highest rates of hypertension, with approximately 20%–30% of the population experiencing the condition.

31. a

Systolic heart failure is defined as the inability of the heart to contract, resulting in decreased cardiac output; likewise, acute heart failure typically presents with dyspnea at rest, wheezing, and frothy cough. Diastolic heart failure also results in decreased cardiac output; however, this is a result of the heart's inability to relax and fill, not contract. Chronic heart failure may also present with dyspnea but tends to produce with more visible symptoms, such as hepatomegaly, dependent edema, and an appearance indicative of chronic illness.

32. b

The enlargement of the aorta on a chest x-ray is more indicative of an aortic aneurysm than right-sided heart failure. Patients with chronic right-sided heart failure may present with Kerley B lines, pulmonary edema, and pleural effusions on a chest x-ray. Kerley B lines, less common in chronic heart failure than in acute heart failure, are less than 2 cm long and reside in the lower left segment of the lungs. Pulmonary edema and pleural effusions are also consistent findings in patients with chronic right-sided heart failure; isolating these findings on a chest x-ray may confirm the diagnosis.

33. b

Fundoscopic changes stemming from malignant hypertension may include flame-shaped retinal hemorrhages, soft exudates, and papilledema. Fundoscopic changes are less common in dissecting aortic aneurysm. Hypertensive urgencies do not normally present with fundoscopic changes. Macular degeneration may present with fundoscopic changes, but these changes typically include retinal pigment epithelium, drusen, and areas of chorioretinal atrophy.

34. d

The cardiac enzymes CK-MB and troponin I are entirely cardioselective and only elevate when myocardial damage is present. Both troponin T and myoglobin may be elevated as a result of regenerative muscular disorders or unstable angina.

35. a

Angiotensin-converting enzyme (ACE) inhibitors act by causing vasodilation and blocking water and sodium retention; side effects of these drugs may include rash, taste disturbances, hyperkalemia, renal impairment, and cough. Although central alpha-2 agonists are known to prevent vasoconstriction and slow the heart rate, they are primarily used for adjunct therapy, not monotherapy. Angiotensin II-receptor blockers are generally reserved for patients who cannot tolerate ACE inhibitors but do not usually produce hyperglycemia and hypokalemia; rather, these drugs are more likely to produce hyperkalemia. Calcium channel blockers may be used to treat angina, arrhythmias, and migraines, but are not associated with dry mouth, sedation, or nausea.

36. a

Mitral regurgitation typically presents with a loud pansystolic murmur that presents at the apex with a blowing, musical, or high-pitched noise. Aortic stenosis likewise usually presents with a systolic "blowing" murmur but typically presents at the second left intercostal space (ICS), not the apex. Aortic regurgitation likewise generally presents with a "blowing" murmur, but this murmur is diastolic in nature and typically presents at the second right ICS. Mitral stenosis often presents with a loud, low-pitched, "rumbling" murmur that is mid-diastolic in nature.

37. a

Stable angina is typically triggered by exertion and can subside with rest or lying down, whereas most myocardial infarctions (MIs) occur at rest. Although pain in an MI is typically more severe than pain experienced during angina, some MIs may present without pain. Both angina and MI may radiate into the jaw and down the left arm. Lastly, whereas pain from an MI is typically characterized as "sharp" or "stabbing," pain from angina often presents as a sensation of discomfort that is hard to qualify.

38. b

Angina, which typically presents with chest discomfort, a positive Levine's sign, and a transient S4 sound, would not be directly treated with a bile acid sequestrant such as cholestyramine, which would be more useful in managing hyperlipidemia. Nitroglycerin, a nitrate, would be one of the first measures in treating anginal symptoms. Beta blockers, such as atenolol, and calcium channel blockers, such as diltiazem, may also see use in the treatment of angina.

39. b

Angiotensin-converting enzyme (ACE) inhibitors are particularly effective for treating hypertension in Caucasians 65 years of age or younger, as well as diabetics. Beta blockers, on the other hand, are most effective for treating hypertensive patients with migraines and angina. Beta blockers are not, however, usually a first-line treatment because use can increase risk of cardiovascular death, myocardial infarction, or stroke. Diuretics work well in African Americans and patients with isolated systolic hypertension, but ACE inhibitors would be better for a Caucasian patient at this time. Lastly, adrenergic inhibitors are common first-line choices for high blood pressure, heart failure, and kidney failure but would not be the best option for a hypertensive diabetic.

40. a

Hypertensive urgencies, as indicated by a patient with a blood pressure reading in excess of 180/110 mmHg who is otherwise asymptomatic, are usually managed with oral therapies such as clonidine. Hypertensive emergencies typically present with additional symptoms, such as papilledema or severe chest pain. Hypertensive emergencies are frequently treated with oral therapies such as nicardipine or sodium nitroprusside. Nitroglycerine is commonly used to relieve chest pain from angina.

DISCUSSION

Cardiovascular Assessment (see figure 14.1)

Overview

A cardiovascular assessment helps to determine the risk of hypertension, angina, myocardial infarctions (MIs), and other cardiac-related conditions. The cardiovascular assessment should include taking the patient's blood pressure (BP) and history, auscultating the patient's chest, and performing an electrocardiogram (ECG).[1]

The cardiac cycle consists of the systolic phase and the diastolic phase. During the systolic phase, the atrioventricular valves close and the semilunar valves open. During the diastolic phase, the aortic and pulmonic valves close, giving way to the opening of the tricuspid and mitral valves. The ventricles are subsequently filled, and the atrium contracts.[2]

Upon auscultation of the precordium, the aortic area is near the second, right intercostal space (ICS) at the right sternal border. The pulmonic area is near the second left ICS at the left sternal border. The tricuspid is near the left lower sternal border at the fifth ICS, and Erb's point is at the third ICS at the left sternal border. The mitral area is near the fifth ICS midclavicular line.[2]

Presentation (see tables 14.1 and 14.2)

Auscultation of the chest involves assessing the timing and normality of each location. The S1 heart sound occurs with the apical and carotid impulses and is heard most easily at the apex. The S2 heart sound signifies the closure of the aortic and semilunar valves near the beginning of diastole. It is most easily heard at the base of the heart.

In some patients, a split S2 heart sound occurs after every fourth heartbeat as the result of the early closure of the aortic valve and the late closure of the pulmonic valve. A split S2 heart sound is only auscultated in the pulmonic auscultatory area.

An S3 heart sound, or ventricular gallop, is the result of blood filling into the left ventricle and is heard early in diastole at the left lower sternal border. This sound produces a galloping rhythm similar in cadence to pronouncing "Kentucky." This is the most common abnormal heart sound in heart failure but is normal during pregnancy. The S4 heart sound, or presystolic gallop, is the result of blood entering the left ventricle during atrial contraction and can be heard at the apex.[2] This sound classically produces a rhythm similar to pronouncing "Tennessee." Patients with an S4 heart sound include those who have previously experienced an MI, left ventricular hypertrophy, or chronic hypertension.

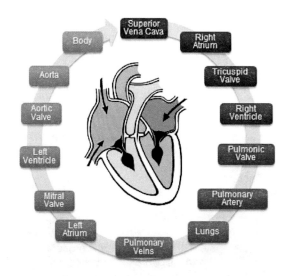

Figure 14.1. Cardiovascular system overview.

Identifying the appropriate heart murmur can help to isolate the underlying cardiac condition. Murmurs are "blowing" or "swooshing" sounds that reflect turbulent blood flow. Important aspects to note include the timing, loudness (classified by grade), pitch, quality, location, radiation, and posture.[2]

Valvular Disease: Major Problems

Overview

Mitral stenosis occurs as a result of the mitral orifice narrowing and thickening, and immobility of the mitral valve leaflets that cause blood flow obstruction from the left atrium to the left ventricle.[3] Mitral stenosis is often distinguished from other valvular diseases by a loud, low-pitched, mid-diastolic murmur with an apical "crescendo" rumble that occurs between S2 and S1 and is best auscultated at the fifth ICS midclavicular line.[4]

Mitral regurgitation is classically characterized by an S3 heart sound with a systolic murmur at the fifth ICS midclavicular line at the apex. This murmur may be musical, blowing, or high-pitched, and may radiate to the base or the left axilla.

Aortic stenosis is evidenced by a systolic "blowing," rough, harsh murmur at the second right ICS that often radiates to the neck. These murmurs are an important factor in confirming a diagnosis of aortic stenosis and determining if an echocardiogram is necessary.[5]

Aortic regurgitation also commonly presents with a "blowing" murmur, but unlike aortic stenosis, this murmur is diastolic and occurs at the second left ICS.

Presentation

Patients with mitral stenosis are typically asymptomatic in the early stages and usually do not develop symptoms until they are in their 30s or 40s. They may experience dyspnea, jugular venous distension, hemoptysis, or an embolic episode. Due to an enlarged left atrium that may put pressure on the laryngeal nerve, patients may complain of hoarseness. Pink or purple patches on the cheek may be indicative of chronic mitral stenosis, which leads to vasoconstriction and decreased cardiac output.[6]

Mild mitral regurgitation may not produce any noticeable symptoms. Patients with more serious cases may complain of chest pain, lightheadedness, and shortness of breath. Patients may also experience palpitations that is exacerbated when lying on their side. Coughing, heart and lung congestion, and swelling of the legs and feet are also common findings.[7]

Acute aortic regurgitation typically presents with sudden shortness of breath and chest pain. Chronic aortic regurgitation is often asymptomatic until tachycardia develops as a compensatory mechanism. Patients with aortic regurgitation may experience palpitations, shortness of breath, and chest pain.[8]

Heart Failure

Overview

Heart failure is a ventricular disorder that results when cardiac output cannot meet the metabolic demands of the body. Heart failure may be classified as systolic or diastolic.

Systolic heart failure occurs when the heart has a decreased ability to contract, which results in a decreased ejection fraction (EF) and reduced cardiac output. Systolic heart failure is often caused by left ventricular dilated cardiomyopathy.

In diastolic heart failure, the heart is unable to relax and fill, resulting in decreased cardiac output. This is often caused by left ventricular hypertrophy related to hypertension, or restrictive or hypertrophic cardiomyopathy. The EF may be normal, but there is a decreased stroke volume.[9,10]

Right-sided heart failure usually occurs as a result of one of these two types of left-sided heart failure.[11] Acute heart failure frequently manifest following an acute MI or valve rupture.[9]

The classifications used to describe heart failure are commonly based on the EF, which is important in determining the patient's survival. In order for patients to be classified as having heart failure with a preserved EF, they must have signs and symptoms of heart failure, a normal or mildly reduced EF, and structural heart disease or diastolic dysfunction. In order for a patient to be diagnosed with heart failure and a reduced EF, the patient must have signs and symptoms of heart failure in addition to a reduced EF. It is important to note that the lower the EF, the poorer the survival rate.[12]

Based on their presentation, patients can be diagnosed according to one of the two guidelines set forth by the American College of Cardiology (ACC)/American Heart Association (AHA) or the New York Heart Association (NYHA).

The ACC/AHA stages of heart failure are classified into four groups. A patient in stage A is at high risk for heart failure but does not have structural heart disease or symptoms. A patient in stage B does not exhibit signs or symptoms of heart failure. In stage C, the patient has previously or is currently experiencing signs or symptoms of heart failure. A patient with refractory heart failure in need of intervention is in stage D.

The NYHA classification divides heart failure assessment into four classes. In class I, there are no limitations of physical activity; the patient is able to carry on normal activity without signs or symptoms. Class II heart failure is characterized by slight limitations to physical activity due to findings such as fatigue, palpitations, dyspnea, or angina. More marked limitations of physical activity are seen in class III heart failure. In both classes II and III, the patient feels comfortable at rest. With class IV, signs and symptoms are severe and persist while the patient is at rest; patients are unable to perform any physical activity without experiencing discomfort.[13]

Presentation

Signs and symptoms of heart failure often manifest insidiously but can appear suddenly if the heart is damaged from acute injury.[14] Patients with left-sided heart failure generally appear healthy except for an acute event but may experience dyspnea at rest and present with a wheezing, frothy cough. Cardiac findings of left-sided heart failure may include the presence of an S3 gallop and coarse rales over all of the patient's lung fields.

Those with right-sided heart failure appear chronically ill.[9] Signs and symptoms include jugular venous distention, hepatomegaly, splenomegaly, and dependent edema.[15,16]

Workup

A basic metabolic panel is usually insignificant unless chronic failure is present.[9] Other tests may include a chest x-ray (CXR), echocardiogram, and ECG.[15] Chest x-ray findings indicative of heart failure may include pulmonary edema, Kerley B lines, and effusions. The echocardiogram shows valve function, wall motion, and EF. A urinalysis and pulmonary function tests may also be ordered.[9,17]

Treatment

Heart failure may be managed by non-pharmacologic and pharmacologic treatments, with the primary goal being to correct or treat the underlying disorder that led to heart failure.[15] Moreover, treatment should be aimed at improving the patient's symptoms and reducing mortality.[12]

Table 14.3	Heart Failure Classification

American Heart Association Stages of Heart Failure

Stage of HF	Definition	Manifestations
Stage A	High risk for HF without structural heart disease	HTN, CAD, DM, obesity, metabolic syndrome
Stage B	Structural heart disease present and strongly associated with HF, but asymptomatic	Previous MI Left ventricular remodeling, including LVH and low EF; asymptomatic valvular disease
Stage C	Structural heart disease with current or prior symptoms	Structural heart disease and symptoms of HF
Stage D	Refractory heart failure	Marked symptoms of HF at rest Recurrent hospitalizations despite guided directed medical therapy

New York Heart Association Heart Failure Functional Classification

Functional Class	Patient Description	Manifestations
Class I	No limitation of activity	Suffer no symptoms from ordinary activities
Class II	Slight, mild limitation of activity	Comfortable at rest or with mild exertion
Class III	Marked limitation of activity	Comfortable only at rest
Class IV	Should be at complete rest, confined to bed or chair	Any activity brings discomfort, and symptoms occur at rest

Note. HF = heart failure; HTN = hypertension; CAD = coronary artery disease; DM = diabetes mellitus; MI = myocardial infarction; LVH = left ventricular hypertrophy; EF = ejection fraction. Used with permission from King J, Fellin R, Barkley TW Jr. Heart Failure. In: Barkley TW Jr, Myers CM, eds. *Practice Considerations for the Adult-Gerontology Acute Care Nurse Practitioner.* West Hollywood, CA: Barkley and Associates; 2015: 169.

Drugs that may be used in the treatment for heart failure include, but are not limited to, angiotensin-converting-enzyme inhibitors, angiotensin II receptor antagonists, diuretics, calcium channel blockers (CCBs) and beta blockers (BBs).[18] Additionally, patients may benefit from lifestyle modifications such as weight reduction and salt restriction, among others.[19]

Hypertension

Overview (see table 14.4)

According to the eighth report of the Joint National Committee in 2014, hypertension is a sustained elevation of systolic BP greater than or equal to 140 mmHg or diastolic BP greater than or equal to 90 mmHg, taken from two or more readings on two different occasions after an initial screening.[20,21] There are two types of hypertension: primary and secondary.

Primary hypertension, also known as essential hypertension, makes up approximately 90%–95% of all cases of hypertension. Secondary hypertension only makes up approximately 2%–10% of cases.[22] The exact cause of primary hypertension is unknown, but exacerbating factors include smoking, obesity, excessive alcohol intake, and the use of non-steroidal anti-inflammatory drugs (NSAIDs).

Factors that may lead to secondary hypertension include estrogen use, renal disease, pregnancy, endocrine disorders (e.g., Cushing's syndrome, pheochromocytoma), and renal artery stenosis, among others.

Presentation

Hypertension is commonly known as the "silent killer," as patients are usually asymptomatic.[9] Most patients are diagnosed with elevated BP upon visiting their nurse practitioner (NP).[23] In cases of severe hypertension, the patient may present with dizziness, lightheadedness, nosebleeds, or an S4 heart sound related to left ventricular hypertrophy. Additionally, a suboccipital pulsating headache may occur early in the morning and resolve throughout the day.[9]

Workup

When diagnosing hypertension, it is essential to measure and interpret the patient's BP properly.[21] Multiple BP measurements should be taken to confirm a diagnosis.[24] In addition to BP readings, other tests used in the workup of hypertension include an ECG, urinalysis, and complete blood count.[24] Initial lab tests include a basic metabolic panel, cholesterol analysis, CXR, and blood urea nitrogen and creatinine determination.[22] Laboratory findings are typically insignificant in uncomplicated hypertension, but other tests may be given to rule out particular causes.[9] Further tests include renovascular disease studies, plasma aldosterone levels to rule out aldosteronism, and morning and evening cortisol levels to rule out Cushing's syndrome.

Treatment (see table 14.5)

The goal of hypertension treatment is to reduce the patient's BP, which begins with therapeutic lifestyle changes, such as relaxing, managing stress, adhering to a low-sodium diet, exercising, and reducing weight.[23,25] The AHA recommends 30–40 minutes of exercise at least 5 days per week for overall health benefits to the heart.[26,27]

Pharmacological treatments may be given if BP cannot be sufficiently reduced by lifestyle modifications.[22] The goal is to use the least amount of medication as possible at the lowest doses to maintain control of BP.[9]

See table 14.5 for the 8th report of the Joint National Committee hypertension treatment recommendations.

Hypertensive Urgencies

Overview

Hypertensive urgencies are indicated by a systolic BP greater than or equal to 180 mmHg or diastolic BP greater than or equal to 110 mmHg.[28] No other signs and symptoms are usually apparent, however, as hypertensive urgencies are classified as severe cases of hypertension in asymptomatic patients.[21] Most patients experiencing a hypertensive urgency are those who are noncompliant with their medication regimen or those inadequately treated for hypertension.[28]

Treatment

Because acute complications are unlikely in patients with hypertensive urgencies, immediate BP reduction is not required as with hypertensive emergencies; instead, patients should be treated with oral therapy, such as clonidine (Catapres), captopril (Capoten), nifedipine (Procardia), or loop diuretics.[24] In addition to selecting an appropriate anti-hypertensive agent, the NP should determine how rapidly the patient's BP needs to be lowered.

Hypertensive Emergencies

Overview

Hypertensive emergencies occur in rare situations and require BP to be lowered aggressively, often within minutes or hours of onset to prevent organ damage.[29] The initial goal of treatment is to reduce mean arterial pressure by no more than 25% within 2 hours.[9] Hypertensive emergencies are classified when the patient has at least a systolic

Table 14.4	JNC 7 Blood Pressure Thresholds		
Classifications	**Systolic BP**		**Diastolic BP**
Normal	< 120	and	< 80
Prehypertension	120 to 139	or	80 to 89
Hypertension			
Stage 1	140 to 159	or	90 to 99
Stage 2	≥ 160	or	≥ 100

Used with permission from Barkley TW Jr, Miley H, Fellin R. Hypertension. In: Barkley TW Jr, Myers CM, eds. *Practice Considerations for the Adult-Gerontology Acute Care Nurse Practitioner*. West Hollywood, CA: Barkley and Associates; 2015: 131.

BP level of 180 mmHg or a diastolic BP level of 120 mmHg.[30]

Malignant hypertension is considered a hypertensive emergency, as it may result in end-organ damage.[31] Malignant hypertension may cause fundoscopic changes, such as flame-shaped retinal hemorrhages, soft exudates, and papilledema.

Hypertensive encephalopathy, another hypertensive emergency, also may cause end-organ damage.[24] Other conditions include intracranial hemorrhages, acute left ventricle failure with pulmonary edema, dissecting aortic aneurysms, and eclampsia, among others. Unstable angina and acute MIs with high BP are also considered hypertensive emergencies.[9]

Treatment

Patients with hypertensive emergencies require immediate hospitalization for treatment with intravenous agents.[32] For instance, hypertensive emergencies are commonly treated by nicardipine (Cardene) or sodium nitroprusside (Nipride).[9,29]

Angina

Overview

Angina pectoris, known simply as angina, is a condition characterized by decreased blood flow through the vessel. Tissue ischemia occurs when there is an imbalance between myocardial blood supply and oxygen demand, resulting in the inability of the coronary arteries to supply an adequate amount of blood to meet myocardial oxygen demands.[33,34]

The most common type of angina is stable angina, which is evidenced by chest discomfort that occurs with physical exertion but subsides at rest.[35] Unstable angina, on the other hand, occurs even during rest, lasts longer than stable angina, and is more severe.[36]

The most common cause of stable angina is coronary artery disease.[37] Prinzmetal's angina, otherwise known as variant or vasospastic angina, occurs at rest, often between midnight and early morning.[38] Microvascular angina is caused by reduced blood flow to the heart due to spasms within the walls of the smallest arterial blood vessels of the heart.[39]

Presentation

Signs and symptoms can vary greatly in severity from patient to patient. Some patients may experience only mild chest discomfort on rare occasions, such as during heavy exertion, whereas others experience severe discomfort during rest or slight exertion. Usually, angina begins with characteristic chest discomfort lasting several minutes.[34] In patients with stable angina, the chest pain is most often precipitated by physical activity and subsides with rest. Chest pain in unstable angina is more severe and is more likely to come with little physical exertion.[40] Physical exam findings may include signs of peripheral arterial disease as well as Levine's sign, characterized by patients clenching a fist over the sternum when describing the discomfort.[33] A transient S4 heart sound is not uncommon during angina.[9]

Workup

Patients with chest pain should receive an ECG to determine if the pain is from angina or an MI.[41] Approximately half of patients with angina present with normal initial ECG findings, but ST or T-wave abnormalities may be seen.[42] If a resting ECG does not show abnormalities, exercise with ECG monitoring should be conducted.[42] If the ECG shows signs of an MI, a cardiology referral is immediately warranted for cardiac catheterization.[41]

Treatment

The central focus of angina management should be to reduce the patient's risk factors through treatments such as statin therapy, weight reduction, and glycemia management for patients with diabetes.[43] Patients should reduce consumption of saturated and unsaturated fats.[44] Common pharmacotherapy options for angina include BBs, nitrates, and CCBs.[45]

Myocardial Infarction (MI)

Overview

Myocardial infarction consists of necrosis resulting from an abrupt reduction of coronary blood flow to the myocardium; necrosis is secondary to prolonged ischemia and is irreversible.[34,46] MI occurs due to a clot that blocks blood flowing from the heart, which may result from a slow buildup of plaque.[47] Furthermore, MI is the leading cause of death in the United States and a leading cause of mortality worldwide.[48]

Presentation

Presentations of MI have a wide range of severity. Some patients present with no signs or symptoms, others may experience sudden cardiac death.[48] Common signs and symptoms of MI include coughing, anxiety, light-headedness with or without syncope, nausea with or without vomiting, or a sense of impending doom.[49] Additional findings may include dysrhythmia, an S4 heart sound, wheezing, tachycardia, pulmonary crackles, and low-grade fever during the first 48 hours of the condition.[9] Chest pain often accompanies the onset of MI and is typically an intense pain within the retrosternal area that may radiate.[46]

Workup

An ECG is the first test ordered for patients suspected of having an MI.[48] ECG changes indicative of MI include peaked T waves, ST elevations, or Q wave development. Changes in leads I and aVL indicate a lateral wall MI, whereas changes in leads II, III, and aVF indicate inferior wall infarction.[50,51] ST segment elevation in V3 and V4, or in all of the V leads (precordial leads), indicates an anterior wall MI. A serum cardiac enzyme panel can also be ordered to find evidence of MI. Post-MI, a patient may exhibit elevated levels of CK-MB, myoglobin, and troponin I and T. Elevated troponin I is always specific for myocardial necrosis.[34]

Treatment

Patients with a suspected MI should be transported to a hospital as soon as possible. Emergency department care management includes ongoing evaluation of ABCs, chewing and swallowing one 325 mg acetylsalicylic acid (i.e., aspirin) tablet, oxygen per nasal cannula, analysis of a twelve-lead ECG, and the use of sublingual nitroglycerin.[52] A cardiology specialist will further derive a plan of care.

Venous Thrombosis

Overview

Venous thrombosis is a partial or complete occlusion of a vein by a thrombus in addition to secondary inflammation to the vessel wall. The two types are known as superficial venous thrombosis (SVT) and deep venous thrombosis (DVT), which is the more severe of the two.[53] Contributing causes of venous thrombosis include hypercoagulability, immobility, prolonged bed rest, and the use of oral contraceptives, particularly with smokers. Venous thrombosis has a higher incidence in females and in patients in the post-operative period.[9]

Table 14.5	Prevention and Treatment of Hypertension Recommendations
Blood pressure measurement	Patient should do the following: • Be seated with feet flat on floor, back and arm supported, and arm at heart level • Rest for 5 minutes before measurement • Wear short sleeves • Not drink coffee or smoke cigarettes 30 min before having blood pressure taken • Go to the bathroom before the reading; having a full bladder can change your blood pressure reading Clinician should do the following: • Use a cuff of appropriate size for the patient; the (cuff) bladder should encircle at least 80% of the upper arm • Use calibrated or mercury manometer
Primary prevention	• Quit smoking to reduce cardiovascular risk • Maintain a healthy weight; lose weight if needed • Restrict sodium intake to no more than 100 mmol/day • Limit alcohol intake to no more than 1–2 drinks per day • Be active; get at least 30–45 minutes of aerobic activity on most days • Maintain adequate potassium intake of about 90 mmol per day • Maintain adequate intakes of calcium and magnesium for general health
Goal	• Set a clear goal of therapy based on patient's risk. Control blood pressure to the levels below: • Less than 140/90 mmHg for patients
Treatment	• Begin with lifestyle modifications for all patients • Be supportive! • Add pharmacologic therapy if blood pressure remains uncontrolled/out of goal • Start with a thiazide type diuretic, but also consider ACE inhibitor, angiotensin receptor blocker, calcium channel blocker, or combination • If no response, try a drug from another class or add a second drug from a different class.
Adherence	• Encourage lifestyle modifications. Be supportive! • Educate the patient and family about the disease. Involve them in measurement and treatment • Maintain communication with patient • Empathy promotes adherence, trust, and motivation • Keep care inexpensive and simple • Consider cultural beliefs, practices, and individual attitudes when treating

Note. Adapted from "The seventh report of the Joint National Committee on prevention, detection, evaluation, and treatment of high blood pressure." National Institutes of Health National Heart, Lung, and Blood Institute. NIH Publication No. 04-5230. 2004.

Table 14.6	JNC 8 Hypertension Treatment Recommendations	
	Population	**Goal BP**
Recommendation 1	Adults ≥ 60 years of age	SBP < 150 mmHg or DBP < 90 mmHg (Grade A)
Recommendation 2	Adults < 60 years of age	DBP < 90 mmHg (Grade A)
Recommendation 3	Adults < 60 years of age	SBP < 140 mmHg (Grade E)
Recommendation 4	Adults ≥ 18 with CKD	SBP < 140 mmHg or DBP < 90 mmHg (Grade E)
Recommendation 5	Adults ≥ 18 with DM	SBP < 140 mmHg or DBP < 90 mmHg (Grade E)
Recommendation 6	Non-African-American	Thiazide type diuretic CCB ACEI ARB (Grade B)
Recommendation 7	African-American	Thiazide diuretics CCB (Grade B) (Grade C for patients with DM)
Recommendation 8	Adults over 18 Adults with CKD	ACEI ARB (Grade B) Regardless of race or other medical conditions
Treatment Goal		
Recommendation 9	• Treatment goal for initial treatment is 1 month • Increase dose or add second drug • Continue to assess monthly until goal is reached • Do not use and ACEI and ARB together • Refer to hypertensive specialist if 3 or more drugs are needed	

Note. JNC = Joint National Committee; BP = blood pressure; SBP = systolic blood pressure; DBP = diastolic blood pressure; CKD = chronic kidney disease; DM = diabetes mellitus; CCB = calcium channel blockers; ACEI = Angiotensin converting enzyme inhibitor; ARB = angiotensin receptor blocker. Grade A = strong recommendation; Grade B = moderate recommendation; Grade C = weak recommendation; Grade E = expert opinion but insufficient evidence for recommendation. Used with permission from Barkley TW Jr, Miley H, Fellin R. Hypertension. In: Barkley TW Jr, Myers CM, eds. *Practice Considerations for the Adult-Gerontology Acute Care Nurse Practitioner.* West Hollywood, CA: Barkley and Associates; 2015: 102.

Superficial Venous Thrombosis (SVT)

Overview

SVT results from a blood clot in a vein just below the surface of the skin, most commonly in the upper or lower extremities.[54] SVT is less severe than DVT and may occur in both inherited and acquired thrombophilic states.[53] SVT is also known as superficial thrombophlebitis because it may result in venous inflammation and/or a clot in the vein.[55]

Presentation

SVT is indicated by acute onset of pain. The patient often feels pain in the limbs or along a vein just below the skin, and inflammation and redness may exist along the vein.[56] The patient may present with a low-grade temperature in addition to experiencing localized heat and erythema.

Workup

While SVT can be diagnosed by the appearance of the affected area, a number of tests can help confirm this diagnosis, including a Doppler ultrasound, duplex ultrasound, and venography.[9,56] After an initial diagnosis of SVT, however, patients should undergo a duplex ultrasonography to rule out DVT.[57]

Treatment

Management of SVT is generally supportive and consists of treatments such as elevating the patient's extremities, applying warm compresses, and using NSAIDs.[55] Additionally, oral contraceptives should be discontinued.[9]

Deep Venous Thrombosis (DVT)

Overview

DVT, however, occurs in a deep vein of the extremities or pelvis as opposed to the veins immediately below the skin.[54] Although DVT can occur at any age, the condition is most common in patients older than 60 years of age.[58]

Presentation

The most specific sign of DVT is edema, which is distal to the occlusion.[9,59] DVT is also indicated by a sudden onset of pain, and the patient's pain may manifest as a dull ache or a tight feeling. Pain and tenderness are especially common while walking. DVT patients may also present with a low-grade temperature, and the patient's skin may be cool to the touch.

Workup

The two tests that are often performed first when diagnosing DVT are an ultrasound and the D-dimer blood test.[58] An ultrasound is an effective tool for evaluating the lower extremities and can help detect thrombi by identifying findings such as abnormal compressibility and abnormal Doppler color flow.[60,61] Venography may be indicated when ultrasound results are normal but the patient is strongly suspected of having DVT.[54] Additionally, thrombi are also commonly detected by the patient's D-dimer levels, which are elevated in conditions that involve clot formation.[62]

Treatment

The mainstay of DVT treatment is anticoagulation therapy, which helps to prevent clots from forming or growing larger.[58,63] Anticoagulation therapy is usually recommended for patients with symptomatic DVT in the lower extremities.[64] Patients should be treated with bed rest with the affected leg elevated until local tenderness subsides, which is typically expected to take 7–14 days; afterward, walking is gradually reintroduced.[9] DVT patients should receive either enoxaparin (Lovenox) in a dose of 1 mg/kg every 12 hours or a heparin infusion for upwards of 7–10 days. In addition, warfarin (Coumadin) therapy is commonly recommended for 12 weeks.

Peripheral Vascular Disease (PVD)

Overview

Peripheral vascular disease (PVD) is an arteriosclerotic narrowing of the lumen of arteries, which results in less blood supply to the extremities. PVD is caused by atherosclerosis, and risk factors include smoking, diabetes mellitus, and increased age.[65]

Presentation

A common finding of PVD is leg pain, which is caused by claudication and occurs most commonly in the calves.[65] Other classic signs and symptoms of PVD include pallor and reduced pulse; the patient may also present with shiny or hairless skin.[66] Furthermore, severe cases of PVD may progress to the point where the patient experiences pain while at rest.[67] Dependent rubor and ulcerations are also common physical findings of PVD, and the patient may additionally experience coldness and numbness in the extremities.[9]

Workup

Of the various imaging tests available to diagnose PVD, the most definitive test is an arteriograph.[9] A Doppler ultrasound generally helps evaluate the patient's blood flow, and an ankle-brachial index may be useful to compare the pressure in the patient's lower extremity to that of the upper extremity.[67]

Treatment

Patients with PVD require risk factor modification, including management of conditions such as diabetes.[67] PVD patients should stop smoking and using tobacco, as these substances narrow the arteries, increase the risk of clot formation, and decrease the ability of the blood to carry oxygen.[68] Patients should lose weight, and it is recommended that patients exercise by walking 1 hour per day. Patients should stop during pain and resume when the pain subsides to develop collateral circulation.[9]

Medications used in PVD treatment commonly include cilostazol and pentoxifylline.[67] Angioplasty, bypass surgery, or amputation may be necessary if the condition is severe and affects the patient's ability to walk or causes pain at rest.[68]

Chronic Venous Insufficiency (CVI)

Overview

Chronic venous insufficiency (CVI) involves venous return that may be associated with varicose veins. This condition commonly occurs when valves in leg veins malfunction, hindering the blood's ability to return to the heart.[69] As a result, patients may experience leg trauma, sustained elevation of venous pressure, and changes due to deep thrombophlebitis.[9] CVI has a higher predominance in women than in men, and CVI is associated with genetic predisposition or a history of leg trauma, among other factors.[70]

Presentation

CVI may present with stasis leg ulcers as well as aching of the lower extremities, which usually worsens when the patient is standing or walking but is often relieved by elevation.[54] Prolonged standing also commonly contributes to edema in the lower extremities, and night cramps may occur in the lower extremities as well. Patients with CVI may exhibit skin hyperpigmentation, including a reddish or brownish discoloration that occurs due to the deposition of hemosiderin from red blood cells.[71]

Workup

Diagnostic testing is recommended to determine the etiology and to localize the anatomic site and severity of the disease.[72] DVT can be reliably excluded by a duplex ultrasonography, which is the diagnostic choice for CVI as well as other venous insufficiency syndromes.[54,70] It is also important to rule out other causes of edema.[9]

Treatment

Treatment of CVI is directed toward relieving the patient's symptoms and correcting the underlying complication.[70] CVI patients should rest in bed with their legs elevated to lessen chronic edema.[54] In addition, heavy-duty elastic support stockings may be used to decrease swelling.[73] Dermatitis and ulcers should be treated as indicated, and treatments for

acute weeping dermatitis include wet compresses and hydrocortisone cream. Systemic antibiotics may also be used to treat dermatitis but are only indicated if an active bacterial infection is present.[9]

Figures

Figure 14.1. Used with permission from Barkley TW Jr. *Adult-Gerontology Primary Care Nurse Practitioner Certification Review/Clinical Update Continuing Education Course.* West Hollywood, CA: Barkley and Associates; 2015.

References

1. Goldberg GD. Basic cardiac assessments: Physical examination, electrocardiography, and chest radiography. Journal of Nursing web site. http://rnjournal.com/journal-of-nursing/basic-cardiac-assessments-physical-examination-electrocardiography-and-chest-radiography. Accessed April 10, 2015.

2. Barkley TW Jr, Myers CM, eds. *Practice Considerations for the Adult-Gerontological Acute Care Nurse Practitioner.* West Hollywood, CA: Barkley and Associates; 2015.

3. Mitral stenosis. In: Porter RS, Kaplan JL, eds. The Merck Manual Online. http://www.merckmanuals.com/professional/cardiovascular_disorders/valvular_disorders/mitral_stenosis.html. Last reviewed July 2014. Accessed April 10, 2015.

4. Pinsky LE, Wipf JE. Technique: Heart Sounds and Murmurs. University of Washington Department of Medicine web site. http://depts.washington.edu/physdx/heart/tech4_diastolic.html. Accessed April 10, 2015.

5. Adegunsoye A, Mundkur M, Nanda NC, Hage FG. Echocardiographic evaluation of calcific aortic stenosis in the older adult. *Echocardiography.* 2011; 28: 117–129. doi: 10.1111/j.1540-8175.2010.01363.x

6. Dima C, Desser KB. Mitral stenosis clinical presentation. In: Lange RA, ed. Medscape. http://emedicine.medscape.com/article/155724-clinical#a0217. Updated November 6, 2014. Accessed April 10, 2015.

7. Problem: Mitral valve regurgitation. American Heart Association web site. http://www.heart.org/HEARTORG/Conditions/More/HeartValveProblemsandDisease/Problem-Mitral-Valve-Regurgitation_UCM_450612_Article.jsp. Reviewed February 18, 2013. Updated January 7, 2015. Accessed April 10, 2015.

8. Wang SS. Aortic regurgitation clinical presentation. In: Lange RA, ed. Medscape. http://emedicine.medscape.com/article/150490-clinical. Updated February 12, 2014. Accessed April 10, 2015.

9. Barkley TW Jr. *Adult-Gerontology Primary Care Nurse Practitioner Certification Review/Clinical Update Continuing Education Course.* West Hollywood, CA: Barkley and Associates; 2015.

10. McPhee S, Papadakis M. *Current Medical Diagnosis and Treatment*. 51st ed. New York, NY: McGraw-Hill; 2012.

11. Types of heart failure. American Heart Association web site. http://www.heart.org/HEARTORG/Conditions/HeartFailure/AboutHeartFailure/Types-of-Heart-Failure_UCM_306323_Article.jsp. Reviewed August 20, 2012. Updated September 9, 2014. Accessed April 10, 2015.

12. Dargie HJ, McDonagh TA. Diagnosing heart failure. In: McDonagh TA, Gardner RS, Clark AL, Dargie HJ, eds. *Oxford Textbook of Heart Failure*. Oxford, UK: Oxford University Press; 2011: 171–176.

13. Yancy C, Jessup M, Bozkurt B, et al. 2013 ACCF/AHA guideline for the management of heart failure. *Circulation*. 2013; 128: e240–e327. doi: 10.1161/CIR.0b013e31829e8776

14. Heart failure. A.D.A.M. Medical Encyclopedia. http://www.ncbi.nlm.nih.gov/pubmedhealth/PMH0001211. Last updated June 11, 2014. Accessed April 10, 2015.

15. Heart failure. In: Porter RS, Kaplan JL, eds. The Merck Manual Online. http://www.merckmanuals.com/professional/cardiovascular_disorders/heart_failure/heart_failure_hf.html. Last reviewed September 2013. Accessed April 10, 2015.

16. Dumitru I, Baker MM. Heart failure overview. In: Ooi HH, ed. Medscape. http://emedicine.medscape.com/article/163062-overview#showall. Updated June 9, 2014. Accessed April 10, 2015.

17. Dumitru I, Baker MM. Heart failure workup. In: Ooi HH, ed. Medscape. http://emedicine.medscape.com/article/163062-workup#showall. Updated June 9, 2014. Accessed April 10, 2015.

18. U.S Department of Health and Human Services, National Institutes of Health (NIH), National Heart, Lung, and Blood Institute (NHLBI). How is angina diagnosed? http://www.nhlbi.nih.gov/health/health-topics/topics/angina/diagnosis.html. Updated June 1, 2011. Accessed April 10, 2015.

19. Colucci WS. Overview of the therapy of heart failure due to systolic dysfunction. In: Basow DS, ed. *UpToDate*. Waltham, MA: UpToDate; 2015. http://www.uptodate.com/contents/overview-of-the-therapy-of-heart-failure-due-to-systolic-dysfunction. Last updated October 29, 2014. Accessed April 10, 2015.

20. James PA, Oparil S, Carter BL, et al. 2014 evidence-based guideline for the management of high blood pressure in adults: Report from the panel members appointed to the Eighth Joint National Committee (JNC 8). *JAMA*. 2014; 311(5): 507–520.

21. Basile J, Bloch MJ. Overview of hypertension in adults. In: Basow DS, ed. *UpToDate*. Waltham, MA: UpToDate; 2015. http://www.uptodate.com/contents/overview-of-hypertension-in-adults. Last updated November 18, 2014. Accessed April 10, 2015.

22. Madhur MS, Riaz K, Dreisbach AW, Harrison DG. Hypertension. In: Maron DJ, ed. Medscape. http://emedicine.medscape.com/article/241381-overview. Updated September 30, 2014. Accessed April 10, 2015.

23. High blood pressure. A.D.A.M. Medical Encyclopedia. http://www.nlm.nih.gov/medlineplus/ency/article/000468.htm. Updated May 13, 2014. Accessed April 10, 2015.

24. Overview of hypertension. In: Porter RS, Kaplan JL, eds. The Merck Manual Online. http://www.merckmanuals.com/professional/cardiovascular_disorders/hypertension/overview_of_hypertension.html. Last reviewed May 2014. Accessed April 10, 2015.

25. Stamm JA, Risbano MG, Mathier MA. Overview of current therapeutic approaches for pulmonary hypertension. *Pulm Circ*. 2011; 1(2): 138–159. doi: 10.4103/2045-8932.83444

26. Physical activity and blood pressure. American Heart Association web site. http://www.heart.org/HEARTORG/Conditions/HighBloodPressure/PreventionTreatmentofHighBloodPressure/Physical-Activity-and-Blood-Pressure_UCM_301882_Article.jsp. Last reviewed August 4, 2014. Updated August 14, 2014. Accessed April 10, 2015.

27. Eckel RH, Jakicic JM, Ard JD, et al. 2013 AHA/ACC guideline on lifestyle management to reduce cardiovascular risk. *Circulation*. 2014; 129 (25 Suppl 2): S76–S99. doi: 10.1161/01.cir.0000437740.48606.d1

28. Barkley TW Jr, Miley H, Fellin R. Hypertension. In: Barkley TW Jr, Myers CM, ed. *Practice Considerations for Adult-Gerontological Acute Care Nurse Practitioner*. West Hollywood, CA: Barkley and Associates; 2015: 100–110.

29. Hopkins C. Hypertensive emergencies. In: Brown DFM, ed. Medscape. http://emedicine.medscape.com/article/1952052-overview#showall. Updated April 2, 2013. Accessed April 10, 2015.

30. Varon J, Elliott WJ. Management of severe asymptomatic hypertension (hypertensive urgencies) in adults. In: Basow DS, ed. *UpToDate*. Waltham, MA: UpToDate; 2015. http://www.uptodate.com/contents/management-of-severe-asymptomatic-hypertension-hypertensive-urgencies-in-adults. Last updated May 6, 2014. Accessed April 10, 2015.

31. Bisognano JD. Malignant hypertension. In: Batuman V, ed. Medscape. http://emedicine.med scape.com/article/241640-overview. Updated September 19, 2014. Accessed April 10, 2015.

32. Mayo Clinic Staff. What's a hypertensive crisis? If I notice a spike in my blood pressure, what should I do? Mayo Clinic web site. http://www.mayoclinic.org/diseases-conditions/high-blood-pressure/expert-answers/hypertensive-crisis/FAQ-20058491. Reviewed August 5, 2014. Accessed April 10, 2015.

33. Alaeddini J, Shirani J. Angina pectoris overview. In: Yang EH, ed. Medscape. http://emedicine.medscape.com/article/150215-overview#showall. Updated March 27, 2014. Accessed April 10, 2015.

34. Overview of coronary artery disease. In: Porter RS, Kaplan JL, eds. The Merck Manual Online. http://www.merckmanuals.com/professional/cardiovascular_disorders/coronary_artery_disease/overview_of_coronary_artery_disease.html. Last reviewed May 2013. Accessed April 10, 2015.

35. Stable angina. A.D.A.M. Medical Encyclopedia. http://www.nlm.nih.gov/medlineplus/ency/article/000198.htm. Updated May 13, 2014. Accessed April 10, 2015.

36. Mayo Clinic Staff. Angina - symptoms. Mayo Clinic web site. http://www.mayoclinic.com/health/angina/DS00994/DSECTION=symptoms. Reviewed February 3, 2015. Accessed April 10, 2015.

37. Unstable angina. A.D.A.M. Medical Encyclopedia. http://www.nlm.nih.gov/medlineplus/ency/article/000201.htm. Updated May 13, 2014. Accessed April 10, 2015.

38. Pinto DS, Beltrame JF, Crea F. (2013). Variant angina. In: Basow DS, ed. *UpToDate*. Waltham, MA: UpToDate; 2015. http://www.uptodate.com/contents/variant-angina. Last updated February 9, 2015. Accessed April 10, 2015.

39. Microvascular angina. American Heart Association web site. http://www.heart.org/HEARTORG/Conditions/HeartAttack/SymptomsDiagnosisofHeartAttack/Microvascular-Angina_UCM_450313_Article.jsp. Updated March 19, 2013. Accessed April 10, 2015.

40. U.S. Department of Health and Human Services, NIH, NHLBI. What are the signs and symptoms of angina? http://www.nhlbi.nih.gov/health/health-topics/topics/angina/signs.html. Updated June 1, 2011. Accessed April 10, 2015.

41. U.S Department of Health and Human Services, NIH, NHLBI. How is angina diagnosed? http://www.nhlbi.nih.gov/health/health-topics/topics/angina/diagnosis.html. Updated June 1, 2011. Accessed April 10, 2015.

42. Alaeddini J, Shirani J. Angina pectoris workup. In: Yang EH, ed. Medscape. http://emedicine.medscape.com/article/150215-workup#showall. Updated March 27, 2014. Accessed April 10, 2015.

43. Kannam JP, Aroesty JM, Gersh BJ. Stable ischemic heart disease: Overview of care. In: Basow DS, ed. *UpToDate*. Waltham, MA: UpToDate; 2015. http://www.uptodate.com/contents/stable-ischemic-heart-disease-overview-of-care. Last updated August 12, 2014. Accessed April 10, 2015.

44. Living with heart disease and angina. A.D.A.M. Medical Encyclopedia. http://www.nlm.nih.gov/medlineplus/ency/patientinstructions/000576.htm. Updated July 12, 2012. Accessed April 10, 2015.

45. Angina pectoris. In: Porter RS, Kaplan JL, eds. The Merck Manual Online. http://www.merckmanuals.com/professional/cardiovascular_disorders/coronary_artery_disease/angina_pectoris.html?qt=angina%20pectoris&alt=sh. Last reviewed May 2013. Accessed April 10, 2015.

46. Zafari AM, Reddy SV, Jeroudi AM, Garas SM. Myocardial infarction overview. In: Yang EH, ed. Medscape. http://emedicine.medscape.com/article/155919-overview#showall. Updated April 1, 2015. Accessed April 10, 2015.

47. Heart attack. A.D.A.M. Medical Encyclopedia. http://www.ncbi.nlm.nih.gov/pubmedhealth/PMH0001246. Updated June 11, 2014. Accessed April 10, 2015.

48. Bolooki HM, Askari A. Acute myocardial infarction. Cleveland Clinic Center for Continuing Education web site. http://www.clevelandclinicmeded.com/medicalpubs/diseasemanagement/cardiology/acute-myocardial-infarction. Published August 2010. Accessed April 10, 2015.

49. Zafari AM, Reddy SV, Jeroudi AM, Garas SM. Myocardial infarction clinical presentation. In: Yang EH, ed. Medscape. http://emedicine.medscape.com/article/155919-clinical#showall. Updated April 1, 2015. Accessed April 10, 2015.

50. Zafari AM, Reddy SV, Jeroudi AM, Garas SM. Myocardial infarction workup. In: Yang EH, ed. Medscape. http://emedicine.medscape.com/article/155919-workup#showall. Updated April 1, 2015. Accessed April 10, 2015.

51. Reeder GS, Kennedy HL. Criteria for the diagnosis of acute myocardial infarction. In: Basow DS, ed. *UpToDate*. Waltham, MA: UpToDate; 2015. http://www.uptodate.com/contents/criteria-for-the-diagnosis-of-acute-myocardial-infarction. Last updated July 1, 2014. Accessed April 10, 2015.

52. Reeder GS, Awtry E, Mahler SA. Initial evaluation and management of suspected acute coronary syndrome (myocardial infarction, unstable angina) in the emergency department. In: Basow DS, ed. *UpToDate*. Waltham, MA: UpToDate; 2015. http://www.uptodate.com/contents/initial-evaluation-and-management-of-suspected-acute-coronary-syndrome-myocardial-infarction-unstable-angina-in-the-emergency-department?source=see_link. Last updated March 18, 2014. Accessed July 7, 2015.

53. Bauer KA, Lip GYH. Overview of the causes of venous thrombosis. In: Basow DS, ed. *UpToDate*. Waltham, MA: UpToDate; 2015. http://www.uptodate.com/contents/overview-of-the-causes-of-venous-thrombosis. Last updated January 30, 2015. Accessed April 10, 2015.

54. Superficial venous thrombosis. In: Porter RS, Kaplan JL, eds. The Merck Manual Online. http://www.merckmanuals.com/professional/cardiovascular_disorders/peripheral_venous_disorders/superficial_venous_thrombosis.html. Last revised May 2014. Accessed April 10, 2015.

55. Fernandez L, Scovell S. Superficial thrombophlebitis of the lower extremity. In: Basow DS, ed. *UpToDate*. Waltham, MA: UpToDate; 2015. http://www.uptodate.com/contents/superficial-thrombophlebitis-of-the-lower-extremity. Last updated November 3, 2014. Accessed April 10, 2015.

56. Superficial thrombophlebitis. A.D.A.M. Medical Encyclopedia. http://www.nlm.nih.gov/medlineplus/ency/article/000199.htm. Updated May 27, 2014. Accessed April 10, 2015.

57. Klever RG, Doss R, Rosh AJ. Superficial thrombophlebitis. In: Rowe VL, ed. Medscape. http://emedicine.medscape.com/article/463256-overview. Updated April 21, 2014. Accessed April 10, 2015.

58. Deep venous thrombosis. A.D.A.M. Medical Encyclopedia. http://www.nlm.nih.gov/medlineplus/ency/article/000156.htm. Updated February 24, 2014. Accessed April 10, 2015.

59. Patel K, Chun LJ. Deep venous thrombosis clinical presentation. In: Brenner BE, ed. Medscape. http://emedicine.medscape.com/article/1911303-clinical#showall. Updated August 28, 2014. Accessed April 10, 2015.

60. Callahan MJ. Musculoskeletal ultrasonography of the lower extremities in infants and children. *Pediatr Radiol*. 2013; 43(Suppl1): S8–S22. doi: 10.1007/s00247-012-2589-6

61. Grant BJB. Diagnosis of suspected deep vein thrombosis of the lower extremity. In: Basow DS, ed. *UpToDate*. Waltham, MA: UpToDate; 2015. http://www.uptodate.com/contents/diagnosis-of-suspected-deep-vein-thrombosis-of-the-lower-extremity. Last updated February 2, 2015. Accessed April 10, 2015.

62. Patel K, Chun LJ. Deep venous thrombosis workup. In: Brenner BE, ed. Medscape. http://emedicine.medscape.com/article/1911303-workup#showall. Updated August 28, 2014. Accessed April 10, 2015.

63. Patel K, Chun LJ. Deep venous thrombosis treatment & management. In: Brenner BE, ed. Medscape. http://emedicine.medscape.com/article/1911303-treatment#aw2aab6b6b2. Updated August 28, 2014. Accessed April 10, 2015.

64. Lip GYH, Hull RD. Overview of the treatment of lower extremity deep vein thrombosis. In: Basow DS, ed. *UpToDate*. Waltham, MA: UpToDate; 2015. http://www.uptodate.com/contents/overview-of-the-treatment-of-lower-extremity-deep-vein-thrombosis-dvt. Last updated March 4, 2015. Accessed April 10, 2015.

65. Mayo Clinic Staff. Peripheral artery disease (PAD). Mayo Clinic web site. http://www.mayoclinic.org/diseases-conditions/peripheral-artery-disease/basics/risk-factors/con-20028731. Reviewed June 22, 2012. Accessed April 10, 2015.

66. Stephens E. Peripheral vascular disease presentation. In: Brown DFM, ed. Medscape. http://emedicine.medscape.com/article/761556-clinical#showall. Updated May 7, 2014. Accessed April 10, 2015.

67. Peripheral arterial disease. In: Porter RS, Kaplan JL, eds. The Merck Manual Online. http://www.merckmanuals.com/professional/cardiovascular_disorders/peripheral_arterial_disorders/peripheral_arterial_disease.html?qt=peripheral%20vascular%20disease&alt=sh. Last reviewed May 2014. Accessed April 10, 2015.

68. Peripheral artery disease. A.D.A.M. Medical Encyclopedia. http://www.ncbi.nlm.nih.gov/pubmedhealth/PMH0001223. Updated June 11, 2014. Accessed April 10, 2015.

69. Cleveland Clinic Staff. Chronic venous insufficiency (CVI). Cleveland Clinic web site. http://my.clevelandclinic.org/disorders/venous_insufficiency/hvi_chronic_venous_insufficiency.aspx. Reviewed December 2010. Accessed April 10, 2015.

70. Weiss R, Izaguirre DE, Lanza J, Lessnau K-D. Venous insufficiency. In: James WD, ed. Medscape. http://emedicine.medscape.com/article/1085412-overview. Updated October 1, 2014. Accessed April 10, 2015.

71. Weiss R, Izaguirre DE, Lanza J, Lessnau K-D. Venous insufficiency clinical presentation. In: James WD, ed. Medscape. http://emedicine.medscape.com/article/1085412-clinical. Updated October 1, 2014. Accessed April 10, 2015.

72. Obermayer A, Garzon K. Identifying the source of superficial reflux in venous leg ulcers using duplex ultrasound. *J Vasc Surg*. 2010; 52(5): 1255–1261. doi: 10.1016/j.jvs.2010.06.073

73. Venous insufficiency. A.D.A.M. Medical Encyclopedia. http://www.nlm.nih.gov/medlineplus/ency/article/000203.htm. Updated May 27, 2014. Accessed April 10, 2015.

Chapter 15

Evidence-Based Practice and Health Care Policy/Issues

QUESTIONS

1. With regard to the Culturally and Linguistically Appropriate Services initiative, which of the following statements regarding health care organizations best defines Standard 5?

   a. Language assistance services, which include bilingual staff and interpreters, must be offered or provided at no cost to patients and consumers who have limited English proficiency.

   b. Healthcare organizations must assure the competency of interpreters and bilingual staff to provide language assistance to patients and consumers with limited English proficiency.

   c. Family and friends should not be used to provide language assistance to patients and consumers with limited English proficiency unless upon request.

   d. Both verbal and written notices must be provided to patients and consumers informing them of their rights to receive language assistance services.

2. Which of the following settings does not typically allow incident-to billing by the nurse practitioner?

   a. Hospitals

   b. Physicians' offices

   c. Home visits

   d. Clinics

3. To qualify as a Medicare provider, a nurse practitioner is usually required to possess all of the following qualifications except:

   a. Master of Science in Nursing or higher degree

   b. Hospital privileges for Advanced Practice Nurses

   c. Certification as a nurse practitioner by a recognized national certifying body

   d. License in the state in which he or she intends to practice

4. In most states, which of the following conditions is not required to be reported by the nurse practitioner to the Department of Health and Human Services?

   a. Chlamydia

   b. Herpes

   c. Tuberculosis

   d. HIV

5. You are a part of a task team charged with evaluating the quality of health care in everyday practice. Since you round on your primary care patients at a community hospital, to accomplish this task, you choose to apply the standards of Quality Improvement, Quality Assurance, and Continuous Process Improvement. These standards would best identify all of the following indicators related to aspects of care <u>except</u>:

a. Establishing thresholds for evaluation

b. Collecting data to identify problems in health care delivery

c. Ensuring that nurses maintain proper licensing

d. Assessing the effectiveness of clinical documentation

6. You are treating Henry, a 21-year-old male diagnosed with anxiety disorder. The patient complains of experiencing panic attacks while attending his college classes and admits to dreading the approaching date of graduation, saying that he is worried about finding a job. In an effort to promote effective therapeutic communication, which of these statements would be best suited for this patient?

a. "Why do you feel anxious about your studies?"

b. "Tell me more about the things that trigger your panic attacks."

c. "It is unusual that someone so young should feel so anxious about his career prospects."

d. "I am concerned that avoidance of anxiety-provoking situations may do more harm than good."

7. To eliminate racial and ethnic disparities in health care, the guidelines of the Culturally and Linguistically Appropriate Services initiative implement all of the following standards <u>except</u>:

a. Healthcare organizations must inform patients of their rights to receive language assistance services.

b. Healthcare organizations must provide language assistance services, including bilingual staff and interpreter services, at no cost to patients with limited English proficiency.

c. Healthcare organizations must ensure that language assistance services are provided at all points of contact in a timely manner during all hours of operation.

d. Healthcare organizations must always rely on qualified interpreters and bilingual staff, and never rely on the patient's family and friends to provide interpretation services even if requested by the patient or consumer.

8. According to Title II of the Health Insurance Portability and Accountability Act, which of the following is protected by the confidentiality provisions of the Patient Safety Rule?

a. Privacy of individually identifiable health information

b. Security of electronic health records

c. Health insurance coverage for workers when they change or lose their jobs

d. Use of identifiable information to analyze patient safety events and improve patient safety

9. What is the aim of Title I of the Health Insurance Portability and Accountability Act?

a. Establishment of national standards for electronic health care transactions

b. Protection of identifiable information being used to analyze patient safety events and improve patient safety

c. Protection of health insurance coverage for workers and their families should they change or lose their jobs

d. Protection of the privacy of individually identifiable health information

10. Which of the following is <u>not</u> typically considered one of the seven key principles governing ethical conduct for nurse practitioners?

    a. Fidelity

    b. Veracity

    c. Justice

    d. Integrity

11. A male patient diagnosed with depression threatens to kill himself. To keep the patient from harming himself, the nurse practitioner may legally perform all of the following actions <u>except</u>:

    a. Order medication to incapacitate the patient to prevent him from harming himself.

    b. Immediately restrain the patient without informing other staff.

    c. Restrain the patient with a reasonable amount of properly checked restraints.

    d. Temporarily commit the patient, then transfer him to care of his relatives regardless of mental state.

12. What is the primary purpose of professional licensure?

    a. To ensure a minimal standard for competency

    b. To ensure high nursing care standards

    c. To standardize nursing programs

    d. To grant prescriptive priority

13. Which of these scenarios best describes the primary component of malpractice?

    a. A nurse practitioner lets slip about a patient's history of gonorrhea, damaging his reputation in the community.

    b. A nurse practitioner acts hastily in treating an aneurysm, resulting in otherwise avoidable partial paralysis.

    c. A nurse practitioner notices symptoms of syphilis but does not work to diagnose or treat the underlying condition, resulting in central nervous system damage.

    d. A nurse practitioner aims to subdue an unruly patient by striking them in the face with a closed fist.

14. Which of these is covered under the auspices of the Danforth Amendment?

    a. A patient's continuity of health care coverage should he or she change jobs

    b. A nurse practitioner's (NP) level of prescriptive authority

    c. A patient's right to refuse care when admitted to a federally-funded institution

    d. An NP's protection from lawsuits when intervening at the site of an accident

15. You are writing a manuscript about an unsolved medical case in which the patient was being treated for heartburn and unexpectedly died. Which of the following would best describe this type of research?

    a. Cross-sectional

    b. Longitudinal

    c. Cohort

    d. Qualitative

16. The Privacy Rule of the Health Insurance Portability and Accountability Act establishes that a patient whose rights are being denied or whose health information is not being protected can file complaints with certain entities. Which of the following is <u>not</u> one of these entities?

    a. Health insurers

    b. Healthcare providers

    c. U.S. government

    d. State agencies

17. You are performing a research study to determine the effects of smoking. You collect data from two sample groups. The first group consists of smokers between the ages of 21 and 45, and the second group consists of smokers between the ages of 65 and 80. Given only this information, which type of research does this study best exemplify?

    a. Experimental

    b. Longitudinal

    c. Cross-sectional

    d. Qualitative

18. What purpose does Cronbach's alpha typically serve in a statistical research analysis?

    a. Measures the differences in means between two groups

    b. Computes the probability of false rejection of the null hypothesis in a statistical test

    c. Finds and measures the interdependence of two random variables which ranges in value from -1 to +1

    d. Determines correlation of values in a survey instrument to assess its reliability

19. A male patient who was admitted to the hospital is diagnosed with a highly contagious, viral illness that could be fatal and potentially cause an epidemic. The decision to keep him in isolation and limit the number of health care providers who come into contact with him would most closely demonstrate which ethical principle?

    a. Nonmaleficence

    b. Beneficence

    c. Utilitarianism

    d. Autonomy

20. Which of the following best delineates the degree to which a nurse practitioner may prescribe medication to patients?

    a. Nurse Practice Acts

    b. Standards of Care

    c. The Health Insurance Portability and Accountability Act

    d. The Patient Safety and Quality Improvement Act

21. Which of these entities is required to comply with HIPAA guidelines?

    a. Law enforcement agencies

    b. Property insurance companies

    c. Value-added networks

    d. Employers

22. James, a 52-year-old male, has just fallen into a diabetic coma. Robert, his domestic partner, arrives at the hospital with a living will from James regarding these particular circumstances. Which component of this will would grant it the strongest standing?

    a. The will outlines that James wishes not to be resuscitated if he is "seriously incapacitated."

    b. The will is preserved as an audio recording without written backup.

    c. The will describes actions to take if James ends up incapacitated by a car crash or stroke, with no specific mention of diabetic coma.

    d. The will names Robert as proxy and grants him authority to do "as he sees fit" in maintaining James's care.

23. Power of attorney must usually meet which of the following criteria before it will be honored by most institutions?

    a. The document must detail the patient's current medical condition.

    b. The document must specify a patient's intent regarding medical treatment.

    c. The document must outline that authority only be granted to a significant other.

    d. The document must form a part of the patient's health care directive.

24. Which of the following is the standard purpose of a t-test?

    a. To measure the average amount of deviation of values from the mean

    b. To measure the interdependence of two random variables which ranges in value from -1 to +1

    c. To evaluate the differences in means between two groups

    d. To determine the limited range in which the interval being measured will most likely fall

25. A nurse practitioner (NP) learns that a female patient's injuries stem from a case of domestic violence involving an argument between the patient and her husband. In accordance with mandatory reporting statutes established in most states, which of the following legal steps should the NP take in this case?

    a. Report the case of domestic violence to the police

    b. Notify the Department of Health and Human Services

    c. Admit the patient for hospital care to prevent further harm from happening

    d. There is no legal obligation to do anything

26. Which of the following actions is not an example of assault, as defined by the literature?

    a. Angrily striking a patient on the shoulder when he or she will not stand still

    b. Brandishing a scalpel and angrily gesturing towards a noncompliant patient

    c. Making the motion to inject a patient against his or her will

    d. Telling a patient, "Sit still and wait, or I will have to have you restrained."

27. Which of the following laws sets national standards for the security of electronic protected health information?

    a. Patient Self Determination Act

    b. Patient Safety and Quality Improvement Act

    c. Health Insurance Portability and Accountability Act

    d. Comprehensive Omnibus Reconciliation Act

28. Respect and spiritual needs are considered components of which of the following principles that the nurse practitioner must often consider in therapeutic communication with a patient?

    a. Cultural competency

    b. Non-judgmental approach

    c. Mutual trust

    d. Confidentiality

29. Which of these statements is true regarding licensure?

    a. It is a voluntary process that acknowledges an individual's mastery of a given skill.

    b. It is acquired through rules and regulations established by a governmental body.

    c. It grants authority to provide services within a given facility.

    d. It evaluates and confirms the qualifications of an NP.

30. In the course of your research study, you determine the measure of the interdependence of two random variables to be -1. What research term best describes this value?

    a. High standard deviation

    b. Low validity

    c. Small confidence interval

    d. Negative correlation

31. What percentage of the patient's bill for physician services is typically covered by Medicare?

    a. 70%

    b. 80%

    c. 85%

    d. 100%

32. The patient safety work product often contains which of the following?

    a. A certified statement of a patient's intent regarding safe medical treatment

    b. Specific findings, procedures, and management methods recorded during a patient safety event

    c. Official documentation regarding the safe and life-prolonging measures that a patient either wants or does not want to be taken if he or she becomes incapacitated

    d. Specifications that outline the requirements for nurse practitioners to report specific health-related information

33. You are treating a patient who has been recently diagnosed with diabetes after undergoing a screening for the condition due to health concerns in the patient's medical history and recent health issues. A cost-effective, quality plan of care that involves monitoring patient progress is developed for the patient. You educate the patient regarding management of the condition prior to implementing that plan. Which process of health care does this scenario most closely resemble?

    a. Quality assurance

    b. Collaborative practice

    c. Continuous quality improvement

    d. Case management

34. For home nurse practitioner (NP) visits billable for Medicare B services, an NP usually does not need a physician's order to bill under the NP's own provider number <u>unless</u>:

    a. The NP and a physician see a patient on the same day.

    b. The NP is billing for an assistant's work.

    c. Services are provided under a physician's direct personal supervision.

    d. The NP is providing nursing services exclusively.

35. What agency or organization enforces the protections safeguarded by the Health Insurance Portability and Accountability Act?

    a. The Office for Civil Rights

    b. U.S. Department of Health and Human Services

    c. The American Medical Association

    d. The Agency for Healthcare Research and Quality

36. A care map identifies all of the following points relevant to the management of a condition <u>except</u>:

    a. Guidelines for planning and managing care delivered by all disciplines

    b. Life-prolonging measures requested by the patient if he or she becomes incapacitated

    c. Common patient-related issues of a specific case type

    d. Day-to-day goals that the patient must achieve, as well as the final desired clinical outcomes

37. A group of researchers are conducting a study that examines insomnia patterns in two groups of males between 20 and 30 years of age. One group consists of subjects that are enrolled in college; the other group contains subjects that are not enrolled in college or any other type of educational institution. What type of research does this study best describe?

    a. Cross-sectional

    b. Cohort

    c. Longitudinal

    d. Qualitative

38. In states that recognize living wills, what condition must be met so that the will is legally recognized?

    a. It must incorporate a written statement of a patient's intent regarding medical treatment.

    b. It must contain specifications regarding durable power of attorney in one or two separate documents.

    c. The will must contain a provision addressing privacy of individually identifiable health information.

    d. The will must be specific enough and address the problem at hand.

39. Which plan of Medicare not only offers coverage for prescriptions but also requires a copay for each as well as a monthly premium?

    a. Medicare A

    b. Medicare B

    c. Medicare C

    d. Medicare D

40. Which scenario most effectively demonstrates a case of negligence?

   a. A nurse practitioner (NP) speeds through the preparation of an intravenous drip, resulting in air bubbles entering the patient's blood stream.

   b. A NP threatens an unruly patient, telling him that if he does not behave, she will "have an orderly wrestle you to the ground."

   c. An elderly patient, who is unable to hear well, is struck by an NP because the patient could not hear the NP's instructions.

   d. An NP waits to administer anticonvulsants to a patient experiencing multiple prolonged, unprovoked seizures, in order to "see if they stop on their own."

RATIONALES

1. d

Standard 5 of the Culturally and Linguistically Appropriate Services (CLAS) initiative requires health care organizations to provide both verbal and written notices to patients with limited English proficiency of their right to receive language assistance services. Standard 4 of CLAS requires that these language assistance services should be provided at no cost to patients and consumers. Standard 6 requires health care organizations to assure the competency of interpreters and bilingual staff, and also states that family and friends of patients or consumers should not be used to provide language assistance services unless upon request.

2. a

Incident-to billing is not allowed in the hospital setting, in which case a nurse practitioner (NP) must bill under his or her provider number. Physicians' offices and clinics are common settings for services often covered under incident-to billing. Home visits billable for Medicare B services also allow for incident-to billing, since the NP does not need a physician's order to bill under his or her provider number unless he or she is providing nursing services exclusively.

3. b

Holding hospital privileges for Advanced Practice Nurses is not usually required for a nurse practitioner (NP) to qualify as a Medicare provider. An NP must typically hold a license in the state in which he or she intends to practice, be certified as an NP by a recognized national certifying body, and hold at least a Master of Science in nursing to qualify as a Medicare provider.

4. b

In most U.S. states, nurse practitioners (NPs) are not required to report diagnoses of herpes to the Department of Health and Human Services. However, many states do require NPs to report a diagnosis of gonorrhea, chlamydia, syphilis, HIV, or tuberculosis.

5. c

Ensuring that registered nurses are properly licensed is a task carried out by the boards of nursing. In the process of identifying indicators related to aspects of health care, management systems such as Quality Assurance, Quality Improvement, and Continuous Process Improvement recommend collecting and organizing data related to the quality of health care, establishing thresholds for evaluation, and assessing the effectiveness of document improvement.

6. b

Effective therapeutic communication presupposes that the nurse practitioner (NP) will listen more than talk. Thus, the NP is advised to make encouraging statements that may begin with "Tell me…" On the other hand, the NP should avoid "why" questions, which call for justification and tend to put the patient on the defensive. Likewise, expressing incredulity about the patient's anxiety over career and education signals a dismissive and judgmental attitude, which should be avoided in therapeutic communication. Lastly, euphemisms and indirect language should be avoided.

7. d

Although Standard 6 of the Culturally and Linguistically Appropriate Services (CLAS) initiative requires health care organizations to use qualified interpreters and bilingual staff to assure the competence of language assistance, the patient may request language interpretation services from family and friends rather than interpreters or bilingual staff. CLAS Standards provide mandates and guidelines for health care organizations that aim to inform patients of their rights to receive language assistance services, to provide language assistance services at no cost to patients with limited English proficiency, and to ensure that language assistance services are provided at all points of contact in a timely manner during all hours of operation.

8. d

Confidentiality provisions under Title II of the Patient Safety Rule of the Health Insurance Portability and Accountability Act (HIPAA) work to protect identifiable information being used to analyze patient safety events. Title II of HIPAA also covers the privacy of individually identifiable health information, as well as national standards for the security of electronically protected health information; these standards are specifically outlined by the HIPAA Security Rule. Title I of HIPAA protects health insurance coverage for workers when they change or lose jobs.

9. c

Title I of the Health Insurance Portability and Accountability Act protects health insurance coverage for workers and their families when they change or lose their jobs. Protection of the privacy of individually identifiable health information, establishment of national standards for electronic health care transactions, and protection of identifiable information being used to analyze patient safety events and improve patient safety are covered under Title II, not Title I.

10. d

Integrity is not typically considered one of the key ethical principles that govern the conduct of nurse practitioners. The typical key ethical principles for governing conduct include nonmaleficence, utilitarianism, beneficence, justice, fidelity, veracity, and autonomy.

11. d

In most states, a nurse practitioner (NP) has a duty to commit someone who is in danger of hurting himself or others as a result of mental illness, and may be held liable if the patient is discharged while still in danger of doing so. Under most circumstances, an NP may legally subdue a mentally ill patient in danger of harming himself through drugs or proper restraints; although the course of intervention will likely need to be documented later, immediately telling other staff of the intended course of action is not necessary if time is of the essence.

12. a

The primary purpose of professional licensure is to ensure that a nurse practitioner (NP) is qualified to perform the roles associated with his or her duty, thus protecting the public by ensuring a minimum standard for competency. The standards of advanced practice aim to provide a standardized measure for nursing programs across the country, whereas credentialing works to establish the minimal levels of acceptable performance for NPs. Prescriptive authority is independent of licensure and is typically determined by state practice acts.

13. b

The core component of malpractice is failing to render services with the degree of care, diligence, and precaution that another practitioner would render under similar circumstances; therefore, an incident in which hasty action results in permanent damage to the patient would best embody malpractice. Failure to act in a reasonable fashion, resulting in injury to the patient, would better define negligence. Releasing a patient's medical records and damaging their reputation falls under defamation, whereas striking a patient or objects on his or her person would count as battery.

14. c

The Danforth Amendment outlines how patients admitted to a federally-funded institution, such as a hospital or nursing home, should be advised of their right to refuse care. A nurse practitioner's (NP) prescriptive authority is typically delineated by state practice acts, whereas Good Samaritan statutes provide protection from lawsuits to NPs who intervene at the scene of an accident. The Comprehensive Omnibus Reconciliation Act (COBRA) seeks to protect a patient's health care when he or she loses or changes jobs.

15. d

A manuscript focusing on a specific case or a small group of cases would best qualify as a case study, which is considered a qualitative type of research. Other types of qualitative studies may include open-ended questioning, field studies, and ethnographic studies. Cross-sectional research assesses the relationship between variables at a specific point in time by examining a population with a very similar attribute that differs in one specific variable. Longitudinal studies aim to find the relationship between variables by taking multiple measures of a group or population over an extended period of time. Lastly, cohort research studies compare a particular outcome in groups of individuals who are alike in many ways but differ in a certain characteristic.

16. d

According to the Privacy Rule of the Health Insurance Portability and Accountability Act (HIPAA), a patient whose rights are being denied or whose health care information is not being protected would not usually need to file a complaint with a state agency; in fact, many state agencies are not required to follow HIPAA. The Privacy Rule of HIPAA allows a patient to file complaints with his or her health care provider, his or her health insurer, or the U.S. government.

17. c

Cross-sectional research seeks to find the relationship between variables by examining a population with a very similar attribute but differs in one specific variable; in this case, both groups in the study are smokers, yet the specific variable that differentiates the two groups is age. Experimental research studies typically involve more than one specific variable, as well as experimental manipulation of variables and a control group to test the effects of an experiment. Longitudinal research studies usually involve taking multiple measures of a group or population over an extended period of time to find relationships between variables. Lastly, qualitative research often takes into account a number of studies in which observations and interview techniques are used to explore phenomena.

18. d

Cronbach's alpha is used to compute correlation of values among questions on a survey instrument to assess its reliability. The probability of a false rejection of the null hypothesis in a statistical test, on the other hand, refers to the level of significance. A measure of the interdependence of two random variables that ranges in value from -1 to +1 is known as perfect correlation. Lastly, the differences in means between two groups is measured by the t-test.

19. c

Utilitarianism is the belief that the right act is the one that produces the greatest good for the greatest number of people. The decision to isolate a patient diagnosed with a highly contagious, viral illness that could be fatal and potentially cause an epidemic, as well as limiting the personnel seeing the patient, most closely adheres to the principles of utilitarianism. This case neither reflects the ethical principle of nonmaleficence, which is the duty to do no harm, nor does it reflect the principle of autonomy, which is the duty to respect an individual's thoughts and actions. Beneficence is the duty to prevent harm and promote good. Although this case may reflect a duty to prevent harm, the decision to isolate the patient to prevent a potential epidemic is one that produces the greatest good for the greatest number of people.

20. a

The extent to which nurse practitioners (NPs) may prescribe medication usually depends on each state's respective Nurse Practice Act. Usually, guidelines establishing the NPs' role in prescribing medication to patients are neither defined by Standards of Care, which establish a process for evaluating quality assurance, nor by the Health Insurance Portability and Accountability Act, which protects health insurance coverage for workers and their families. The Patient Safety and Quality Improvement Act seeks to establish a voluntary reporting system to enhance the data available to assess and resolve patient safety and health care quality issues.

21. c

Value-added networks and other health care clearinghouses are covered entities under the Health Insurance Portability and Accountability Act (HIPAA) and are required to follow all guidelines of the act. Property insurance companies, state agencies, and employers may hold patient personal information, but are not required to comply with HIPAA guidelines.

22. d

Living wills typically grant durable power of attorney to a significant other to serve as the patient's proxy and articulate his or her advance care directive; although the course of this particular directive is left in the hands of the proxy, it would still be relatively valid. A living will may run into trouble if it does not specifically address the problem at hand or uses uncertain terminology such as "seriously incapacitated," which may be interpreted differently between different practitioners. A living will granting power of attorney must usually be in writing, meaning one that only exists as an audio recording may not be considered valid.

23. d

Power of attorney may be incorporated into a health care directive, which is a type of advance directive that may also include a living will. Most institutions recognize living wills as long as they are specific and address the current issue, without necessarily applying the same requirement to power of attorney documents. Although power of attorney is frequently granted to a significant other, this specification is not necessary for power of attorney to be honored by institutions. Lastly, a patient's intent regarding medical treatment is typically specified by an advance directive, not by power of attorney.

24. c

A t-test is a statistical test that evaluates the differences in means between two groups. A measure of the average amount of deviation of values from the mean, on the other hand, is known as standard deviation. The term for a measure of the interdependence of two random variables that ranges in value from -1 to +1 is perfect correlation. Lastly, a confidence interval establishes a range of values, with limits at either end, in which the parameter being measured will most likely fall.

25. d

In most states, a nurse practitioner (NP) is not legally required to report cases of domestic violence. Therefore, the NP is not legally obligated to report cases of domestic violence to the police, notify the Department of Health and Human Services, or detain the patient's husband to prevent him from further harming the patient.

26. a

Angrily grabbing a patient's shoulder when he or she will not stand still would typically be classified as battery, not assault, as it involves the willful, angry striking of a person. Assault is usually defined as an intentional act by a person that creates an apprehension in another person of an imminent harmful or offensive contact. Hence, threatening offensive contact to a patient awaiting care, using a scalpel to angrily gesture at a noncompliant patient, and making a motion to inject a person against his or her will are all standard examples of assault, rather than battery.

27. c

The Health Insurance Portability and Accountability Act sets national standards for the security of electronic protected health information. The Patient Self-Determination Act does not aim to protect information; rather, it requires hospitals to inform all patients of their right to execute an advance directive. The Patient Safety and Quality Improvement Act establishes a voluntary reporting system to enhance the data available to assess and resolve patient safety and health care quality issues. The Comprehensive Omnibus Reconciliation Act is federal legislation that protects health insurance coverage and allows employees to keep their information consistent while they change jobs and health plans.

28. a

In therapeutic communication between the nurse practitioner (NP) and a patient, respect and spiritual needs are considered two components of the principle of cultural competency. Although mutual trust, confidentiality, and a non-judgmental approach are important principles for an NP to follow in therapeutic communication with a patient, respect and spiritual needs are not subsumed under these principles.

29. b

Licensure, the accrediting and legitimizing of a nurse practitioner's (NP's) ability in a specific scope of practice, is achieved and maintained by following the rules and regulations laid out by a governmental body, such as a state board of nursing. Certification, on the other hand, is a voluntary process granted by nongovernmental agencies that acknowledges an NP's mastery in a certain skill within his or her practice area. Credentialing is the process of evaluating and confirming the qualifications of an NP, whereas privileging is the process of evaluating and confirming the qualifications of an NP.

30. d

A measure of the interdependence of two random variables is known as a perfect correlation, with a value of -1 indicating a negative correlation between the two variables. Standard deviation, on the other hand, determines the average amount of deviation of values from the mean. Low validity indicates a low degree of correspondence between a variable and what this variable is intended to measure. Lastly, a confidence interval does not measure the interdependence of two random variables, but designates an interval with a specific probability of including the parameter being estimated, with a small confidence interval implying a very precise range of values.

31. b

Medicare usually covers 80% of the patient's bill for physician services; the patient usually pays the remaining 20%. In regards to a procedure, Medicare can pay 80%–85% of the Physician Fee Schedule (PFS) rate, whereas incident-to billing can reimburse the physician 100% of the PFS. Under Medicare, prospective payment systems and skilled nursing facilities are paid 70% of a patient's bad debt.

32. b

Under the Patient Safety and Quality Improvement Act (PSQIA), information that is collected or created during a patient safety event, such as findings recorded or procedures or courses of management undertaken, is typically classified as a patient safety work product; this product is then covered under federal privilege and confidentiality protections meant to encourage the reporting of medical errors. A written statement of a patient's intent regarding medical treatment would be considered an advance directive. A living will, on the hand, is typically an official document specifying the life-prolonging measures that a patient either wants or does not want to be taken should the patient become incapacitated. The health-related information each nurse practitioner is required to report is often specified in his or her state's particular nursing statutes.

33. d

The scenario most closely resembles the process of case management, which utilizes a comprehensive, systematic approach to provide quality care by mobilizing, monitoring, and controlling patient resources during illness while balancing the quality and costs of these resources. The quality assurance process typically involves evaluating patient care according to established standards of care. Collaborative practice, on the other hand, exists to enhance the quality of care and improve patient outcomes. The process of continuous quality improvement often involves an environment in which management and staff strive to constantly improve quality health care.

34. d

The nurse practitioner (NP) would typically require a physician's order to bill home visits to the NP's own provider number if the NP is providing nursing services exclusively. Seeing a patient on the same day as a physician would require the NP to coordinate billing with the physician, but the NP would not necessarily be required to obtain a physician's order to bill under his or her own provider number. The rules of incident-to billing typically allow the NP to bill for an assistant's work and provide services under a physician's direct personal supervision; however, neither of these circumstances usually requires that the NP obtain a physician's order before billing.

35. a

The Office for Civil Rights enforces the protections safeguarded by the Health Insurance Portability and Accountability Act (HIPAA). Although the function of the Department of Health and Human Services (HHS) is to protect the health of all Americans and provide essential human services, it does not usually enforce the protections safeguarded by HIPAA. The HHS also encompasses the Agency for Healthcare Research and Quality, which contains listings of patient safety organizations that collect and analyze data regarding patient safety information. The American Medical Association is a professional organization associated with promoting the best interests of patients and physicians alike.

36. b

A care map does not typically identify life-prolonging measures requested by the patient if he or she becomes incapacitated; these life-prolonging measures would more often be outlined in a living will. The care map typically establishes guidelines for planning and managing care delivered by all disciplines, identifies common patient-related problems of a specific case type, and sets out day-to-day goals that the patient must achieve as well as the final desired clinical outcomes.

37. b

A cohort study compares a particular outcome in groups of individuals who share many characteristics but differ in a particular characteristic; in this case, the effects of insomnia are looked at in two separate groups of males in their 20s, with one group comprised of subjects attending college, while the other group is comprised of subjects not attending college or any other institution of higher learning. A cross-sectional study is designed to find relationships between different variables at a specific point in time by focusing on a population rather than a group of individuals. A longitudinal study involves taking multiple measures of a group or population over an extended period of time to find relationships between variables. Lastly, a qualitative study would not compare specific outcomes in groups of individuals; qualitative studies incorporate case studies, open-ended questions, field studies, participant observation, and ethnographic studies in which observations and interview techniques are used to explore phenomena through detailed descriptions of people, events, situations, or observed behavior.

38. d

Most states will recognize living wills that are specific enough and address the problem at hand. A written statement of a patient's intent regarding medical treatment, on the other hand, is more often defined as an advance directive. A health care directive typically includes a living will and specifications regarding durable power of attorney in one or two separate documents. Lastly, privacy of individually identifiable health information is not a required component of a living will; instead, it is protected by the Health Insurance Portability and Accountability Act.

39. d

Medicare D not only offers coverage for prescriptions but also requires a monthly premium and a co-pay for each prescription. Medicare A does not require a monthly premium, but it does require individuals to be 65 years of age in order to qualify. Medicare B recipients may have to pay a premium for supplemental medical insurance, but it does not place a limit on prescription drug coverage. Medicare C, also known as "Medicare Advantage," is available to patients enrolled in Medicare B who are also eligible for Medicare A.

40. d

Negligence often involves cases in which a nurse practitioner (NP) fails to do what a reasonable person would do, resulting in further injury to the patient; as such, an NP waiting to administer anticonvulsants to a seizing patient would qualify as negligence. Malpractice is considered a form of negligence, but usually centers on an active action by the NP that falls below the accepted standard of care, such as professional misconduct, demonstrating unreasonable lack of skill, or illegal or immoral conduct. Hence, a case where an NP's faulty preparation results in air bubbles entering the blood stream and would most closely resemble malpractice. Threatening to have another individual subdue a patient with brute force would most closely resemble assault, as the NP threatens the patient with bodily harm while possessing the apparent ability to do so. Battery, on the other hand, would most closely resemble a case involving an NP striking a patient, as the threat of harm to the patient is actually carried out.

DISCUSSION

Evidence-based Practice and Research Methods

Major Steps in the Research Process

Evidence-based practice is an interdisciplinary approach used to evaluate and incorporate published research into the clinical setting.

The initial step in conducting a research study is formulating a research question that addresses a particular problem or topic in need of further exploration. The researcher must review the preexisting literature related to the research problem and in cases of quantitative research designs, formulate a hypothesis. Decisions such as selecting the research design, identifying the population to be studied, specifying methods of data collection, and

Table 15.1	Types of research
Non-experimental	A "no experiment" design; usually includes two broad categories of research: descriptive and ex-post facto/correlational research. Includes: *Descriptive research*: aims to describe situations, experiences, and phenomena as they exist *Ex-post-facto (correlational) research*: examines relationships among variables
Cross-sectional[1]	Study of a population that has very similar attributes but differs by one specific variable (such as age); designed to find relationships between variables at a specific point in time or "surveys." Example: observing the population a small mining town and examining the prevalence of respiratory diseases
Cohort[2]	A research study that compares a particular outcome (such as lung cancer) in groups of individuals who are alike in many ways but differ by a certain characteristic. Example: female nurses who smoke compared with those who do not smoke
Longitudinal[3]	A study that involves taking multiple measures of a group/population over an extended period of time to find relationships between variables. Example: studying monozygotic twins from birth into adulthood to compare their personalities
Experimental	Includes experimental manipulation of variables utilizing randomization and a control group to test the effects of an intervention or experiment Example: studying the effect of the newest beta-blocker drug in hypertensive patients compared to hypertensive patients not taking medication *Quasi-experimental research*: includes the manipulation of variables but lacks a control group or randomization
Qualitative[4]	Includes case studies, open-ended questions, field studies, participant observation and ethnographic studies, where observations and interview techniques are used to explore phenomena through detailed descriptions of people, events

designing the study must all be addressed. Once the study has been conducted, the data must be analyzed and interpreted so that the findings can be communicated. The evidence-based research process is a critical component in continuously improving nurse practitioner (NP) practice, as well as patient and health care outcomes.

Research Terms

The most essential research terms that assist with quantifying findings include confidence intervals, standard deviation, level of significance, perfect correlation, t-tests, reliability, and validity. A confidence interval is an estimated range that predicts the probability of including a specific parameter being assessed.[5] The smaller the confidence interval, the more precise the sample size is when compared to the total population. The standard deviation measures the degree to which individual results deviate from the mean of the sample population. For example, in a sample population that has a relatively normal distribution, about 68% of the sample falls within one standard deviation of the mean, and 95% of the sample falls within two standard deviations.[6] The level of significance is expressed as the p (probability) value of falsely rejecting the null hypothesis.[7] A t-test evaluates two sample populations by evaluating the differences in means between the two groups.

The correlation coefficient is a measure ranging from -1 to 1 that analyzes the linear relationship between two variables. If the coefficient is -1, the two variables have a negative correlation and create a negative linear slope. This means that if the value of variable x increases, then the value of variable y decreases. If the coefficient is 1, the two variables have a positive correlation and create a positive slope, which indicates that if the value of variable x increases, then the value of *y* increases as well. If the coefficient is 0, there is no correlation between the *x* and *y* variables.[8]

Reliability is the consistency of a measurement and the likelihood that the same results will be yielded if the test is repeated again with the same factors. Reliability can be tested using either the test/retest method, which involves repeating the same test after a period of time and expecting the same results, or the internal consistency method, which involves repeating a different but comparable test that assesses the same topic to analyze the consistency of the results. The correlation value that indicates reliability is commonly measured with Cronbach's alpha. The closer Cronbach's alpha is to 1, the more reliable the results of the experiment are. Validity is the degree to which a study reflects the specific focus being researched.[9]

Advance Directives vs. Living Wills

An advance directive is a written statement of a patient's intent regarding medical treatment. The Patient Self Determination Act of 1990 requires that all patients entering a hospital should be advised of their right to execute an advance directive.[10] A health care advance directive may, or may not, include a living will and/or specifications regarding durable power of attorney in one or two separate documents.

A living will is a written compilation of statements in document format that specifies which life-prolonging measures one does and does not want to be taken if one becomes incapacitated. In addition, living wills often include granting durable power of attorney to an individual, often a significant other, to act as a proxy/agent/attorney-in-fact for the patient in making health care decisions should the patient become incapacitated.[11] Essentially, the proxy is responsible for articulating the patient's advance directive. Power of attorney must usually be in writing before it will be honored by most institutions such as hospitals, banks, etc. In the United States, most states recognize living wills as long as the will is specific enough and addresses the issue at hand.

Privacy and Confidentiality

Health Insurance Portability and Accountability Act (HIPAA)

There are several titles of the Health Insurance Portability and Accountability Act (HIPAA). Title I of HIPAA protects health insurance coverage for workers and their families when they change or lose their jobs. Such is the Comprehensive Omnibus Reconciliation Act (COBRA), which offers a temporary extension of coverage to eligible employees and their families who have undergone voluntary or involuntary job loss.

Title II of HIPAA, known as the Administrative Simplification (AS) provisions, required the U.S.

Department of Health and Human Services to set national standards for electronic health care transactions and national identifiers for providers, health insurance plans, and employers. The title also speaks to specifics about the security and privacy of health data. As a result, it is posed that improved efficacy and effectiveness will encourage widespread use of electronic data in health care. The Office for Civil Rights enforces the HIPAA, which protects the (a) privacy of individual and identifiable health information; (b) sets national standards for the security of electronically protected health information via the HIPAA Security Rule; and (c) protects identifiable information being used to analyze patient safety events and improves patient safety, via the confidentiality provisions outlined in the Patient Safety Rule.

In general, the following are referred to as "covered entities" with regard to HIPAA regulations: (a) health plans, including health insurance companies, HMOs, company health plans, and certain government programs that pay for health care such as Medicare and Medicaid; (b) most health care providers, especially those who use electronic billing to health insurers; and (c) health care clearinghouses that process nonstandard health information data received from another entity into a standard, such as standard electronic formats.

Specific examples of HIPAA protected information include (a) written information in the medical record; (b) conversations among health care providers about one's care or treatment; (c) patient information stored in a health insurer's computer system; and (d) patient billing information stored at a clinic.

A patient's health information cannot be used or shared without written permission, unless this law allows it. Without a patient's written authorization, a provider usually cannot disclose information to one's employer, use or share a patient's information for marketing or advertising purposes, or share private notes about a patient's health care.

The HIPAA Privacy Rule protects medical records and other information from being inappropriately shared. Further, patients have the right to see or receive a copy of their health records and request corrections to their health information. Additionally, the HIPAA Privacy Rule permits patients to receive notification of how their health information may be used and shared, decide if they want to give permission before their health information can be used or shared for certain purposes (e.g., marketing), and receive a report outlining when and why their health information was shared for certain purposes. Patients may also file complaints with their health care provider, health insurer, and/or the United States government if their rights are being denied or if their health information is not being protected.[12]

In contrast, there are numerous situations in which health information is allowed to be viewed or shared without notifying the patient. For example, health information can be shared to ensure proper treatment and coordination of care and payment of health care services (e.g., physicians, NPs, hospitals, etc.). The patient's family, relatives, friends, or others the patient identifies as being involved with their health care or bill payment may also receive health information, unless the patient objects. Health information can also be disclosed in order to protect the health of the public (e.g., reporting disease outbreaks) and comply with reporting statutes (e.g., reporting gunshot wounds).

It should be noted that some entities are not formally required to follow HIPAA regulations. Examples include life insurers, employers, workers compensation carriers, many schools and school districts, many state agencies like child protective service agencies, many law enforcement agencies, and many municipal offices, among others.

Confidentiality vs. "Duty to Warn"

The duty to warn another health care provider supersedes the patient's right to confidentiality if the patient's mental condition puts the patient or others in danger. That is, the duty to protect a patient from self-harm and harm to others supersedes the right to confidentiality.[4]

Defamation

Defamation is a common law tort involving damaging a patient's reputation as a result of information being shared without the patient's permission. NPs will not be held liable for defamation if the patient consented to the release of the information or the information was accurate.[13]

Invasion of Privacy

Under the common law tort of invasion of privacy, NPs can be held liable for public disclosure of private facts about a patient if the information disclosed would be considered highly offensive to a reasonable person.[14] If the private facts concern a legitimate public interest, the patient may need to show the NP acted with malice, depending on the circumstances. Because NPs need to disclose private information in order for treatment, this tort typically comes into play when the private facts are disclosed to improper sources.

Health Care Delivery

"Healthy People 2020"

Healthy People 2020 is a national health promotion and disease prevention initiative bringing together many individuals and agencies to improve the health of all Americans, eliminate disparities in health, and improve years and quality of life.[15] The initiative is a continuation of Healthy People 2000, a 1990 initiative by the United States Department of Health and Human Services. Healthy People 2020 contains hundreds of health objectives relating to equal access, availability, cost, and quality of care, among others. The initiative is used to understand the health status of the nation and plan prevention programs accordingly, but individuals, communities, and organizations are responsible for determining how to meet the goals of Healthy People 2020.

"Reporting" Statutes

Reporting statutes are state laws that require NPs to report specific health-related information to the police, Department of Health and Human Services, animal control, or social services.[16] Incidences in which a case must be reported include violent criminal activity with a dangerous weapon that poses a threat to self and others; animal bites that may lead to infectious disease; suspected or confirmed child or elder abuse; and certain infectious diseases (e.g., gonorrhea, chlamydia, syphilis, HIV, tuberculosis). Despite universal reporting statutes regarding violence, most states do not require NPs to report domestic violence.[4]

Health Care Financing

Evaluation and Management (E&M) coding is a medical billing practice used in the United States for health care providers to be reimbursed by private insurance, Medicare, or Medicaid. The codes identify and match the level of service provided with the complexity of the presenting patient's problems. NPs are reimbursed by a variety of third-party payers that include Medicare, Medicaid, commercial indemnity insurers, and health maintenance organizations, among others.

Medicare sets the standard for reimbursement. For most codes, Medicare pays 80% of the amount listed and the patient is responsible for the remaining 20%. Medicare reimburses NPs 85% of the physician fee delineated in Medicare's Physician Fee Schedule.

The four types of Medicare are A, B, C, and D. Medicare A covers inpatient hospitalization, skilled nursing facility services, home health services, and/or hospice associated with the inpatient event. Most individuals qualify to receive benefits at 65 years of age.

Medicare B covers physician and NP services, as well as the following services and equipment: outpatient hospital services, laboratory and diagnostic procedures, medical equipment, and some home health services. Medicare B is a supplemental medical insurance requiring patients to pay a premium.

Medicare C, known as Medicare Advantage, is available for those who qualify for Medicare A and enroll in Medicare B. This benefit allows eligible patients to receive all of their Medicare services health care services through one of the provider organizations under Part C which include private health insurance companies (e.g., health maintenance organizations, preferred provider organizations, etc.)

Medicare D provides limited drug coverage to those who join. Patients must pay a monthly premium and a copay on each prescription.

To qualify to be a Medicare provider, an NP must hold a state license as a nurse practitioner, be certified as an NP by a recognized national certifying body, and hold at least a master's degree in nursing.

While Medicare reimburses NPs 85% of the physician fee delineated in the Medicare's Physician Fee Schedule, in special circumstances, the NP may bill under the physician's Medicare provider number and receive 100% reimbursement. This is known as "incident-to" billing or "Incident to the Physician" billing. However, the following rules regarding provided services apply and must be strictly followed: (1) The services are an integral, although incidental, part of the physician's professional service; (2) furnished in a physician's office; and (3) furnished under the physician's direct supervision. (4) Direct supervision does not require the physician's presence in the same room but the physician must be present in the same office suite and he or she must be immediately available. (5) The physician must perform "the initial service and subsequent services of a frequency which reflects his or her active participation in the management of the course of treatment." (6) The physician under whose name and number the bill is submitted must be the individual present in the same office suite when the service is provided.

Medicaid

Medicaid is a federally supported, state-administered program to assist low-income families and individuals with medical costs. Eligibility requirements and benefits vary from state to state. Medicaid payments are made after all other insurance and third-party payments have been made.[4]

Professional Responsibility

Scope of Practice

The scope of practice, which provides guidelines for nursing practice, varies according to the legal allowances in each state. Basic elements of scope of practice include clinical leadership, research-based clinical practice, and integration of care across the acute illness continuum through collaboration and coordination of care, family assessment, and discharge planning.[4]

Standards of Professional Nursing Practice

The American Nurses Association defines standards of professional nursing practice as "authoritative statements of the duties that all registered nurses, regardless of role, population, or specialty, are expected to perform competently."[17] The standards set out in the latest edition of the American Nurses Association Nursing: Scope and Standards of Practice combine standards of practice and standards of professional performance. The standards of practice include assessment, diagnosis, outcomes identification, planning, implementation, and evaluation. The standards of professional performance consist of ethics, education, evidence-based practice and research, quality of practice, communication, leadership, collaboration, professional practice evaluation, resource utilization, and environmental health.[17]

State Practice Acts

Every state legislature enacts a nurse practice act to protect the health and welfare of patients. Each state's act establishes the board of nursing to develop administrative rules and regulations.[18] Each act also specifies the standards for education programs, scope of nursing practice, prescriptive authority, specific practice requirements, types and requirements of titles and licenses, and violation and disciplinary action rules.[19]

Prescriptive Authority

Prescriptive authority is the NP's ability to prescribe drugs, medical services, or goods. The Drug Enforcement Agency permits nurses in advanced practice to obtain registration numbers, but the specifics of an NP's prescriptive authority vary according to the laws of each state. The laws cover the independent authority to prescribe, the controlled substances that may be prescribed, and whether collaboration with an attending physician is necessary.[20]

Credentials

Credentials allow for the enforcement of professional standards of practice and compliance with advanced practice laws. Credentials for NPs include an education, licensure, and certification to legally practice in their respective states. Credentials facilitate the enforcement of professional standards by establishing minimum levels of acceptable performance, mandating accountability, and acknowledging the NP's scope of practice.[4]

Licensure

Licensure establishes that a person is qualified to perform in a particular professional role. Licensure is acquired and maintained by conforming to the rules and regulations established by a governmental body, known as the state board of nursing.[21]

Certification

Certification is a voluntary process that is granted by nongovernmental agencies (i.e., American Nurses Credentialing Center; American Academy of Nurse Practitioners Certification Program; Pediatric Nursing

Certification Board; American Association of Critical Care Nurses; National Certification Corporation for the Obstetric, Pediatric Nursing Certification Board; Gynecologic and Neonatal Nursing Specialties). Obtaining a certification acknowledges an individual's mastery of specialized knowledge and skills within a practice area.[21]

Credentialing and Privileging

Credentialing is the process of evaluating and confirming NP qualifications. Credentialing with hospital privileges is granted by a hospital credentialing committee comprised of physicians, and occasionally other credentialed providers, who hold privileges at the given hospital where the NP has made the request. Privileging is the process through which an NP is granted the authority to furnish services within a facility.[22] Privileges may be partly granted, with supplemental privileges granted by a credentialing committee.[4]

Informed Consent and Obtaining Informed Consent

Informed consent is a process that includes discussing with the patient the risks and benefits of a certain treatment or other treatment options, including refusal of treatment. The patient must have the opportunity to ask questions and have questions answered by the NP, as well as be given the time needed to discuss the decision with his or her family. Patients usually sign consent forms after discussing the treatment or procedure but may choose to refuse part or all of the treatment at any time, regardless of previously signing a consent form.[23] Patients must be advised at the time of their admission to a federally funded institution of this right to refuse care.

In obtaining informed consent, patients are required to demonstrate competency in making decisions about their own treatment. Generally, a patient is considered incompetent if he or she is unable to respond intelligently and knowingly to questions regarding treatment. Patients are also deemed incompetent if they are unable to participate in treatment decisions by means of rational thought processes or are unable to understand minimum basic medical treatment information. Consent is presumed in emergency cases in which the patient is incapacitated or if there is no surrogate decision maker present for the patient to state otherwise.[24]

Key Ethical Principles

The practice of ethics is based on the study of the moral rules and standards governing the conduct of individuals, including NPs and all health care professionals. NPs should keep in mind the key ethical principles of health care: nonmaleficence, utilitarianism, beneficence, justice, fidelity, veracity, and autonomy.[4]

Nonmaleficence is the avoidance of harm, such as prescribing a drug with a lower risk of side effects than an alternative, but equally therapeutic, drug. Utilitarianism is a philosophy that reflects making decisions based on what is right for the most amount of people, or in other words, providing the greatest good for the greatest number of people. The triage system is an example of utilitarianism. Beneficence refers to doing what is good and in the best interest of the patient, such as providing pain medication. Justice is a principle ensuring fair and equal treatment and distribution of resources. Fidelity is the principle of being faithful and committed to the patient. NPs practice fidelity by keeping their promises to their patients, such as respecting a patient's wishes to not disclose the diagnosis to the patient's mother. Veracity, the principle of being truthful, refers to both the duty to disclose and the obligation to respect confidentiality. The principle of veracity would dictate not using a patient's medical information in a research study without receiving consent first. The principle of autonomy reflects the NP's duty to respect an individual's choices regarding care.[25]

NPs often encounter ethical principles in conflict with each other. For example, the principle of beneficence may call for a patient with cancer to receive chemotherapy. The patient, however, has expressed his wishes to not receive treatment. The principle of autonomy requires the NP to respect the patient's wishes and not administer chemotherapy.

History of the NP Role

The NP's role arose out of a demand for primary health care services, particularly in rural areas. Specialization in medicine drove many physicians out of primary care, and advanced practice nurses were able to fill their shoes. The first NP program was established in 1965 by Loretta Ford and Henry Silver; it was a pediatric NP program aimed at health promotion and disease prevention.[26] The growth of NP programs followed, with NPs eventually working in specialized scopes of practice. Federal funding for education allowed an increase in the presence of NPs in primary care. Managed care, hospital restructuring, and decreases in medical residency programs allowed for the expansion of NPs to the inpatient setting. Currently, the NP may practice as an expert clinician, consultant, educator, or researcher.[4]

Legal Terms

Liability

Liability, in a medical context, is the legal responsibility of the NP's actions or omissions that fail to meet the standard of care and cause actual or potential harm to the patient. An NP may be held liable for any harm caused to the patient in their care regardless of whether or not the harm was inflicted by the NP. Standards of care provide benchmarks in determining liability or negligence.[27]

Negligence

The tort of negligence is the failure of the NP to provide care as any reasonable NP would that results in harm to the patient. Negligence can also be applied to an action that the NP takes that any reasonable NP would not take.[28]

Malpractice

Medical malpractice, a negligence tort, occurs when a health care professional's actions fall below the appropriate standard of care and hurt the patient. Malpractice claims frequently concern diagnosis, treatment, medication, patient assessment, or monitoring. Malpractice insurance does not cover advanced practice NPs from practicing outside their scope without a license.[4]

Assault

The tort of assault is either an attempt to commit a battery or an intentional act performed by one individual that produces apprehension in another individual of imminent harm or offensive contact. The attacker must be aware and capable of carrying out the attack. If the victim is touched, the act is battery, not assault. Some states allow some assault charges with deadly weapons without the victim's awareness of the attack.[29,30] Examples of assault include shaking a fist in the air in the direction of another person and making the motion to inject someone against his will.

Battery

The tort of battery is an unlawful act of contact with another person resulting in either bodily injury or offensive touching. The force need not be applied directly. Unlike assault, battery does not require that the victim be aware of the attack.[30]

Involuntary Commitment

Involuntary commitment is admitting individuals into a mental health unit against their will. Although specific laws vary state to state, every state requires a hearing and due process for involuntary commitment. Generally, patients are admitted due to developmental disability, substance abuse, or mental illness. Individuals with mental illness are likely to be involuntarily committed if they have become a danger to themselves or others.[31] An NP is potentially liable for discharging patients who are in danger of hurting themselves or others.

Use of Restraints

Restraint use is regulated by national and state agencies. NPs are within their legal scope to use restraints when attempting to control or prevent harmful behavior by the patient. The use of restraints must be based on an individual order. If the NP initiated the order, the attending physician must be notified as soon as possible. Restraints are to be used as a last resort and only until the harmful behavior ceases.[32] The NP may be liable if restraints are used excessively, if the exact reason and rationale for the use of restraints is not documented, or if safety checks of the restraints are not charted.[4]

Good Samaritan Statutes

Outside of the workplace, health care professionals may be called upon to act as first responders to care for injured individuals due to accidents or disasters. In states that have enacted Good Samaritan statutes, NPs and other health care professionals are exempt from liability for ordinary negligence when the injured person's status worsens after the care.[33] However, NPs and other health care professionals can be found liable for gross negligence.

References

1. Study designs. Center for Evidence-Based Medicine web site. http://www.cebm.net/study-designs. Accessed April 3, 2015.

2. Healy P, Devane D. Methodological considerations in cohort study designs. *Nurse Res.* 2011; 18(3): 32–36.

3. Longitudinal studies. The BMJ web site. http://www.bmj.com/about-bmj/resources-readers/publications/epidemiology-uninitiated/7-longitudinal-studies. Accessed April 3, 2015.

4. Barkley TW Jr. Practice issues, trends, and health policy. In: Barkley TW Jr, ed. *Adult-Gerontology Primary Care NP: Certification Review/Clinical Update Continuing Education Course*. West Hollywood, CA: Barkley & Associates; 2015: 158–171.

5. United States Department of Commerce, National Institute of Standards and Technology. What are confidence intervals? Engineering Statistics Handbook web site. http://www.itl.nist.gov/div898/handbook/prc/section1/prc14.htm. Last updated October 30, 2013. Accessed April 3, 2015.

6. Standard deviation. Laerd Statistics web site. https://statistics.laerd.com/statistical-guides/measures-of-spread-standard-deviation.php. Accessed April 3, 2015.

7. Hypothesis testing. Laerd Statistics web site. https://statistics.laerd.com/statistical-guides/hypothesis-testing-3.php. Accessed April 3, 2015.

8. Correlation coefficient. Stat Trek web site. http://stattrek.com/statistics/correlation.aspx. Accessed April 3, 2015.

9. Basic concepts: Reliability and validity. Florida Center for Instructional Technology web site. http://fcit.usf.edu/assessment/basic/basicc.html. Accessed April 3, 2015.

10. Health care advance directives: What is the Patient Self-Determination Act? American Bar Association web site. http://www.americanbar.org/groups/public_education/resources/law_issues_for_consumers/patient_self_determination_act.html. Accessed July 20, 2015.

11. Irving S. Types of health care directives. Nolo web site. http://www.nolo.com/legal-encyclopedia/living-will-power-attorney-advance-directive-30023.html. Accessed July 20, 2015.

12. Fact sheet 8c: The HIPAA Privacy Rule: Patients' rights. Privacy Rights Clearinghouse web site. https://www.privacyrights.org/content/hipaa-privacy-rule-patients-rights. Accessed July 20, 2015.

13. Doskow E. Defamation law made simple. Nolo web site. http://www.nolo.com/legal-encyclopedia/defamation-law-made-simple-29718.html. Accessed July 20, 2015.

14. Mroczek JM. Legal issues in nursing. National Center of Continuing Education, Inc. web site. https://www.nursece.com/courses/92-legal-issues-in-nursing. Accessed July 20, 2015.

15. About Healthy People. HealthyPeople.gov web site. http://www.healthypeople.gov/2020/About-Healthy-People. Accessed July 20, 2015.

16. Lo B. Resolving Ethical Dilemmas: A Guide for Clinicians. 5th ed. Philadelphia, PA: Wolters Kluwer Health/Lippincott Williams & Wilkins; 2013: 41–51.

17. American Nurses Association. Nursing: Scope and Standards of Practice. 2nd ed. Silver Spring, MD: Nursesbooks.org; 2010.

18. Contact a board of nursing. National Council of State Boards of Nursing web site. https://www.ncsbn.org/47.htm. Accessed April 2, 2015.

19. Nurse Practice Act, rules & regulations. National Council of State Boards of Nursing. https://www.ncsbn.org/1455.htm. Accessed April 2, 2015.

20. Von Gizycki C. APRN prescribing law: A state-by-state summary. Medscape. http://www.medscape.com/viewarticle/440315. Published July 25, 2013. Accessed April 2, 2015.

21. Certification v. licensure. National Registry of Emergency Medical Technicians web site. https://www.nremt.org/nremt/about/Legal_Opinion.asp. Accessed April 2, 2015.

22. Nurse practitioner FAQs: What is credentialing and privileging for nurse practitioners? Michigan Nurses Association web site. http://minurses.org/nursing-practice/resources/advanced-practice#credentialing. Accessed April 2, 2015.

23. American Cancer Society. Informed consent. American Cancer Society web site. http://www.cancer.org/acs/groups/cid/documents/webcontent/003014-pdf.pdf. Last revised July 28, 2014. Accessed April 2, 2015.

24. Competency to make medical decisions. Stanford School of Medicine Psychiatry & Law web site. forensicpsychiatry.stanford.edu/Files/Medical%20Competency.doc. Accessed April 2, 2015.

25. Short definitions of ethical principles and theories. American Nurses Association web site. http://www.nursingworld.org/MainMenuCategories/EthicsStandards/Resources/Ethics-Definitions.pdf. Accessed April 3, 2015.

26. Kohler, S. Case 31: The development of the nurse practitioner and physician assistant professions. Duke Sanford Center for Strategic Philanthropic & Civil Society web site. https://cspcs.sanford.duke.edu/sites/default/files/descriptive/nurse_practitioners_and_physician_assistants.pdf. Accessed April 3, 2015.

27. Hill G, Hill K. Liability. In: Hill G, Hill K, eds. The People's Law Dictionary. http://dictionary.law.com/Default.aspx?selected=1151. Accessed April 3, 2015.

28. Hill G, Hill K. Negligence. In: Hill G, Hill K, eds. The People's Law Dictionary. http://dictionary.law.com/Default.aspx?selected=1314. Accessed April 3, 2015.

29. Hill G, Hill K. Assault. In: Hill G, Hill K, eds. The People's Law Dictionary. http://dictionary.law.com/Default.aspx?selected=2444. Accessed April 3, 2015.

30. Hill G, Hill K. Battery. In: Hill G, Hill K, eds. The People's Law Dictionary. http://dictionary.law.com/Default.aspx?selected=43. Accessed April 3, 2015.

31. Slobogin C, Hafemeister TL, Mossman D, Reisner R. Law and the Mental Health System: Civil and Criminal Aspects. 6th ed. St. Paul, MN: West Academic Publishing; 2013: 704–705.

32. Use of restraints. A.D.A.M. Medical Encyclopedia. http://www.nlm.nih.gov/medlineplus/ency/patientinstructions/000450.htm. Updated February 4, 2014. Accessed April 3, 2015.

33. Good Samaritans law & legal definition. US Legal web site. http://definitions.uslegal.com/g/good-samaritans. Accessed April 3, 2015.

Chapter 16

Special Considerations in Gerontology

1. All of the following are typical physiologic changes in the central nervous system of the elderly population <u>except</u>:

   a. Decreased beta-adrenergic responsiveness

   b. Increased alpha responses

   c. Decreased dopamine receptors

   d. Increased muscarinic parasympathetic responses

2. Which of the following is attributed to decreased renal function in the elderly with regard to prescription medication?

   a. Decreased drug metabolism

   b. Inhibited drug absorption

   c. Impaired drug elimination

   d. Limited drug distribution

3. Which of the following most closely resembles an instrumental activity of daily living for the geriatric population?

   a. Going to work

   b. Paying bills

   c. Going to the bathroom

   d. Reading the newspaper

4. Alice, an 87-year-old female, arrives at your clinic complaining of fatigue during the day. After looking up some of her symptoms on the Internet, she thinks she may have hypersomnia. In evaluating Alice's medical history, which of the following would you be <u>least</u> likely to associate with hypersomnia?

   a. Sleep apnea as a cause

   b. Chronic use of hypnotic medications as a cause

   c. Unusual daytime sleepiness as a symptom

   d. Nocturnal confusion as a complaint

5. A 79-year-old patient with chronic hypertension comes to your practice with complaints of dizziness and feeling like the inside of his head is spinning. He adds that these symptoms began about a week after being diagnosed with and prescribed medication for congestive heart failure 2 months prior. Which of the following is the best first line treatment choice to prescribe for this patient's condition?

   a. Enalapril

   b. Atenolol

   c. Hydralazine

   d. Furosemide

6. Which of the following would <u>least</u> qualify as an advanced activity of daily living?

    a. Routine phone calls and visits with neighbors

    b. Grocery shopping and making dinner

    c. Teaching music at the community center

    d. Reading poetry

7. Which of the following age groups is the fastest-growing segment of the total population?

    a. Late middle age – 55–64 years

    b. Young old – 65–74 years

    c. Old – 75–84 years

    d. Oldest old – 85 years and older

8. You are assessing a patient who has just spent several weeks in a body cast. The patient has complained of a very "sore spot" on his lower back. Upon physical examination, you notice an area of skin breakdown presenting as a crater on the patient's sacrum that is dark red in the middle; however, bone is not visible. How should you chart this patient's pressure ulcer?

    a. Unclassifiable

    b. Stage 2

    c. Stage 3

    d. Stage 4

9. Immunosenescence refers to:

    a. The gradual decline of overall immune system function due to chronic disease

    b. The decline in innate immune system function

    c. The gradual decline of overall immune system function due to age

    d. The waning of vaccine-induced antibody response

10. You are prescribing niacin to one of your geriatric patients as a treatment for hyperlipidemia. Knowing the potential interactions of niacin, you review the patient's history. Which of these medications would warrant the most caution for adverse interactions?

    a. Phenylephrine

    b. Naproxen

    c. Levothyroxine

    d. Methyldopa

11. You are treating a patient who has developed a pressure ulcer characterized by intact skin with erythema that does not blanch. You apply transparent film to the area. Using the standard system of the National Pressure Ulcer Advisory Panel, which stage is your patient's pressure ulcer?

    a. Stage 1

    b. Stage 2

    c. Stage 3

    d. Stage 4

12. Pharmacokinetics is defined as the study of:

    a. How genes explain different responses to drugs

    b. How drugs interact with the body

    c. Single-gene genetic variations in drug variations

    d. How the body interacts with drugs

13. Of the following, which is the <u>least</u> common condition in older adults?

    a. Diabetes mellitus

    b. Osteoarthritis

    c. Atherosclerosis

    d. Parkinson's disease

14. Which of these statements is <u>not</u> true regarding aging skin?

    a. Skin loses sensation and immune response.

    b. The amount of cell layers in the skin decreases.

    c. Skin is not as resistant to the development of pressure ulcers.

    d. No warning signs may precede pressure ulcer formation.

15. You are evaluating 81-year-old Luther's nutritional status. Which of the following levels would most indicate nutritional risk?

    a. Albumin: 3.5 g/dl

    b. Prealbumin: 15 mg/dl

    c. Transferrin: 250 mg/dl

    d. Total lymphocyte count: 1,350 cells/mm³

16. A drug is introduced to a group of patients of Middle Eastern heritage, with the goal of searching for details in their family histories that may explain different responses to the drug within their ethnic group. Which subfield of pharmacology would be most relevant to this study?

    a. Pharmacogenetics

    b. Pharmacokinetics

    c. Pharmacogenomics

    d. Pharmacodynamics

17. William, a 68-year-old, had been suffering from shingles and complained of extreme continual burning pain on his head and legs. He was given medication to treat the intense burning sensations, but has now returned to the clinic with complaints of blurry vision and the inability to urinate or have a bowel movement. Which of the following drugs is most likely the cause of his latest complaints?

    a. Phenytoin

    b. Acyclovir

    c. Ibuprofen

    d. Amitriptyline

18. Oxidative stress, as a factor of aging, most closely demonstrates which of the following biological theories of aging?

    a. Biological programming theory

    b. Cross-linkage theory

    c. Wear and tear theory

    d. Free radical theory

19. Which of the following is <u>least</u> true regarding the physiologic changes and findings in the immune systems of the elderly?

    a. Innate immunity functions decline while adaptive immune responses remain constant

    b. Decreased thymic hormone production results in a decreased number of functioning T-cells

    c. Decreased antibody production and response to antigens occurs

    d. Vaccine-induced antibody response wanes

20. Which of the following types of retirement communities is defined as one that provides a continuum of care, ranging from 24/7 independent living care to special nursing home care?

    a. Board and care

    b. Adult congregate communities

    c. Assisted living communities

    d. Continuing care communities

21. As adults get older, all of the following physiological changes typically present <u>except</u>:

    a. Decreased maximum urine osmolality

    b. Increased blood pressure

    c. Decreased percentage of body water

    d. Increased thirst drive

22. Of the following, which is the <u>least</u> common gram-negative pathogen responsible for pneumonia in the elderly population?

    a. *Haemophilus influenzae*

    b. *Klebsiella pneumoniae*

    c. *Moraxella catarrhalis*

    d. *Neisseria meningitidis*

23. A man and his elderly father come to the clinic because the father has been continuously coughing for the past few days. After examination of the patient, the son pulls you aside to tell you that he fears that his father cannot continue to watch after himself in old age. The son is looking into the possibility of putting his father into a continuing care community. Which of the following is most likely required for the father to enter a continuing care community?

   a. He must have a serious health condition not requiring hospitalization.

   b. He must buy property and pay monthly fees for utilities and services.

   c. He must be independent when he enters the community.

   d. He must be admitted by prescription of a physician.

24. It is recommended that older patients take at least 0.8 grams/kg of protein a day. Which of the following findings is most often directly linked to low protein intake?

   a. Decreased healing ability

   b. Decreased calcium absorption

   c. Decreased heat production

   d. Decreased percentage of body water

25. Julie, a 72-year-old female, comes to see you because of complaints of memory loss, extreme drowsiness, and dizziness. Which of the following drugs would most likely lead to these side effects?

   a. Paromomycin

   b. Furosemide

   c. Phenytoin

   d. Doxazosin

26. Social Security is the sole income for about what percentage of the elder population?

   a. About 15%

   b. About 25%

   c. About 35%

   d. About 45%

27. Which of the following types of drugs should elderly patients take 1 hour before or 4 hours after other medications?

   a. Beta-blockers

   b. Antacids

   c. Benzodiazepines

   d. Diuretics

28. Which of these is least representative of typical chest X-ray findings of pneumonia in the elderly population?

   a. Bacterial pneumonia presenting with bronchopneumonia

   b. Aspiration pneumonia localized to the right middle lobe

   c. Viral pneumonia showing diffuse involvement

   d. Bacterial pneumonia presenting with lobar pneumonia

29. Which of the following over-the-counter agents is best known for decreasing renal blood flow, further reducing elimination of many drugs?

   a. Cimetidine

   b. Naproxen

   c. Niacin

   d. Magnesium hydroxide

30. You are considering prescribing furosemide to an elderly patient, believing it to be the drug best-suited for treatment. After looking over the patient's recent lab tests, however, you notice decreased serum albumin levels. Which of the following choices would be the best course of treatment at this time?

   a. Treat the underlying cause of decreased albumin

   b. Decrease the dosage of furosemide

   c. Switch to torsemide

   d. Start the patient on metolazone

31. Which of these statements is least attributable to the error theory of aging?

    a. Aging is due to internal or external assaults that affect cells or organs so they can no longer function properly.

    b. Aging produces changes in DNA.

    c. Aging is responsible for increased amounts of error in the RNA transcription or protein synthesis.

    d. Aging is mostly determined by the inherited amount of adaptability used to deal with stress.

32. A nurse practitioner is assessing an elderly patient who has just entered her care. The examination employs the Barthel Index. Which of the following types of assessments is she most likely performing?

    a. Environmental

    b. Functional

    c. Sexual

    d. Nutritional concerns and risk

33. According to the free radical theory, which of the following is not a result of free radicals escaping the neutralizing process?

    a. DNA damage

    b. Cross-linking of proteins

    c. Abnormal cells may double an infinite amount of times

    d. Formation of age pigments

34. You are prescribing medication to Ethel, a 72-year-old female who has a history of cardiac disease. Which of the following effects on the efficiency of the drug is most likely to occur due to Ethel's heart condition?

    a. Increased receptor regulation, leading to increased drug affinity

    b. Decreased perfusion of tissues, leading to inhibited drug delivery

    c. Increased tissue absorption, leading to prolonged drug effects

    d. Decreased receptor regulation, leading to decreased drug affinity

35. Joe, a 65-year-old patient, arrives at your clinic complaining of trouble "performing" in the bedroom. You decide to examine his medical history for a possible cause. Which of the following events in his history would most likely be responsible for Joe's erectile dysfunction?

    a. Myocardial infarction

    b. Hyperthyroidism

    c. Prescription for atenolol

    d. Ulcer treatment with histamine H2 antagonists

36. In performing a spiritual assessment on an elder, which of these questions would be least important to ask?

    a. "What are your views on death and dying?"

    b. "What is your religion?"

    c. "Do you have any rituals you would like performed before death?"

    d. "How can we assist you with your spiritual needs?"

37. Although the average age of onset for reduced inability to maintain homeostasis is 30 years, this is not usually seen in organs until which age?

    a. 50

    b. 60

    c. 70

    d. 80

38. When reviewing an older patient for any nutritional concerns, you assess his calcium intake. Which of the following conditions is least likely to be associated with abnormal calcium levels?

    a. Nephrolithiasis

    b. Hyperparathyroidism

    c. Hashimoto's disease

    d. Prostate cancer

39. Which of these contexts best illustrates the disengagement theory?

    a. A former CEO removes herself from company affairs and shifts her focus to her social circle.

    b. A retired man has experienced a minor financial crisis and feels ashamed that he is no longer self-sufficient.

    c. An introvert who's always felt more at home in books spends the vast majority of her retirement years in her home or in bookstores by herself.

    d. A veteran teacher receives mandatory retirement; he feels somewhat relieved, but is not entirely sure how to implement his plans for old age.

40. Which of the following is <u>least</u> likely to be associated with subsidized housing for the elderly?

    a. Two meals per day are usually provided.

    b. Monthly fees are not required.

    c. Daily blood pressure and basic check-ups are available.

    d. Services are only available to elderly patients in good health.

RATIONALES

1. a

Decreased beta-adrenergic responsiveness is a typical physiologic change in the peripheral nervous system of the elderly population, not the central nervous system. Decreased dopamine receptors, and increased alpha response and muscarinic parasympathetic responses, are typical physiologic changes in the central nervous system in the elderly.

2. c

Renal insufficiency in elderly patients typically results in the inability to properly eliminate medication, which results from a decrease in renal blood flow, glomerular filtration, tubular secretion, and creatinine clearance; thus, the practitioner must establish an appropriate dose. Decreased drug metabolism in elderly patients is attributed to changes in the liver, not the kidneys. Drug absorption typically remains unaffected in the aging process, unless an elderly patient takes an adsorbent medication that inhibits the stomach's ability to absorb properly. This process is attributed to the gastrointestinal tract, rather than the kidneys. Changes in the fluid and tissue compartments occur during the aging process, but the distribution of medication remains constant, except in patients with a cardiovascular disease.

3. b

Paying bills, as well as any other activity involved with managing one's own financial matters, is considered an instrumental activity of daily living. Going to work and reading the newspaper—the latter of which would be considered a recreational activity—are both advanced activities of daily living, whereas going to the bathroom would simply be an activity of daily living.

4. d

Nocturnal confusion is not an expected finding of hypersomnia. Sleep apnea, chronic use of hypnotic medications, and unusual daytime sleepiness are all associated with hypersomnia.

5. a

Enalapril would be the best choice because it is an ACE inhibitor and is appropriate treatment for hypertension itself and heart failure. Although furosemide would normally be the first choice, this is contraindicated by the vertigo symptoms the patient experiences. Atenolol is a beta blocker and hydralazine is a vasodilator, both which are also contraindicated by vertigo symptoms in the elderly.

6. b

Grocery shopping and making dinner are considered instrumental activities of daily living, as these are more pertinent to basic functional independence than the other choices. Routine phone calls and visits with neighbors indicate maintaining a connection with peers and community, an advanced activity of daily living. Teaching music at the community center, as a volunteer or employee, would qualify as an advanced activity of daily living. Reading poetry would be considered a recreational activity, which would also be an advanced activity of daily living.

7. d

The fastest growing segment of the total population is the oldest old, individuals aged 85 years and older. Their growth rate is twice that of those who are 65 years of age and older. While the old, those aged 75–84 years, may grow as life expectancy increases, the oldest old are growing at a faster rate. The late middle-age population segment is not growing as fast as the oldest old segment of the population.

8. c

Stage 3 pressure ulcers involve full-thickness skin loss, often involving subcutaneous tissue, and typically present as a crater. An unclassifiable pressure ulcer would be covered by scabby, dead tissue, and look dark brown. A stage 2 pressure ulcer may present as a fresh opening blister with only a shallow sore. A stage 4 pressure ulcer is a deep open sore, in which muscle, bone, or tendon may be visible.

9. c

Immunosenescence refers to the gradual decline in overall immune system function due to age. Because both the innate and adaptive immune systems are affected, the immune system's ability to respond to infection is reduced. Consequently, chronic disease may be exacerbated, and elderly patients may require new administration of prior vaccines because of waning vaccine-induced antibody response.

10. d

Methyldopa would warrant caution in prescribing niacin, as niacin exacerbates the effects of antihypertensives, and methyldopa is an antihypertensive. Phenylephrine is a decongestant, which, like niacin, may exacerbate antihypertensive symptoms, but would not warrant specific reaction from the niacin itself. Naproxen would warrant some caution, as NSAIDs can reduce the elimination of niacin; it would not warrant as much caution as methyldopa, however, especially as lower doses of medication are already encouraged for elderly patients, due to metabolic and renal changes. Levothyroxine has no interactions with niacin.

11. a

Stage 1 pressure ulcers, characterized by intact skin with erythema that does not blanch, can be treated with transparent film. Stage 2 pressure ulcers, characterized by partial-thickness loss of skin, should be treated with dressings that maintain a moist environment. Stage 3 and 4 pressure ulcers may require surgical interventions.

12. d

Pharmacokinetics is the study of how the body interacts with drugs, including absorption, distribution, metabolism, and excretion. Pharmacodynamics is the study of how drugs interact with the body, while pharmacogenetics is the study of single-gene genetic variations in drug variations. Pharmacogenomics is the study of how genetic differences explain different responses to drugs.

13. b

Although osteoarthritis is one of the more common reasons for older adults to be hospitalized, Parkinson's disease, diabetes mellitus, and atherosclerosis are more common conditions in older adults.

14. b

With age, the epidermis grows thinner, though the amount of layers within it remains unchanged. As the skin ages, the number of sebaceous glands, sweat glands, melanocytes, and Langerhans' cells are reduced, which leads to an inhibited natural immune response. Aging leads to a decrease in Meissner's and Pacinian corpuscles, which are the mechanisms responsible for sensory perception in the skin. The appearance of pressure ulcers in the elderly population is more common because the skin is less resistant to unrelieved external pressure and less able to repair itself. Restricted mobility increases the chance of developing pressure ulcers, which may or may not be preceded by warning signs.

15. b

Of the choices, the prealbumin level would most strongly indicate nutritional risk, as it is slightly below the normal index. Normal prealbumin levels range from 16–35 mg/dl. All of the other values fall within their respective normal ranges. Normal albumin levels range from 3.5–5 g/dl; normal transferrin levels are greater than 200 mg/dl; and a normal total lymphocyte count would fall in the range from 1,200–1,800 cells/mm^3.

16. c

Pharmacogenomics is the study of how different genetic differences can explain varying responses to a drug, often focusing on precise differences in a defined population. Pharmacogenetics, on the other hand, begins with an unexplained drug response and then looks for a genetic rationale. Pharmacokinetics focuses on how the drug is internalized by the body, whereas pharmacodynamics examines how the drug affects the body.

17. d

Amitriptyline would most likely be the reason for the patient's latest complaints as it is a tricyclic antidepressant, a class of drug which causes anticholinergic adverse effects, especially in the elderly. The patient most likely would have been taking this for the neuropathic pain associated with shingles. Phenytoin, an anticonvulsant, acyclovir, an antiviral medication, and ibuprofen, an NSAID, are all appropriate forms of treatment for shingles, and may yield constipation as a side effect, but would not yield the blurry vision and urinary retention problems experienced by the patient.

18. d

Oxidative stress, as a factor of aging, would most likely serve as a model for the free radical theory of aging. Oxidative stress occurs from an imbalance favoring free radicals over antioxidants. The free radical theory states that aging occurs due to free radicals that escape the neutralization process, resulting in DNA damage, cross-linking of proteins, and formation of age pigments. The biological programming theory claims a hereditary basis in aging. The cross-linkage theory claims that proteins, DNA, and other molecules develop detrimental bonds to each other, leading to decreased mobility and functionality of the proteins. The wear and tear theory states that age is determined by accumulated stress to the body.

19. a

Both innate immunity functions and adaptive immunity responses typically decline with age. It is true that decreased thymic hormone production results in a decreased number of functioning T-cells. Decreased antibody production does lead to a decreased response to antigens, while vaccine-induced antibody response also typically decreases with age.

20. d

Continuing care communities are retirement communities provide a continuum of care, from 24/7 independent living care to special nursing home care. Adult congregate communities are different in that residents buy condominiums in an adult community that includes a medical center and 24/7 nursing services. Assisted living communities are rental retirement communities for seniors who need assistance with complex instrumental activities of daily living. Board and care communities are similar to assisted living communities but focus on converted single-family homes.

21. d

Thirst drive tends to decrease, not increase, with age, along with percentage of body water and antidiuretic hormone response to dehydration. Maximum urine osmolality also decreases as age impairs renal function. Blood pressure typically does increase with age.

22. d

Of the choices, *Neisseria meningitidis*—though a gram negative bacteria that can cause pneumonia—is the least common gram negative pathogen responsible for pneumonia in elderly patients. *Haemophilus influenza, Moraxella catarrhalis,* and *Klebsiella pneumoniae* are the most common gram negative pathogens in pneumonia in the elderly.

23. c

An individual must be independent when he or she enters a continuing care community. Skilled nursing facilities are for people with serious health issues not requiring hospitalization and require a physician-prescribed admission. Though continuing care communities do require monthly fees, it is not required for the individual to buy property, as is common in adult congregate communities.

24. a

Low protein intake retards healing. Calcium absorption and percentage of body water are two things that decrease with age. Body temperature also decreases with age, as there is decreased muscle activity which leads to a decrease in heat production.

25. b

Of the agents listed, furosemide is most likely to lead to sedation, memory loss, and dizziness, as it is a diuretic. Paromomycin is an aminoglycoside, which would be more likely to cause adverse effects on balance and movement. Phenytoin, though an anticonvulsant, would also be more likely to cause adverse effects on balance and movement. Doxazosin is an alpha-adrenergic blocker and may cause drowsiness or dizziness, but would not likely cause memory loss.

26. b

For about 25% of elderly beneficiaries, Social Security is the sole source of retirement income. For about 35% of elders, Social Security provides more than 90% of their income. Social Security provides about half the total income for about 65% of elderly beneficiaries.

27. b

Elderly patients should be instructed to take antacids 1 hour before or 4 hours after other medications, as the adsorbent properties of antacids may affect drug absorption. Beta-blockers, benzodiazepines, and diuretics may all affect absorption of certain drugs, but do not generally interfere with absorption on as wide a scale as antacids.

28. c

Aspiration pneumonia may be localized to the right middle lobe or show diffuse involvement; viral pneumonia, however, typically presents as bilateral interstitial infiltrates. Bacterial pneumonia may present with bronchopneumonia or lobar pneumonia.

29. b

Non-steroidal anti-inflammatory drugs, such as naproxen, decrease renal blood flow, further reducing elimination of many drugs. Cimetidine can reduce renal blood flow, but is better known for inhibiting cytochrome P450 in the liver, prolonging the effects of other drugs in the body. Niacin may exacerbate the effects of antihypertensives, but does not typically decrease renal blood flow. Although magnesium hydroxide is an antacid and would reduce absorbance of other drugs, it would not decrease renal blood flow and disrupt drug elimination.

30. b

The dosage of furosemide should be decreased, as the natural decline of serum albumin levels in elderly patients may experience greater effects from highly protein-bound drugs. These effects occur as a result of such drugs distributing through the body in a clinically significant free drug concentration. Looking for an underlying cause is not the top priority, as serum albumin levels typically decrease naturally with age. Switching to torsemide, another protein-binding loop diuretic, will not address the concerns that come with prescribing furosemide. Although metolazone is a thiazide diuretic and is not highly protein-bound, there is no need to abandon protein-bound drugs in the presence of low serum albumin levels.

31. d

The concept that each person has an inherited amount of adaptability to deal with stress to the body is associated with the wear and tear theory of aging, not the error theory of aging. The error theory of aging hangs on the idea that aging is due to internal or external assaults that affect cells or organs so they can no longer function properly. These assaults produce increased amounts of error in the RNA transcription or protein synthesis, producing changes in DNA.

32. b

The Barthel Index is used in the functional assessment of an older patient. The environmental assessment must be conducted by addressing the personal competence and physical limitations of the individual, not through pre-established tests. Similarly, a review of the patient's self-view of sexual relations is part of a sexual assessment. Lastly, risk assessment and identifying nutritional concerns relies on key laboratory indices that measure for substances such as prealbumin or transferrin.

33. c

The theory that abnormal cells may double an infinite amount of times is a reflection of the biological programming theory of aging, not the free radical theory. DNA damage, cross-linking of proteins, and formation of age pigments all result from free radicals escaping the neutralizing process.

34. b

Cardiac disease can potentially impact the perfusion of tissues and the delivery of a drug, which may result in inhibited distribution of the medication. Cardiac disease is not commonly attributed to affecting receptors in the body; however, receptors do change during the aging process. Increased receptor regulation leads to increased sensitivity to medication, whereas decreased receptor regulation leads to decreased sensitivity to medication. Cardiac disease would not produce increased tissue absorption that leads to prolonged drug effects.

35. a

Myocardial infarction and other sources of vascular damage are common causes of erectile dysfunction (ED), associated with 50% of all cases of the condition. Although endocrine disorders may be associated with the condition, hyperthyroidism rarely produces ED. Antihypertensives are also associated with ED, but beta blockers such as atenolol are less likely to produce the condition. Some histamine H2 antagonists, such as cimetidine, may likewise cause ED, but others, such as ranitidine and famotidine, are less likely to cause sexual dysfunction.

36. b

Although religion may be a concern, some patients may not necessarily hold to a particular religion but still hold spiritual views; therefore, the patient's spiritual needs should be addressed, but not necessarily through the filter of any particular religion. The patient should also be assessed for their views on death and dying, the potential necessity of any rituals before death, and how the nurse practitioner can aid in any spiritual needs the patient may have.

37. a

Although the average onset of the reduced ability to maintain homeostasis is at age 30, it does not tend to manifest in the organs until age 50. From then on, the ability of the body to regulate temperature and acidity continues to worsen with age.

38. c

Hashimoto's disease is the least likely of the choices to be associated with abnormal calcium levels, as this disease attacks thyroid function and metabolism. Nephrolithiasis commonly occurs because of calcium deposits in the kidneys. Hyperparathyroidism is an excess of parathyroid hormone in the bloodstream, which may affect the maintenance of balance of calcium. Although it is not definite, some studies suggest that high calcium intake can increase the risk of some cancers, such as prostate cancer.

39. d

The disengagement theory is best illustrated by the scenario of an elder teacher who is given mandatory retirement and is both relieved and uncertain about what to do next. As the disengagement theory is often focused on the idea of a mutual "disengagement" between older persons and society, it rests on the idea that the retiree will be relieved by the lapse of societal roles, but does not put much stock in the activity and contributions of older adults. A former CEO who transfers attention from her company to her social circle may be an example of either the continuity or activity theory, depending on whether she devotes the same attention or increased attention to her circle. An elderly man who fears he is no longer self-sufficient would be classified under the continuity theory as a defended personality, somebody who holds on to middle-aged values and frets as those values are challenged by age. The continuity theory would also apply to an introvert who maintains the same hobbies and social presence in old age as she did in middle age, such as the woman who spends her retirement in bookstores.

40. a

Subsidiary housing for the elderly does not typically provide two meals per day; this option is more often found in assisted living communities. Subsidiary housing is subsidized by the Department of Housing and Urban Development, and does not require monthly fees. Basic check-ups and blood pressure tests are available daily from on-site nurses; however, subsidiary housing is only for low-income elderly in good health.

DISCUSSION

Gerontology Health Assessment

Functional Assessment

A standard functional assessment of a patient includes reviews and evaluations of the patient's social and economic resources, physical and mental health, and cognitive status. Changes in a geriatric patient's ability to function in everyday activities are often related to changes in health and further result in adjustments in a patient's living status.[1] Examples of functional assessment tools include the Katz ADL Scale, the Barthel Index, the Kenny Self-Care Scale, the IADL Scale, the Timed Manual Performance, the Performance Test of ADL, the Framingham Disability Scale, and the Lawton Scale.[2]

Advanced Activities of Daily Living (AADLs) are complex measures of functional status, which include assessments of working, volunteering, social activities, recreational activities, and connection with peers and community.[1] Losing competency in these activities may indicate a major decline in the patient's overall health. Instrumental Activities of Daily Living (IADLs), on the other hand, are activities that contribute to independent functioning. IADLs are listed under the acronym "SHAFT," which consists of Shopping; Housekeeping (e.g., cooking, laundry, and vacuuming) and health maintenance activities (e.g., medical appointments and medications); Accounting (i.e., managing financial matters); Food preparation; and Transportation and telephone use and skills.[3]

In contrast to AADLs or IADLs, Activities of Daily Living (ADLs) are basic self-care activities. Older adults with functional decline generally lose the ability to do their IADLs prior to losing ADL function. ADLs are categorized under the acronym "DEATH," which consists of Dressing; Eating; Ambulating; Transferring and toileting (i.e., being able to sit down on, rise from, and properly use a toilet); and Hygiene.[1]

Environmental Assessment

An environmental assessment is conducted by addressing the patient's personal competence and physical limitations.[4] Because normal lower body temperature and a decreased amount of natural insulation generally make elderly patients more sensitive to lower temperatures, the recommended room temperature for elderly adults is 75 °F. The nurse practitioner (NP) should also be mindful that room temperatures less than 70 °F can cause hypothermia in the elderly.[5] Certain conditions can influence the safety of the elderly; for instance, good sources of lighting help to enhance the patient's mood and behavior, and may assist to maintain orientation. Nightlights are often helpful, whereas fluorescent lights may produce eyestrain. Warm colors such as red, orange, and yellow can be stimulating. Conversely, cool tones such as blues and greens may have a relaxing effect.

Scattered and area rugs should be avoided, as they are common sources for falls. Bold floor designs are also discouraged as they can cause dizziness and confusion during ambulation. A single solid color and non-glare surface are preferable. Floor treatments that provide a non-slip surface are also particularly useful. Finally, furnishings should be appealing, functional, and comfortable, and those with cognitive impairments should have simple environments.[1,6]

Furthermore, because many accidental injuries occur in the bathroom, the NP should pay particular attention to reducing the risk of bathroom hazards. The bathroom should be kept lit at all times, and potential sources of falls (e.g., bathmats, throw rugs, leaks) should be mitigated. Lever-shaped faucet handles are easier to use than round ones, and color-coding faucet handles makes it easier to differentiate between hot and cold water. In tubs and shower stalls, nonslip surfaces should be used, as should grab bars on the wall. Grab bars or support frames also aid in the difficult task of sitting down and rising from a toilet seat. Storage of cleaning supplies and other toxins should be reviewed, and clear labels should be made for products that appear similar. Lastly, it is important to clearly label medications and set up a workable system for taking them.[1]

Nutritional Assessment

In a nutritional assessment, the NP should ask if the patient takes a multivitamin daily. The recommended daily protein intake for adults is at least 0.8 grams/kg per day. Low protein intake and albumin levels are indicative of malnutrition.[7,8] Medications associated with an increase in appetite include antidepressants, tranquilizers, beta adrenergic agents, narcoleptics, hormones, and steroids.[1] Calcium absorption decreases with age, so calcium intake needs to be individualized. Additional conditions that should be considered in elderly patients include nephrolithiasis, hyperparathyroidism, and certain cancers.[1]

When measuring the patient's body mass index (BMI), keep current standards in mind. By these standards, a BMI between 18.5% and 24.9% is considered normal weight. A patient with a BMI of less than 18.5% is considered underweight, whereas a BMI between 25% and 29.9% indicates the patient is overweight. Lastly, patients with a BMI above 30% are considered obese.[9]

In a nutritional risk assessment, the patient's history should be considered, including involuntary weight loss, changes in appetite, and how well the patient's clothing fits his or her body. Common indicators of nutritional risk include weight loss at a rate of 5 lb in 1 month, 5% of body weight in 1 month, 7.5% of body weight in 3 months, or 10% of body weight in 6 months.[10,11]

Measurements of serum protein levels are often used to determine the patient's nutritional status. Serum proteins such as albumin, prealbumin, and transferrin, as well as a total lymphocyte count, are frequently assessed to evaluate protein status.[12] Normal albumin levels are 3.5–5 g/dl, normal prealbumin levels are 16–35 mg/dl, and normal transferrin levels are greater than 200 mg/dl.[13] Additionally, a normal total lymphocyte count ranges between 1,200 and 1,800 cells/mm³.[1]

Sexual Assessment

It is a widely held belief that people over a certain age do not engage in sexual activity. In many cases, this myth interferes with comprehensive health assessments and treatment. Although there is a general decline in sexual libido as one gets older, the amount of sexual activity varies from person to person, and some people experience little to no decline in sexual activity. Male sexual dysfunction is considered the primary reason for reducing or discontinuing sexual activity.[1] The NP should, however, assess the patient's history of and outlook on sexual activity.

Living arrangements can interfere with privacy required for sexual relations. It is also important to be aware of situations contributing to lack of respect for the patient's sexuality. These situations may include forgetting to fasten clothing, denying same gender attendants for bathing, and discussing incontinence issues and other medical conditions in front of the patient's peers.[1]

The patient's medical history should be assessed for factors that may impair sexual desire or performance, such as certain medications (e.g., pharmacotherapy for hypertension), diagnoses/ conditions (e.g., myocardial infarction), or surgeries (e.g., mastectomy, prostatectomy).[14,15] Further, the NP should assess for sexual dysfunction.[1,16] The NP should also review and screen for sexually transmitted diseases and infections.

Physiology and Aging

Overview

Certain changes that come with aging are responsible for atypical disease presentations,

such as impaired thermoregulation, fluid volume regulation, immune alterations, and changes in the cardiac and nervous systems. Impaired thermoregulation is a frequent occurrence in older adults, resulting in lower than normal basal body temperatures. Possible causes of impaired thermoregulation include decreased diet-induced thermogenesis, decreased heat production per kilogram of body weight, and reduced activity in muscles that influence heat production. Normal oral temperatures in the aged are 35.8–36.8 °C (96.4–98.2 °F), and normal rectal temperatures are 36.8–37.2 °C (98.2–98.9 °F). The general rule is that the body temperatures of older adults are, on average, about 1–2 °F lower than those of younger adults.[17]

Fluid volume regulation is also a potential concern, as older adults present with decreased percentages of body water, thirst drive, and antidiuretic hormone response to dehydration. Older adults may also experience renal dysfunction, which results in decreased maximum urine osmolality and impaired renin-angiotensin-aldosterone responsiveness. As a result, less water is taken in, which in turn causes less water on reserve. Moreover, since many patients are able to retain less water, they are predisposed to earlier and faster dehydration.[18]

Infections/Sepsis

Overview

Approximately 40% of all deaths in those over the age of 65 are attributable to infections.[19] With sepsis infections, however, the mortality rate increases 9 times when compared to other adults.[1] Infections may be caused by an immune system decline from lack of cell proliferation, especially interleukin-2 and T cells.[20] Infections may also stem from drying and thinning of the skin and mucous membranes, inefficient mucociliary clearance, and malnutrition.[20,21] Several comorbidities (e.g., malignancy, diabetes mellitus, immunocompromised states, etc.) increase the risk of infection, as does a decreased ability to produce antibodies.[22] Sepsis is characterized by inflammation that occurs in tissues remote from the infection.[23] Systemic inflammatory response syndrome (SIRS) is the beginning of the sepsis continuum that can lead to severe septic shock. Sepsis can occur with any infection or from inflammation.

Presentation

Among adults over 65 years of age, 30%–60% display both protein and calorie malnutrition.[24] As a result of these types of malnutrition, patients may respond inefficiently to vaccines, as well as exhibit an increased risk of infection and impaired wound healing. Up to 50% of all older adults with infection present without fever.[24] Many older adults have a core temperature that is 1–2 °F lower, so a fever can easily go unnoticed by both patient and NP. This lack of fever possibly stems from altered thermoregulation in general, coupled with decreased heat production by adipose tissue.[25] Tachycardia, hypotension, and tachypnea are all signs of sepsis and SIRS, and call for immediate evaluation.

The American Medical Directors Association's Clinical Practice Guidelines for Infections provide three long-term care criteria for fever in the elderly. The first criterion is an increasing temperature of equal to or greater than 2 °F (1.1 °C) from the baseline. The second criterion is two or more measurements of either the patient's oral temperature that are equal to or greater than 99 °F (37.2 °C), or the patient's rectal temperature equal to or greater than 99.5 °F (37.5 °C). The final criterion is a single measurement of temperature that is equal to or greater than 100 °F (37.8 °C).[26] Furthermore, infected or septic older adults can present with other atypical findings such as diminished or low oral intake, fatigue, and withdrawal from activities of interest. Patients may have alterations in mental status that range from agitation to confusion and even delirium. Sepsis may also be indicated by falls, triggered by the patient's dehydration, fatigue, and altered mental status.[27,28]

Aging Demographic

Overview

There are increasing numbers of older adults, with older adulthood being defined as 65 years of age or greater. The "young old" are 65–74 years of age and consist of the first wave of aging Baby Boomers who have reached full retirement age. Over the next 20 years, it is anticipated that 74 million Boomers will retire. The "old" age group, on the other hand, ranges from 75 to 84 years of age. During the next decade, the wave of aging Boomers will steadily increase due to increased life expectancy. Lastly, the "Oldest Old" age group is comprised of individuals aged 85 years and over and is the most rapidly-growing segment of the total population. This group's growth rate is twice that of individuals aged 65 and over and almost 4 times that of the total population, with the greatest increase being in women.[29]

Caring for the Aging and Elderly

Overview

When caring for the aging and elderly, it is important to remember that age regularly heightens the complexity of diagnosis and treatment. The current life expectancy in the United States is 81.2 years for females and 76.4 years for males.[29] Organ system decline is usually due to diseases, not the aging process. The NP must recognize the difference between unnatural aging and normal age-related changes.[30]

Elderly patients who are particularly immunocompromised are at an increased risk of complications and atypical presentations. Furthermore, the patient's ability to maintain homeostasis shows a general decrease with age; on average, changes to homeostasis start at 30 years of age, with such changes manifesting in the organs by 50 years of age.[31] Key organ systems at greatest risk for disease in the elderly include the circulatory and musculoskeletal systems, the central nervous system (CNS), and the lower urinary tract.[32]

Presentation

Common findings indicating disease in the elderly include incontinence, functional decline, and syncope. Other potential indications for disease include delirium, dementia, and a vulnerability to falls.[33] The organ system associated with a particular finding, such as the musculoskeletal system in cases of loss of balance, is less likely to cause that particular finding in older adults when compared to younger adults.[34] Many compensatory mechanisms are compromised concurrently, and drug side effects can be pronounced at low doses due to alterations in absorption, a decline in drug metabolism by the liver, and reduced kidney function to excrete the drug.[35]

Principles

Overview

The American Nurses Association's Scope and Standards of Gerontological Practice highlights the importance of the following critical gerontology functions for assessment: health promotion, health maintenance, disease prevention, and facilitation of self-care.[36]

Presentation

The top nine most common conditions in older adults are Parkinson's disease, hypertension, heart disease, respiratory disease, diabetes mellitus, cancer, cerebrovascular disease, atherosclerosis, and Alzheimer's disease. Further, the top ten most likely reasons for older adults to be hospitalized are heart disease, cancer, cerebrovascular disease, pneumonia, fractures, bronchitis, osteoarthritis, prostate hyperplasia, diseases of the nervous system or sense organs, and diabetes mellitus. Lastly, the top twelve most common causes of death among older adults are heart disease, cancer, cerebrovascular disease, chronic obstructive pulmonary disease, pneumonia, influenza, diabetes mellitus, accidents, Alzheimer's disease, septicemia, atherosclerosis, and hypertension.[36]

Adjustments in Aging

Many aging adults face a decline in their health and functional status, which may be difficult to accept as they become increasingly aware of their mortality.[37] As older adults become more cognizant of their own death, they tend to develop interests in fulfilling their own dreams, deepening their religious convictions, strengthening family ties, and leaving a legacy.[1]

Adjustment to retirement can prove to be challenging since a person's sense of worth and identity are frequently associated with productivity, and individuals tend to define themselves by what they do for work rather than their personal characteristics. In addition to these adjustments, older patients may also have income issues, as many elderly are poor, with approximately one in six living below the poverty line.[38] Moreover, retirement income is generally much less than one's working salary, resulting in older adults making major lifestyle changes such as relocating to less expensive housing, changing their social practices and diet, and lowering their independence.[39] Social Security is the primary source of income for many elderly people, with an average monthly retirement benefit of under $1,300.[40] For 36% of all older adults, Social Security supplies over 90% of their income. Furthermore, for 24% of all elderly beneficiaries, Social Security is the only source of income during retirement.[41]

The family is traditionally seen as a major source of satisfaction and provides a vital source of support by helping older adults cope with multiple losses and changes in life.[42] Adjustments are traditionally made with regard to the independence of children, as there is limited extended family interaction in today's society, and children are generally less responsible for aging parents. The elderly likewise tend to experience shrinkage in their social world due to the loss of a spouse and friends, as well as children being grown and living away; this shrinking social world often causes loneliness and desolation. The death of a spouse, however, typically affects women more than men.

The declining health of an older adult coupled with the loss of a spouse can raise the question of how safely one can live independently. Signs of danger that indicate an elderly person needs extra assistance or a change in living environment include sudden weight loss, burns or injury marks, and general forgetfulness. Patients may also need changes in their living environment or extra help if they exhibit peculiar behavior of any kind, fail to take medication or overdose, or are involved in an increasing number of car accidents. If danger signals are apparent, alternative housing options should be considered.

Aging in place is defined as the elderly person continuing to live in his or her own place of residence with additional resources for support.[43] In particular, assisted living allows older adults to enjoy adequate levels of care without having to leave their communities.

Settings of Care

There are several types of retirement communities, such as adult congregate communities, in which residents buy condominiums and pay a monthly fee for grass mowing, leaf raking, and other services. Many adult congregate communities may also feature on-site medical facilities with 24/7 nursing service.[42,44]

Assisted living communities, on the other hand, are rental retirement communities for seniors who need help with important aspects of daily living, such as cooking, shopping, and money management. Many assisted living communities also provide three meals per day, housekeeping, and laundry service, as well as a 24/7 registered nurse on call as per the rental agreement. Board and care is another type of retirement option, similar to assisted living, and frequently consists of a single-family house that has been converted into a residence for elderly and disabled residents.[42,44]

Continuing care communities provide a continuum of care, from 24/7 independent living care to special nursing home care. A long term contract regularly establishes that care will be given on this continuum for the remainder of a person's life; as such, these housing options are expensive. Individuals must be independent when they enter this type of community. For low-income elderly in good health, however, options exist for subsidized housing, usually overseen by the Department of Housing and Urban Development. Although 24/7 nursing care is not a standard feature of subsidized housing, on-site nursing care may be available.[42,44]

In skilled nursing facilities, 24-hour nursing for people with serious health care needs that can be managed outside of the hospital, such as those needing extensive physical therapy, is typically provided. Admission to these facilities is generally determined by a physician. Intermediate care facilities, by comparison, are a less involved health care alternative compared to skilled nursing facilities. These facilities are mainly for people unable to live alone who require minimal medical assistance and help with personal and social care.[42,44]

System-Specific Considerations in Gerontology

Hematologic

Gerontology considerations in the hematologic system involve several physiologic changes. These changes include immunosenescence, which is the diminished function of the immune system with age that commonly results in a lessened response to infection. Likewise, functions of innate immunity, such as macrophages, natural killer cells, and neutrophils, decline. Adaptive immune responses also decline. Decreased thymic hormone production will likewise occur, resulting in fewer functioning

T-cells. Decreased antibody production and response is another physiologic change, as well as diminished response to antigens.[45]

Thus, hematologic changes in the elderly result in overall increased susceptibility to infection, poor wound healing, exacerbation of chronic diseases, and waning vaccine-induced antibody response.[45]

Neurologic

As one ages, the nervous system undergoes a number of physical changes. The number of active neurons and neurotransmitters diminishes, and cerebral dendrites, glial support cells, and synapses all undergo changes that result in altered function.[46,47] Elderly patients likewise experience a general impairment of thermoregulation, which leads to decreased temperature sensitivity and a blunted or absent fever response. A decreased sense of touch is another common finding, along with an increased pain tolerance. As such, many elderly patients may be slow to recognize or report injuries such as wounds or ulcers. Specific manifestations present in the various parts of the nervous system. In the peripheral nervous system, a general decrease is seen in baroreflex responses, beta-adrenergic responsiveness, signal transduction, and muscarinic parasympathetic responses; alpha responses, however, are typically preserved.[48] In the central nervous system, there is a decrease in the number of dopamine receptors, but alpha responses and muscarinic parasympathetic responses are generally increased.[49]

As a result of these changes, elderly patients exhibit diminished muscle strength and deep tendon reflexes, as well as delayed nerve conduction velocity. Cognitive processing may also slow, resulting in a cognitive decline in some patients; in most patients, however, memory functions are satisfactory in later life. A decrease in motor skill ability, balance, and coordination can result in an increased risk for falls in elderly patients.[50]

Gastrointestinal

Physiological changes must be taken into consideration when a geriatric patient presents with gastrointestinal complaints. The elderly have decreased strength of jaw muscles for chewing, as well as decreased thirst and taste perception. In addition, the elderly experience decreased gastric motility with delayed emptying, increased intestinal transit time, and an impaired defecation signal. Elderly patients also have decreased liver size and decreased liver blood flow, which can result in altered drug absorption and decreased or impaired metabolism of drugs.[50]

Other common gastrointestinal risks in elderly patients include poor nutrition, dysphagia, NSAID-induced ulcers, and constipation. Constipation is not a normal finding in elderly patients, but most commonly stems from lack of fiber, decreased exercise, poor dentition, history of laxative abuse, and impaired mental status.[50]

Respiratory

The effects of the aging process on the respiratory system cause physiological changes that may affect the health and well-being of the elderly patient. Some changes, such as rounding of the chest wall and enlargement of the cartilaginous airways, do not have much of an impact on the pulmonary system. Skeletal changes related to aging also cause the anteroposterior (AP) diameter to become larger. The risk of pulmonary complications associated with surgery or lower respiratory tract illness increases in these patients. Elderly patients are also at an increased risk of atelectasis, infection, and bronchospasms.[51]

Older adults may exhibit increased exercise intolerance and less effective exhalation. Further, there is a decreased cough reflex and a diminished response to hypoxia and hypercapnia. Also, the number of mucous-producing cells increases as the number of cilia diminishes, resulting in decreased mucus clearance.[50]

Respiratory muscle strength and endurance also diminish with age. Although total lung capacity remains constant, pulmonary function diminishes as the lungs stiffen, resulting in decreased lung expansion—vital capacity decreases as residual volume increases. The alveolar surface area decreases up to 20%, which reduces maximal oxygen uptake.[52]

Elderly patients are highly susceptible to pneumonia; at least 50% of all reported pneumonia cases occur in adults 65 years of age or older. For those living in long-term care facilities, the risk of developing pneumonia over the next 2 years is increased by 30%.[19] The most common pathogens include *Streptococcus pneumoniae, Staphylococcus aureus*, and gram-negative bacilli (e.g., *Haemophilus influenzae, Moraxella catarrhalis, Klebsiella*).[53]

Clinical findings of pneumonia among the elderly may include weakness, anorexia, shortness of breath, tachypnea, tachycardia, and confusion, among others.[33,53]

Cardiovascular

The aging process causes a number of physiological changes to the cardiovascular system. High blood pressure may lead to arteriosclerosis and atherosclerosis, resulting in decreased arterial compliance.[54] Hypertension may also cause left ventricular hypertrophy or atrial hypertrophy.[55] The increase in atrioventricular conduction time causes a loss of pacemaker cells.

The overall physical findings of an exam are most likely to include diminished peripheral pulses and cool extremities. Heart murmurs are common, and dysrhythmias may occur because of systemic illness or as a side effect of medications.[56] The intrinsic and maximum heart rates decrease, but the resting heart rate and cardiac output are unaffected. The NP should also note decreased cardiac reserve, which increases the risk for orthostatic hypotension or syncope.[57]

Pharmacology Considerations in Gerontology

Pharmacokinetics

Pharmacokinetics is the study of how the body interacts with drugs, including absorption, distribution, metabolism, and excretion. Distribution relies on blood flow, lipid or water solubility, and protein binding to deliver and distribute the drug, all of which can be problematic in an older adult. Older adults exhibit a decrease in total body water, increase in fat, and decreased muscle mass. In elderly patients, a decrease in serum albumin produces uneven distribution of protein-bound drugs, which rely on albumin for binding and transport. Those with nutritional deficiencies have a low serum albumin concentration, resulting in an increased drug concentration.[58,59]

Metabolism can be significantly reduced in geriatric patients, particularly if there is liver impairment. Thus, dosage adjustments should be taken into consideration. In elderly patients, a natural decrease in hepatic blood flow occurs, and is associated with potential decreased first pass effects.[58,59]

Pharmacokinetics also encompasses the patient's excretion or elimination, and largely focuses on renal clearance. Glomerular filtration declines with aging, producing a subsequent decline in creatinine clearance. In addition, blood flow to the kidneys is decreased. Thus, drug elimination changes in the elderly are often due to overall decreased renal function. As a result, many drugs can be therapeutic at dosages lower than those for a younger adult. The Cockcroft-Gault equation is often used to estimate creatinine clearance.[58,59]

Pharmacodynamics

Pharmacodynamics is the study of how drugs interact with the body. Receptors can up-regulate or down-regulate with age, causing an increased or decreased sensitivity to certain agents. Homeostasis changes include a decreased capacity to respond to physiological challenges and the adverse side effects of drug therapy, such as orthostatic hypotension.[60]

Pharmacogenetics

Pharmacogenetics is the study of single-gene genetic variations in drug responses. The goal of pharmacogenetics is to understand the role that an individual's genetic make-up plays in how well a drug works, including any likely side effects. Pharmacogenetics produces many benefits, including more accurate methods of determining dosages, drugs that are prescribed specifically for a patient's genetic profile, and the development of drugs that maximize therapeutic effects.[61]

Pharmacogenetics vs. Pharmacogenomics

The terms pharmacogenetics and pharmacogenomics are frequently used interchangeably. The differences between the two lie in the initial approach of the science. Pharmacogenetics begins with an unexpected drug response, and then searches for a genetic cause. Pharmacogenomics, on the other hand, begins with looking for genetic differences within a population that explain certain observed responses to a drug.[62]

Adverse Reactions

In elderly patients, adverse reactions closely associated with medication use include CNS effects such as sedation, memory loss, dizziness, depression, and confusion. Also common are anticholinergic effects, which may include blurred vision, urinary retention, constipation, and dry mouth. Moreover, elderly patients may also experience adverse effects on their movement and balance, as well as their bone and supporting structures.[63,64]

Drugs most likely to cause adverse reactions in the geriatric patient are those with CNS adverse effects, such as benzodiazepines, antipsychotics, beta blockers, steroids, cimetidine, narcotics, and diuretics, among others. Agents with anticholinergic adverse effects include cholinergic agonists, tricyclic antidepressants, and antipsychotics, among others. Furthermore, certain drugs may have adverse effects on the patient's balance and movement, such as neuroleptics, metronidazole, phenytoin, aspirin, aminoglycosides, furosemide, beta blockers, vasodilators, and metoclopramide, among others.[65] Finally, regimens with adverse effects on bone and supporting structures include steroids, lithium, and long-term heparin use, among others.[66]

Promoting Safe Drug Use

Approximately 45% of all older adults do not adhere to drug regimens, especially in light of the common use of multiple medications.[67] The NP should also recognize that self-medication can be a problem, as the patient may be using medications that belongs to someone else. Likewise, alternative or herbal medications or therapies can interact adversely with prescription medicines. Patients should be given a rationale for why a particular drug is or is not indicated. Since some geriatric patients are incapable of managing a medication regimen, functional assessment tools such as a Mini-Mental State Examination (MMSE) and the Geriatric Depression Scale can serve as good indicators of patients' decision-making abilities.[68,69] The Beers Criteria for Potentially Inappropriate Medication Use in Older Adults should also be used to measure the safety of prescribing medications for patients over 65 years of age.

Polypharmacy in the Elderly

Polypharmacy, defined as the use of more medicines than are clinically indicated, is a regular occurrence in geriatric patients. Promoting factors include the presence of comorbid conditions, the use of multiple prescribers, overuse of non-prescription and alternative medicines, and the prevalence of the concept of a "pill for every ill." Prevention of polypharmacy requires recognizing the underlying problem; clinical consultation with a pharmacist may be helpful as well. Communication between pharmacists and prescribers is key, and the NP should take an "essential medicines only" approach. Patients should avoid combination products and start with lowest effective doses, if possible.[1] The patient should also be encouraged to bring in a list of current mediations for review by the NP. Education of the patient should include discussion of all over-the-counter and herbal medications.

Polypharmacy puts elderly patients at increased risk for morbidity, medical expense, and adverse reactions.[70] Certain over-the-counter agents complicate polypharmacy, such as cimetidine, which can prolong the effects of other liver-metabolized drugs in the body.[71] Decongestants and other drugs with anticholinergic effects commonly antagonize the activity of antihypertensives.[72] NSAIDs can decrease renal blood flow, further reducing the elimination of many drugs.[73] Niacin, in turn, may exacerbate the effect of antihypertensives.[74] Antacids can adsorb other oral agents, reducing their absorbance across the gut wall.[75] Laxatives can likewise reduce absorbance of some drugs, as well as increase gut motility and chelate other drugs so they cannot be absorbed.[76] Calcium products can decrease absorbance of thyroid hormones.[77] Lastly, herbal agents may complicate polypharmacy by interacting with prescribed medications and producing adverse side effects.[78]

Pressure Ulcers

Overview

Pressure ulcers are lesions that are caused by unrelieved external pressure, resulting in the occlusion of blood flow, tissue ischemia, and cell death. Impaired or restricted mobility is an important agent in the development of pressure ulcers, which are one of the most common conditions that develop in patients receiving prolonged hospital care.[79]

Patients over 65 years of age are also at increased risk for pressure ulcers, possibly due to reduced subcutaneous fat and capillary blood flow.[80] Additionally, the skin of older patients is drier and more fragile than that of younger adults; thus, aging skin tends to be more vulnerable to damage and less resistant to the development of pressure ulcers.[81] Malnutrition and comorbidities (e.g.,

diabetes mellitus, anemia) also increase the risk of ulcer development.[82] The rate of mortality increases four-fold for people with pressure ulcers and six-fold for people with non-healing ulcers.[1,83]

Presentation

Pressure ulcers are identified by discoloration and their location over a bony prominence.[79] Patients frequently exhibit red, nonblanchable skin that develops into lesions over time; the affected area tends to first manifest as a blister, then as an open sore.[84] In dark-skinned people, however, ulcers may be difficult to see. Pressure ulcers are classified in stages depending on their presentation. Although there are several staging systems used for pressure ulcers, the standard system is that of the National Pressure Ulcer Advisory Panel, which consists of four stages and classifies ulcers according to the depth of soft-tissue damage.[80] The patient's skin is still intact in stage 1 and presents with erythema that does not blanch. Stage 2 ulcers are partial-thickness lesions extending into the epidermis and dermis. Stage 3 ulcers progress to full-thickness skin loss involving the subcutaneous tissue. Lastly, in stage 4 lesions, extensive tissue damage occurs and extends to the muscles, bones, and underlying structures.[80]

Staging of pressure ulcers is difficult when eschar is present. Staging can only be done once the devitalized tissue is removed via debridement and the base of the wound can be seen. Further, the purpose of staging is to describe the anatomic status of an ulcer at the time of assessment.[85]

Treatment

Treatment of pressure ulcers consists of removing the source of the ischemic injury by relieving pressure. Additionally, the NP should consult a wound care specialist. When treating stage 1 and 2 pressure ulcers, non-operative options are used. Stage 1 ulcers should be protected by transparent films, and stage 2 ulcers require dressings that maintain a moist environment around the wound.[86] Stage 3 and 4 ulcers may require surgical interventions and potential antimicrobial treatment.

Approximately 70%–90% of all pressure ulcers are superficial and heal by secondary intention. As soon as pressure is relieved on otherwise healthy and vascularized skin, clinical improvement may be evident within 48 hours.[1,87]

Elder Abuse

Overview

Elder abuse encompasses various forms of mistreatment of the older adult, including physical and psychological abuse, neglect, and financial exploitation.[88,89] Ninety percent of the time, the victim knows the abuser.[90] Older adults at risk for abuse exhibit factors such as increasing age, lack of close family ties, and physical or mental impairment. Other potential contributing factors in elder abuse include caregiver stress, unsafe housing, and poverty or financial distress. Additionally, women are at higher risk than men and make up the majority of abuse victims.[91]

Approximately 6% of all elderly people report being abused, and it is estimated that five times as many cases are unreported.[92] Factors that contribute to the underreporting of elder abuse cases may include the patient's emotional response (e.g., fear, shame, guilt, ignorance, embarrassment) or dependency upon the abuser as a caregiver.[93]

Presentation

Elder abuse is a frequent problem in the United States and can be physical, psychological, or financial.[94,95] Older adults are suspected of being abused based on their history, physical examination, and responses to screening questions.[96] The patient should receive a complete examination to detect signs of abuse, preferably upon his or her first visit.[88] Laboratory tests such as a complete blood count and urinalysis are ordered to evaluate for findings that would suggest abuse (e.g., infection, dehydration, etc.).[93]

Physical abuse is defined as any type of violence that results in physical pain or injury, such as pushing, slapping, hitting, or improper use of physical restraints, among other forms. Emotional or psychological abuse, on the other hand, encompasses any type of abuse that bestows mental anguish, such as intimidation, threatening, shunning, isolation, insulting, and yelling. Sexual abuse is defined as forced or non-consensual sexual activities, such as rape, sexual harassment, forced viewing of pornography, and molestation. Demented, delusional, and sedated individuals cannot give consent to sexual activity; thus, they are at risk for sexual abuse.[1]

Furthermore, financial exploitation of older adults, characterized by misappropriating funds, withdrawing money from accounts, removing valuable possessions, or signing over assets, is widespread.[91] Caregivers can also neglect older adults by disregarding or ignoring their needs, which may include isolating the individual, giving the individual an unhealthy diet, oversedation of the individual, and failure to pay attention to the individual's physical state. Moreover, abused older adults may live in a poorly kept home environment with non-hygienic living conditions.[97]

Management

Cases of elder abuse should be evaluated, referred, and reported. Most states have mandatory statutes for reporting, and all states have protection from civil and criminal liability for those who report abuse. Potential consequences for the NP not reporting abuse include fines, damages, and the loss of professional licenses, among other penalties.

Medical, social, and legal interventions should be offered to geriatric patients who are determined to be abuse victims and given to those who accept aid.[96] In most circumstances, abuse victims should help determine their own intervention if they have decision-making capability.[97] Early intervention should consist of addressing caregiver stress through education and counseling.[93]

Sleep Disorders

Overview

More than one-half of all older adults report at least one recurring sleep complaint.[98] Many sleep disorders manifest with insomnia, which causes difficulties going to sleep, difficulties maintaining sleep, or early awakening.[99] Other types of sleep disorders include hypersomnia, parasomnias (strange behaviors during sleep), and nocturnal movement disorders such as restless leg syndrome.[100,101,102]

Presentation

Insomnia is a recurring difficulty with sleep that can result in daytime impairment.[103,104] Standard complaints of insomnia include inability to fall asleep, recurrent awakenings, inability to return to sleep, and difficulty staying asleep. In contrast to insomnia, hypersomnia causes recurrent episodes of excessive daytime sleepiness or prolonged nighttime sleep.[100] Patients with hypersomnia generally feel excessively sleepy at a time when they should be awake, resulting in poor sleep at night; these patients, however, may feel that their sleeping habits are fine. Fatigue, weakness, memory impairment, and learning difficulties are common associated findings of hypersomnia patients. Sleep apnea is a regular cause of hypersomnia that results in unusual daytime sleepiness and consists of snoring and interrupted breathing for at least 10 seconds. Chronic use of hypnotic medications such as cough suppressants and over-the-counter preparations frequently results in daytime sleepiness.[100]

Lastly, parasomnias are strange or unusual behaviors during sleep, such as nightmares, nocturnal confusion, and talking and walking in one's sleep. These conditions can be exacerbated by drugs or medications such as caffeine, alcohol, and beta blockers, among others. Patients may also experience sleep-related leg cramps as well as REM sleep behavior disorder, which frequently presents with behaviors such as verbalization and violent behavior during REM sleep. REM sleep behavior disorder is more common among elderly patients, especially those with CNS disorders such as Parkinson's or Alzheimer's disease.[99,101]

Management

Management of sleep disorders consists of primary and secondary prevention methods. In primary prevention, the patient should sleep only as much as needed and exercise daily. Additionally, the patient should be discouraged from reading or watching TV in bed, or from consuming caffeine in the afternoon or evening. Education on the adverse effects of drugs that contain caffeine and other stimulants is important. Secondary prevention strategies are aimed at reducing the problem once it exists, and are determined by asking the patient questions such as how well he or she sleeps at home, how many times each night he or she awakes, and what rituals are performed at bedtime. NPs should also ask what amount and type of exercise patients get and how much room ventilation the patient needs to feel comfortable. Interventions should aim to maintain conditions conducive to sleep and to help the patient relax with treatments such as bedtime snacks and massages.[105]

Pain

Overview

The leading reason that patients seek health care is pain, which is classified as either acute or chronic.[106] Acute pain begins suddenly and is an important protective mechanism against potential dangers to the body, as it is a standard early warning sign of disease.[107] Chronic pain, on the other hand, remains active for at least 6 months and can persist even after injuries heal.[108] Moreover, chronic pain is a common symptom of a pathological process and not a normal part of aging.[1]

Presentation

Patients should receive a precise and systematic pain assessment using a multidimensional approach to properly diagnose pain and determine the best treatment plan for the patient's circumstances.[109] The NP should evaluate the patient's level of function in a variety of settings and assess the severity of pain before any interventions.[106]

The NP should be aware that the patient might also be unable to express pain due to poor cognitive or mental functioning; regarding medication, the patient could also be concerned about addiction or have a fear of side effects. Patients may believe that reporting pain will not be taken seriously, or withhold reporting pain out of a desire to be a good, non-complaining patient.

Management

Pharmacologic treatments are the most frequently used method of managing pain.[110] Mild or moderate pain is treated effectively by acetaminophen or NSAIDs, whereas opioid analgesics are better suited for managing severe acute or chronic pain.[110] Multimodal therapy should be taken into consideration for postoperative pain management, as this method aims to produce maximum pain relief through a mixture of opioid and nonopioid pharmacologic agents.[111] The NP should, however, be mindful that family members may suggest that the patient not take pain medication based on the belief that these medications can cause dependence or respiratory depression.[1] Non-pharmacologic options such as massage, positioning, distraction therapy, and application of heat and cold should also be considered.

Falls

Overview

Falls are the leading cause of injury-related deaths and nonfatal injuries among older adults, and the risk of falls increases significantly with age.[112] Moreover, falls contribute to up to approximately 40% of all nursing home admissions.[113] Intrinsic factors that cause falls include medical and neuropsychiatric conditions, impaired vision and hearing, and age-related changes in neuromuscular function, gait, posture, and reflexes.[114] Falls can also be caused by extrinsic factors, which include medications, environmental hazards, and improper use of assistive devices for ambulation.[115]

Presentation

When a fall occurs, NPs should inquire into the following: what the patient was doing at the time of the fall, whether there was a loss of consciousness, and in what direction the patient fell, either forward or backward. The NP should also ask if the patient broke the fall and whether or not any assistive devices were being used appropriately. Further assessment should include determining whether the fall was a first occurrence or whether falls have increased in number. The NP needs to differentiate between a mechanical fall versus a syncopal fall, as a syncopal event will need further workup to determine if there was a physiologic cause. The patient's medical history should be reviewed thoroughly, with a focus on drug use. Specifically, the NP will need to ask about anticoagulation medications to evaluate for excessive bleeding or hemorrhage post-fall. Additionally, environmental assessment will determine if the patient should stay at home or be moved to a health facility.[115]

Elderly patients who have experienced a fall should undergo a comprehensive exam with special focus on the cause and sequelae. This includes assessing the patient for visual or hearing impairments as well as cardiovascular disorders such as dysrhythmias and murmurs. The patient should also receive blood pressure checks to assess for orthostatic hypotension, which is a common cause.[116]

Management

Patients' risk of falling should be assessed annually. In particular, regular assessment of cognitive status and mental health is a key component of fall prevention in cognitively impaired older adults. The patient's cognitive status is best evaluated by an MMSE, whereas the Geriatric Depression Scale serves to evaluate the patient's mood.[68,69] The Functional Reach Test evaluates the risk of falls based on how far patients are able to reach, first by raising their arm sitting behind a line perpendicular to and adjacent to a wall, then by leaning as far forward as possible without losing balance. Additionally, the timed up-and-go test evaluates a patient's gait and balance by timing how long it takes for him or her to get up out of an armchair, walk 10 feet, and then sit back down again.[114] The Berg balance test, which assigns scores to patients based on how well they are able to perform a series of tasks, can also be used.[117]

Family members must be included in education and intervention planning. There should be targeted interventions for risk factors, and the patient should be considered for weight training and an exercise program, as needed. Physical therapy is aimed at balance and gait training, as well as strengthening. Assistive devices such as a cane or walker may help to provide additional stability. Other general interventions include minimizing medications and dosages, preventing and treating osteoporosis, recommending proper footwear, and maintaining a well-lit environment. It is also important to raise toilet seat and chair heights, as well as remove home hazards. Grab bars should be installed in places such as the bathroom and shower, and rails should be installed at entrances to the home as well.[1]

Patients' home settings can be modified to remove risk factors for falls, such as clutter and poor lighting.[114] For instance, removing throw rugs can prove critical in preventing falls. If a provider or nurse is not able to visit the patient's home, a Home Safety Checklist provides a helpful rubric for examining one's surroundings for risks. In addition to changes in the patient's home setting, the patient's stability can be improved by footwear with flat heels with some ankle support.[113]

Palliative Care

Overview

Palliative care is specialized medical care for people with a life-threatening illness. This standard of care serves to provide relief from symptoms, pain, and the stress of disease. Palliative care teams regularly consist of physicians, NPs, social workers, and clergy.[118] The focus of palliative care is on improving the patient's quality of life by preventing or treating signs and symptoms of the patient's condition, as well as any emotional, social, spiritual, or practical issues that the illness may cause.[119,120,121]

Palliative care should be initiated as soon as patients are identified as seriously ill.[122]

Presentation

Complex diseases resulting in palliative care include cancers, congestive heart failure, chronic pulmonary diseases, and dementia. The single most common problem for patients needing palliative care is pain. Moreover, during the last months of life, many patients report chronic, unrelieved pain.[123] After pain, the next most common issue is dyspnea, which is associated with chronic obstructive pulmonary disease, among other conditions. Further health concerns common in those receiving palliative care include loss of appetite, sleeplessness, drowsiness, constipation, depression, vomiting, and feelings of sickness.[1,124]

Management

When treating a patient needing palliative care, the NP should review the patient's living will, advance health care directive, or durable power of attorney. Knowing the laws and policies that govern these documents will help the NP to ensure that care is administered according to the patient's wishes, even when he or she is no longer able to make decisions regarding care.[122] The NP should also facilitate access to palliative care and hospice care, respect the patient's right to refuse treatment, and promote clinical, evidence-based research on providing care at the end of the patient's life.[125]

Furthermore, the NP should respect the dignity of both the patient and caregivers, as well as help alleviate the patient's pain and other physical symptoms, both of which are widely adopted core principles for end-of-life care.[126] Under these principles, the NP should offer continuity so that patients are able to continue to be cared for, if desired, by their primary care and specialist providers.

The NP should perform a spiritual assessment, including the patient's religious and spiritual beliefs, views on death and dying, and any rituals that the patient desires to be performed before death. The Faith, Importance, Community, and Address tool for spiritual assessment addresses the patient's spiritual issues, as well as the importance of faith in his or her life. The patient's participation in a spiritual or religious community should also be assessed, along with the benefits the patient receives from the community. The NP should also discuss and evaluate how other healthcare professionals can assist the patient with spiritual needs.[126]

The final hours of the patient's life are known as the terminal phase or active dying. This phase is an extremely stressful time for the patient and his or her family. During the terminal phase, the NP should attend to the patient's personal hygiene, assess and treat pain, and be mindful not to force fluids, which can worsen symptoms. The patient should also receive lubricating gels for the lips, eyes, and nares as needed. Further, the NP should remind caregivers and family that the semi-comatose patient may hear and understand what is being said. Caregivers and family should also be educated that loss of the ability to swallow and changes in breathing patterns are normal, and do not generally indicate discomfort or pain.[127]

Biology Theories of Aging

Immunity Theory

Biological theories try to explain how individuals differ in the aging process, and how aging affects the person physically. According to the immunity theory, the thymus stimulates the production of lymphocytes, increasing resistance to infection. The immunity theory also suggests a link between aging and the disappearance of the thymus gland by late middle age. The absence of this gland thus tends to result in weakening of the body's natural defense against foreign bodies.[128]

Cross-linkage Theory

The cross-linkage theory states that an individual's proteins, DNA, and other molecules often develop inappropriate attachments or cross-links to one another as a result of aging. Inappropriate cross-linkages result in decreased mobility of proteins and other molecules; problems can also be caused by damaged or inhibited proteins. Additionally, cross-linking of the skin protein, collagen, is partially responsible for wrinkling.[128]

Free Radical Theory

According to the free radical theory, free radicals are one of the toxic byproducts of normal cell metabolism. Substances within a person's cells generally contain or neutralize dangerous free radicals. Free radicals that escape the neutralization process can result in DNA damage, cross-linking of proteins, and the formation of age pigments.[128]

Wear and Tear Theory

The wear and tear theory states that age is not chronological, but is determined by the amount of stress to the body and the resulting damage. This theory states that each person has an inherited amount of adaptability that can be used in dealing with stress to the body. Exercise is viewed as a source of stress; however, this part of the theory is not widely accepted, and it is acknowledged that exercise is generally beneficial to overall health.[128]

Nutrition Restriction Theory

According to the nutrition restriction theory, reduction of food intake, rather than decreased body mass or decreased metabolic rate, contributes to an anti-aging process. There is a potential connection between reduction of food intake and metabolic changes controlling the aging process, as well as decline in protein synthesis and reduction in reactive oxygen molecules (free radicals).[1]

Error Theory

The error theory states that aging is due to internal or external assaults that affect cells or organs so they can no longer function properly. These assaults may include changes in the DNA and increased amounts of error in the RNA transcription or protein synthesis. These resulting cell mutations are thought to be the result of exposure to radiation.[1]

Biological Programming Theory

According to the biological programming theory, there is a hereditary basis in aging as shown by similar life spans of blood relatives. Twin studies show that identical twins have more similar life spans than non-identical twins. Researchers also point to cell division studies, which show that normal in vitro cells multiply finitely most of the time. Conversely, abnormal cells can double an infinite amount of times.[128]

Psychosocial Theories of Aging

Disengagement Theory

The disengagement theory of aging states that older people and society frequently partake in a mutual "disengagement" or withdrawal. This disengagement can be instigated by the older adult or others in society. Potential benefits to the individual include being relieved from societal roles and being able to reflect and be centered on oneself.[129]

The ascribed value of this theory to society is that it provides an orderly means to transfer power and authority from the previous generation to the next. However, issues with the disengagement theory include that the theory does not consider activity and contributions of older adults. Moreover, although disengagement is posited to be a universal practice, it does not account for the valued status placed on older adults in some cultures.[129]

Activity Theory

According to the activity theory, people who remain socially active are more likely to adjust well to becoming older. Social activity is commonly needed for ongoing role enactment and positive self-image, and people with multiple roles tend to have a broad spectrum to endorse a positive self-image. The activity theory is supported by a number of studies. In this theory, older adults should think of middle-age lifestyle activity as the norm, and replacement of discontinued activities should be encouraged. For example, a person may move into volunteering after retirement. Activities with close personal contacts generally yield the greatest benefit.[129]

Continuity Theory

According to the continuity theory, adjustment to aging can be ameliorated by previously developed adaptive coping skills, as well as the maintenance of previous roles and activities. There are four common patterns of personality and coping. Integrated personalities are characteristically mature and happy, with varied activity levels. Defended personalities, on the other hand, show a tendency to hold on to middle-age values and fret over changes that occur with age. Passive-dependent personalities may have high dependency needs or are apathetic. Lastly, un-integrated personalities typically have a history of mental illness.[130]

Maintaining some level of involvement is thought to lead to optimum adjustment to aging. In general, shy, quiet individuals who prefer solitude should not be encouraged to become more active. Conversely, extremely active individuals should be encouraged to stay active and not "watch life pass by from the rocking chair."[1] The greatest chances of adjustment for people continuing middle-life activities into old age are for activities such as gardening, where mobility and agility are not too complex. People who like to mountain bike or kick-box, on the other hand, may have more problems adjusting. According to the continuity theory, older adults utilize strategies based on their past experiences to preserve and maintain their existing structures.[129] However, the continuity theory is criticized as being too simplistic, on the grounds of ignoring issues of power and inequality in society.[130]

References

1. Barkley TW Jr. *Adult-Gerontology Primary Care NP Certification Review/Clinical Update Continuing Education Course.* West Hollywood, CA: Barkley and Associates; 2015.

2. Granger CV, Brownscheidle CM, Carlin M, et al. Functional assessment. In: Stone JH, Blouin M, eds. *International Encyclopedia of Rehabilitation.* 2010. http://cirrie.buffalo.edu/encyclopedia/en/article/44/. Accessed April 3, 2015.

3. Goldbaum E. Aging in place: Does a loved one need a geriatric assessment? University of Buffalo Web site. http://www.buffalo.edu/news/releases/2014/10/021.html. Released October 22, 2014. Accessed April 3, 2015.

4. Gitlin LN. Environmental adaptations for individuals with functional difficulties and their families in the home and community. In: Söderback I, ed. *International Handbook of Occupational Therapy Interventions.* 2nd ed. Cham, Switzerland: Springer International Publishing; 2015: 165–176.

5. Miller CA. Thermoregulation. In *Nursing for Wellness in Older Adults.* 6th ed. Philadelphia, PA: Wolters Kluwer Health/Lippincott Williams and Wilkins; 2012: 513–524.

6. Paveza GJ. Assessment of the elderly. In: Holosko MJ, Dulmus CN, Sowers KM, eds. *Social Work Practice with Individuals and Families.* Hoboken, NJ: John Wiley & Sons; 2013: 177–196.

7. Dent E, Chapman IM, Piantadosi C, Visvanathan R. Performance of nutritional screening tools in predicting poor six-month outcome in hospitalised older patients. *Asia Pac J Clin Nutr.* 2014; 23(3): 394–399. http://search.informit.com.au/documentSummary;dn=573644469760811;res=IELHEA. Accessed April 3, 2015.

8. Durán AP, Milà VR, Formiga F, Virgili CN, Vilarasau FC. Assessing risk screening methods of malnutrition in geriatric patients: Mini-nutritional assessment (MNA) versus geriatric nutritional risk index (GNRI). *Nutr Hosp.* 2012; 27(2): 590–598. doi: 10.1590/S0212-16112012000200036.

9. United States Department of Health and Human Services, Centers for Disease Control and Prevention. About adult BMI. http://www.cdc.gov/healthyweight/assessing/bmi/adult_bmi/. Updated May 15, 2015. Accessed May 18, 2015.

10. State Government of Victoria, Department of Health and Human Services. Indicator 5: Unplanned weight loss. http://docs2.health.vic.gov.au/docs/doc/4AAA31437FD57FE5CA257DCE00195903/$-FILE/Section%203%20Indicator%205%20Unplanned%20weight%20loss.pdf. Published January 15, 2015. Accessed April 3, 2015.

11. Krishnan K, Taylor MD. Nutrition assessment and monitoring. In: Cresci GA, ed. *Nutrition Support for the Critically Ill Patient: A Guide to Practice.* 2nd ed. Boca Raton, FL: CRC Press; 2015: 77–92.

12. Bernstein M, Munoz N. *Nutrition for the Older Adult.* Burlington, MA: Jones & Bartlett Learning; 2014.

13. Kokkinos P, Tsimploulis A, Faselis C. PDE-5 inhibitors for the treatment of erectile dysfunction in patients with hypertension. In: Viigimaa M, Vlachopoulos C, Doumas M, eds. *Erectile Dysfunction in Hypertension and Cardiovascular Disease.* Cham, Switzerland: Springer International Publishing; 2015: 185–193.

14. Seliger S. Loss of libido in men. WebMD Web site. http://www.webmd.com/sex-relationships/features/loss-of-libido-in-men?page=2. Accessed April 3, 2015.

15. Mayo Clinic Staff. Low sex drive in women. Mayo Clinic Web site. http://www.mayoclinic.org/diseases-conditions/low-sex-drive-in-women/basics/causes/con-20033229. Updated December 17, 2014.

16. Mayo Clinic Staff. Erectile dysfunction. Mayo Clinic Web site. http://www.mayoclinic.org/diseases-conditions/erectile-dysfunction/basics/treatment/con-20034244. Updated February 4, 2015.

17. Atypical presentation of disease in the elderly. Southern Care University Web site. http://www.mysoutherncare.com/scu/files/modules/Atypical%20Presention%20of%20Disease%20in%20the%20Elderly%20-%20Nurse,%20SW,%20CHAP%20-%203.14.13.pdf. Published March 2013. Accessed April 12, 2015.

18. Lewis JL III. Overview of disorders of fluid volume. In: Porter RS, Kaplan JL, eds. The Merck Manual Online. http://www.merckmanuals.com/professional/endocrine_and_metabolic_disorders/fluid_metabolism/overview_of_disorders_of_fluid_volume.html. Last revised August 2014. Accessed April 12, 2015.

19. McDonald M. Infectious disease in older adults. University of Kansas Medical Center Web site. http://classes.kumc.edu/coa/Education/AMED900/InfectiousDiseaseOlderAdults.htm. Accessed April 3, 2015.

20. Azar A, Ballas ZK. Immune function in older adults. In: Basow DS, ed. *UpToDate*. Waltham, MA: UpToDate; 2015. http://www.uptodate.com/contents/immune-function-in-older-adults. Last updated January 5, 2015. Accessed April 12, 2015.

21. Aging changes in skin. A.D.A.M. Medical Encyclopedia. http://www.nlm.nih.gov/medlineplus/ency/article/004014.htm. Updated September 4, 2012. Accessed April 12, 2015.

22. Blomberg BB, Frasca D. Quantity, not quality, of antibody response decreased in the elderly. *J Clinical Invest*. 2011; 121(8): 2981–2983. doi:10.1172/JCI58406

23. Neviere R. Sepsis and the systemic inflammatory response syndrome: Definitions, epidemiology, and prognosis. In: Basow DS, ed. *UpToDate*. Waltham, MA: UpToDate; 2015. http://www.uptodate.com/contents/sepsis-and-the-systemic-inflammatory-response-syndrome-definitions-epidemiology-and-prognosis. Last updated March 13, 2015. Accessed April 12, 2015.

24. Hayley D, Twenter K. Infectious disease of the elderly. University of Kansas Medical Center Web site. http://classes.kumc.edu/coa/Education/AMED900/InfectiousDisease.htm. Revised 2009. Accessed April 12, 2015.

25. Sloane PD, Kistler C, Mitchell CM, et al. Role of body temperature in diagnosing bacterial infection in nursing home residents. *J Am Geriatr Soc*. 2014; 62(1): 135–140. doi: 10.1111/jgs.12596

26. American Medical Directors Association. *Common Infections in the Long-Term Care Setting*. Columbia, MD: American Medical Directors Association; 2011.

27. Rubenstein LZ, Dillard D. Falls. In: Ham RJ, Sloane PD, Warshaw GA, Potter JF, Flaherty E, eds. *Ham's Primary Care Geriatrics: A Case-Based Approach*. 6th ed. Philadelphia, PA: Elsevier Health Sciences; 2014: 235–242.

28. Dellinger RP, Levy MM, Rhodes A, et al. Surviving sepsis campaign: International guidelines for management of severe sepsis and septic shock: 2012. *Crit Care Med*. 2013; 41(2): 580–637. DOI: 10.1097/CCM.0b013e31827e83af

29. United States Department of Health and Human Services Centers for Disease Control and Prevention. Life expectancy. http://www.cdc.gov/nchs/fastats/life-expectancy.htm. Reviewed January 20, 2015. Updated April 29, 2015. Accessed May 3, 2015.

30. Taffet GE. Normal aging. In: Basow DS, ed. *UpToDate*. Waltham, MA: UpToDate; 2015. http://www.uptodate.com/contents/normal-aging. Last updated January 8, 2015. Accessed April 12, 2015.

31. Goodman CC, Snyder TEK. Interviewing as a screening tool. In *Differential Diagnosis for Physical Therapists: Screening for Referral*. 5th ed. St. Louis, MO: Elsevier Saunders; 2013: 31–95.

32. Clegg A, Young J, Iliffe S, Olde Rikkert M, Rockwood K. Frailty in elderly people. *Lancet*. 2013; 381(9868): 752–762. doi: 10.1016/S0140-6736(12)62167-9

33. Besdine RW. Unusual presentations of illness in the elderly. In: Porter RS, Kaplan JL, eds. The Merck Manual Online. http://www.merckmanuals.com/professional/geriatrics/approach-to-the-geriatric-patient/unusual-presentations-of-illness-in-the-elderly. Last reviewed July 2013. Accessed April 12, 2015.

34. Besdine RW. Evaluation of the elderly patient. In: Porter RS, Kaplan JL, eds. The Merck Manual Online. http://www.merckmanuals.com/professional/geriatrics/approach-to-the-geriatric-patient/evaluation-of-the-elderly-patient. Last reviewed July 2013. Accessed April 12, 2015.

35. Katzung BG. Special aspects of geriatric pharmacology. In: Katzung BG, Trevor AJ, eds. *Basic and Clinical Pharmacology*. 13th ed. New York, NY: McGraw-Hill Education; 2015: 1024–1032.

36. American Nurses Association. *Gerontological Nursing: Scope and Standards of Practice*. Silver Spring, MD: American Nurses Association; 2010.

37. Von Humboldt S, Leal I. Adjustment to aging in late adulthood: A systematic review. *Int J Gerontol*. 2014; 8(3): 108–113. doi: 10.1016/j.ijge.2014.03.003

38. American Psychological Association. Fast facts on poverty. https://www.apa.org/pi/ses/poverty-facts.pdf. Published 2014. Accessed April 12, 2015.

39. United States Department of Health and Human Services, National Institutes of Health (NIH), National Institute on Aging. Global health and aging. http://www.nia.nih.gov/sites/default/files/global_health_and_aging.pdf. Published October 2011. Accessed April 12, 2015.

40. United States Social Security Administration. Monthly statistical snapshot, May 2015. http://www.ssa.gov/policy/docs/quickfacts/stat_snapshot/. Released June 2015. Accessed June 8, 2015.

41. Social Security Administration. Fast facts & figures about Social Security, 2013. http://www.ssa.gov/policy/docs/chartbooks/fast_facts/2013/fast_facts13.pdf. Released August 2013. Accessed April 12, 2015.

42. Morris V, Chin Hansen J. *How to Care for Aging Parents*. 3rd ed. New York, NY: Workman Publishing; 2014.

43. Older adults' health and age-related changes. American Psychological Association web site. http://www.apa.org/pi/aging/resources/guides/older.aspx?item=1. Accessed April 12, 2015.

44. Long term care options. Assisted Living Federation of America web site. https://www.alfa.org/alfa/Senior_Living_Options.asp. Accessed April 12, 2015.

45. Azar A, Ballas ZK. Immune function in older adults. In: Porter RS, Kaplan JL, eds. *UpToDate*. Waltham, MA: UpToDate; 2015. http://www.uptodate.com/contents/immune-function-in-older-adults. Updated January 5, 2015. Accessed March 25, 2015.

46. Shippee-Rice RV, Long JV, Fetzer SJ. Neurological. In: Shippee-Rice RV, Fetzer S, Long JV, eds. *Gerioperative Nursing Care: Principles and Practice in Surgical Care of the Older Adult*. New York, NY: Springer Publishing Company; 2012: 265–286.

47. Ojo JO, Rezaie P, Gabbott PL, Stewart MG. Impact of age-related neuroglial cell responses on hippocampal deterioration. *Front Aging Neurosci*. 2015; 7: 57. Doi: 10.3389/fnagi.2015.00057

48. Lipsitz LA, Novak V. Aging and the autonomic nervous system. In: Robertson D, Biaggioni I, Burnstock G, Low PA, Paton JFR, eds. *Primer on the Autonomic Nervous System*. 3rd ed. San Diego, CA: Academic Press; 2012: 271–274.

49. Besdine RW. Physical changes with aging. In: Porter RS, Kaplan JL, eds. The Merck Manual Online. http://www.merckmanuals.com/professional/geriatrics/approach-to-the-geriatric-patient/physical-changes-with-aging. Last reviewed July 2013. Accessed April 12, 2015.

50. Smith CM, Cotter VT. Age related changes in health. Hartford Institute for Geriatric Nursing Web site. http://consultgerirn.org/topics/normal_aging_changes/want_to_know_more#item_9. Updated July 2012. Accessed April 12, 2015.

51. Vaz Fragoso CA. Physiologic changes in the aging lung. In: Pisani M, ed. *Aging and Lung Disease: A Clinical Guide*. New York, NY: Humana Press; 2012: 3–24.

52. Hawkins KA, Kalhan R. Pulmonary changes in the elderly. In: Katlic MR, ed. *Cardiothoracic Surgery in the Elderly*. New York, NY: Springer Science and Business Media; 2011: 271–278.

53. Kamanagar N, Harrington A. Bacterial pneumonia. In: Byrd RP Jr, ed. Medscape. http://emedicine.medscape.com/article/300157-overview. Updated May 19, 2015. Accessed May 21, 2015.

54. Klodas E. High blood pressure and atherosclerosis. WebMD Web page. http://www.webmd.com/hypertension-high-blood-pressure/guide/atherosclerosis?page=2. Reviewed June 12, 2015. Accessed June 15, 2015.

55. Cardiac hypertrophy. University of Southern California Web site. http://www.cts.usc.edu/zglossary-cardiachypertrophy.html. Accessed April 12, 2015.

56. United States Department of Health and Human Services, National Institutes of Health, National Heart Lung and Blood Institute. Who is at risk for an arrhythmia? Updated July 1, 2011. Accessed April 12, 2015.

57. Jarvis C. Heart and neck vessels. In: *Physical Examination and Health Assessment*. 7th ed. St. Louis, MO: Elsevier; 2015: 459-508.

58. Miller SW. Therapeutic drug monitoring in the geriatric patient. In: Murphy JE, ed. *Clinical Pharmacokinetics*. 5th ed. Bethesda, MD: American Society of Health-System Pharmacists; 2012; 46–72.

59. Wooten JM. Pharmacotherapy considerations in elderly adults. *South Med J*. 2012; 105(8): 437–445.

60. DiPiro JT, Spruill WJ, Wade WE, Blouin RA, Pruemer JM. Introduction to pharmacokinetics and pharmacodynamics. In: *Concepts in Clinical Pharmacokinetics*. 5th ed. Bethesda, MD: American Society of Health-System Pharmacists; 2010: 1–18. http://www.ashp.org/DocLibrary/Bookstore/P2418-Chapter1.aspx

61. Scott SA. Personalizing medicine with clinical pharmacogenetics. *Genet Med*. 2011; 13(12): 987–995. doi: 10.1097/GIM.0b013e318238b38c.

62. Pharmacogenomics. American Medical Association Web site. http://www.ama-assn.org/ama/pub/physician-resources/medical-science/genetics-molecular-medicine/current-topics/pharmacogenomics.page?. Accessed April 3, 2015.

63. Haider SI, Ansari Z, Vaughan L, Matters H, Emerson E. Prevalence and factors associated with polypharmacy in Victorian adults with intellectual disability. *Res Dev Disabil*. 2014; 35(11): 3071–3080. doi: 10.1016/j.ridd.2014.07.060

64. Petrovic M, van der Cammen T, Onder G. Adverse drug reactions in older people. *Drugs Aging*. 2012; 29(6): 453–462. doi: 10.2165/11631760-000000000-00000

65. Ruscin JM, Linnebur SA. Drug categories of concern in the elderly. In: Porter RS, Kaplan JL, eds. The Merck Manual Online. http://www.merckmanuals.com/professional/geriatrics/drug-therapy-in-the-elderly/drug-categories-of-concern-in-the-elderly. Last reviewed June 2014. Accessed April 12, 2015.

66. Medications that may cause bone loss. National Osteoporosis Foundation Web site. http://nof.org/articles/6. Accessed April 12, 2015.

67. Kocurek B. Promoting medication adherence in older adults... and the rest of us. *Diabetes Spectr.* 2009; 22(2): 80–84. doi: 10.2337/diaspect.22.2.80

68. Factsheet: The Mini Mental State Examination (MMSE). Alzheimer's Society web site. http://www.alzheimers.org.uk/site/scripts/download_info.php?fileID=2414. Last reviewed January 2012. Accessed April 12, 2015.

69. Bienenfeld D, Stinson KN. Screening tests for depression. In: Bienenfield D, ed. Medscape. http://emedicine.medscape.com/article/1859039-overview#aw2aab6b9. Last updated February 14, 2014. Accessed April 12, 2015.

70. Maher RL, Hanlon J, Hajjar ER. Clinical consequences of polypharmacy in elderly. *Expert Opin Drug Saf.* 2014; 13(1): 57–65. doi: 10.1517/14740338.827660

71. Lee H-C, Huang KTL, Kuang-Win S. Use of antiarrhythmic drugs in elderly patients. *J Geriatr Cardiol.* 2011; 8(3): 184–194. doi: 10.3724/SP.J.1263.2011.00184

72. Steinbaum SR. High blood pressure and drug safety. WebMD Web site. http://www.webmd.com/hypertension-high-blood-pressure/high-blood-pressure-medication-safety?page=2. Reviewed July 27, 2014. Accessed April 12, 2015.

73. MacKichan JJ, Lee MWL. Factors contributing to drug-induced disease. In: Tisdale JE, Miller DA, eds. *Drug-Induced Diseases: Prevention, Detection, and Management.* 2nd ed. Bethesda, MD: American Society of Health-System Pharmaceuticals; 2010: 23–30.

74. Duggett A. Niacin drug interactions. Drugsdb Web site. http://www.drugsdb.com/sup/niacin/niacin-drug-interactions/. Published June 19, 2012. Accessed April 12, 2015.

75. Woo TM. Drugs affecting the gastrointestinal system. In: Woo TM, Wynne AL, eds. *Pharmacotherapeutics for Nurse Practitioner Prescribers.* 3rd ed. Philadelphia, PA: F. A. Davis Company; 2011: 523–570.

76. Brenner GM, Stevens CW. Drug development and safety. In *Pharmacology.* 4th ed. Philadelphia, PA: Elsevier Saunders; 2013: 34–44.

77. Nippoldt TB. Can calcium supplements interfere with hypothyroidism treatment? Mayo Clinic Web site. http://www.mayoclinic.org/diseases-conditions/hypothyroidism/expert-answers/hypothyroidism-faq-20058536. Published October 22, 2014. Accessed April 12, 2015.

78. Ruscin JM, Linnebur SA. Drug-related problems in the elderly. In: Porter RS, Kaplan JL, eds. The Merck Manual Online. http://www.merckmanuals.com/professional/geriatrics/drug-therapy-in-the-elderly/drug-related-problems-in-the-elderly. Last reviewed June 2014. Accessed April 12, 2015.

79. Berlowitz D. Epidemiology, pathogenesis, and risk assessment of pressure ulcers. In: Basow DS, ed. *UpToDate.* Waltham, MA: UpToDate; 2015. http://www.uptodate.com/contents/epidemiology-pathogenesis-and-risk-assessment-of-pressure-ulcers. Last updated September 8, 2014.

80. Kroshinsky D, Strazzula L. Pressure ulcers. In: Porter RS, Kaplan JL, eds. The Merck Manual Online. http://www.merckmanuals.com/professional/dermatologic_disorders/pressure_ulcers/pressure_ulcers.html. Last reviewed March 2013. Accessed April 12, 2015.

81. Mayo Clinic Staff. Bedsores (pressure sores). Mayo Clinic web site. http://www.mayoclinic.com/health/bedsores/DS00570/DSECTION=risk-factors. Updated December 13, 2014. Accessed April 12, 2015.

82. Salcido R, Popescu A. Pressure ulcers and wound care. In: Geibel J, ed. Medscape. http://emedicine.medscape.com/article/190115-overview. Updated April 1, 2015. Accessed April 12, 2015.

83. Serra R, Caroleo S, Buffone G, et al. Low serum albumin level as an independent risk factor for the onset of pressure ulcers in intensive care unit patients. *Int Wound J.* 2014; 11(5): 550–553. doi: 10.1111/iwj.12004

84. Pressure ulcer. A.D.A.M. Medical Encyclopedia. http://www.nlm.nih.gov/medlineplus/ency/article/007071.htm. Updated November 20, 2012. Accessed April 12, 2015.

85. National Pressure Ulcer Advisory Panel. NPUAP pressure ulcer stages/categories. http://www.npuap.org/resources/educational-and-clinical-resources/npuap-pressure-ulcer-stagescategories. Accessed April 12, 2015.

86. Berlowitz D. Clinical staging and management of pressure ulcers. In: Basow DS, ed. *UpToDate.* Waltham, MA: UpToDate; 2015. http://www.uptodate.com/contents/clinical-staging-and-management-of-pressure-ulcers. Last updated September 9, 2014. Accessed April 12, 2015.

87. Flanagan M. Principles of wound management. In: Flanagan M, ed. *Wound Healing and Skin Integrity: Principles and Practice.* Chichester, West Sussex, UK: Wiley-Blackwell; 2013: 66–86.

88. Kaplan DB. Elder abuse. In: Porter RS, Kaplan JL, eds. The Merck Manual Online. http://www.merckmanuals.com/professional/geriatrics/elder_abuse/elder_abuse.html?qt=elder%20abuse&alt=sh. Last reviewed July 2013. Accessed April 12, 2015.

89. Patient information: Elder abuse (the basics). In: Basow DS, ed. *UpToDate*. Waltham, MA: UpToDate; 2015. http://www.uptodate.com/contents/elder-abuse-the-basics. Accessed April 12, 2015.

90. What is elder abuse? National Council on Aging Web site. https://www.ncoa.org/public-policy-action/elder-justice/elder-abuse-facts/. Accessed April 12, 2015.

91. United States Department of Health and Human Services, NIH, National Institute on Aging. Elder abuse. http://www.nia.nih.gov/health/publication/elder-abuse. Published May 2011. Last updated January 27, 2015. Accessed April 12, 2015.

92. National Committee for the Prevention of Elder Abuse, MetLife Mature Market Institute. The essentials: preventing elder abuse. MetLife web site. https://www.metlife.com/assets/cao/mmi/publications/essentials/mmi-preventing-elder-abuse-essentials.pdf. Published 2013. Accessed April 12, 2015.

93. Mills TJ. Elder abuse. In: Brenner BE, ed. Medscape. http://emedicine.medscape.com/article/805727-overview. Updated February 25, 2015. Accessed April 12, 2015.

94. Ernst JS, Brownell P. United States of America. In: Phelan A, ed. *International Perspectives on Elder Abuse*. New York, NY: Routledge; 2013: 206–221.

95. Abid A, Kayani N, Jencius A. Financial abuse of the elderly: Risk factors. In: Factora RM, ed. *Aging and Money: Reducing Risk of Financial Exploitation and Protecting Financial Resources*. New York, New York: Springer; 2014: 39–52.

96. Halphen JM, Dyer CB. Elder mistreatment: Abuse, neglect, and financial exploitation. In: Basow DS, ed. *UpToDate*. Waltham, MA: UpToDate; 2015. http://www.uptodate.com/contents/elder-mistreatment-abuse-neglect-and-financial-exploitation. Last updated January 20, 2015. Accessed April 12, 2015.

97. Reyes-Ortiz CA, Burnett J, Flores DV, et al. Medical implications of elder abuse: Self-neglect. *Clin Geriatr Med*. 2014; 30(4): 807–823. Doi: 10.1016/j.cger.2014.08.008

98. Ratini M. Sleep and aging. WebMD Web site. http://www.webmd.com/healthy-aging/guide/sleep-aging. Reviewed October 14, 2014. Accessed April 12, 2015.

99. Doghramji K. Insomnia and excessive daytime sleepiness (EDS). In: Porter RS, Kaplan JL, eds. The Merck Manual Online. http://www.merckmanuals.com/professional/neurologic_disorders/sleep_and_wakefulness_disorders/insomnia_and_excessive_daytime_sleepiness_eds.html?qt=insomnia%20and%20excessive%20daytime&alt=sh. Last reviewed October 2014. Accessed April 12, 2015.

100. United States Department of Health and Human Services, NIH, National Institute of Neurological Disorders (NINDS). NINDS hypersomnia information page. http://www.ninds.nih.gov/disorders/hypersomnia/hypersomnia.htm. Last updated July 25, 2014. Accessed April 12, 2015.

101. Ahmed SMS, Anklesaria A, Bienenfeld D. Sleepwalking. In: Benbadis SR, ed. Medscape. http://emedicine.medscape.com/article/291931-overview#showall. Updated October 21, 2013. Accessed April 12, 2015.

102. United States Department of Health and Human Services, NIH, NINDS. Restless leg syndrome fact sheet. http://www.ninds.nih.gov/disorders/restless_legs/detail_restless_legs.htm. Last updated February 23, 2015. Accessed April 12, 2015.

103. Chawla J, Park Y, Passaro EA. Insomnia. In: Benbadis SR, ed. Medscape. http://emedicine.med scape.com/article/1187829-overview. Updated September 10, 2014. Accessed April 12, 2015.

104. United States Department of Health and Human Services, NIH, National Heart, Lung, and Blood Institute. What is insomnia? http://www.nhlbi.nih.gov/health/health-topics/topics/inso. Updated December 13, 2011. Accessed April 12, 2015.

105. Sleep hygiene. University of Maryland Medical Center web site. Last updated July 31, 2013. Accessed April 12, 2015.

106. Markman J, Narasimhan SK. Overview of pain. In: Porter RS, Kaplan JL, eds. The Merck Manual Online. http://www.merckmanuals.com/professional/neurologic_disorders/pain/overview_of_pain.html. Last reviewed April 2014. Accessed April 12, 2015.

107. Macintyre PE, Schug SA. *Acute Pain Management: A Practical Guide*. 4th ed. Boca Raton, FL: CRC Press; 2015.

108. Diseases & conditions: Acute pain vs. chronic pain. Cleveland Clinic web site. http://my.clevelandclinic.org/services/Pain_Management/hic_Acute_vs_Chronic_Pain.aspx

109. Kishner S, Ioffe J, Cho SR. Pain assessment. In: Schraga ED, ed. Medscape. http://emedicine.medscape.com/article/1948069-overview. Updated April 25, 2014. Accessed April 12, 2015.

110. Rosenquist EWK. Overview of the treatment of chronic pain. In: Basow DS, ed. *UpToDate*. Waltham, MA: UpToDate; 2015. http://www.uptodate.com/contents/overview-of-the-treatment-of-chronic-pain. Last updated April 7, 2015. Accessed April 12, 2015.

111. Pasero C, Stannard D. The role of intravenous acetaminophen in acute pain management: a case-illustrated review. *Pain Manag Nurs*. 2012; 13(2): 107–124. Doi: 10.1016/j.pmn.2012.03.002

112. United States Department of Health and Human Services, Centers for Disease Control and Prevention. Falls among older adults: An overview. http://www.cdc.gov/homeandrecreationalsafety/falls/adultfalls.html. Updated March 19, 2015. Accessed April 12, 2015.

113. Rubenstein LZ. Falls in the elderly. In: Porter RS, Kaplan JL, eds. The Merck Manual Online. http://www.merckmanuals.com/professional/geriatrics/falls_in_the_elderly/falls_in_the_elderly.html?qt=falls%20in%20the%20elderly&alt=sh. Last reviewed November 2013. Accessed April 12, 2015.

114. Ponce M. How to prevent falls among older adults in outpatient settings. *Am Nurse Today*. 2012; 7(4). http://www.medscape.com/viewarticle/762687

115. United States Department of Health and Human Services, Centers for Disease Control and Prevention. STEADI (Stopping Elderly Accidents, Deaths, & Injuries) tool kit for health care providers. http://www.cdc.gov/homeandrecreationalsafety/Falls/steadi/index.html#info. Last updated April 10, 2015. Accessed April 12, 2015.

116. Mayo Clinic Staff. Orthostatic hypotension (postural hypotension). Mayo Clinic web site. http://www.mayoclinic.com/health/orthostatic-hypotension/DS00997. Updated May 13, 2014. Accessed April 12, 2015.

117. Rehab measures: Berg Balance Scale. Rehabilitation Measures Database Web site. http://www.rehabmeasures.org/Lists/RehabMeasures/PrintView.aspx?ID=888. Accessed April 7, 2015.

118. What is palliative care? Get Palliative Care web site. http://getpalliativecare.org/whatis/. Accessed April 12, 2015.

119. Dy S, Gran M. *UNIPAC 1: The Hospice and Palliative Care Approach to Serious Illness*. Glenview, IL: American Academy of Hospice and Palliative Medicine; 2012. http://digitaleditions.walsworthprintgroup.com/publication/?i=102688

120. Nash RR, Nelson LJ. *UNIPAC 6: Ethical and Legal Issues*. Glenview, IL: American Academy of Hospice and Palliative Medicine; 2012. http://digitaleditions.walsworthprintgroup.com/publication/?i=102718

121. What is palliative care? A.D.A.M. Medical Encyclopedia. http://www.nlm.nih.gov/medlineplus/ency/patientinstructions/000536.htm. Updated May 11, 2014. Accessed April 12, 2015.

122. Cobbs EL. The dying patient. In: Porter RS, Kaplan JL, eds. The Merck Manual Online. http://www.merckmanuals.com/professional/special_subjects/the_dying_patient/the_dying_patient.html.

123. Weinstein S, Portenoy RK, Harrington SE. UNIPAC 3: Assessing and Treating Pain. Glenview, IL: American Academy of Hospice and Palliative Medicine; 2012. http://digitaleditions.walsworthprintgroup.com/publication/?i=102749

124. Krause RS. Palliative care in the acute care setting. In: Kulkarni R, ed. Medscape. http://emedicine.medscape.com/article/1407757-overview. Updated April 16, 2013. Accessed April 12, 2015.

125. American Academy of Hospice and Palliative Medicine. Hospice and palliative medicine competencies project toolkit of assessment methods. http://aahpm.org/uploads/education/competencies/Toolkit%20Intro%202014.pdf. Published 2010. Accessed April 12, 2015.

126. Saguil A, Phelps K. The spiritual assessment. *Am Fam Physician*. 2012; 86(6): 546–550. http://www.aafp.org/afp/2012/0915/p546.html

127. Bailey FA, Harman SM. Palliative care: The last hours and days of life. In: Basow DS, ed. *UpToDate*. Waltham, MA: UpToDate; 2015. http://www.uptodate.com/contents/palliative-care-the-last-hours-and-days-of-life. Last updated March 26, 2015. Accessed April 12, 2015.

128. Jin K. Modern biological theories of aging. *Aging Dis*. 2010; 1(2): 72–74.

129. Padilla RL, Byers-Connon S, Lohman H. *Occupational Therapy with Elders: Strategies for the COTA*. 3rd ed. Maryland Heights, MO: Elsevier Mosby; 2011.

130. Lange J, Grossman S. Theories of aging. In: Mauk KL, ed. *Gerontological Nursing: Competencies for Care*. 3rd ed. Burlington, MA: Jones & Bartlett Learning; 2014: 63–94.

SECTION TWO
Pediatric Curriculum Review

Chapter 1

Growth and Development

QUESTIONS

1. The mother of a 2-month-old patient says that their family is relocating to Japan to pursue a long-term business opportunity. You know that the majority of Japan does not practice water fluoridation. You recommend that the mother incorporate fluoride supplementation of 0.25 mg/day into her child's diet, starting at what age?

   a. Three months

   b. Six months

   c. One year

   d. Three years

2. When treating a child prone to seizures, a nurse practitioner should primarily keep which childhood anatomical feature in mind?

   a. Smaller circulating blood volume

   b. Large tongue compared to the oropharynx

   c. A thin cranium

   d. Large head in comparison to body proportion

3. A newborn is born weighing 9 lb. After 2 weeks, what would be the expected weight of the newborn?

   a. Eight lb

   b. Eight lb 5 oz

   c. Nine lb

   d. Nine lb 10 oz

4. The Denver II assessment test commonly measures a child for all of the following except:

   a. Personal-social development

   b. Language

   c. Fine motor development

   d. Intelligence

5. Kasey, age 7 months, is brought to the clinic by her concerned parents. They have been talking to other parents in their parenting group and need reassurance that Kasey is keeping up developmentally. As you observe Kasey, you notice that she responds to her name, consistently babbles, crawls around on the floor, and is able to pick up objects. Which of the following additional milestones would also be expected in a child her age?

   a. Supports weight on feet

   b. Holds head steady

   c. Equal coordination of hands

   d. Plays independently

6. Isaac, age 6 months, has been brought to your practice by his parents for a routine check-up. As you enter the interview phase, you would know all of these methods would be well-suited for the interview except:

    a. Carefully phrasing potential health and safety concerns to respect the cultural practices of Isaac's parents

    b. Breaking from the assessment regularly to ensure the parents have accurately expressed their concerns

    c. Phrasing your questions in an open-ended fashion to ensure a non-judgmental approach

    d. Using play to keep the patient engaged, regularly putting the assessment on hold to ensure to a proper response

7. Which of the following does not commonly impact temperature stability and regulation in a child?

    a. Increased subcutaneous tissue with increased evaporative heat loss

    b. Decreased body surface area to mass ratio

    c. Thinner skin

    d. Increased energy expenditure

8. You ask Samuel, a toddler, to point to one body part and he points directly to his elbow. Samuel's mother states that he just started correctly pointing to body parts last week. If Samuel is properly reaching expected developmental milestones, he would most likely be:

    a. About 13 months old

    b. About 18 months old

    c. About 20 months old

    d. About 2 years old

9. Holly, age 4, is at a well-child visit. During the visit, her weight is recorded as being 40 lb. Assuming expected growth parameters, how much will Holly most likely weigh in 2 years?

    a. Sixty lb

    b. Fifty-two lb

    c. Forty-five lb

    d. Forty-two lb

10. All of the following accurately reflect the typical well-child care visit except:

    a. After age 4 years, a child should have a well-child care visit yearly.

    b. Children on ADHD medication should see a physician or nurse practitioner every 6 months.

    c. Well-child care visits are arranged around immunization schedules, which are the key purpose of the visit.

    d. If the parents are experienced, their newborn does not commonly need to have a check-up until 1–2 weeks after birth.

RATIONALES

1. b

The American Academy of Pediatrics recommends that in areas with little to no water fluoridation, children should be started on fluoride supplementation at 6 months, with a daily dose of 0.25 mg. Supplementation is not required for the first 6 months of life, meaning 3 months of age is too early to introduce fluoride. By 1 year of age, the patient should already be receiving 0.25 mg/day. From 3 to 6 years of age, children should receive 0.50 mg/day of supplementary fluoride.

2. b

Developmentally, the tongue of a child is often comparatively larger than the oropharynx, which can potentially cause obstruction during a seizure and may lead to severe repercussions attributed to oxygen loss. Children have a smaller circulating blood volume in absolute terms, but this is primarily a concern in cases of blood loss or bacterial infection, not seizures. Children have thinner craniums, which would place them at a greater risk of head injury if the skull is penetrated; this may present a concern during convulsions, but is less of a concern than the risk of obstruction. Lastly, a child's large head, in comparison to the child's body, accounts for a smaller body surface area when compared with an adult, but this does not greatly influence potential complications from seizures.

3. c

The normal weight gain progression of an infant indicates that, at the 1–2 week mark, the weight will be approximately the same as it was at birth. The infant will typically lose 10% of the birth weight in the days after birth, weighing a little over 8 lb, and then gain that weight back within 7–14 days. By 5 months, the infant's weight should be doubled. The weight will usually be tripled by the first year and will be four times the birth weight by the second year.

4. d

Although the Denver II assessment test measures several aspects of child development, it is not an intelligence test. The Denver II measures the fields of language, personal-social development, and fine and gross motor development.

5. a

A child exhibiting the milestones of a 6–9 month old, as evidenced by crawling, babbling, picking up objects, and responding to her name, is likely to be able to support her weight on her feet. The ability to hold her head steady is an age milestone that typically occurs around 2–5 months; as such, the patient should already be able to do this. At around 10–12 months, she should be able to play independently and exhibit equal coordination in her hands.

6. c

Although a non-judgmental approach should be utilized at all times during the interview, questions should be directed and purposeful, not open-ended, to ensure that key details of the patient's history are not missed. Other proper techniques to utilize during an interview include ensuring cultural sensitivity, ensuring accurate perception of the parents' concerns, using play to enhance the patient's comfort, and pausing to allow adequate time for a response.

7. a

Temperature stability in children is commonly impacted by their limited, not increased, subcutaneous tissue with evaporative heat loss, as well as a smaller body surface area to mass ratio, thinner skin, and increased energy expenditure. Due to the fact that more energy is needed to facilitate proper growth, less energy is available for thermoregulation. These factors are important because they put children at an increased risk of hypothermia.

8. b

A properly-developing toddler would be expected to point to his body parts at 15–18 months old. A 13-month-old can typically walk and understand a few words, but would not be expected to point to body parts. A 20-month-old and a 2-year-old would already be expected to be able to properly indicate parts of their body.

9. b

School-age children typically gain around 5–7 lb annually, so a 40 lb, normally-developing child would often weigh between 50 and 54 lb in 2 years; as such, 52 lb is the only answer choice that falls within that range. Gaining only 5–8 lb within 2 years, as indicated by a final weight of 45 lb or 48 lb, may suggest a developmental deficiency or malnutrition. A child who gains 16 or more pounds within 2 years exceeds the normal weight gain progression, and may indicate obesity in later childhood.

10. c

Well-child care visits commonly include physical exams to assess the physical well-being of a child; preventative care (i.e., immunizations), communication with the parents, developmental tracking, and personal family issues are all equally important aspects of a well-child care visit. If there are no complications in development, a child should have a well-child care visit yearly after the age of 4. However, a child taking medication for ADHD should see a health care professional every 6 months. After a baby is born, it is recommended that the newborn receive a check-up within 2–4 days; however, if the parents have experience with newborns, they may not need to see a health care provider for 1–2 weeks.

DISCUSSION

Overview

A child's growth and development progresses across four stages: infancy, preschool, school age, and adolescence.[1] Knowing the major growth and development landmarks for each stage will allow the nurse practitioner (NP) to determine a patient's expected developmental progression, in addition to providing anticipatory guidance measures. Moreover, being knowledgeable about the various stages will help to identify developmental warning signs or red flags in a child's development.[2]

A child's growth and development is monitored during regular health maintenance visits. Developmental surveillance occurs in three main domains: physical, cognitive, and psychosocial.

Primary guidelines for growth and development are contained in the American Academy of Pediatrics' (AAP) *Bright Futures: Guidelines of Health Supervision of Infants, Children, and Adolescents*.[3]

The Physical Domain

Overview

Physical growth occurs in an orderly sequence. Children progress at different rates through this sequence depending on a number of factors, such as genetics, culture, nutrition, and individual variability.[2] Serial measurements are important for assessing a pediatric patient's physical growth. The Centers for Disease Control and Prevention (CDC) recommend assessing the patient's growth using standardized growth charts. The World Health Organization (WHO), in conjunction with the CDC and the National Center of Health Statistics, have created standardized growth charts that allow health care providers to collect serial growth data in order to develop an overall clinical impression of the child's growth and development.[4]

Nutritional Factors

Caloric requirements for children vary according to the child's age. From birth to 6 months of age, children should consume 120 kcal/kg/day. Some sources suggest 110 kcal/kg/day through 1 year of age, with a decrease to 100 kcal/kg/day from 1 to 3 years of age. The daily caloric requirement decreases to 100 kcal/kg for children 7 months to 1 year of age. Children 2–10 years of age may consume a daily caloric intake from 70 to 100 kcal/kg. Lastly, adolescents should consume 45 kcal/kg daily.[2]

Typical weight gain progression consists of rapid decelerating growth, followed by consistent growth. Neonates may initially lose 5%–10% of their weight within the first few days of life, and then regain their birth weight by 14 days.[2] An infant's weight usually doubles by 6 months of age, triples by 1 year of age, and quadruples by 2 years of age. Furthermore, young children tend to grow 2.5 inches and gain about 4 lb annually from 3 years of age to school age, and school-age children commonly grow 2 inches and gain 6.5 lb annually.[7]

Breastfeeding is the evidence-based standard for infant feeding, as breast milk is the best source of nutrition during the first 6 months of a child's life.[5,6] The AAP recommends, in its policy statement on breastfeeding, that women with no health problems should breastfeed infants for a minimum of 6 months.[7] During these 6 months, infants should be exclusively breastfed on demand.

Furthermore, the AAP recommends that breastfeeding continue for the first 12 months of life, if possible. Breastfeeding offers numerous health benefits for both mothers and children, such as improving gastrointestinal function and decreasing the incidence of acute illnesses.[2,8] Breastfeeding may also decrease the risk of allergic diseases and prevent inflammatory diseases.[6] Additionally, breastfeeding may help prevent childhood problems of being overweight or obese, regardless of parental education or socioeconomic status. Consequently, the longer the mother breastfeeds, the less likely the child will become overweight. In mothers, potential benefits of breastfeeding include analgesia during painful procedures, more rapid involution of the uterus, and a decreased risk of both ovarian and breast cancer.[2,7,8]

Adequate intake is confirmed by six to eight wet diapers per day in a newborn or young infant, and is associated with satiety and appropriate weight gain. Well-nourished infants may also produce four or more stools per day by 2 weeks of age.[9] The AAP recommends that daily vitamin D supplements of 400 international units (IU) begin a few days after delivery and continue until the child is weaned to whole milk at about 1 year of age.[2,10,11] Mothers of breastfed infants who are vegan or who have vitamin B12 deficiency should receive B12 supplementation to prevent neurological abnormalities in the infant.[12] Term infants typically have sufficient iron stores for up to 6 months. However, breast milk contains little iron, and premature breastfed infants or infants with anemia should receive iron supplementation and multivitamins to ensure proper growth.[12] At around 6 months of age, infants should begin eating iron-fortified, single-grain cereals.[12]

The AAP recommends that fluoride supplements be given to patients over 6 months of age whose local drinking water supply has less than 0.3 parts per million of fluoride; however, supplementation is not needed during the first 6 months of life.[12] For low- to moderate-risk fluoride deficiency, bottled water and toothpaste with fluoride may be recommended. For children who are at high risk for developing dental caries, the dosage of fluoride supplementation depends on the patient's age: Children 6 months to 3 years of age should receive 0.25 mg per day, children 3–6 years of age should receive 0.5 mg per day, and 1 mg per day is recommended for patients 6–16 years of age.[13]

Eruption of the teeth begins with the central incisor, followed by the lateral incisor, canine, first molar, and second molar. This sequence is usually completed by the time the child is 3 years of age (see figures 1.1–1.2).[17]

Cognitive Domain

Overview

Jean Piaget's theory of the development of the cognitive domain assigns various stages to the cognitive development of a child. The sensorimotor stage, which lasts from birth to about 2 years of age, is characterized by rapid cognitive growth and learning through trial and error. A primary component

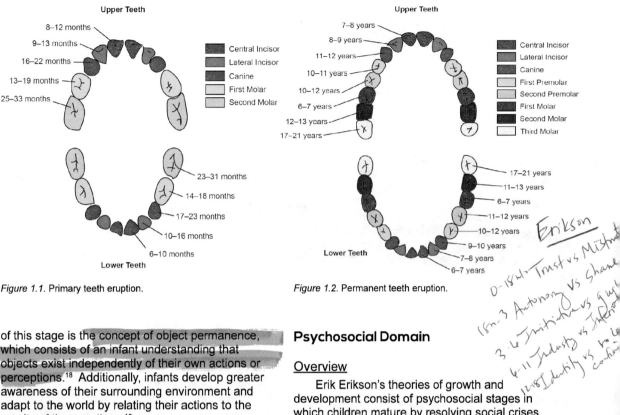

Figure 1.1. Primary teeth eruption.

Figure 1.2. Permanent teeth eruption.

of this stage is the concept of object permanence, which consists of an infant understanding that objects exist independently of their own actions or perceptions.[18] Additionally, infants develop greater awareness of their surrounding environment and adapt to the world by relating their actions to the results of those actions.[18]

The preoperational and preconceptual stage lasts from approximately 2 to 4 years of age. During this stage, the child can focus on a single aspect of a situation and begin developing intuitive thought; however, children at this stage are not yet capable of cause-and-effect reasoning. The preoperational stage is also marked by egocentrism, manifested as the inability to see situations from another person's point of view.[18] Additionally, children also exhibit animism, which is the belief that inanimate objects have human feelings.[18] The intuitive and preoperational thinking stage lasts from 4 to 7 years of age and marks the beginning of causation, with the child beginning to make logical assumptions about how one phenomenon produces another.[2]

When children reach roughly 7 years of age, they enter the concrete operational stage, which lasts until about 11 years of age. During the concrete operational stage, the child becomes capable of solving problems logically and gains the ability to conserve numbers and liquid, understanding that quantity may remain the same despite disparities in presentation.[18] Finally, formal operational thought lasts from around 11 to 15 years of age. Children in this stage become capable of thinking abstractly, solving complex problems, and reaching logical conclusions.[18]

Psychosocial Domain

Overview

Erik Erikson's theories of growth and development consist of psychosocial stages in which children mature by resolving social crises and developing a series of life skills.[18] As with all of Piaget's cognitive theories, the age ranges listed are approximate, beginning with the trust versus mistrust stage, which begins at birth and lasts until 18 months of age. During this stage, the infant learns that the world is an uncertain place and seeks some measure of stability from caregivers and the environment. Afterward, the child enters the autonomy versus shame and doubt stage, which lasts until 3 years of age and is characterized by self-assertion and developing confidence in one's own skills and abilities. Next, the initiative versus guilt stage lasts from 3 to 6 years of age, wherein the child begins interacting with peers and develops confidence in his or her ability to make decisions. This is followed by the industry versus inferiority stage, which lasts from 6 to 11 years of age and involves the child learning to be productive in his or her particular competencies. The final Erikson stage before young adulthood is the identity versus role confusion stage, which lasts from 12 to 18 years of age and focuses on defining one's own place in society.[18]

According to Sigmund Freud's psychosexual theory, three components of personalities are developed by experiences in particular stages of a child's development. These three components are the id, the principle of pleasure; the ego, the principle of reality and self-interest; and the superego, the principle of morality or conscience. Freud's stages of psychosexual development begin with the oral stage, which lasts from birth to 18 months of age and is marked by focus on the sensations of feeding, which can lead to the development of a sense of trust and comfort between child and mother. This is followed by the anal stage, which begins at 18 months of age, lasts until 3 years of age, and involves the child developing a sense of independence by mastering control of his or her bodily needs.[19] The phallic stage lasts until the child is 6 years of age and is marked by the development of the ego, love of the opposite sex, and the Oedipus complex, which is characterized by an increased attachment towards the opposite sex parent and resultant jealously towards the same sex parent. The latency stage lasts from 6 to 12 years of age and is marked by socialization, repression of sexual drive, and development of the child's superego and morality. Lastly, the genital stage occurs during adolescence, from 12 to 18 years of age; during this stage, adolescents direct their sexual urges onto their peers.[19]

Growth and Development Landmarks

Overview

Growth measurements are the gold standard by which the NP can assess a child's health and well-being.[20] Individual stages of growth and development, with a comprehensive outline of developmental milestones, follow in the subsequent sections. Assessment of developmental milestones should be determined using corrected age for premature infants; this is especially true when performing the Denver Developmental Screening Test, second edition (Denver II) assessment.[2] The corrected gestational age is the adjustment of developmental expectations for premature infants through 2 years of age, at which point most infants catch up developmentally.[21]

Workup

Every well-child visit requires a physical examination to assess the child's growth in relation to expected growth and developmental milestones. The growth parameters of pediatric patients are measured by growth charts, with norms expressed as percentiles of height, weight, and head circumference in accordance with the patient's age. Serial measurements should be examined; historically, any child whose measurement cross over two or more percentile lines needs further evaluation. Although this remains true, the issue of further workup is much more complex. Other factors to consider for further investigation include, but are not limited to, growth out of proportion to expected norms for ethnicity, body type, and familial trends and nutrition. Body mass index (BMI) uses a baseline of height and weight to measure a patient's body fat. The CDC and AAP recommend BMI screenings for overweight and obese children as early as 2 years of age.[22]

The Denver II test does not measure intelligence, but serves as a generalized assessment tool that can be used from birth to 6 years of age. This test assesses a child's development by measuring his or her growth, use of language, personal-social skills, and gross and fine motor skills.[23] Although normal development is widely variable, any child who is unable to meet the majority of developmental milestones during the well-child visit should be referred for a full developmental assessment.

Growth and Development Milestones (see table 1.1)

Well Child Checks (WCC)

Workup

Well Child Checks (WCCs) are stage appropriate screenings in which specific tools are used to screen the health of children. In the initial screening, a comprehensive health and development history is taken. Subsequent visits include interval histories to update the patient's records. These screenings also consist of a complete physical examination, developmental screening, and questions about the child's well-being.[2] The AAP recommends a screening schedule that begins at birth and continues at regular intervals throughout childhood and adolescence.[24]

A WCC measures a child's health by both objective and subjective data. Subjective data consists of an interval history that evaluates the child's nutrition, appetite, elimination, sleep, and development, among other factors.[25] Furthermore, this stage of the WCC should include discussion of any concerns the child's parents or caregivers may have. Objective data of a WCC includes the physical examination, laboratory testing, and developmental screening, which may include the Ages and Stages questionnaire (ASQ) or the Denver II test. The management plan of a WCC should include health promotion strategies with anticipatory guidance and the initiation of the primary series of immunizations.[2]

The Interview

Overview

The NP's general approach to interviewing a pediatric patient should begin with ascertaining who will be present and ensuring that privacy is maintained. It is important to use a non-judgmental approach during an interview and ensure accurate perceptions of the concerns of the child's parents. Additionally, the NP should phrase his or her questions purposefully, use non-threatening words, convey interest and attention, allow adequate time for response, and employ cultural sensitivity. The NP should play with the child and engage the child, as well as the parents, during the interview process.

Table 1.1 | Developmental Milestones and Warning Signs

Age	What Most Children Do At This Age				Developmental Warning Signs
	Social/Emotional	Language/Communication	Cognitive	Movement/Physical Development	
2 months	-Begins to smile at people -Briefly calms him or herself -Tries to look at parent	-Coos, gurgling sounds -Turns head towards sounds	-Pays attention to faces -Follows things with eyes, recognizes people at a distance -Begins to act bored if activity doesn't change	-Can hold head up, pushes up when lying on tummy -Smoother arm and leg movement	-Doesn't respond to loud sounds -Doesn't watch things that move -Doesn't smile at people -Doesn't bring hands to mouth -Can't hold head up when lying on tummy
4 months	-Smiles spontaneously -Likes to play with people, cries when playing stops -Copies movements and facial expressions	-Babbles -Copies sounds -Cries in different ways to demonstrate hunger, pain, being tired, etc.	-Lets you know if he or she is happy, sad, etc. -Responds to affection -Reaches with one hand -Uses hands and eyes together -Follows moving things with eyes from side to side -Watches faces closely -Recognizes familiar people at a distance	-Holds head steady when unsupported -Pushes down on legs when feet are on a surface -Roll over from tummy to back -Holds, shakes, and swings toys -Brings hands to mouth -Pushes up to elbows when lying on stomach	-Doesn't watch things that move -Doesn't smile at people -Can't hold head steady -Doesn't coo or make sounds -Doesn't bring things to mouth -Doesn't push down with legs when feet are on hard surface -Has trouble moving one or both eyes in all directions
6 months	-Knows familiar faces and begins to know if someone is a stranger -Likes to play with others, especially parents -Responds to other people's emotions and often seems happy -Likes to look at self in a mirror	-Responds to sounds by making sounds -Strings vowels together when babbling ("ah," "eh," "oh") and likes taking turns with parent while making sounds -Responds to own name -Makes sounds to show joy and displeasure -Begins to say consonant sounds (jabbering with "m," "b")	-Looks around at things nearby -Brings things to mouth -Shows curiosity about things and tries to get things that are out of reach -Begins to pass things from one hand to the other	-Rolls over in both directions (front to back, back to front) -Begins to sit without support -When standing, supports weight on legs and might bounce -Rocks back and forth, sometimes crawling backward before moving forward	-Doesn't try to get things that are in reach -Shows no affection for caregivers -Doesn't respond to sounds around him/her -Has difficulty getting things to mouth -Doesn't make vowel sounds ("ah", "eh", "oh") -Doesn't roll over in either direction -Doesn't laugh or make squealing sounds -Seems very stiff with tight muscles -Seems very floppy like a rag doll

Table 1.1	Developmental Milestones and Warning Signs				
	What Most Children Do At This Age				**Developmental Warning Signs**
Age	**Social/Emotional**	**Language/ Communication**	**Cognitive**	**Movement/Physical Development**	
9 months	-May be afraid of strangers -May be clingy with familiar adults -Has favorite toys	-Understands "no" -Makes a lot of different sounds -Copies other's sounds and gestures -Uses fingers to point	-Watches the path of something as it falls -Looks for things he/she sees you hide -Plays peek-a-boo -Puts things in his/her mouth -Moves things smoothly from one hand to the other -Picks up things like cereal o's between thumb and index finger	-Stands, holding on -Can get into sitting position -Sits without support -Pulls to stand -Crawls	-Doesn't bear weight on legs with support -Doesn't sit with help -Doesn't babble -Doesn't play back-and-forth games -Doesn't respond to own name -Doesn't recognized familiar people -Doesn't look where you point -Doesn't transfer toys from one hand to the other
1 year	-Is shy or nervous with strangers -Cries when mom or dad leaves -Has favorite things and people -Shows fear in some situations -Hands you a book when he/she wants to hear a story -Repeats sounds or actions to get attention -Puts out arm or leg to help with dressing -Plays games such as "peek-a-boo" and "pat-a-cake"	-Responds to simple spoken requests -Uses simple gestures, like shaking head "no" or waving "bye-bye" -Makes sounds with changes in tone (sounds more like speech) -Says "mama" and "dada" and exclamations like "uh-oh!" -Tries to say words you say	-Explores things in different ways, like shaking, banging, throwing -Finds hidden things easily -Looks at the right picture or thing when it's named -Copies gestures -Starts to use things correctly; for example, drinks from a cup, brushes hair -Bangs two things together -Puts things in a container, takes things out of a container -Lets things go without help -Pokes with index (pointer) finger -Follows simple directions like "pick up the toy"	-Gets to a sitting position without help -Pulls up to stand, walks holding on to furniture ("cruising") -May take a few steps without holding on -May stand alone	-Doesn't crawl -Can't stand when supported -Doesn't search for things that he/she sees you hide -Doesn't say single words like "mama" or "dada" -Doesn't learn gestures like waving or shaking head -Doesn't point to things -Loses skills he/she once had

Table 1.1 | Developmental Milestones and Warning Signs

Age	What Most Children Can Do At This Age				Developmental Warning Signs
	Social/Emotional	Language/Communication	Cognitive	Movement/Physical Development	
18 months	-Likes to hand things to others as play -May have temper tantrums -May be afraid of strangers -Shows affection to familiar people -Plays simple pretend, such as feeding a doll -May cling to caregivers in new situations -Points to show others something interesting -Explores alone but with parent close by	-Says several single words -Says and shakes head "no" -Points to show someone what he/she wants	-Knows what ordinary things are for; for example, telephone, brush, spoon -Points to get the attention of others -Shows interest in a doll or stuffed animal by pretending to feed -Points to one body part -Scribbles on his/her own -Can follow 1-step verbal commands without any gestures; for example, sits when you say "sit down"	-Walks alone -May walk up steps and run -Pulls toys while walking -Can help undress him/herself -Drinks from a cup -Eats with a spoon	-Doesn't point to show things to others -Can't walk -Doesn't know what familiar things are for -Doesn't copy others -Doesn't gain new words -Doesn't have at least 6 words -Doesn't notice or mind when a caregiver leaves or returns -Loses skills he/she once had
2 years	-Copies others -Gets excited when around other children -Shows increasing independence -Shows defiant behavior -Plays beside other children, begins to include other children	-Points to things/pictures when named -Knows names of familiar people and body parts -Says 2–4 word sentences -Repeats words overheard in conversation -Points to things in a book	-Finds things, even when hidden under 2 or 3 items -Sorts shapes and colors -Completes sentences and rhymes in familiar books -Plays make-believe games -Builds towers with 4 or more blocks -May use one hand more than the other -Follows two-step instructions -Names items in a picture book	-Stands on tiptoes -Kicks a ball -Begins to run -Climbs up and down furniture while holding on -Walks up and down stairs -Throws ball overhand -Makes/copies straight lines and circles	-Doesn't use 2-word phrases -Doesn't know what to do with common things (i.e., brush, phone, fork) -Doesn't copy actions and words -Doesn't follow simple instruction -Doesn't walk steadily -Loses skills he/she once had

Table 1.1 Developmental Milestones and Warning Signs

Age	What Most Children Can Do At This Age				Developmental Warning Signs
	Social/Emotional	Language/Communication	Cognitive	Movement/Physical Development	
3 years	-Copies adults and friends -Shows affection for friends without prompting -Takes turns in games -Shows concern for a crying friend -Understands the idea of "mine" and "his" or "hers" -Shows a wide range of emotions -Separates easily from mom and dad -May get upset with major changes in routine -Dresses and undresses self	-Follows instructions with 2 or 3 steps -Can name most familiar things -Understands words like "in," "on," and "under" -Says first name, age, and sex -Names a friend -Says words like "I," "me," "we," and "you" and some plurals (cars, dogs, cats) -Talks well enough for strangers to understand most of the time -Carries on a conversation using 2–3 sentences	-Can work toys with buttons, levers, and moving parts -Plays make-believe with dolls, animals, and people -Does puzzles with 3 or 4 pieces -Understands what "two" means -Copies a circle with pencil or crayon -Turns book pages one at a time -Builds towers of more than 6 blocks -Screws and unscrews jar lids or turns door handle	-Climbs well -Runs easily -Pedals a tricycle (3-wheel bike) -Walks up and down stairs, one foot on each step	-Falls down a lot or has trouble with stairs -Drools or has very unclear speech -Can't work simple toys (such as peg boards, simple puzzles, turning handle) -Doesn't speak in sentences -Doesn't understand simple instructions -Doesn't play pretend or make-believe -Doesn't want to play with other children or with toys -Doesn't make eye contact -Loses skills he/she once had
4 years	-Enjoys doing new things -Plays "mom" and "dad" -Is more and more creative with make-believe play -Would rather play with other children than by him/herself -Cooperates with other children -Can't tell what's real and what's make believe -Talks about what he/she likes and is interested in	-Knows some basic rules of grammar, such as correctly using "he" and "she" -Sings a song or says poem from memory -Tells stories -Can say first and last name	-Names some colors and numbers -Understands counting -Starts to understand time -Remembers parts of stories -Understands idea of "same" and "different" -Draws a person with 2–4 body parts -Uses scissors -Starts to copy capital letters -Plays board or card games -Tells you what he/she things is going to happen next in book	-Hops and stands on one foot up to 2 seconds -Catches bounced ball most of the time -Pours, cuts with supervision, and mashes own food	-Can't jump in place -Has trouble scribbling -Shows no interest in interactive games or make-believe -Ignores other children or doesn't respond to people outside of family -Resists dressing, sleeping, using toilet -Can't retell favorite story -Doesn't follow 3-part commands -Doesn't understand "same" and "different" -Doesn't use "me" and "you" correctly -Speaks unclearly -Loses skills he/she once had

Table 1.1	Developmental Milestones and Warning Signs			
	What Most Children Can Do At This Age			**Developmental Warning Signs**
Age	**Social/Emotional**	**Language/ Communication**	**Cognitive**	**Movement/Physical Development**	
5 years	-Wants to please friends -Wants to be like friends -More likely to agree with rules -Likes to sing, dance, act -Is aware of gender -Can tell what's real and what's make believe -Shows more independence -Sometimes demanding, sometimes cooperative	-Speaks clearly -Tells a simple story using full sentences -Uses future tense -Says name and address	-Counts 10 or more things -Can draw a person with 6 body parts -Can print letters or numbers -Copies a triangle and other shapes -Knows about things used every day (i.e., food, money)	-Stands on one foot for 10 seconds or longer -Hops, may be able to skip -Can do a somersault -Uses fork and spoon -Can use toilet on his/her own -Swings and climbs	-Doesn't show wide range of emotions -Shows extreme behavior -Usually withdrawn, inactive -Easily distracted -Doesn't respond to people or responds superficially -Can't tell what's real or make believe -Doesn't play a variety of games -Can't give first and last name -Doesn't use plurals or tenses properly -Doesn't talk about daily activities or experiences -Doesn't draw pictures -Can't brush teeth, wash and dry hands, or get undressed without help -Loses skills he/she once had

Note. Adapted from: Developmental milestones. CDC. http://www.cdc.gov/ncbddd/actearly/milestones/index.html. Published 2014. Accessed April 2015. Reproduced with permission.

When seeing an infant or toddler, the conversation will be mostly with the parents; however, as the child grows, he or she should be increasingly included in the interview process. Finally, the child should be kept clothed during an interview until the physical examination or until it is otherwise necessary to remove clothing. In some cases, it is wise to unclothe the child piece by piece during the exam, only removing clothing when an area needs to be examined (e.g., only removing the shirt when the chest needs to be assessed).[2]

Injury Prevention (see table 1.2)

Overview

Injury prevention is particularly important in pediatric patients, as injuries are a leading cause of death in infants and children in the United States and worldwide.[26] Unintentional injury is one of the major types of injuries in children and includes poisonings, motor vehicle accidents, drownings, and falls, among others.[27] To prevent poisoning in children, it is important to have poison control numbers nearby at all times and keep all poisons locked and out of reach.[2] Firearms are another major cause of injury to children; proper storage and safety concerns should be discussed with parents and children when appropriate.[28]

It is important that children be properly placed in adequate restraint systems in passenger vehicles, as motor vehicle accidents are the leading cause of death in children 4 years of age and older.[29] The child's home should likewise be fitted to protect against injuries resulting from fires and other unintentional injuries.[30]

Domestic violence and other types of child maltreatment are a common source of injuries. NPs play a key role in minimizing the risk of child maltreatment by promoting awareness of the issue in the community, engaging in home visits, and educating parents in proper techniques to ensure a positive environment for their child.[31] If child abuse is identified, most states have mandatory reporting statutes that require NPs to report the incident to the proper authorities, such as child protective services, a law enforcement agency, or a state's toll-free child abuse reporting hotline.[32]

Developmental Considerations

During a child's growth and development, the NP must be mindful that children cannot be treated as small adults due to many unique anatomical, physiological, cognitive, and psychological differences.[33]

Anatomic Differences

Size

Because their bodies are not fully mature, children are at increased risk from environmental hazards. Body surface area (BSA) to body mass ratio is highest at birth and diminishes with age.[34] Because children have a higher BSA to body mass ratio, they may absorb larger doses of pollutants than adults.[35]

Small Body Mass

The body mass of a child typically has less fat, less elastic connective tissue, and a closer proximity of the chest to the abdominal organs. Because of these anatomic differences, flying objects, falls, and blunt or blast trauma may result in increased injury to multiple organs.[33] Young children have a very large head size in comparison to their body size, which causes them to be more likely to fall on their head. This predisposes a child to an increased incidence of head injuries. As brain development continues through 20 years of age, any head injuries sustained by children or young adults can have deleterious effects and result in long term sequelae.

Table 1.2	Leading Causes of Unintentional Injury Death Among Children 0–19 Years, by Age Group, United States				
	Age Group (in years)				
Rank	**Younger than 1**	**1–4**	**5–9**	**10–14**	**15–19**
1	Suffocation	MVT-related	MVT-related	MVT-related	MVT-related
2	MVT-related	Drowning	Other injuries	Other injuries	Other injuries
3	Drowning	Other injuries	Fires or burns	Drowning	Poisoning
4	Other injuries	Fires or burns	Drowning	Fires or burns	Drowning
5	Fires or burns	Suffocation	Suffocation	Suffocation	Falls
6	Poisoning	Falls	Falls	Poisoning	Fires or burns
7	Falls	Poisoning	Poisoning	Falls	Suffocation

Note. MVT = motor vehicle traffic. Adapted from CDC childhood injury report: Patterns of unintentional injuries among 0–19 year olds in the United States, 2000–2006. CDC. http://www.cdc.gov/safechild/images/CDC-childhoodinjury.pdf. Published 2008. Accessed April 2015. Reproduced with permission.

Smaller Circulating Blood Volume/Less Fluid Reserve

Blood loss of even a small amount can be considered significant in children. A 5 kg child who has a hemorrhage of 100 ml will lose approximately 10% of their total blood volume.[33]

Skeletal

Children's bones are more susceptible to fractures and offer less protection to the internal organs.[37] Moreover, cervical vertebrae are cartilaginous in an infant and slowly become replaced by bone; thus, childhood cervical spine injuries occur at a higher rate than adult cervical spine injuries. Other injuries are then more likely to result, which may include damage to cartilaginous-osseus structures and surrounding ligaments, as well as spinal cord compression or transection.[37] Due to the increased elasticity of children's bones, they are most prone to having greenstick fractures, which occur when a bone bends before cracking.[38]

Head

Children have larger head-to-body ratios than adults. Because of their larger head sizes, children are more vulnerable to head and spine injuries as well as heat loss and hypothermia.[33] Furthermore, the brain, which typically doubles in size by 6 months and is 80% of adult size by 2 years of age, continues to perform functions such as myelination, synapse formation, neuronal plasticity, and biochemical stability, all of which are at risk for arrest and resultant permanent changes.[2]

Chest

Children's chests are mobile and pliable, and their abdominal walls are relatively thin. Additionally, their small size leads to closer proximity of organs, resulting in an increased likelihood of multiple organs being injured during a given traumatic event.[33]

Airway

The anatomy of the pediatric respiratory system is significantly different from that of an adult. Children have a smaller trachea, smaller lung volumes, a more compliant chest wall, and a smaller forced residual capacity than adults. Thus, they are more vulnerable to respiratory distress during life-threatening injuries.[33,39]

Physiological Differences

Circulatory System

Depending on their stage of development, children may have smaller absolute blood volume, lower systemic vascular resistance, smaller blood vessels, and more subcutaneous tissue than adults.[33]

Furthermore, children are vulnerable to certain types of shock, most commonly hypovolemic shock. This occurs from a decreased preload from extravascular or intravascular fluid loss, which subsequently results in decreased cardiac output.[40] A rapid deterioration with little warning may follow.[2]

Temperature Stability and Regulation

Because of their larger head size and increased BSA, children are at increased risk for heat loss and hypothermia.[33] Additional factors that affect the temperature stability and regulation of children include thin skin, evaporative heat loss due to lack of subcutaneous tissue, and increased caloric and energy expenditures. The use of thermal blankets, as well as warmed resuscitation rooms, fluids, and inhaled gases, may be required for treatment while undergoing resuscitative measures.[2]

Ventilation

When managing a child's ventilation, the NP should consider the anatomic differences of pediatric patients' airways when compared to those of adults. For instance, children have a shorter trachea, a larger tongue, and a glottic opening that is anterior and superior to that of an adult.[33] The Broselow-Hinkle measuring tape is recommended for selecting drug doses and equipment sizes during pediatric resuscitation. This tape has drug dosages and equipment sizes printed directly on the apparatus, thus eliminating the need for the practitioner to perform calculations during resuscitation efforts.[41] Meticulous fluid management is critical in pediatric patients, and normal saline or lactated Ringer's solution should be administered to restore intravascular volume.[42]

Glycogen (Energy) Stores

A limited store of glycogen with higher relative metabolism puts children at risk for hypoglycemia. Hypoglycemia is most common in newborns and may also appear in older children as a complication of insulin therapy for diabetes.[43]

Immunologic Differences

An immature immunologic system creates a greater risk of infection for children. As a result, certain conditions can be magnified or are more likely to appear in pediatric patients than adults. One example is eczema, which can manifest over the child's entire body. As children grow older, the manifestation of these conditions becomes more similar to that of an adult.

Developmental Differences

Because of limited verbal abilities, children may not be able to describe symptoms or localize pain. As children are often dependent on caretakers for food, children may be more vulnerable to food source limitations when potential sources are unavailable or contaminated. Children have limited motor skills to escape injury, as well as limited cognitive abilities to conceptualize their way out of danger, follow directions from others, or recognize threatening circumstances. Moreover, children are often emotionally labile due to their developing brain, which is especially taxed during stressful encounters. Reactions to danger and threats may be dictated by the child's developmental stage, and there are additional concerns when the child has special health care needs.[2]

Psychological Differences

Developmental stages alter the child's emotions in specific ways. Hyperactive startle responses may begin to occur during the newborn stage and last up to 2 months of age. A child may begin to cry more around the third month of life, whereas separation anxiety is developmentally appropriate around 9–12 months of age. Toddlers and preschool age children may exhibit regressive behaviors, such as temper tantrums, clinginess, and problems with separation or sleep.[2] These regressive behaviors may be exacerbated by a major change in a child's life.

Mental health problems tend to particularly manifest in late childhood and early adolescence and can have a detrimental impact on school, relationships, and overall health. The WHO suggests that depression is the leading health care concern among children and adolescents.[44] Depression does not have a single cause, but a number of factors may contribute to depression in children, including genetics, stressful situations, and the child's home environment.[45] Furthermore, depression may manifest in the form of risk-taking behaviors such as alcohol and drug use, unplanned pregnancies, and violent behavior.[44]

Figures

Figure 1.1. Primary teeth eruption. Barkley & Associates, Inc. Published 2015.

Figure 1.2. Permanent teeth eruption. Barkley & Associates, Inc. Published 2015.

References

1. Normal growth and development. A.D.A.M. Medical Encyclopedia. http://www.nlm.nih.gov/medlineplus/ency/article/002456.htm. Updated February 26, 2014. Accessed April 3, 2015.

2. Barkley TW Jr. *Pediatric Primary Care Nurse Practitioner Certification Review/Clinical Update Continuing Education Course*. West Hollywood, CA: Barkley and Associates; 2015.

3. Hagan JF, Shaw JS, Duncan P. (Eds.). *Bright Futures: Guidelines for Health Supervision of Infants, Children, and Adolescents, Pocket Guide*. 3rd ed. Elk Grove Village, IL: American Academy of Pediatrics; 2008.

4. United States Department of Health and Human Services, Centers for Disease Control and Prevention. Growth charts. http://www.cdc.gov/growthcharts. Last updated September 9, 2010. Accessed April 3, 2015.

5. Wagner CL. Counseling the breastfeeding mother. In: Rosenkrantz T, ed. Medscape. http://emedicine.medscape.com/article/979458-overview. Updated February 5, 2015. Accessed April 3, 2015.

6. Fleischer DM. The impact of breastfeeding on the development of allergic disease. In: Basow DS, ed. *UpToDate*. Waltham, MA: UpToDate; 2015. http://www.uptodate.com/contents/the-impact-of-breastfeeding-on-the-development-of-allergic-disease. Last updated September 24, 2014. Accessed April 3, 2015.

7. American Academy of Pediatrics. Breastfeeding and the use of human milk. *Pediatrics*. 2012; 129(3): e827–e841. http://pediatrics.aappublications.org/content/129/3/e827.full.pdf+html

8. Schanler RJ. Infant benefits of breastfeeding. In: Basow DS, ed. *UpToDate*. Waltham, MA: UpToDate; 2015. http://www.uptodate.com/contents/infant-benefits-of-breastfeeding. Last updated March 22, 2015. Accessed April 3, 2015.

9. Hellings PJ. Breastfeeding. In: Burns CE, Dunn AM, Brady MA, Starr NB, Blosser CG, Garzon DL, eds. *Pediatric Primary Care*. 5th ed. Philadelphia, PA: Elsevier Saunders; 2013: 186–201.

10. Vitamin D supplementation for infants. American Academy of Pediatrics web site. http://www.aap.org/en-us/about-the-aap/aap-press-room/Pages/Vitamin-D-Supplementation-for-Infants.aspx. Published March 22, 2010. Accessed April 3, 2015.

11. Pettifor JM. Nutritional rickets. In: Glorieux FH, Pettifor JM, Jüppner H. *Pediatric Bone*. 2nd ed. London: Elsevier/Academic Press; 2012: 625–654.

12. Bright Futures. American Academy of Pediatrics. Nutrition supervision. In: Holt K, Wooldridge N, Story M, Sofka D, eds. *Bright Futures: Nutrition*. 3rd ed. Elk Grove, IL: American Academy of Pediatrics; 2011: 17–111. https://brightfutures.aap.org/pdfs/BFNutrition3rdEditionSupervision.pdf

13. Oral health topics: Fluoride supplements. American Dental Association web site. http://www.ada.org/en/member-center/oral-health-topics/fluoride-supplements.

14. Boom JA. Normal growth patterns in infants and prepubertal children. In: Basow DS, ed. *UpToDate*. Waltham, MA: UpToDate; 2015. http://www.uptodate.com/contents/normal-growth-patterns-in-infants-and-prepubertal-children. Last updated March 13, 2014. Accessed April 3, 2015.

15. American Academy of Pediatrics. Physical appearance and growth: Your 2 year old. Healthy Children web site. http://www.healthychildren.org/English/ages-stages/toddler/Pages/Physical-Appearance-and-Growth-Your-2-Year-Od.aspx. Last updated August 6, 2013. Accessed April 3, 2015.

16. American Academy of Pediatrics. Physical changes during puberty. Healthy Children web site. http://www.healthychildren.org/English/ages-stages/gradeschool/puberty/Pages/Physical-Development-of-School-Age-Children.aspx. Last updated December 19, 2014. Accessed April 3, 2015.

17. Domino FJ. Teething. In: Domino FJ, Baldor RA, Golding J, Grimes JA, eds. *The 5-Minute Clinical Consult 2015*. 23rd ed. Philadelphia, PA: Wolters Kluwer Health; 2014: 1156–1157.

18. Jarvis C. *Physical Examination and Health Assessment*. 6th ed. St. Louis, MO: Elsevier Saunders; 2012.

19. Felluga D. Modules on Freud: On psychosexual development. Introductory Guide to Critical Theory web site. http://www.purdue.edu/guidetotheory/psychoanalysis/freud.html. Last updated January 31, 2011. Accessed April 3, 2015.

20. Phillips SM, Shulman RJ. Measurements of growth in children. In: Basow DS, ed. *UpToDate*. Waltham, MA: UpToDate; 2015. http://www.uptodate.com/contents/measurement-of-growth-in-children. Last updated February 10, 2014. Accessed April 3, 2015.

21. American Academy of Pediatrics. Corrected age for preemies. Healthy Children web site. http://www.healthychildren.org/English/ages-stages/baby/preemie/pages/Corrected-Age-For-Preemies.aspx. Last updated January 8, 2015. Accessed April 3, 2015.

22. United States Department of Health and Human Services, Centers for Disease Control and Prevention. About BMI for children and teens. http://www.cdc.gov/healthyweight/assessing/bmi/childrens_bmi/about_childrens_bmi.html. Last updated July 11, 2014. Accessed April 3, 2015.

23. Willacy H, Tidy C. Denver Developmental Screening Test. Patient web site. http://www.patient.co.uk/doctor/denver-developmental-screening-test. Reviewed December 3, 2014. Accessed April 3, 2015.

24. Health supervision of the well child. In: Porter RS, Kaplan JL, eds. The Merck Manual Online. http://www.merckmanuals.com/professional/pediatrics/approach_to_the_care_of_normal_infants_and_children/health_supervision_of_the_well_child.html#v1077060. Last reviewed April 2014. Accessed April 3, 2015.

25. Haupt M. 4 Month Well Child visit. University of Chicago Department of Pediatrics web site. http://pediatrics.uchicago.edu/chiefs/ClinicCurriculum/documents/4MonthWellChild.pdf. Accessed April 3, 2015.

26. Norton R, Kobusingye O. Injuries. *N Engl J Med*. 2013; 368(18): 1723–1730. doi: 10.1056/NEJMra1109343.

27. Kelly NR. Prevention of poisoning in children. In: Basow DS, ed. *UpToDate*. Waltham, MA: UpToDate; 2015. http://www.uptodate.com/contents/prevention-of-poisoning-in-children. Last updated December 9, 2014. Accessed April 3, 2015.

28. Gill AC, Wesson DE. Firearm injuries in children: Prevention. In: Basow DS, ed. *UpToDate*. Waltham, MA: UpToDate; 2015. http://www.uptodate.com/contents/firearm-injuries-in-children-prevention. Last updated October 30, 2014. Accessed April 3, 2015.

29. Committee on Injury, Violence, and Poison Prevention, Durbin DR. Child passenger safety. *Pediatrics*. 2011; 127(4): 788–793. doi:10.1542/peds.2011-0213

30. Protecting children in your home. Safe Kids Worldwide web site. http://www.safekids.org/infographic/protecting-children-your-home. Accessed April 3, 2015.

31. Merrick MT, Latzman NE. Child maltreatment: A public health overview and prevention considerations. *Online J Issues Nurs*. 2014; 19(1): 2. doi: 10.3912/OJIN.Vol19No01Man02

32. United States Department of Health and Human Services, Administration for Children and Families, Administration on Children Youth and Families, Children's Bureau. Mandatory reporters of child abuse and neglect. https://www.childwelfare.gov/pubPDFs/manda.pdf#page=1&view=Professionals Required to Report. Published 2014. Accessed April 29, 2015.

33. How are children different? Royal Children's Hospital Melbourne web site. http://www.rch.org.au/paed_trauma/manual/11_How_are_children_different. Accessed April 3, 2015.

34. Brandt BL. Household environmental toxins and neurodevelopment in children [professional paper]. Bozeman, MT: Montana State University; 2012. http://scholarworks.montana.edu/xmlui/bitstream/handle/1/966/BrandtB0512.pdf?sequence=1&isAllowed=y

35. United States Department of Health and Human Services, Centers for Disease Control and Prevention, Agency for Toxic Substances and Disease Registry. Principles of pediatric environmental health: How are newborns, infants, and toddlers exposed to and affected by toxicants? http://www.atsdr.cdc.gov/csem/csem.asp?csem=27&po=9. Issued February 15, 2012. Renewed February 15, 2014. Accessed April 3, 2015.

36. American Academy of Pediatrics. Curriculum for managing infectious diseases in early education and child care settings: Module 1, understanding infectious diseases. Healthy Child Care American web site. http://www.healthychildcare.org/PDF/InfDiseases/Module1.pdf. Published 2010. Accessed April 3, 2015.

37. Thompson GH, Stern LC, Wilber JH, Son-Hing JP. The multiply injured child. In: Mencio GA, Swiontkowski MF, eds. *Green's Skeletal Trauma in Children*. 5th ed. Philadelphia, PA: Elsevier Saunders; 2015: 59–85.

38. Mayo Clinic Staff. Greenstick fractures. Mayo Clinic web site. http://www.mayoclinic.org/diseases-conditions/greenstick-fractures/basics/definition/con-20027302. Reviewed June 18, 2013. Accessed April 3, 2015.

39. Kache S. Pediatric airway and respiratory physiology. Stanford School of Medicine Pediatric Housestaff web site. http://peds.stanford.edu/Rotations/picu/pdfs/10_Peds_Airway.pdf. Accessed April 3, 2015.

40. Pomerantz WJ, Roback MG. Physiology and classification of shock in children. In: Basow DS, ed. *UpToDate*. Waltham, MA: UpToDate; 2015. http://www.uptodate.com/contents/physiology-and-classification-of-shock-in-children?source=search_result&search=shock+children&selectedTitle=4~150#H8. Last updated December 17, 2014. Accessed April 3, 2015.

41. Jevon P. Paediatric advanced life support: A practical guide for nurses. 2nd ed. Chichester, West Sussex: John Wiley & Sons; 2012.

42. Pomerantz WJ, Roback MG. Hypovolemic shock in children: Initial evaluation and management. In: Basow DS, ed. *UpToDate*. Waltham, MA: UpToDate; 2015. http://www.uptodate.com/contents/hypovolemic-shock-in-children-initial-evaluation-and-management?source=see_link#H13. Last updated September 18, 2014. Accessed April 3, 2015.

43. Hypoglycemia and low blood sugar in children. Boston Children's Hospital web site. http://www.childrenshospital.org/health-topics/conditions/hypoglycemia-and-low-blood-sugar. Accessed April 3, 2015.

44. Adolescents and mental health. World Health Organization web site. http://www.who.int/maternal_child_adolescent/topics/adolescence/mental_health/en. Accessed April 3, 2015.

45. Continuing medical education: Frequently asked questions. American Academy of Child & Adolescent Psychiatry web site. http://www.aacap.org/aacap/Families_and_Youth/Resource_Centers/Depression_Resource_Center/FAQ.aspx. Accessed April 3, 2015.

Chapter 2
Immunization Recommendations

1. Which of the following vaccines should not be given to patients who are pregnant?

   a. The inactivated polio vaccine

   b. The measles, mumps, rubella vaccine

   c. The influenza vaccine

   d. The tetanus, diptheria, and acellular pertussis vaccine

2. If a newborn's mother is HBsAg-positive, when should the nurse practitioner order the hepatitis B vaccine for the newborn?

   a. Within 12 hours after birth

   b. Prior to home discharge

   c. One week after birth

   d. Not until 1 year of age

3. By the age of 3, a child should have received the third dose of all of the following immunizations except:

   a. Hepatitis B

   b. Diptheria, tetanus, and acellular pertussis

   c. *Haemophilus influenzae*

   d. Varicella

4. The measles, mumps, and rubella vaccine (MMR) may be given simultaneously with tuberculosis testing and the purified protein derivative (PPD) skin test, but it is commonly recommended to postpone the PPD for 4–6 weeks for which reason?

   a. To avoid unwanted protein binding to the MMR vaccine

   b. To avoid adverse effects

   c. To allow the MMR vaccine to form antibodies

   d. To avoid possible false negative on the PPD test

5. You are treating a 24-month-old infant who has completed her PCV13 series. All of the following are possible preexisting conditions that would require administration of one dose of the 23PS formulation except:

   a. Chronic cardiac disease

   b. Hepatitis B

   c. Renal failure

   d. Asplenia

6. Which of the following is not a typical minor adverse reaction to a vaccine?

   a. Low-grade temperature

   b. Local tenderness

   c. Local pallor

   d. Local muscle soreness

7. At least how many months apart should hepatitis A doses of vaccines be administered?

   a. At least 1 month apart

   b. At least 3 months apart

   c. At least 6 months apart

   d. At least 12 months apart

8. Sharon, age 16, has just received her first meningococcal conjugate vaccine. How long should she ideally wait before receiving the booster dose?

   a. Eight weeks

   b. Six months

   c. One year

   d. The patient does not require a booster dose.

9. Jason, age 8 years, is going to South America on vacation with his parents. His parents want to know which vaccinations he needs to keep from getting sick. Assuming he is caught up on all of his other vaccinations, which of the following vaccines would be least necessary for Jason?

   a. Hepatitis A vaccine

   b. Typhoid vaccine

   c. Malaria vaccine

   d. Tetanus, diptheria, acellular pertussis vaccine

10. Jack, a school-aged child, has a 4-year-old brother who has just been diagnosed with acute lymphocytic leukemia. Jack should receive which of the following flu vaccine preparations?

    a. Inhaled influenza vaccine

    b. Quadrivalent inactivated influenza vaccine

    c. Trivalent inactivated influenza vaccine

    d. The child should not receive any influenza vaccine at risk of shedding the virus to the sibling.

RATIONALES

1. b

The measles, mumps, and rubella (MMR) vaccine should not be given to patients who are pregnant or immunosuppressed, as it is a live virus vaccine. It is recommended that women should not become pregnant within 4 weeks after receiving the MMR vaccine, but they can typically be vaccinated after giving birth or while breastfeeding, as the risk to the fetus has passed. The tetanus, diptheria, and acellular pertussis vaccine is usually safe to give to pregnant patients, and the ideal time to vaccinate is between 27 and 36 weeks of gestation. The inactivated poliovirus may be given to pregnant women if clearly needed. The influenza vaccine is commonly recommended for pregnant women to protect both the mother and unborn child.

2. a

Infants who are born to HBsAg-positive mothers should be given the hepatitis B vaccine within 12 hours of being born. Pregnancy is not a contraindication to vaccination, so pregnant mothers can receive the hepatitis B vaccine. However, a newborn born to a hepatitis B carrier would still typically need to receive a vaccination shortly after birth. If the mother tests positive for HBsAg when her status was previously unknown, hepatitis B immune globulin should be given to the infant no later than 1 week of age. The hepatitis A vaccine is commonly given at 1 year of age.

3. d

By the age of 3, a child should have received only one dose of the varicella vaccine, with the subsequent dose administered between the ages of 4 and 6. By 3 years of age, children should have received all three doses of the hepatitis B vaccine, ideally administered at 0, 2, and 6 months of age. The three primary immunizations for diphtheria, tetanus, and acellular pertussis would typically be administered at 2, 4, and 6 months of age, followed by boosters at 15 months and 6 years of age. The *Haemophilus influenzae* vaccine would likewise usually be administered at 2, 4, and 6 months of age, followed by one booster at 12 months.

4. d

The measles, mumps, and rubella (MMR) vaccine may be given simultaneously with tuberculosis testing and the purified protein derivative (PPD) skin test, but it is recommended to postpone the PPD for 4–6 weeks to avoid a possible suppressive response to the PPD, which may potentially yield a false negative response. Unwanted protein binding to MMR and risk of adverse effects are not common contraindications to supplying the vaccine simultaneously. Furthermore, the formation of antibodies from MMR typically has no effect on the efficacy of the PPD test.

5. b

A 24-month-old with hepatitis B who has completed the PCV13 series would not typically need a 23PS vaccination. Chronic cardiac disease, renal failure, and asplenia are all conditions for which the nurse practitioner should consider administering a dose of 23PS, so long as the patient is 24 months of age and has completed the PCV13 series. Other conditions that would typically call for necessary administration of a 23PS dose include splenic dysfunction, HIV, nephrotic syndrome, pulmonary diseases, and diabetes.

6. c

Local pallor is not a typical minor adverse reaction to a vaccine; rather, many vaccines produce localized redness and swelling as common minor side effects. Other typical adverse reactions to vaccines may include local muscle soreness, low-grade temperature, and local tenderness.

7. c

The two doses of the hepatitis A vaccine should ideally be administered at least 6 months apart between 1 and 2 years of age. The first booster dose protects against hepatitis A for 1 year and allows the body to make antibodies against the virus. The subsequent dose, given after 6 months, acts to protect against hepatitis A for 20 years. Giving the second vaccine after 1 or 3 months does not typically allow the body enough time to make antibodies to the virus. Although waiting 12 months for the second vaccination is not recommended because the efficacy of protection from the first vaccine might dwindle, the second vaccination should still be received as soon as possible.

8. d

If the meningococcal conjugate vaccine is given at the age of 16 or older, a booster dose is not considered necessary. However, it is recommended that patients receive the first dose between 11 and 12 years of age. Patients who receive the first vaccination prior to age 16 should require a booster at age 16, at least 8 weeks after the first dose was administered. Although 6 months is the recommended time frame between hepatitis A vaccines, the meningococcal conjugate vaccine requires a different time frame based on the patient's age. The time frame of 1 year would only be relevant if the patient received her first dose of meningococcal conjugate vaccine at age 15, as she would require a booster at age 16.

9. d

Patients who are current on their vaccinations would not typically require a subsequent tetanus, diptheria, and acellular pertussis vaccine, as the vaccine commonly protects for 10 years and is not particularly indicated for foreign travel. Because hepatitis A can be acquired through contaminated food and water, the hepatitis A vaccine is recommended for all travelers. Similarly, the typhoid vaccine is recommended for people travelling to rural areas. The malaria vaccination is recommended to travelers visiting foreign countries that pose a risk of encountering infected mosquitos.

10. c

The sibling should definitely receive a flu vaccine and the trivalent influenza vaccine is the preferred formulation, as the quadrivalent product is commonly recommended after the age of 18. The inhaled influenza vaccine is a live virus and not recommended for families of immunocompromised patients.

DISCUSSION

Hepatitis B Vaccination

Overview

The hepatitis B (HepB) vaccination is given to newborns in a series of three intramuscular (IM) injections that should be completed by 18 months of age.[1] All newborns should receive the first dose prior to hospital discharge. The second and third doses are usually administered 1 month and 6 months after the initial dose. For the initial dose at birth, only a monovalent HepB vaccine should be administered. Either a monovalent or combination vaccine may be used for the second and third doses.[2] Pediatric patients younger than the age of 18 who have not received the vaccine should be vaccinated as soon as possible.[1]

The Centers for Disease Control and Prevention (CDC) recommends that infants born to mothers who are positive for the hepatitis B surface antigen (HBsAg) should receive a HepB vaccine and a 0.5 ml dose of hepatitis B immune globulin (HBIG) within 12 hours of birth. These two injections should be administered at separate sites. The second dose of HepB should then be given at 1–2 months of age, and the last dose should be administered by 6 months of age. An additional HBsAG titre should be drawn at 9–12 months of age, and one additional dose of HepB should be given if the child does not demonstrate immunity.[3]

If the HBsAg status of the mother is unknown, the nurse practitioner (NP) should determine her status, assess the baby's status immediately after birth, and administer HepB within 12 hours of birth. If the mother is positive for the antigen, HBIG should be administered to the newborn by no later than 1 week of age.[3]

Rotavirus Vaccine (Rota)

Overview

The rotavirus vaccine is given as a series of three doses to newborns at 6 and 32 weeks of age. The NP may order the first dose at a minimum 6 weeks of age, and each subsequent dose is given at a minimum of 4-week intervals. The rotavirus vaccination series should be completed by 8 months of age.[4]

Diphtheria/Tetanus/Acellular Pertussis Vaccines (DTaP)

Overview

The DTaP vaccine is given in a series of three primary doses and two boosters. The three primary doses are given at 2 months, 4 months, and 6 months of age. Once this series is completed, the first booster is administered at 15–18 months of age and the second at 4–6 years of age.[5]

Tetanus, Diphtheria, Acellular Pertussis Vaccines (Tdap)

Overview

The Tdap vaccine is administered in a single dose at 11 or 12 years of age. After this dose is given, tetanus-diphtheria (Td) boosters are currently recommended to be given every 10 years.[6]

Children older than 7 years of age who have not received the DTaP series should receive the Tdap vaccine as the first dose of their catch-up series.[7] Due to a resurgence of pertussis, Tdap boosters

should also be considered for adults who will be around infants.

Haemophilus Influenzae Type B (Hib) Conjugate Vaccine

Overview

The *Haemophilus influenzae* type b (Hib) conjugate vaccine is given in a series of three primary doses and one booster. The primary doses are administered at 2 months, 4 months, and 6 months of age, and the booster is given at 12–15 months of age. The first dose of the Hib vaccine should not be given before 6 weeks of age, and no dosage of the Hib vaccine is recommended for children at 5 years of age or later.[8]

Pneumococcal Vaccine (PCV13 or PPSV23)

Overview

The pneumococcal vaccine consists of two different types: the 13-valent pneumococcal conjugate vaccine (PCV13) and the 23-valent pneumococcal polysaccharide vaccine (PPSV23).[9]

The PCV13 vaccine (Prevnar) is recommended for children younger than 5 years of age and is given as a series that consists of three primary doses and one booster. The three primary doses of PCV13 should be given at 2 months, 4 months, and 6 months of age, and the booster is given at 12–15 months of age.[10]

The PPSV23 vaccine (Pneumovax) series is recommended for children older than 2 years of age who are at high risk of disease due to immuno-compromising conditions.[11] These conditions may include HIV infection, renal failure, nephrotic syndrome, and diabetes.[10]

Polio Vaccine (IPV)

Overview

The polio vaccine is administered in a series of four doses. The first three are given at 2 months, 4 months, and 6–18 months of age, and a booster is administered at 4–6 years of age.[5] The inactivated polio vaccine is recommended for all four of these scheduled vaccines. The CDC no longer recommends the oral polio vaccine because this formulation is strongly correlated with the onset of paralysis in rare instances.[12]

Influenza Vaccine

Overview

The influenza vaccine should be administered to children 6 months of age and older.[13] In children 6–35 months of age, the recommended annual dose is 0.25 ml IM. The dose increases to 0.50 ml IM for children 3 years of age and older.[11] Children younger than 9 years who have not yet received the influenza vaccine should receive two doses administered 1 month apart. Once children reach 9 years of age, they only need a single dose annually.[13,14]

Inactivated influenza vaccines are offered in either quadrivalent or trivalent formulations.[15] The quadrivalent formulation covers four strains, whereas the trivalent formulation covers three. Additionally, a live attenuated virus can be distributed via FluMist and may serve as an alternative to trivalent vaccines in healthy children older than 2 years.[11]

Measles, Mumps, and Rubella (MMR)

Overview

The MMR vaccine is given in a series of two doses. The first dose should be administered at 12–15 months of age, and the second dose should be administered at 4–6 years of age.[16] Children aged 4–6 years who have not yet received the first dose must wait at least 4 weeks between doses. If a patient is exposed to measles or is travelling to endemic areas, the NP can order the MMR vaccine as early as 6 months of age; however, the primary series must be resumed at the appropriate time.

Varicella

Overview

The varicella vaccine is given in a series of two doses: The first should be administered between 12–15 months of age, and the second should be administered at 4–6 years of age.[17] According to the CDC, these two doses should be a minimum of 3 months apart when administered to children younger than the age of 13.[5] Both doses should be administered after the age of 12 months if no evidence of immunity is available and the parents cannot recall a history of chicken pox. Moreover, it is preferable to separate the varicella vaccine from the MMR vaccine by 1 month, as concomitant administration of the vaccines has been associated with rash and a higher rate of fever.[17]

Hepatitis A Vaccine

Overview

The CDC recommends that two doses of the hepatitis A vaccine should be administered to all children between 1 and 2 years of age.[18] Both of these doses should be given at a minimum of 6 months apart, although these may be separated by up to 18 months.[5]

Meningococcal Vaccine

Overview

The meningococcal vaccine is available as a conjugate vaccine and as a polysaccharide vaccine. The meningococcal conjugate vaccine is recommended for children who are at an increased risk of meningococcal disease and is administered between 2 months and 10 years of age. Booster doses may be given under certain circumstances or conditions that increase the risk of meningococcal disease. For older children and adolescents, the initial dose of the meningococcal polysaccharide vaccine is administered at 11 or 12 years of age with a booster given from age 16 to 18.[19] It is important to adhere to this schedule because incidence of meningococcal disease peaks in patients between the ages of 16 and 21 years.[5] No booster is necessary if an adolescent receives his or her first dose at 16 years of age or later.[19]

Human Papillomavirus Vaccine (HPV)

Overview

HPV is the most common sexually transmitted disease and males and females are both recommended to be vaccinated against HPV.[14] The human papillomavirus (HPV) vaccine is administered in a series of three doses, the first of which is recommended for all adolescents at 11 or 12 years of age. The second dose is then given 1–2 months after the first dose, with the third dose administered 6 months after the initial dose.[5] Adolescents are advised to remain seated for at least 15 minutes after receiving the HPV vaccine, as the vaccine may produce postural hypotension, labile syncope, and vasovagal responses shortly after administration.[11]

Two preparations of the HPV vaccine are commercially available: the HPV quadrivalent vaccine (HPV4), distributed as Gardasil, and the HPV bivalent vaccine (HPV2), which is distributed as Cervarix. Females may be given either HPV2 or HPV4, but males may only be administered HPV4.[5] Both HPV2 and HPV4 protect against oncologic strains of HPV (e.g., types 16 and 18), which cover cancerous lesions of the cervix, anus, penis, and oropharynx, as well as genital warts and recurrent papillomatosis. The HPV4 protects against cancerous lesions and HPV types 6 and 11, which cause the majority of genital warts in both females and males.[20]

Table 2.1   Recommended immunization schedule for persons 0–18 years, United States, 2015

Vaccine	Birth	1 mo	2 mos	4 mos	6 mos	9 mos	12 mos	15 mos	18 mos	19–23 mos	2–3 yrs	4–6 yrs	7–10 yrs	11–12 yrs	13–15 yrs	16–18 yrs
Hepatitis B	1st dose	2nd dose			3rd dose											
Rotavirus			1st dose	2nd dose												
DTap: < 7 yrs			1st dose	2nd dose	3rd dose			4th dose				5th dose				
Tdap: ≥ 7 yrs														Tdap		
***Haemophilus influenzae* type b**			1st dose	2nd dose	See footnote		3rd or 4th dose									
PCV13			1st dose	2nd dose	3rd dose		4th dose									
PPSV23																
IPV (< 18 yrs)			1st dose	2nd dose	3rd dose		3rd dose					4th dose				
Influenza (IIV; LAIV)					Annual vaccine (IIV only) 1 or 2 doses						Annual vaccine (LAIV or IIV) 1 or 2 doses		Annual vaccine (LAIV or IIV) 1 dose only			
MMR							1st dose					2nd dose				
VAR							1st dose					2nd dose				
Hep A							2 dose series, see footnote									
HPV2: females; HPV4: males and females)														3-dose series		
Meningococcal														1st dose		Booster

Key

Range of recommended ages for all children	Range of recommended ages for catch-up immunization	Range of recommended ages for certain high-risk groups	Range of recommended ages during which catch-up is encouraged and for certain high-risk groups	Not routinely recommended

Note. DTap = Diptheria, tetanus, & acellular pertussis; Tdap = Tetanus, diphtheria, & acellular pertussis, PCV13 = Pneumococcal conjugate; PPSV23 = Pneumococcal polysaccharide; IPV = Inactivated polio virus; MMR = Measles, mumps, & rubella, VAR = Varicella; Hep A = Hepatitis A; HPV = Human papillomavirus *Note.* Adapted with permission from *Recommended immunization schedule for persons 0–18 years, United States, 2015*, The Centers for Disease Control and Prevention. http://www.cdc.gov/vaccines/schedules/downloads/child/0-18yrs-schedule.pdf. Published 2015. Accessed April 2015.

References

1. Centers for Disease Control and Prevention. Hepatitis B in short. http://www.cdc.gov/vaccines/vpd-vac/hepb/in-short-adult.htm#who. Last updated August 21, 2012. Accessed April 3, 2015.

2. Centers for Disease Control and Prevention. Hepatitis B vaccination. http://www.cdc.gov/vaccines/vpd-vac/hepb. Last updated February 3, 2014. Accessed April 3, 2015.

3. CDC recommendation for infant vaccination. Hepatitis B Foundation web site. http://www.hepb.org/patients/infant_vaccination_cdc_summary.htm. Accessed April 3, 2015.

4. Centers for Disease Control and Prevention. Rotavirus vaccine – Questions and answers. http://www.cdc.gov/vaccines/vpd-vac/rotavirus/vac-faqs.htm. Last updated September 14, 2012. Accessed April 3, 2015.

5. Centers for Disease Control and Prevention. Recommended immunization schedules for persons age 0 through 18 years. http://www.cdc.gov/vaccines/schedules/hcp/imz/child-adolescent.html. Last updated January 28, 2015. Accessed April 3, 2015.

6. Centers for Disease Control and Prevention. Tdap vaccine: What you need to know. http://www.cdc.gov/vaccines/hcp/vis/vis-statements/tdap.pdf. Published February 24, 2015. Accessed April 3, 2015.

7. DTaP vaccine. A.D.A.M. Medical Encyclopedia. http://www.nlm.nih.gov/medlineplus/druginfo/meds/a682198.html. Last revised May 15, 2014. Accessed April 3, 2015.

8. Haemophilus influenzae type b (Hib) vaccine. A.D.A.M. Medical Encyclopedia. http://www.nlm.nih.gov/medlineplus/druginfo/meds/a607015.html. Last revised April 15, 2014. Accessed April 3, 2015.

9. Centers for Disease Control and Prevention. Pneumococcal vaccination. http://www.cdc.gov/VACCINES/VPD-VAC/pneumo/default.htm#vacc. Last updated February 10, 2015. Accessed April 3, 2015.

10. Healthwise, Inc. Pneumococcal vaccine. WebMD. http://children.webmd.com/vaccines/pneumococcal-vaccine-1?page=2. Reviewed May 26, 2014. Accessed April 3, 2015.

11. Live attenuated influenza vaccine [LAIV] (The nasal spray flu vaccine). Centers for Disease Control and Prevention web site. http://www.cdc.gov/flu/about/qa/nasalspray.htm. Last updated September 9, 2014. Accessed April 3, 2015.

12. A look at each vaccine: Polio vaccine. Children's Hospital of Philadelphia Vaccine Education Center web site. http://www.chop.edu/service/vaccine-education-center/a-look-at-each-vaccine/polio-vaccine.html. Reviewed May 2013. Accessed April 3, 2015.

13. Influenza vaccine, inactivated or recombinant. A.D.A.M. Medical Encyclopedia. http://www.nlm.nih.gov/medlineplus/ency/article/002025.htm. Last reviewed September 15, 2014. Accessed April 3, 2015.

14. Barkley TW Jr. *Pediatric Primary Care Nurse Practitioner Certification Review/Clinical Update Continuing Education Course.* West Hollywood, CA: Barkley and Associates; 2015.

15. Grohskopf LA, Shay DK, Shimabukuro TT, et al. Prevention and control of seasonal influenza with vaccines: recommendations of the Advisory Committee on Immunization Practices — United States, 2013–2014. *MMWR Morb Mortal Wkly Rep.* 2013; 62(RR07): 1–43. http://www.cdc.gov/mmwr/preview/mmwrhtml/rr6207a1.htm.

16. MMR vaccine (measles, mumps, rubella). A.D.A.M. Medical Encyclopedia. http://www.nlm.nih.gov/medlineplus/druginfo/meds/a601176.html. Last reviewed July 18, 2012. Accessed April 3, 2015.

17. Centers for Disease Control and Prevention. Routine varicella vaccination. http://www.cdc.gov/vaccines/vpd-vac/varicella/hcp-routine-vacc.htm. Last updated April 5, 2012. Accessed April 3, 2015.

18. Healthwise, Inc. Hepatitis A and B vaccines. WebMD. http://children.webmd.com/vaccines/hepatitis-a-and-b-vaccines?page=2. Reviewed May 26, 2014. Accessed April 3, 2015.

19. Meningococcal vaccine. Vaccines.gov. http://www.vaccines.gov/diseases/meningitis/#. Accessed April 3, 2015.

20. Centers for Disease Control and Prevention. HPV vaccine - Questions and answers. http://www.cdc.gov/vaccines/vpd-vac/hpv/vac-faqs.htm. Last updated August 6, 2014. Accessed April 3, 2015.

Chapter 3
Genetic Evaluation

1. Which of these couples in the early stages of their pregnancy would least require a genetic screening for mutations in the HEXA gene?

   a. An Inuit mother and a Louisiana Cajun father

   b. An African-American mother and a Druze father

   c. An Ashkenazi Jewish mother and a Scots-Irish father

   d. A Pinoy mother and a French Canadian father

2. Seizures and dementia can manifest in infants and young pediatric patients as a typical result of which of the following hereditary disorders?

   a. Klinefelter's syndrome

   b. Tay-Sachs disease

   c. Turner's syndrome

   d. Marfan syndrome

3. Alex, an 11-year-old male, comes to your clinic for a physical examination. During the examination, you notice that his spine is severely curved in the lumbar and thoracic areas. Although the diagnosis is concurrent, you also know that this finding is most consistent with which of the following genetic conditions?

   a. Marfan syndrome

   b. Down syndrome

   c. Turner's syndrome

   d. DiGeorge syndrome

4. Which of these factors is not a typical indication to recommend a prenatal evaluation for genetic disorders?

   a. The mother has experienced two stillbirths.

   b. The father has a brother with Down syndrome.

   c. The father worked with pesticides 3 years ago.

   d. The mother is of African descent.

5. Which of these genetic disorders is not associated with cardiac defects?

   a. DiGeorge syndrome

   b. Marfan syndrome

   c. Turner's syndrome

   d. Tay-Sachs disease

6. Which of these factors is most likely to increase the risk of Down syndrome in infants?

   a. Advanced maternal age

   b. Intrauterine infection during the second trimester

   c. Alcoholism during pregnancy

   d. Smoking during pregnancy

7. Which of the following is true regarding Turner syndrome?

   a. It presents as a result of mutations in the HEXA gene.

   b. It is the most common sex-chromosome anomaly found in females.

   c. It typically presents with tall stature and kyphoscoliosis.

   d. It typically presents with increased risk of infection due to thymus aplasia.

8. Which of these conditions is <u>least</u> likely to be inherited through genetics or other parental factors?

  a. Down syndrome

  b. Marfan syndrome

  c. Klinefelter's syndrome

  d. Tay-Sachs disease

9. Which of these genetic disorders is most likely to lead to blindness in later life?

  a. Turner's syndrome

  b. DiGeorge syndrome

  c. Kleinfelter's syndrome

  d. Marfan syndrome

10. You are counseling one of your pregnant patients on the prevalence of genetic disorders. If the baby has no predisposition for a specific genetic disorder, his chance of being born with a major malformation is most likely:

  a. Approximately 2%

  b. Approximately 5%

  c. Approximately 8%

  d. Approximately 10%

RATIONALES

1. b

The mutations in the HEXA gene that result in Tay-Sachs disease are not particularly common in either African-American or Druze populations. Tay-Sachs disease is closely linked to Ashkenazi Jewish populations; however, the mutations that produce the condition are also common in French Canadian and Louisiana Cajun populations.

2. b

Tay-Sachs disease is a progressive disorder that destroys nerve cells in the brain and spinal cord, commonly producing symptoms such as dementia in pediatric patients diagnosed with the disease and eventually leading to death. Some cases of Klinefelter's syndrome may lead to seizures due to hypocalcemia; however, dementia is not typically associated with the condition, and patients with Klinefelter's are more likely to present with learning disabilities and personality impairment. Turner's syndrome and Marfan syndrome are not degenerative disorders affecting neurological development; however, some patients with Turner's syndrome may develop learning disabilities. Marfan syndrome is not typically known to produce dementia.

3. a

Kyphoscoliosis, a combination of both kyphosis and scoliosis, is a common phenotypic presentation of Marfan syndrome. Children with Down syndrome or DiGeorge syndrome may develop scoliosis, but rarely present with kyphoscoliosis. Turner syndrome may likewise present with scoliosis; however, this condition only presents in females as the result of a missing X chromosome.

4. c

Exposure to toxic chemicals is a common indicator for genetic evaluation if the fetus itself is exposed; as it was the father, not the fetus, who experienced prior exposure to toxic chemicals, this scenario does not strongly indicate the need for genetic evaluation. A history of miscarriages and stillbirths, as well as a family history of mental retardation, are common indicators for genetic evaluation. Depending on circumstances, ethnic background may be an indicator as well, as the gene responsible for sickle cell anemia is more likely to present in individuals with African or African-American ancestry.

5. d

Tay-Sachs disease is an irreversible condition associated with neurological degeneration, not cardiac defects. DiGeorge syndrome often results in congenital heart defects such as aortic arch anomalies, resulting in significant morbidity and mortality in pediatric patients. Patients with Marfan syndrome may present with aortic regurgitation and mitral valve prolapse at birth, and coarctation of the aorta is a common congenital heart defect in patients with Turner's syndrome.

6. a

Advanced maternal age is a strong risk factor for Down syndrome. As the disorder typically occurs as a result of trisomy that develops at conception, intrauterine infection during the second trimester is not viewed as a risk factor. Some studies suggest a link between alcohol intake and smoking during pregnancy and Down syndrome; results, however, are inconclusive.

7. b

Turner's syndrome, also known as XO karyotype, is the most common sex-chromosome anomaly found in females occurring as a result of a missing or altered X chromosome. Tay-Sachs disease, a genetic disorder particular to the Ashkenazic Jewish population and other ethnic groups, is not a sex-chromosome anomaly. Although Turner's syndrome may present with scoliosis, tall stature and kyphoscoliosis are more common indicators of Marfan's syndrome. DiGeorge syndrome often manifests with cardiac malformations, thymus aplasia, and an associated increased susceptibility to infection; Turner's syndrome, on the other hand, is more likely to produce increased risk of autoimmune disorders later in life.

8. c

Klinefelter's syndrome is not an inherited condition, since one of its mainstay characteristics is infertility; rather, it is commonly attributed to the failure of chromosomal separation during meiosis. Although maternal age may be a factor for the onset of the condition, Klinefelter's is not inherited via the genetic pool. Down syndrome may typically be attributed to parental age or presence of the genetic translocation for Down syndrome. Marfan syndrome is an inherited condition caused by mutations in the FBN1 gene. Tay-Sachs disease primarily presents among populations with common mutations in the HEXA gene, which primarily appear in Ashkenazi Jews, but have been seen in Louisiana Cajuns and Quebecois French-Canadians.

9. d

Patients with Marfan syndrome often exhibit ectopia lentis and have an increased chance of experiencing retinal detachment and glaucoma, which can lead to blindness. Patients with Turner's syndrome are more likely to experience strabismus, cataracts, and red-green color blindness. DiGeorge syndrome may produce strabismus and ambylopia but does not significantly increase the risk of blindness. Although patients with Klinefelter's syndrome have presented with myopia and bilaterial retinal detachment, structural eye abnormalities are not a common feature of the condition.

10. a

Approximately 2% of all live births are affected by a major genetic malformation. About 40%–45% of these accountable genetic disorders are usually diagnosed during the neonatal period and 80% are commonly diagnosed before the child is 6 months old.

DISCUSSION

Genetic Evaluation

Overview

Genetic disorders are basically uncommon, with major malformations occurring in approximately 2% of all live births.[1,2] Genetic disorders include single gene disorders, chromosomal abnormalities, and multifactorial disorders.[3] Single gene disorders occur after a mutation in the DNA sequence of a single gene. This mutation can occur within the sperm or egg, or can be passed on to a child from either parent. Single gene disorders can be autosomal (e.g., sickle cell disease) or X-linked (e.g., fragile X syndrome).[3]

Chromosomal abnormalities occur when the normal 23 pairs of chromosomes are altered to be more or less than 23 pairs. Conditions that derive from this kind of abnormality include such problems as Down syndrome and Turner's syndrome.[3] Multifactorial disorders involve variations in multiple genes and environmental factors.[3] Alzheimer's disease and hypothyroidism are two multifactorial disorders.

Only 40%–45% of all genetic disorders are diagnosed in the neonatal period, but about 80% are identified before the age of 6 months.[1]

Presentation

A genetic evaluation should be conducted if certain risk factors are present. Some indications include advanced parental age, which is classified as about 35 years or older,[4] and a maternal history of miscarriages or stillbirths.[5] Genetic testing is warranted if the mother has abnormal tests during pregnancy, has been exposed to teratogenic substances (e.g., x-rays, chemicals, drugs), has had difficulty with conception, or has experienced a genetic condition with a previous pregnancy.[6] Finally, many conditions in a patient's family history may necessitate a genetic evaluation, such as a history of birth defects, mental retardation, growth retardation, neurologic conditions, or familial conditions.[7]

Routine newborn screening tests vary from state to state; however, all states screen for phenylketonuria, congenital hypothyroidism, and galactosemia, in addition to other metabolic or genetic-associated disorders. Parents in specific ethnic groups that are at higher risk for certain genetically-acquired conditions (e.g., sickle cell anemia, 1 per 600 people of African descent; Tay-Sachs, 1 per 3,500 Ashkenazi Jews) may choose to be evaluated for carrier status.[8,9]

When evaluating a child for genetically-acquired conditions, a child's phenotype and genotype should be considered. Phenotypic indications for genetic evaluation include: dysmorphic features, developmental delay, below average intelligence, short stature, failure to thrive, progressive deterioration of health status, and seizures.[3]

A genogram is a genetic family history used to assess a child's genotype. Family members' histories of miscarriages, stillbirths, and other abnormalities should also be obtained. If the child's pedigree is concerning, a prenatal screening and diagnosis should be conducted for subsequent pregnancies.[4,10]

Trisomy 21 (Down Syndrome)

Overview

A variety of chromosomal abnormalities, collectively known as "syndromes," may develop spontaneously or as a result of either parent's genetic influence. Trisomy 21, or Down syndrome, occurs if a third chromosome 21 is present. The condition occurs in approximately 1:691 births.[11] The incidence of Down syndrome is greater when the maternal parent is of advanced age; however, recent studies have found advanced paternal age is also a contributing factor.[12] Down syndrome can be diagnosed prenatally via blood and fetal cell sampling or morphologically after birth.[13] Although a high percentage of patients with Down syndrome die within the first year of life, recent health care advancements have increased the median life expectancy to approximately 49 years.[13]

Presentation

Children with Down syndrome often display delayed growth and development. The degree of retardation may range from mild to severe. Facial features characteristic of Down syndrome include a flat facial profile or abnormal head shape, a flattened nasal bridge, a protruding tongue, inner epicanthal folds, and slanted palpebral fissures. Other physical manifestations may include short broad hands with a single palmar crease, short broad fingers, and hypotonia. Down syndrome infants may also have small ears, a short neck, tiny white spots on the iris, and unstable joints.[6]

Those affected are more likely to have epilepsy, congenital heart disease, endocrine abnormalities, esophageal and duodenal atresia, and hearing and vision impairment. Children with Down syndrome are also at increased risk of leukemia and early dementia.[13,14]

XXY Syndrome (Klinefelter's Syndrome)

Overview

Klinefelter's syndrome, the most common sex-linked chromosomal abnormality in males, is characterized by an extra X chromosome.[15] Although the mortality rate of those with Klinefelter's syndrome is over half, those that do survive do not have a significantly increased rate of mortality compared to healthy individuals.[16]

Presentation

Patients are typically born with no apparent abnormalities. The condition is often diagnosed later in life when the patient experiences infertility.[3] Klinefelter's syndrome is the most common cause of hypogonadism, gynecomastia, and infertility in men.[17]

Phenotypic manifestations of Klinefelter's syndrome include osteoporosis, subnormal libido, and reduction in gross and fine motor skills. Individuals may also have behavioral or mental health problems, poor muscle tone, tremors, and an increased incidence of vascular, endocrine, and autoimmune diseases.[16]

XO Karyotype (Turner's Syndrome)

Overview

Turner's syndrome, or XO karyotype, is the most common sex-chromosome anomaly in females. This syndrome occurs in about 1 in every 2,000 live births. Fetuses with the XO karyotype account for about 10% of all miscarriages.[1,18] Approximately 95% of all embryos affected by Turner's syndrome do not survive to term.[1,19] Although there is limited conclusive data, it is suggested that the life expectancy of an individual is shortened by about ten years.[18]

Presentation

Although karyotype testing may diagnose the condition in early childhood, Turner's syndrome is usually diagnosed around puberty when there is a lack of common signs of sexual maturation.[18] A patient with Turner's syndrome may present with a webbed neck, low hairline, scoliosis, and a "shield"-shaped chest with widely spaced nipples. Other presentations may include learning disabilities, lack of secondary sexual characteristics, and strabismus. Congenital heart disease and urinary tract anomalies are also prevalent concerns in patients with Turner's syndrome.[20,18]

Marfan Syndrome

Overview

Marfan syndrome is an inherited connective tissue disorder in which there is a mutation on the gene that produces the protein fibrillin-1. This results in an increase of the transforming growth factor beta protein, which subsequently causes complications within the connective tissue.[21] These complications affect the skeletal, cardiac, and ophthalmic body systems.[22] Due to these complications, most commonly cardiovascular, Marfan syndrome results in a slightly lower life expectancy than that of a person without Marfan syndrome.[22] Marfan syndrome occurs in approximately 1:5,000 births.[21]

Presentation

The phenotypic presentation of Marfan syndrome may include tall stature, long and thin extremities and fingers, pectus carinatum or excavatum, hyperextension of joints, genu recurvatum, and kyphoscoliosis. Manifestations specific to the head may include a long narrow face and a high-arched, narrow palate.[21] Pediatric patients with Marfan's syndrome may also exhibit cardiovascular issues, such as aortic regurgitation and mitral valve prolapse.[23] Ophthalmic complications may include ectopia lentis and iridodonesis.[21,24,25] The most severe complications may include aortic dissection resulting in sudden death, as well as blindness from lens complications.[21]

Tay-Sachs Disease

Overview

Tay-Sachs disease is a condition occurring from the absence of the enzyme hexosaminidase-A.[26] The disease is mostly found in the Ashkenazic Jewish population and occurs in approximately 1:2,500 live births.[27] Approximately 1 in every 27 Ashkenazic Jews in the United States is a carrier. Other populations that have an increased incidence of the condition include French Canadians and Louisiana Cajuns.[26] Patients with Tay-Sachs disease present normally at birth, but they begin to deteriorate typically between 3 and 6 months of age.[26]

Presentation

Around three to six months of age, those with Tay-Sachs begin to regress while fatty enzymes begin to build up in the brain.[26] Patients may experience decreased muscle tone, listlessness, blindness, deafness, seizures, and dementia. Regression to a vegetative state typically occurs, with death usually occurring around the age of 5.[26]

DiGeorge (Velocardiofacial) Syndrome

Overview

DiGeorge (velocardiofacial) syndrome is a congenital defect involving the parathyroid glands, thymus, and the conotruncal region of the heart[28] that affects 1 out of every 2,000–4,000 individuals in the United States.[29] Although infants with DiGeorge syndrome have an increased risk of mortality, those that live past infancy may live a similar lifespan to that of an individual without DiGeorge syndrome.[29]

Presentation

DiGeorge syndrome often presents with phenotypic manifestations, such as increased susceptibility to infection due to thymic aplasia. Abnormal facies are common as well, such as lateral displacement of inner canthi, short palpebral fissures, short philtrum, micrognathia, and ear anomalies.[29] Pediatric patients with DiGeorge syndrome are often born with congenital heart defects, such as aortic arch anomalies, resulting in significant neonatal morbidity and mortality.[30] DiGeorge syndrome may cause cognitive and behavioral psychiatric problems, such as attention-deficit/hyperactivity disorder or anxiety.[29] Additionally, pediatric patients may be afflicted with hypoparathyroidism and hypocalcaemia, which can cause seizures in infancy.[31,32]

References

1. Barkley TW Jr. Genetic evaluations. In: Barkley TW Jr, ed. *Pediatric Primary Care Nurse Practitioner Certification Review.* West Hollywood, CA: Barkley and Associates; 2015: 24–28.

2. Centers for Disease Control and Prevention, National Center on Birth Defects and Developmental Disabilities. Birth defects: Data and Statistics. http://www.cdc.gov/ncbddd/birthdefects/data.html. Last updated October 20, 2014. Accessed April 3, 2015.

3. Centers for Disease Control and Prevention, National Center on Birth Defects and Developmental Disabilities. Family health history and genetics: Genetics basics. http://www.cdc.gov/ncbddd/genetics/basics.html. Last updated March 3, 2015. Accessed April 3, 2015.

4. Genetic Alliance & The New York-Mid-Atlantic Consortium for Genetic and Newborn Screening Services. Indications for a genetic referral. In *Understanding Genetics: A New York, Mid-Atlantic Guide for Patients and Health Professionals.* Washington, DC: Genetic Alliance; 2009: 29–32. http://www.ncbi.nlm.nih.gov/books/NBK115554/

5. Fretts RC. Stillbirth: diagnosis and management. In: Basow DS, ed. *UpToDate*. Waltham, MA: UpToDate; 2015. http://www.uptodate.com/contents/diagnosis-and-management-of-stillbirth. Last updated June 13, 2014. Accessed April 3, 2015.

6. Centers for Disease Control and Prevention, National Center on Birth Defects and Developmental Disabilities. Family health history and genetics: Genetic counseling. http://www.cdc.gov/ncbddd/genetics/genetic_counseling.html. Last updated March 3, 2015. Accessed April 3, 2015.

7. Interpreting family history. National Coalition for Health Professional Education in Genetics Web site. http://www.nchpeg.org/index.php?option=com_content&view=article&id=170&Itemid=64. Accessed April 3, 2015.

8. Wiener DL. Inborn errors of metabolism. In: Kemp S, ed. Medscape. http://emedicine.medscape.com/article/804757-overview. Updated February 18, 2015. Accessed April 3, 2015.

9. U.S. Department of Health and Human Services, Health Resources, and Services Administration, Discretionary Advisory Committee on Heritable Disorders in Newborns and Children. Newborn screening: Towards a uniform screening panel and system. http://www.hrsa.gov/advisorycommittees/mchbadvisory/heritabledisorders. Chartered April 24, 2013. Accessed April 3, 2015.

10. U.S. Department of Health and Human Services, National Institutes of Health (NIH), U.S. National Library of Medicine, Lester Hill National Center for Biomedical Communications. Handbook: Help me understand genetics. http://ghr.nlm.nih.gov/handbook.pdf. Published March 30, 2015. Accessed April 3, 2015.

11. Down syndrome facts. National Down Syndrome Society Web site. http://www.ndss.org/Down-Syndrome/Down-Syndrome-Facts. Accessed April 3, 2015.

12. Centers for Disease Control and Prevention, National Center on Birth Defects and Developmental Disabilities. Facts about Down syndrome. http://www.cdc.gov/ncbddd/birthdefects/DownSyndrome.html. Last updated October 20, 2014. Accessed April 3, 2015.

13. Chen H, Down syndrome. In: Descartes M, ed. Medscape. http://emedicine.medscape.com/article/943216-overview#showall. Updated August 18, 2014. Accessed April 3, 2015.

14. U.S. Department of Health and Human Services, NIH, Eunice Kennedy Shriver National Institute of Child Health and Human Development. What conditions or disorders are commonly associated with Down syndrome? http://www.nichd.nih.gov/health/topics/down/conditioninfo/Pages/associated.aspx. Last updated April 9, 2014. Accessed April 3, 2015.

15. Frühmesser A, Kotzot D. Chromosomal variants in Klinefelter syndrome. *Sex Dev.* 2011; 5(3): 109–123. doi: 10.1159/000327324

16. Chen H. Klinefelter syndrome clinical presentation. In: Rohena LO, ed. Medscape. http://emedicine.medscape.com/article/945649-clinical#showall. Updated August 20, 2014. Accessed April 3, 2015.

17. Larner AJ. *Neuropsychological Neurology: The Neurocognitive Impairments of Neurological Disorders.* 2nd ed. Cambridge, UK: Cambridge University Press; 2013: 110–144.

18. Overview. Turner Syndrome Society of the United States Web site. http://www.turnersyndrome.org/#!overview/ctzx. Accessed April 3, 2015.

19. Davenport ML, Ross J, Backeljauw PF. Turner syndrome. In: Radovick S, MacGillivray MH, eds. *Pediatric Endocrinology: A Practical Clinical Guide.* 2nd ed. Heldelberg, Germany. Springer; 2013; 109–136.

20. U.S. Department of Health and Human Services, NIH, U. S. National Library of Medicine, Lester Hill National Center for Biomedical Communications. Genetics home reference: Conditions: Turner syndrome. http://ghr.nlm.nih.gov/condition/turner-syndrome. Reviewed January 2012. Published March 30, 2015. Accessed April 3, 2015.

21. What is Marfan syndrome? The Marfan Foundation Web site. http://www.marfan.org/about/Marfan. Accessed April 3, 2015.

22. U.S. Department of Health and Human Services, NIH, National Heart, Lung, and Blood Institute (NHLBI). What is Marfan syndrome? http://www.nhlbi.nih.gov/health/health-topics/topics/mar. Updated October 1, 2010. Accessed April 3, 2015.

23. U.S. Department of Health and Human Services, NIH, NHLBI. What are the signs and symptoms of Marfan syndrome? http://www.nhlbi.nih.gov/health/health-topics/topics/mar/signs.html. Updated October 1, 2010. Accessed April 3, 2015.

24. Eifrig CW. Ectopic lentis clinical presentation. In: Roy H Sr, ed. Medscape. http://emedicine.medscape.com/article/1211159-clinical. Updated March 10, 2015. Accessed April 3, 2015.

25. Hoang QV, Leong JA, Gallego-Pinazo R. Myopia: Ocular and systemic disease. In: Spaide RF, Ohno-Matsui K, Yannuzzi LA. *Pathologic Myopia.* New York, NY: Springer; 2014: 333–344.

26. U.S. Department of Health and Human Services, NIH, National Human Genome Research Institute. Learning about Tay-Sachs disease. http://www.genome.gov/10001220. Last reviewed March 17, 2011. Accessed April 3, 2015.

27. Tegay DH. GM2 gangliosidoses: Introduction and epidemiology. In: Rohena LO, ed. Medscape. http://emedicine.medscape.com/article/951943-overview. Updated December 11, 2014. Accessed April 3, 2015.

28. Horenstein MS, Ardinger R Jr, Ardinger H. Velocardiofacial syndrome. In: Weber HS, ed. Medscape. http://emedicine.medscape.com/article/892655-overview. Updated February 13, 2014. Accessed April 3, 2015.

29. Bawle EV. DiGeorge Syndrome. In: Jyonouchi H, ed. Medscape. http://emedicine.medscape.com/article/886526-overview. Updated March 12, 2014. Accessed April 3, 2015.

30. Chin AJ. Interrupted aortic arch. In: Neish SR, ed. Medscape. http://emedicine.medscape.com/article/896979-overview#showall. Updated August 29, 2013. Accessed April 3, 2015.

31. Immune Deficiency Foundation. DiGeorge syndrome. In: Blaese RM, Stiehm ER, Bonilla FA, Younger ME, eds. *Patient and Family Handbook for Primary Immunodeficiency Diseases.* 5th ed. Towson, MD: Immune Deficiency Foundation; 2013: 72–76. http://primaryimmune.org/idf-publications/patient-family-handbook/

32. Pitukcheewanont P. Pediatric hypoparathyroidism. In: Kemp S, ed. Medscape. http://emedicine.medscape.com/article/922204-overview#showall. Updated March 6, 2014. Accessed April 3, 2015.

Chapter 4
Prenatal Assessment/ Screening

QUESTIONS

1. You are examining a newborn in the nursery. As part of your examination, you stimulate the Moro reflex. How would you do this, and what reaction would you look for in the patient?

   a. Turn his head to one side and watch for contralateral upper extremity to extend.

   b. Release your support of the newborn's head to observe nervous system response.

   c. Stroke the infant's lower foot to observe an upward curling of his big toe.

   d. Hold the baby aloft to see if he extends his arms towards the ground.

2. During a physical examination, a newborn is found to have length, width, and head circumference all at less than the 10th percentile for her age. All of the following factors are likely be considered as potential sources for her condition except:

   a. Residing at high altitudes

   b. Bacterial intrauterine infection

   c. Inborn errors of metabolism

   d. Congenital or chromosomal abnormalities

3. Which of the following skin variations that occurs in newborns would be of most concern?

   a. Milia

   b. Hemangioma

   c. Erythema toxicum

   d. Port wine stain

4. While examining a newborn infant, which of the following would be most indicative of a neuromuscular problem?

   a. Arms and legs flexed over abdomen

   b. Inability to track with eyes

   c. No response to clapping of hands

   d. Three café au lait spots on back

5. In the correct method for assessing an infant for developmental hip dysplasia, the nurse practitioner would have the baby on his back with knees flexed and:

   a. Abduct knees, listening for click as femoral head slips into acetabulum

   b. Adduct knees, listening for click as femoral head slips into acetabulum

   c. Abduct knees, feeling femoral head enter acetabulum

   d. Adduct knees, feeling femoral head slip into acetabulum

6. Which of these abdominal findings would be of most concern in newborns?

   a. Umbilical hernia

   b. Diastasis recti

   c. Flat abdomen

   d. Abdomen rising with inspiration, falling with expiration

7. Which of the following findings in a newborn would be <u>least</u> likely to indicate an abnormality?

    a. Heart murmurs

    b. White forelocks

    c. Wide fontanels

    d. Four junctional nevi clustered on trunk

8. You are examining the newborn child of a recovering alcoholic. During the interview, she mentions she was still drinking early into her pregnancy and did not know she was pregnant for some time. You examine the newborn's mouth. Which of the following findings would most strongly indicate fetal alcohol syndrome?

    a. Shrunken, contracted mouth

    b. Enlarged tongue

    c. Triangular upper lip

    d. Whitish-yellow cysts on gums

9. You are performing an eye exam on a newborn child. When you perform the red reflex test, a black spot presents instead. Which of these conditions would this finding typically indicate?

    a. Optic nerve hypoplasia

    b. Retinoblastoma

    c. Heterochromia

    d. Absence of a clear retinal pathway

10. According to the normal stage of primitive reflex development, which of the following reflexes is expected to <u>not</u> disappear by about 12 months of age?

    a. The head turning towards anything that strokes the cheek or mouth

    b. The arms spreading or contracting in response to loss of balance

    c. Sucking in response to objects touching the roof of the mouth

    d. Toes fanning out in response to stroking of the sole

RATIONALES

1. b

The Moro reflex is best tested by releasing the newborn's head in order to observe the nervous system's response to surprise; most infants will respond by abducting or adducting their arms in an attempt to regain balance. An impaired or absent response may indicate motor or neurologic disorders. Turning the head to one side with ipsilateral arm extension is the fencing reflex. Stroking the infant's lower foot tests the Babinski reflex, which, barring pathology, commonly vanishes by 2 years of age. Holding the infant aloft and rotating him or her forward to test the response to a simulated fall is part of the parachute test and should not typically stimulate the startle reflex.

2. a

Symmetric intrauterine growth retardation (IUGR) presents with length, weight, and head circumference at less than the 10th percentile; residing at high altitudes is more likely to produce asymmetric IUGR, due to decreased oxygen available to the fetus, than symmetric IUGR. Bacterial intrauterine infection, inborn errors of metabolism, and congenital or chromosomal abnormalities are known factors that may contribute to symmetric IUGR.

3. d

Port wine stains are vascular birthmarks consisting of superficial and deep dilated capillaries that cause permanent reddish to purplish discoloration of the skin and may signify neurologic concerns. Milia are pinpoint white papules on the face that spontaneously disappear within 3–4 weeks of life. A hemangioma is characterized by raised, soft, red lumps on the skin and is not usually a concern. Erythema toxicum is a benign newborn rash.

4. c

A newborn should respond to a loud sound with a startle; failure to elicit this response could indicate hearing damage or other neuromuscular challenges. The normal posture of a newborn is flexion of extremities over trunk. Newborns may look at an object or face, but are not commonly expected to track. Café au lait spots are often counted and measured, and could be indicative of a problem if larger than 5 or 6 mm in size.

5. a

Ortolani's click, commonly used to assess for developmental hip dysplasia, is performed by abducting the knees, then listening and feeling for the femoral head to re-enter the acetabulum. Barlow's maneuver, which also assesses for developmental hip dysplasia, is done by adducting the knees and feeling the femoral head pop out of, not into, the acetabulum.

6. c

A flat contour to the abdomen is abnormal in infants and may indicate malnutrition or intrauterine growth retardation. Reduction in nutrients to the fetus can cause a decrease in intra-abdominal fat. This can be caused by poor blood flow, decreased transplacental concentration of amino acids, or impairment of the ability of the placenta to transfer nutrients. Slight distension is normal and the nurse practitioner should see a slight protuberance in a healthy infant. A rounded, symmetrical contour to the abdomen that rises with inspiration is normal in infants; an asymmetrical abdomen may indicate an abdominal mass. An umbilical hernia may present in the infant, but this condition is fairly harmless and often resolves itself by 1 year of age. Likewise, diastasis recti may present in newborns, but this condition typically resolves.

7. a

Heart murmurs may present in 85%–90% of all newborns; despite this high percentage, structural heart disease typically only presents in 8–10 live births out of 1000. White forelocks may indicate Waardenburg syndrome, whereas wide fontanels may indicate hydrocephalus, Down syndrome, or hypothyroidism. Although junctional nevi may be present in newborns, groupings of the spots may signal a precursor tuberous sclerosis or generalized neurofibromatosis.

8. c

A triangular upper lip with fish-like mouth, or the fish mouth deformity, is commonly observed in neonates and pediatric patients born with fetal alcohol syndrome. Microstomia, on the other hand, presents as a shrunken, contracted mouth and is usually observed in trisomy 18 and trisomy 21. Macroglossia, or enlarged tongue, may be due to hypothyroidism or mucopolysaccharidoses. Epstein pearls present as whitish-yellow cysts on the gums and roof of the mouth; these pearls are common in newborns and are not considered an abnormal sign because they typically disappear within 1–2 weeks of birth.

9. d

The red reflex replaced by a black spot commonly indicates that there is no clear pathway from the lens to the retina and is a crucial finding for congenital cataracts, corneal scar, or ocular hemorrhage. Optic nerve hypoplasia, on the other hand, is a midline defect of the central nervous system and may present with colobomas. Heterochromia simply refers to a difference in coloration of the iris and usually does not indicate an underlying condition. Further, retinoblastoma and congenital cataracts may be indicated by the red reflex being replaced by a whitish color, not a black spot.

10. d

The Babinski reflex, or fanning of the toes upon stroking of the sole, is expected to disappear after 12 months or when the infant starts walking, but may last for up to 2 years; if it persists past this point, it may indicate a nervous system disorder. The turning of the head towards anything that strokes the cheek is a sign of the rooting reflex, whereas sucking on anything that touches the roof of the mouth demonstrates the sucking reflex; both these reflexes are expected to disappear at 3–4 months of age. The Moro reflex, indicated by stretching or contracting the arms upon perceiving a loss of balance, is also expected to disappear during this window.

DISCUSSION

The Newborn Assessment: History

Prenatal History

A newborn assessment should begin with a prenatal history. The prenatal history should consist of a review of the pregnancy, past pregnancies, and mother's and father's medical and genetic histories.[1] When reviewing the pregnancy, the nurse practitioner (NP) should determine if the mother used any foreign substances.[2,3] Any health problems the mother experienced during pregnancy (e.g., placenta previa, abruptio placentae, gestational diabetes, hypertension) should also be documented. The NP should review the results of any prenatal screening tests performed and determine if there are any abnormal findings that warrant further evaluation.

A review of past pregnancies should include a history of congenital anomalies, still births, and genetic conditions. When reviewing the mother's medical and genetic history, maternal illnesses prior to and during pregnancy should be discussed.[4] Any maternal medications should also be discussed, and medications should be reviewed for intrauterine effects or the potential for excretion in breast milk.[1] The father's medical and genetic history should also be included in the prenatal history.

Perinatal History

The perinatal history should include a record of events surrounding labor, the newborn's weight and length, and the Apgar score. A review of the events of labor should include the duration of labor, the duration of rupture of membranes, and the use of analgesia or anesthesia.[1] The type of delivery and whether the labor was spontaneous or induced should also be included in the report. Any complications (e.g., prolonged labor, meconium staining or aspiration, or use of forceps or vacuum) should be noted.[3] Resuscitative measures used on the newborn should be included in the history as well.

Apgar scores, which assess the clinical status of infants immediately after delivery, should be recorded at 1 minute and 5 minutes after birth. The Apgar score contains five areas of assessment for a total of 10 points, as displayed in table 4.1.

Each component of the test receives a score of 0, 1, or 2. If the newborn scores below 7 at 5 minutes, the test should be repeated every 5 minutes for 20 minutes or until the newborn scores above 7 in two consecutive tests.[3,5,6]

The birth weight and length of the newborn should also be recorded. Low birth weight (LBW) is characterized as less than 2,500 grams, very low birth weight (VLBW) is less than 1,500 grams, and extremely low birth weight (ELBW) is less than 1,000 grams.[7,8,5]

Postnatal History

The NP should review any maternal problems, such as bleeding, anesthesia reactions, breastfeeding complications, and depression.[3,9] The NP should also review any infant problems, such as ABO/Rh blood type incompatibilities, hyperbilirubinemia, hip dysplasia, murmurs, or talipes equinovarus congenita (i.e., club feet).[10,11,12,13]

The Newborn Assessment: Physical Examination

Measurements

The newborn's weight, length, and head circumference should be plotted on standard growth curves. The average length of a newborn is 51 cm, the average weight is 3.6 kg for males and 3.5 kg for females, and the average head circumference is 35 cm.[1] The newborn's length should be measured by using a measurement board or standard tape measure and measuring from the crown to the heel. Newborns should be unclothed and quiet while being weighed to ensure an accurate reading.[6]

Gestational Age

Gestational age is frequently assessed using the New Ballard Score. The New Ballard Score can estimate the gestational age of full term and extremely premature newborns alike, but the score tends to overestimate the gestational age of extremely premature newborns. To increase accuracy, the assessment should be conducted within 12 hours of birth.[6]

The New Ballard Score maturational assessment consists of six neuromuscular and six physical characteristics.[14] The six portions of the neuromuscular section are posture, square window, arm recoil, popliteal angle, scarf sign, and heel–to-ear. The NP should assess the newborn's posture at rest, noting the position of arms and legs. Square window refers to the newborn's wrist flexibility. The NP should estimate the angle measurement between the palm of the newborn's hand and forearm. Arm recoil is the measurement of the angle of recoil following brief extension of the upper extremity. The popliteal angle assesses the maturation of the passive flexor tone around the knee point. The scarf sign tests the passive tone of flexors around the shoulder girdle. The heel to ear maneuver tests for passive flexion or resistance to extension of posterior hip flexor muscles.[15]

Table 4.1	APGAR Sign		
	2	1	0
Appearance (skin coloration)	Pink color all over (hands and feet are pink)	Pink color (but hands and feet are bluish)	Bluish-gray or pale all over
Pulse	Normal (above 100 beats per minute)	Below 100 beats per minute	Absent (no pulse)
Grimace (responsiveness or "reflex irritability")	Pulls away, sneezes, or coughs with stimulation	Facial movement only (grimace) with stimulation	Absent (no response to stimulation)
Activity (muscle tone)	Active, spontaneous movement	Arms and legs flexed with little movement	No movement, "floppy" tone
Respirations	Normal rate and effort (30–60 breaths per minute), good cry	Slow or irregular breathing, weak cry	Absent (no breathing)

Used with permission from Barkley TW Jr. Prenatal/newborn assessment and newborn screening. In: Barkley TW Jr, ed. *Pediatric Primary Care Nurse Practitioner Certification Review/Clinical Update Continuing Education Course.* West Hollywood, CA: Barkley and Associates; 2015: 30.

The six portions of the physical section are skin, lanugo, plantar surface, breast, ear, and genitals. The maturation level of fetal skin, the amount of lanugo covering the body, and the amount of major foot creases are noted. Palpating the breast tissue beneath the skin and holding it between the thumb and forefinger helps to estimate the amount of tissue. The ear examination consists of assessing the cartilage thickness and folding forward the pinna. If the pinna does not recoil, the eyelid development should be assessed. In males, the descent of testes and amount of rugae is assessed. In females, the prominence of clitoris and labia minora is noted.[15]

Each of the 12 sections is scored based on the degree of development. Gestational age is determined based upon the sum of these scores. Low scores indicate immaturity, whereas high scores indicate a mature or post-mature infant.[3,14]

Newborns born at 37–41 weeks gestation are considered at term and have the best health outcomes. Newborns born prior to 37 weeks gestation are premature, and newborns born after 42 weeks are post-term.[16,17,18]

Newborns whose weight is within the 10th and 90th percentiles for their gestational age are considered appropriate for gestational age (AGA).[19] Infants large for gestational age (LGA) are born with a weight above the 90th percentile for gestational age.[20,21] Genetic risk factors for LGA include genetic syndromes (e.g., Beckwith-Wiedemann syndrome, Simpson-Golabi-Behmel syndrome) and race and ethnicity (e.g., Caucasian, American Indian, Samoan). Maternal risk factors include maternal diabetes and maternal obesity.[22]

Infants small for gestational age (SGA) are born with a weight below the 10th percentile for their gestational age.[20,21] Some SGA infants may also have experienced intrauterine growth restriction (IUGR), which is diminished growth velocity in the fetus. IUGR can be caused by maternal, placental, or neonatal factors. Maternal factors include severe maternal starvation, medical disorders, substance abuse, and intrauterine infection.[22,23] Placental factors include placental injuries and structural anomalies.[22] Neonatal factors include inborn errors of metabolism, genetic syndromes, and karyotypic abnormalities.[3,22]

Fifty-five percent of all SGA newborns have asymmetric IUGR. Asymmetric IUGR newborns typically have a head circumference and length within normal limits and weight below the 10th percentile.[22,24,25,26] Asymmetric IUGR is often caused by a reduction in fetal nutrients.[22] Other causes include chronic hypertension, pre-eclampsia, renal or cyanotic heart disease, hemoglobinopathies, abruptio placentae, multiple gestation, or high altitude.[3] Symmetric IUGR is characterized by a reduction in both body and head growth. Symmetric IUGR is usually caused by intrinsic factors, such as congenital infections or chromosomal abnormalities.[6]

Vital Signs

Vital signs should be recorded every 30–60 minutes during the first 4–6 hours, and then every 8–12 hours. A normal temperature ranges from 36.1– 37 °C (97–98.6 °F). A normal respiratory rate falls between 30 and 60 breaths per minute. The newborn's heart rate should be between 120 and 160 beats per minute (bpm).[1,27,28] Newborns suspected of cardiovascular or renal abnormalities should also have their blood pressure monitored. A reading less than 112/74 mmHg is normal.[3]

Skin

Within 2–3 days, a newborn's skin usually becomes dry and flaky. The skin turns red when the newborn cries. When cold, the extremities typically turn bluish with a mottled tint.[29]

Skin abnormalities that may indicate an underlying disorder include abnormal pigmentation, macular stains, and hemangiomas.[1] Congenital nevi often begin as flat, evenly pigmented patches but later may become uneven and speckled. There is a small risk that congenital nevi will develop into melanoma.[30] Macular stains are blanchable, pink-red patches. Macular stains may be associated with extracutaneous disorders, such as spinal dysraphism or Beckwith-Wiedemann syndrome.[31] Hemangiomas (i.e., strawberry marks) are vascular neoplasms that typically present as red or crimson macules. Although most hemangiomas are benign and disappear by age 5, some, depending on placement, may interfere with vital functions. Large cutaneous or visceral hemangiomas, in particular, may result in high-output cardiac failure and structural abnormalities.[32]

Some common, benign skin findings in newborns are milia, erythema toxicum, Mongolian spots, and miliaria. Milia (i.e., milk spots) are white papules frequently found on the nose and cheeks. Milia tend to disappear within 3–4 weeks.[1,29,33] Erythema toxicum are white papules on an erythematous base commonly found on the face and trunk. Erythema toxicum usually resolves within 2 weeks.[1,29,33] Mongolian spots, more common in African-American and Asian newborns, are blue-black macules with indefinite borders. Mongolian spots are usually located on the buttocks and gradually disappear within the first year of life.[1,6] Miliaria are thin-walled vesicles with a nonerythematous and nonpigmented base caused by blockage of sweat glands. The rash usually resolves when the newborn is removed from the warm, humid environment.[6]

Port wine stains and café au lait spots are usually benign. Port wine stains are low flow capillary malformations. Port wine stains are initially pink in color with sharply delineated borders. Over time, the pink color progresses to dark red or purple. Port wine stains may sometimes be associated with structural anomalies (e.g., Sturge-Weber

Table 4.2	Primitive Reflexes in Newborn Neurological Development	
Reflex	**Appears**	**Disappears**
Rooting	Newborn	3–4 months
Sucking	Newborn	3–4 months
Moro	Newborn	3–4 months
Grasp (palmar, plantar)	Newborn	3–6 months; 4 months
Pacing/stepping	Newborn	1–2 months
Tonic neck	Newborn	3 months
Babinski	Newborn	12 months or when walking

Used with permission from Barkley TW Jr. Prenatal/newborn assessment and newborn screening. In: Barkley TW Jr, ed. *Pediatric Primary Care Nurse Practitioner Certification Review/Clinical Update Continuing Education Course*. West Hollywood, CA: Barkley and Associates; 2015: 32.

syndrome).[1,6,31] Café au lait spots are light brown macules with well-defined borders. Six or more café au lait spots may indicate neurofibromatosis.[6]

Neurological Exam

A neurological exam consists of a general assessment and an assessment of motor function, cranial nerves, reflexes, senses, and behavior. A general assessment examines the newborn's vital signs, levels of alertness, and skin, head, and spine. A neurological exam is best conducted when the newborn is quiet and awake because portions of the exam, such as motor function, are difficult to assess when the newborn is asleep. Altered levels of alertness (e.g., mild stupor, moderate stupor, deep stupor, coma) are seen in infants with cortical dysfunction.[34]

In a healthy newborn, muscle function should be symmetric, smooth, and spontaneous. Sustained tremulousness beyond the fourth day may indicate cortical dysfunction.[34] When at rest, a term newborn should present with hips abducted and partially flexed with knees flexed, arms abducted, elbows flexed, and fists clenched.[35]

All 12 cranial nerves can be assessed, but the olfactory nerve very rarely needs to be assessed in newborns. The optic nerve is assessed by examining the fundi. A term infant should be able to turn toward soft lights. The oculomotor, trochlear, and abducens nerves can be assessed by observing spontaneous eye movements. To assess the trigeminal nerve, observe the newborn's response to tactile stimuli. The facial nerve can be assessed by noting whether the newborn closes both eyelids during vigorous crying. The vestibulo cochlear nerve can be assessed by examining the newborn for a startle or blink response to sudden loud noises. When the glossopharyngeal or vagus nerves are impaired, the newborn will have difficulty swallowing. Impairment of the hypoglossal nerve is indicated by the tongue resting to one side.[34,35]

The reflex portion of the exam should include an assessment of superficial and developmental reflexes. The abdominal reflex can be assessed by gently stroking each of the four quadrants in an axial to peripheral direction. This should result in contraction of the abdominal wall.[34] The anal wink reflex can be exhibited by gently stroking the perianal region. The perianal muscle should contract. The lack of a contraction may indicate a spinal cord lesion.[34] Developmental (i.e., primitive) reflexes are generally present at birth and resolve with maturation. The developmental reflexes are presented in the chart below.[35,36]

The sensory examination is rarely performed because it is challenging to determine an infant's response to sensory stimuli. The rooting reflex, however, can be used to detect perioral tactile sensation.[34,35]

Two key elements of the behavioral evaluation are consolability and habituation. Healthy newborns can be consoled within about fifteen seconds. Infants with brain injury typically are more difficult to console. Habituation measures the newborn's ability to diminish response to repetitive stimuli. A lack of habituation is associated with cortical dysfunction and prenatal substance abuse exposure.[34]

Head/Neck

An inspection of the newborn's head should include an examination of size, shape, and symmetry.[1,6] Bony abnormalities, such as frontal bossing, should be noted and may indicate a hormonal or skeletal disorder.[37,38] Microcephaly, a head circumference smaller than two standard deviations, and macrocephaly, a head circumference larger than two standard deviations, may be detected at the newborn screening but would require further examination over the coming weeks.[3,39,40,41]

The newborn's hair should be uniform in color and distribution.[1] White forelocks may indicate deafness.[1,42,43] Multiple hair whorls may indicate Down syndrome. The scalp should also be examined for defects, unusual lesions, or protuberances.

The head should be palpated to detect

fontanelles, which should be flat and soft.[6] In normal newborns, the anterior fontanelle is diamond shaped and persists until about 18 months. The posterior fontanelle is triangle-shaped, and closes by 2–3 months. The posterior fontanelle is not always palpable at birth, however. Tense or bulging fontanelles may indicate intracranial pressure. Sunken fontanelles may indicate dehydration. Fontanelles that are smaller than expected are a potential indicator for premature fusion of skull bones and should be investigated. Wide fontanelles may indicate underlying conditions, such as IUGR, hydrocephalus, Down syndrome, or hypothyroidism.[44,45] Sutures should also be palpated. An asymmetric skull after birth is normal, but may indicate craniosynostosis if it remains after 2 or 3 days.[1]

Caput succedaneum, edema that crosses the midline, should resolve within a few days.[1,46] Cephalohematoma, blood under the periosteum that does not cross the midline, requires closer examination, however.[1,47,48]

The face should be examined for shape, symmetry, and bruises or dysmorphic features.[1] Facial palsies, such as loss of nasolabial fold, partial closing of the eye, or the appearance of a "drooping" mouth, typically resolve within a few weeks.[34] Asymmetric crying facies are the congenital absence or hypoplasia of the depressor angularis muscle. Asymmetric crying facies are benign and become less noticeable as the child gets older. The condition may be associated with a cardiovascular anomaly.[34]

The position, spacing, and symmetry of the newborn's eyes should be noted.[1] Abnormally wide interpupillary distance may indicate trisomy 13 or Apert syndrome. Asymmetry due to epicanthal folds usually suggests a genetic syndrome, such as trisomy 21. Sclera should be white and clear.[1] Blue sclera may indicate osteogenesis imperfecta.[49] Pupils should be round and equal in diameter. The pupils should constrict in response to the light from an ophthalmoscope.[6] An infant may present with colobomas, which are an embryonic fissure defect. Mild forms of colobomas may only affect the iris.[50] In more severe cases, the choroid and optic nerve may be involved; these severe cases may also indicate central nervous system midline defects, such as optic nerve hypoplasia.[51] The newborn should have a normal red reflex.[52,53] Dark spots or a white reflex justify a referral to an ophthalmologist.[6]

The position of the ears should be similar bilaterally.[6] The size and appearance should also be inspected.[1] The ears should be examined for branchial cleft cysts, sinuses, and skin tags. Any external ear abnormalities increase the risk of abnormalities in the middle and inner ear.[1]

The shape and patency of the nose should be examined. The birth process may cause the nose to be abnormally shaped, but this should correct itself within a few days. The patency of each naris should be checked because newborns are predominantly nose breathers.[6]

The mouth should be symmetric and in proportion to the chin and tongue. Mucous membranes should be pink and moist. Oral secretions should be thin and clear. The NP should also check for any clefts.[1,6]

The newborn examination should reveal a relatively short neck that is symmetric with the head. The newborn should have full range of motion.[6] Any excess skin, such as webbing, may indicate a genetic disorder, such as Turner syndrome.[1] The NP should palpate the clavicle. Tenderness or swelling may indicate a fracture.[1]

Pulmonary/Chest

A full-term newborn's chest circumference should be about two centimeters smaller than the head circumference.[6] A small or malformed thorax may indicate pulmonary hypoplasia or a neuromuscular disorder. The newborn's chest should be symmetrical. An asymmetrical chest may be from an absent pectoralis muscle or abscess. Pectus excavatum (i.e., funnel chest) and pectus carinatum (i.e., pigeon breast) should also be noted.[1,54,55]

The newborn's breast size and nipples should be noted. The breast size can be used in determining the gestational age because a newborn's breast tissue may hypertrophy as a result of maternal hormones.[1,6] Supernumerary nipples are a common finding, especially among African-American newborns.[1,34] A newborn's breast may secrete a milky fluid (i.e., witch's milk) for several weeks, but this will resolve on its own.[6]

The majority of newborn lung examinations do not require the use of a stethoscope. At rest, the newborn should exhibit unlabored breathing without grunting, nasal flaring, or intercostal retractions. Auscultation may reveal rales or decreased breath sounds, which may indicate disease (e.g., pulmonary edema, neonatal pneumonia).[56]

Cardiovascular

A cardiovascular examination of a newborn includes an examination of rate, rhythm, quality of heart sounds, murmurs, and femoral pulses. In the first few days of life, the point of maximal impulse is located at the fourth intercostal space at or to the left of the midclavicular line. The NP should auscultate at the second and fourth intercostal spaces, cardiac apex, and axilla.[6] The normal heart rate for a newborn is 120–160 bpm but may dip to 85–90 bpm while the newborn is sleeping.[1,6]

Asymptomatic rhythms are relatively common in preterm infants. Sinus bradycardia and tachycardia are the two most common benign dysrhythmias. Premature atrial or ventricular contractions are also common. An electrocardiogram is needed to properly identify the condition.[6]

Heart sounds should be auscultated to evaluate

the quality. The split second heart sound, which should be expected, indicates the presence of two semilunar valves. Any gallops detected would require further evaluation. Ejection clicks, which also require further evaluation, may indicate pulmonary or aortic valve stenosis or a bicuspid aortic valve.[56]

About 85% of all newborns have murmurs.[57,58] Many cases of slight murmurs cease once the ductus arteriosus closes, but innocent murmurs may present in infants, children, and adolescents. However, murmurs still require examination to rule out the possibility of congenital heart defects (CHDs).[59] Pulse oximetry is often performed at birth to determine the possibility of CHD in the newborn.[60]

The femoral pulses should be palpated when the infant is quiet. Diminished femoral pulses may indicate coarctation of the aorta.[1] Blood pressure of the upper and lower extremities should be measured if there is still doubt about detecting the femoral pulses at the time of discharge.[34] Increased femoral pulses may occur with patent ductus arteriosus.[1]

Blood pressure should be assessed at birth as well. Hypotension should be recognized and treated in order to avoid complications such as intraventricular hemorrhage. Hypertension should also be noted and may indicate several abnormalities, but frequently presents with bronchopulmonary dysplasia.[61]

Abdomen

The NP should examine the newborn's abdomen while the newborn is quiet because it will make palpation easier. The abdomen should be slightly protuberant. Distention may indicate intestinal obstruction, organomegaly, or ascites.[1] Palpation should reveal a liver that is soft with a smooth edge.[1,6] The NP may also be able to locate the tip of the spleen.[6] The kidneys should be smooth and firm to the touch.[6] Enlarged kidneys may indicate hydronephrosis or cystic renal disease.[1] Any other masses that the NP detects would be considered abnormal.[1]

The umbilical cord should have two arteries and one vein. It should be bluish-white in color, shiny, and moist.[6] An erythema or odorous discharge may indicate omphalitis.[1] The average diameter of the umbilical cord in a normal term infant is 1.5 cm; poor nutritional status may result in a small cord.[1,62] Umbilical hernias may present in newborns and young children but are generally benign and resolve spontaneously.[34,63]

Genitourinary

The newborn should be inspected immediately after birth to identify the gender.[1] Female newborns should have their labia minora and labia majora examined.[56] A pre-term newborn will present with a prominent labia minora and clitoris.[1] A term newborn, however, will present with a prominent labia majora. The labia majora may be reddened and swollen.

Clear and white vaginal discharge, sometimes tinged with blood, may occur within the first few days.[56,64] The hymen should also be inspected. An imperforate hymen should prompt a referral to a pediatric gynecologist.[56]

The penis and scrotum should be examined in male newborns. The penis should be stretched to assess the length.[1] Phimosis is normal in newborns.[6] The degree of hypospadias, if apparent, should be noted. Circumcision should be postponed if hypospadias is present.[56] The scrotum should be palpated for testes. The testes should be firm, smooth, and comparatively equal in size.[6] Blue testes visible through the scrotal skin is a sign of torsion.[56] Undescended testes are not a cause for concern unless the testes have not descended by 6 months of age.[56]

In both males and females, the anus should be checked for patency, position, and size.[56]

Musculoskeletal

The spine should be examined for curvature, patency, and presence of structural abnormalities. The spine should be straight and flexible with no visible defects.[6] Both sides of the back should be symmetrical.[6] The NP should palpate along the spine to check for any abnormal growths. Soft tissue masses covered with normal skin may be lipomas or myelomeningocele.[1] Sacral dimpling is not a cause for concern unless the dimples are larger than 0.5 cm or located more than 2.5 cm from the anal verge.[56] If this is the case, the newborn should be screened for a neural tube defect.[1] The lower back should also be examined for tufts of hair or skin tags, which may indicate spina bifida.[65]

The hands and feet should be inspected for syndactyly and polydactyly.[1] Newborns should also be examined for palmar creases. A single palmar crease may suggest trisomy 21. Newborns with talipes equinovarus genita (i.e., clubfoot) require orthopedic intervention as soon as possible.[56] Limbs should be proportional and equal in length and exhibit full range of motion.[6]

Every newborn should be observed for developmental dysplasia of the hips (DDH).[56] The Barlow maneuver and Ortolani maneuver are two common maneuvers for assessing newborns for DDH. The Barlow maneuver causes posterior dislocation of an unstable hip.[12,43,56] The Ortolani maneuver makes a click sound with reduction of dislocation.[12,43,56] Newborns with suspected DDH should be referred to an orthopedic surgeon.[66]

The Newborn Assessment: Selected Screening Tests

Screening Principles

The goal of newborn screening is to detect life-threatening disorders while the disorders are asymptomatic.[67] Screening can detect inborn errors of metabolism, endocrine disorders, hemoglobinopathies, immunodeficiencies, cystic fibrosis, and CHDs. Not all diseases that can be screened will become part of a mass screening program. When determining which conditions to screen for, several principles are considered: if a lack of treatment for the disease can result in significant morbidity or death, if effective treatment is readily accessible, if early treatment leads to better outcomes, if the test has a low false-negative rate, and if the test is simple and inexpensive. Results should be received in a timely manner, and a definitive follow-up test should be available.[67,68]

Mandatory Screening Program

The Recommended Uniform Screening Panel created by the Secretary's Advisory Committee on Heritable Disorders in Newborns and Children includes 32 core conditions and 26 secondary conditions.[69] Each state has its own mandated screening program.[70] Some conditions that every state screens for are phenylketonuria (PKU), galactosemia, sickle cell disease, and congenital hypothyroidism.[3,60]

Considerations for Newborn Screening

Overview

Screening typically occurs while the newborn is still in the hospital. The blood spot specimen is collected as close to discharge as possible so abnormal compounds have time to accumulate. If the specimen is collected while the newborn is younger than 24 hours old, a repeat test should be conducted. If the test is positive, a confirmatory test should be performed as soon as possible. Hearing loss and critical CHD should also be screened for prior to discharge.[67]

Screened Considerations

A newborn's hearing can be screened by observing the infant's response to loud noises and voices, also known as the startle reflex. Hearing screening can also be conducted via the brain stem auditory evoked response test (BSAER). The BSAER measures the auditory brainstem response to click stimuli. Delayed or absent waves may indicate neurologic or cochlear deficit.[71] If hearing loss is indicated, treatment should begin by 6 months of age.

Critical CHDs can be screened through pulse oximetry screening, an effective, noninvasive, and inexpensive test. The seven critical CHDs are hypoplastic left heart syndrome, pulmonary atresia, tetralogy of Fallot, total anomalous pulmonary venous return, transposition of the great arteries, tricuspid atresia, and truncus arteriosus. Critical CHDs must be diagnosed and treated shortly after birth to prevent death or disability.[72]

Inborn errors of metabolism, such as PKU and galactosemia, are screened using dried blood

spots from a heel prick. PKU occurs in 1 out of every 10,000–25,000 infants and may produce developmental delay, seizures, aggression, autism, and hyperactivity. When galactosemia is present, liver dysfunction and coagulopathies will often manifest. Galactosemia occurs in 1 out of every 60,000–80,000 infants; 25% of all infants who carry the condition unrecognized run the risk of developing sepsis.[3]

Dried blood spots are also used to screen for hemoglobinopathies, including sickle cell disease and thalassemia. Certain hemoglobinopathies are more common in certain populations, with sickle cell disease occurring in 1 out of every 400 African-American infants. Hemoglobinopathies commonly result in anemia.[3]

Cystic fibrosis can also be screened using a dried blood spot. Most newborns who have a positive screen do not have cystic fibrosis, however. Therefore, a confirmatory sweat test is required.[3,73]

References

1. McKee-Garrett TM. Assessment of the newborn infant. In: Basow DS, ed. *UpToDate*. Waltham, MA: UpToDate; 2015. http://www.uptodate.com/contents/assessment-of-the-newborn-infant?source=search_result&search=assessment+of+the+newborn+infant&selectedTitle=1~150. Last updated February 19, 2015. Accessed May 6, 2015.

2. Prouillac C, Lecoeur S. The role of the placenta in fetal exposure to xenobiotics: importance of membrane transporters and human models for transfer studies. *Drug Metab Dispos*. 2010; 38(10): 1623–1635. doi: 10.1124/dmd.110.033571

3. Barkley TW Jr. Prenatal/newborn assessment and newborn screening. In: Barkley TW Jr, ed. *Pediatric Primary Care Nurse Practitioner Certification Review/ Clinical Update Continuing Education Course*. West Hollywood, CA: Barkley and Associates; 2015: 29–37.

4. Sackey JA. The preconception office visit. In: Basow DS, ed. *UpToDate*. Waltham, MA: UpToDate; 2015. http://www.uptodate.com/contents/the-preconception-office-visit. Last updated March 19, 2015. Accessed April 3, 2015.

5. Wheeler BJ. Health promotion of the newborn and family. In: Hockenberry MJ, Wilson D, eds. *Wong's Essentials of Pediatric Nursing*. 9th ed. St. Louis, MO: Elsevier Mosby; 2012: 185–227.

6. Cavaliere TA, Sansoucie DA. Assessment of the newborn and infant. In: Kenner C, Wright Lott J, eds. *Comprehensive Neonatal Nursing Care*. 5th ed. New York, NY: Springer Publishing Company; 2014: 71–112.

7. Ogawa M, Matsuda Y, Kanda E, et al. Survival rate of extremely low birth weight infants and its risk factors: Case-control study in Japan. *ISRN Obstet Gynecol*. 2013; 2013: 873563. doi: 10.1155/2013/873563.

8. Subramanian KNS, Seo SC, Barton AM, Montazami S. Extremely low birth weight infant. In: Rosenkrantz T, ed. Medscape. http://emedicine.medscape.com/article/979717-overview#showall. Updated December 17, 2014. Accessed April 3, 2015.

9. Pregnancy complications. Centers for Disease Control and Prevention Web site. http://www.cdc.gov/reproductivehealth/maternalinfanthealth/pregcomplications.htm. Last updated January 22, 2014. Accessed April 3, 2015.

10. Krauspe R, Weimann-Stahlschmidt K, Westhoff B. The current state of treatment for clubfoot in Europe. In: Bentley G, ed. *European Instructional Lectures, Vol. 11.* Copenhagen, Denmark: Springer; 2011: 47–66.

11. Wong RJ, Bhutani VK. Patient information: Jaundice in newborn infants (Beyond the Basics). In: Basow DS, ed. *UpToDate.* Waltham, MA: UpToDate; 2015. http://www.uptodate.com/contents/jaundice-in-newborn-infants-beyond-the-basics. Last updated February 28, 2014. Accessed April 3, 2015.

12. Infant and child hip dysplasia: Infant signs and symptoms. International Hip Dysplasia Institute Web site. http://hipdysplasia.org/developmental-dysplasia-of-the-hip/infant-signs-and-symptoms. Accessed April 3, 2015.

13. U.S. Department of Health and Human Services, National Institutes of Health (NIH), National Heart, Lung, and Blood Institute. How is a heart murmur diagnosed? http://www.nhlbi.nih.gov/health/health-topics/topics/heartmurmur/diagnosis.html. Updated September 20, 2012. Accessed April 3, 2015.

14. Smith VC. The high-risk newborn: Anticipation, evaluation, management, and outcome. In: Cloherty JP, Eichenwald EC, Hansen AR, Stark AR, eds. *Manual of Neonatal Care.* 7th ed. Philadelphia, PA: Lippincott, Williams, & Wilkins; 2012: 74–90.

15. New Ballard Score Maturational Assessment of Gestational Age. The New Ballard Score Web site. http://www.ballardscore.com/. Accessed May 6, 2015.

16. Lissauer T. Physical examination of the newborn. In: Martin RJ, Fanaroff AA, Walsh MC, eds. *Neonatal-Perinatal Medicine: Diseases of the Fetus and Infant.* 9th ed. St. Louis, MO: Elsevier Mosby; 2011: 485–500.

17. Premature infant. A.D.A.M. Medical Encyclopedia. http://www.nlm.nih.gov/medlineplus/ency/article/001562.htm. Updated November 14, 2011. Accessed April 3, 2015.

18. Donahue SMA, Kleinman KP, Gillman MW, Oken E. (2010).Trends in birth weight and gestational length among singleton term births in the United States. *Obstet Gynecol.* 2010; 115(2 Pt 1): 357–384. doi: 10.1097/AOG.0b013e3181cbd5f5

19. Appropriate for gestational age (AGA). A.D.A.M. Medical Encyclopedia. http://www.nlm.nih.gov/medlineplus/ency/article/002225.htm. Updated December 4, 2013. Accessed April 3, 2015.

20. Resnik R, Creasy RK. Intrauterine growth restriction. In: Creasy RK, Resnik R, Iams JD, Lockwood CJ, Moore T, Greene MF, eds. *Creasy and Resnik's Maternal-Fetal Medicine: Principles and Practice.* 7th ed. Philadelphia, PA: Elsevier Saunders; 2013: 743–755.

21. Small for gestational age. A.D.A.M. Encyclopedia. http://www.nlm.nih.gov/medlineplus/ency/article/002302.htm. Updated August 11, 2013. Accessed April 6, 2015.

22. Mandy GT. Small for gestational age infant. In: Basow DS, ed. *UpToDate.* Waltham, MA: UpToDate; 2015. http://www.uptodate.com/contents/small-for-gestational-age-infant. Last updated January 20, 2015. Accessed April 6, 2015.

23. Mandy GT. Large for gestational age newborn. In: Basow DS, ed. *UpToDate.* Waltham, MA: UpToDate; 2015. http://www.uptodate.com/contents/large-for-gestational-age-newborn?source=search_result&search=large+for+gestational+age&selectedTitle=1~45. Last updated September 3, 2014. Accessed May 6, 2015.

24. Carlo WA. Prematurity and intrauterine growth restriction. In: Kliegman RM, Stanton BF, Schor NF, St. Geme JW III, Behrman RE, eds. *Nelson Textbook of Pediatrics.* 19th ed. Philadelphia, PA: Saunders Elsevier; 2011: 532–535.

25. Soliman AT, ElAwwa A. Catch-up growth: Role of GH-IGF-I axis and thyroxine. In: Preedy VR, ed. *Handbook of Growth and Growth Monitoring in Health and Disease, Vol. 1.* New York, NY: Springer Science and Business Media; 2011: 935–962.

26. Brown JE, Isaacs JS, Krinke UB, et al. *Nutrition Through the Life Cycle.* 5th ed. Stamford, CT: Cengage Learning; 2013: 87–137.

27. American Academy of Pediatrics, American College of Obstetricians and Gynecologists. Care of the newborn. In: Riley LE, Stark AR, eds. *Guidelines for Perinatal Care.* 7th ed. Elk Grove Village, IL: American Academy of Pediatrics; 2012: 265.

28. Lo MD, Mazor SS. Neonatal resuscitation. In: Marx JA, Hockberger RS, Walls RM, et al., eds. *Rosen's Emergency Medicine: Concepts and Clinical Practice.* 8th ed. Philadelphia, PA: Elsevier Saunders; 2013: 112–118.

29. Skin characteristics in newborns. A.D.A.M. Medical Encyclopedia. http://www.nlm.nih.gov/medlineplus/ency/article/002301.htm. Updated December 4, 2013. Accessed April 6, 2015.

30. Schaffer JV, Bolognia JL. Congenital melanocytic nevi. In: Basow DS, ed. *UpToDate*. Waltham, MA: UpToDate; 2015. http://www.uptodate.com/contents/congenital-melanocytic-nevi?source=search_result&search=congenital+melanocytic+nevus&selectedTitle=1~11. Last updated October 14, 2014. Accessed May 6, 2015.

31. Pielop JA. Vascular lesions in the newborn. In: Basow DS, ed. *UpToDate*. Waltham, MA: UpToDate; 2015. http://www.uptodate.com/contents/vascular-lesions-in-the-newborn?source=search_result&search=vascular+lesions+in+the+newborn&selectedTitle=1~150. Last updated May 4, 2015. Accessed May 6, 2015.

32. Antaya RJ. Infantile hemangioma. In: James WD, ed. Medscape. http://emedicine.medscape.com/article/1083849-overview#showall. Updated March 31, 2014. Accessed April 6, 2015.

33. Lewis ML. A comprehensive newborn examination: Part II. Skin, trunk, extremities, neurologic. *Am Fam Physician*. 2014; 90(5): 297–302. http://www.aafp.org/afp/2014/0901/p297.html

34. Kotagal S. Neurologic examination of the newborn. In: Basow DS, ed. *UpToDate*. Waltham, MA: UpToDate; 2015. http://www.uptodate.com/contents/neurologic-examination-of-the-newborn?source=search_result&search=neurologic+examination+of+the+newborn&selectedTitle=1~150. Last updated May 28, 2014. Accessed May 6, 2015.

35. Khan OA, Garcia-Sosa R, Hageman JR, Msall M, Kelley KR. Core concepts: Neonatal neurological examination. *Neoreviews*, 2014; 15(8): e316–e324. http://pediatrics.uchicago.edu/Research/Publications/Khan.Hageman%20NeonatalNeuroExam%20NeoReviews%2008.2014.pdf

36. Infant reflexes. A.D.A.M. Medical Encyclopedia. http://www.nlm.nih.gov/medlineplus/ency/article/003292.htm. Updated December 4, 2013. Accessed April 6, 2015.

37. What causes frontal bossing? Healthline Web site. http://www.healthline.com/symptom/frontal-bossing. Accessed May 6, 2015.

38. Dibas B, Srivastava T. Vitamin D in health and bone disease. In: Vijayakumar M, Nammalwar BR, eds. *Principles and Practices of Pediatric Nephrology.* 2nd ed. New Delhi, India: Jaybee Brothers Medical Publishers; 2013: 785–794.

39. Ul Hassan A. *Platinum Notes USMLE Step-2: The Complete Preparatory Guide.* New Delhi, India: Jaypee Brothers Medical Publishers; 2013: 304–306.

40. Kinsman SL, Johnston MV. Congenital anomalies of the central nervous system. In: Kliegman RM, Stanton BF, St. Geme JW III, Schor NF, Behrman RE, eds. *Nelson Textbook of Pediatrics.* 19th ed. Philadelphia, PA: Elsevier Saunders; 2011: 2007.

41. Increased head circumference. A.D.A.M. Medical Encyclopedia. http://www.nlm.nih.gov/medlineplus/ency/article/003305.htm. Updated May 10, 2013. Accessed April 7, 2015.

42. U.S. Department of Health and Human Services, NIH, U.S. National Library of Medicine, Lister Hill National Center for Biomedical Communications, Genetics Home Reference. Waardenburg syndrome. http://ghr.nlm.nih.gov/condition/waardenburg-syndrome/show/print. Reviewed October 2012. Published April 6, 2015. Accessed April 8, 2015.

43. Benjamin K, Furdon SA. Physical assessment. In: Verklan MT, Walden M, eds. *Core Curriculum for Neonatal Intensive Care Nursing.* 5th ed. St. Louis, MO: Elsevier Saunders; 2014: 110–145.

44. Gallagher ER, Hing AV, Cunningham ML. Evaluating fontanels in the newborn skull. *Contemp Pediatr.* 2013, November 1. http://contemporarypediatrics.modernmedicine.com/contemporary-pediatrics/content/tags/cerebrospinal-fluid-dynamics/evaluating-fontanels-newborn-skull?page=full

45. Carlo WA. Physical examination of the newborn infant. In: Kliegman RM, Stanton BF, Schor NF, St. Geme JW III, Behrman RE, eds. *Nelson Textbook of Pediatrics.* 19th ed. Philadelphia, PA: Saunders Elsevier; 2011: 541–544.

46. Newborn head molding. A.D.A.M. Medical Encyclopedia. http://www.nlm.nih.gov/medlineplus/ency/article/002270.htm. Updated December 4, 2013. Accessed April 6, 2015.

47. Cephalohematoma. Stanford School of Medicine: Newborn Nursery at LPCH Web site. http://newborns.stanford.edu/PhotoGallery/Cephalohematoma1.html. Accessed April 7, 2015.

48. Doerr S. Newborn jaundice (neonatal jaundice). In: Mersch J, ed. MedicineNet. http://www.medicinenet.com/newborn_jaundice_neonatal_jaundice/page3.htm. Reviewed March 24, 2014. Accessed April 7, 2015.

49. Ramachandran M, Achan P, Jones DHA, Panchbhavi VK. Osteogenesis imperfecta. In: Gellman H, ed. Medscape. http://emedicine.medscape.com/article/1256726-overview#showall. Updated November 24, 2014. Accessed April 8, 2015.

50. Olitsky SE, Hug D, Plummer LS, Stass-Isern M. Abnormalities of pupil and iris. In: Kliegman RM, Stanton BF, Schor NF, St. Geme JW III, Behrman RE, eds. *Nelson Textbook of Pediatrics.* 19th ed. Philadelphia, PA: Elsevier Saunders; 2011: 2154–2156.

51. Warner-Rogers J. Clinical neuropsychological assessment of children. In: Goldstein LH, McNeil JE, eds. *Clinical Neuropsychology: A Practical Guide to Assessment and Management for Clinicians.* 2nd ed. Chichester, West Sussex, UK: Wiley-Blackwell; 2013: 317–346.

52. Blosser CG, Woo TM. Eye disorders. In: Burns CE, Dunn AM, Brady MA, Starr NB, Blosser CG, eds. *Pediatric Primary Care*. 5th ed. Philadelphia, PA: Elsevier Saunders; 2012: 622–651.

53. Tuli SY, Giordano BP, Kelly M, Fillipps D, Tuli SS. Newborn with an absent red reflex. *J Pediatr Health Care.* 2013; 27(1): 51–55. doi: 10.1016/j.pedhc.2011.10.010

54. Lesnick BL, Davis SD. Infant pulmonary function testing: Overview of technology and practical considerations – new current procedural terminology codes effective 2010. *Chest.* 2010; 139(5): 1197–1202. doi:10.1378/chest.10-1423

55. Wanger J. *Pulmonary Function Testing: A Practical Approach.* 3rd ed. Sudbury, MA: Jones & Bartlett Learning; 2012: 263–280.

56. Johnson L, Cochran WD. Assessment of the newborn history and physical examination of the newborn. In: Cloherty JP, Eichenwald EC, Hansen AR, Stark AR, eds. *Manual of Neonatal Care.* 7th ed. Philadelphia, PA: Lippincott, Williams, & Wilkins; 2012: 91–102.

57. Blundell A, Harrison R. *OSCEs at a Glance.* 2nd ed. Hoboken, N.J.: John Wiley & Sons; 2013: 304–306.

58. Parikh AS, Mitchell AL. Congenital anomalies. In: Martin RJ, Fanaroff AA, Walsh MC, eds. *Fanaroff and Martin's Neonatal-Perinatal Medicine: Diseases of the Fetus and Infant.* 10th ed. St. Louis, MO: Elsevier Saunders; 2014: 577–596.

59. Frank JE, Jacobe KM. Evaluation and management of heart murmurs in children. *Am Fam Physician.* 2011; 84(7): 793–800. http://www.aafp.org/afp/2011/1001/p793.html

60. Pulse oximetry screening for critical congenital heart defects. Centers for Disease Control and Prevention Web site. http://www.cdc.gov/Features/CongenitalHeartDefects. Last reviewed August 29, 2014. Accessed April 8, 2015.

61. Department of Health and Human Services, State Government of Victoria, Australia. Blood pressure – neonates. http://www.health.vic.gov.au/neonatal-handbook/procedures/blood-pressure.htm. Accessed April 8, 2015.

62. Palazzi DL, Brandt ML. Care of the umbilicus and management of umbilical disorders. In: Basow DS, ed. *UpToDate.* UptoDate: Waltham, MA; 2015. http://www.uptodate.com/contents/care-of-the-umbilicus-and-management-of-umbilical-disorders?source=search_result&search=care+of+the+umbilicus+and&selectedTitle=1~150. Last updated February 20, 2015. Accessed May 6, 2015.

63. Drutz JE. The pediatric physical examination: Chest and abdomen. In: Basow DS, ed. *UpToDate.* UptoDate: Waltham, MA; 2015. http://www.uptodate.com/contents/the-pediatric-physical-examination-chest-and-abdomen. Last updated October 14, 2013. Accessed April 8, 2015.

64. Bowden VR, Greenberg CS. *Children and Their Families: The Continuum of Care.* 2nd ed. Philadelphia, PA: Wolters Kluwer Health/Lippincott Williams & Wilkins; 2010: 860–935.

65. Mayo Clinic Staff. Sacral dimple: complications. Mayo Clinic Web site. http://www.mayoclinic.org/diseases-conditions/sacral-dimple/basics/complications/con-20025266. Reviewed October 24, 2012. Accessed April 9, 2015.

66. Rosenfeld SB. Developmental dysplasia of the hip: Clinical features and diagnosis. In: Basow DS, ed. *UpToDate.* UptoDate: Waltham, MA; 2015. http://www.uptodate.com/contents/developmental-dysplasia-of-the-hip-clinical-features-and-diagnosis?source=search_result&search=developmental+dysplasia+of+the+hip&selectedTitle=1~33. Last updated April 14, 2015. Accessed May 6, 2015.

67. Kemper AR. Newborn screening. In: Basow DS, ed. *UpToDate.* UptoDate: Waltham, MA; 2015. http://www.uptodate.com/contents/newborn-screening?source=search_result&search=newborn+screening&selectedTitle=1~146. Last updated July 14, 2014. Accessed May 6, 2015.

68. Anderson R, Rothwell E, Botkin JR. Newborn screening: Ethical, legal, and social implications. In: Pepper GA, Wysocki KJ, eds. *Annual Review of Nursing Research, Vol. 29: Genetics.* New York, NY: Springer Publishing Company; 2012: 113–132.

69. The Recommended Uniform Screening Panel. Baby's First Test Web site. http://babysfirsttest.org/newborn-screening/the-recommended-uniform-screening-panel. Accessed may 6, 2015.

70. Lewis JA. Human genetics and genomics: Impact on neonatal care. In: Kenner C, Wright Lott J, eds. *Comprehensive Neonatal Nursing Care.* 5th ed. New York, NY: Springer Publishing Company; 2014: 829–848.

71. Adcock LM, Freysdottir D. Screening the newborn for hearing loss. In: Basow DS, ed. *UpToDate.* UptoDate: Waltham, MA; 2015. http://www.uptodate.com/contents/screening-the-newborn-for-hearing-loss?source=search_result&search=screening+the+newborn+for+hearing+loss&selectedTitle=1~150. Last updated April 20, 2015. Accessed May 6, 2015.

72. Riley C, Spencer B, Prater LS. Normal term newborn. In: Kenner C, Wright Lott J, eds. *Comprehensive Neonatal Nursing Care.* 5th ed. New York, NY: Springer Publishing Company; 2014: 113–132.

73. What are the chances my baby has CF? Cystic Fibrosis Foundation Web site. http://www.cff.org/AboutCF/Testing/NewbornScreening/UnderstandingtheResults/. Last updated January 27, 2014. Accessed May 6, 2015.

Chapter 5
Infant Health and Issues

QUESTIONS

1. You are conducting a Well Child Check on a 5-month-old boy, as per the Bright Futures guidelines. At this point in time, which of the following would <u>least</u> qualify as a concerning finding?

   a. Undescended testes

   b. Galactorrhea

   c. Head lag when pulled to sitting position

   d. Failure to hold head up when lying on stomach

2. A mother brings her 3-month-old male child to your office with complaints of sudden difficulty feeding the child, as well as an inability to console his screaming. Although the child shows a response to her efforts, his crying and agitation have not decreased. The mother also notes that she noticed a bump on his head, which she assumed was from him hitting his head during one of his screaming fits. Which of the following would be the best initial course of action?

   a. Lumbar puncture

   b. Administration of ceftriaxone

   c. Immediate admission to hospital

   d. Blood count and culture

3. A mother brings her 7-month-old infant daughter to your office because, over the past week, she's felt the daughter's lymph nodes in the neck "getting harder." Upon physical examination, you notice that the lymph nodes feel small, round, and slightly hardened. Which of the following is the most likely cause?

   a. Pyelonephritis

   b. Lymphoma

   c. Respiratory infection

   d. Leukemia

4. According to the psychosocial development model, at which age would an infant be <u>least</u> likely to cry when she is handed to her new babysitter?

   a. Four months

   b. Six months

   c. Eight months

   d. Ten months

5. Which of the following standardized tests may be performed by parents with no formal training?

   a. Denver Developmental Screening Test II

   b. Ages and Stages Questionnaire

   c. Bayley Scales of Infant Development

   d. Newborn Behavioral Assessment Scale

6. A 9-month-old infant presents to the clinic fussy, with decreased appetite and a fever of 102.3 °F. Upon examining the patient, you find it difficult to find a localized site of infection. Which of the following is the most likely condition?

    a. Otitis media

    b. Group B streptococcal infection

    c. Occult bacteremia

    d. Urinary tract infection

7. Which of the following findings would most strongly indicate that a febrile infant is moderately ill?

    a. The infant has a temperature of 101.8 °F but smiles often.

    b. The infant is fussy but calms quickly when offered support.

    c. The infant appears listless and does not feed well.

    d. The infant has a temperature of 103 °F but appears alert and active.

8. During the examination of a 3-month-old patient, you place the infant in the supine position with the hips flexed 90° and abducted. You then grab the patient's legs by the thigh and gently adduct the leg while applying downward, lateral pressure. What is the name of the supplementary exam that is commonly performed in conjunction with the exam you are performing on your patient?

    a. Klisic

    b. Barlow

    c. Ortolani's

    d. Galeazzi

9. What is the name of the condition in which the foreskin is not retractable over the tip of the penis?

    a. Epispadias

    b. Chordee

    c. Hypospadias

    d. Phimosis

10. You are consulting a mother who is worried about her 8-month-old male infant. She states that he has a fever, and she wants to give him ibuprofen. You recommend giving him 90 mg of ibuprofen every 6 hours. Based on the above treatment guidelines, what is the most likely weight of this infant?

    a. 7.5 kg

    b. 8.18 kg

    c. 9 kg

    d. 10 kg

RATIONALES

1. c

Although infants should mostly maintain head control by 4 months of age, it is still normal for an infant to reach this developmental milestone anywhere between 4 and 6 months of age. The inability to raise the head when lying on the stomach, galactorrhea, and undescended testes are all considered to be developmental warning signs starting at 3 months of age.

2. c

The signs that the child is displaying—persistent screaming with no evidence of fever and a soft, bulging fontanel—are indicative of intracranial pressure in the infant, which warrants immediate hospital admission. A bulging fontanel typically occurs when fluid builds up in the brain, causing increased intracranial pressure. A lumbar puncture would be appropriate if the aim was to measure the intracranial pressure. Administering ceftriaxone would be warranted in cases of bacterial infection, which is often indicated by a temperature change in the infant. Performing a blood count test and obtaining cultures are often used to detect bacteremia in infants.

3. c

The most likely cause is a respiratory infection because the infant is presenting with shotty lymph nodes, which often indicate a past infection. Although pyelonephritis is an infection, it is less likely than a respiratory infection to cause shotty lymph nodes in the neck. Lymphoma would be more strongly indicated by enlarged lymph nodes, as opposed to shotty lymph nodes. Leukemia would be characterized by generalized lymphadenopathy, not localized to one area.

4. a

An infant would be least likely to cry when introduced to a stranger at around 4 months, as stranger anxiety typically develops at around 6 months. Thus, the 6-month-old, the 8-month-old, and the 9-month-old are more likely than the 4-month-old to have developed a fear of strangers, and would be more likely to cry when introduced to a new babysitter.

5. b

The Ages and Stages Questionnaire is a standardized test that may be utilized by parents or care takers and does not require a professional. The Denver Developmental Screening Test II and the Bayley Scales of Infant Development test typically require the employment of professionals. The Newborn Behavioral Assessment Scale may be performed by Brazelton-certified individuals.

6. d

A diagnosis of urinary tract infection (UTI) should be considered if a local site of infection cannot be found in a febrile infant. Typically, an unexplained fever is the most characteristic symptom in an infant with a UTI. Pneumonia and otitis media are also associated with causing fever in infants, but both conditions would likely present with other findings as well, such as tachypnea or respiratory distress in pneumonia and irritability and vertigo in otitis media. Gastroenteritis in infants would also cause other symptoms and would not be the most likely diagnosis.

7. a

Moderately ill infants typically display irritable or fussy behavior and have a fever temperature below 102 °F, yet are easy to console, may smile, and continue to feed normally. Infants that present with a temperature above 100.4 °F but smile, feed normally, and appear alert and active are typically classified as mildly ill. Severely ill infants normally present with a temperature higher than 104 °F; these infants often appear listless, may not feed at all or feed poorly, and are typically recommended for hospital admission.

8. c

The scenario describes the Barlow test, which is used to assess for developmental dysplasia of the hip (DDH); the Ortolani test is typically performed with the Barlow test and is also used to assess for developmental dysplasia of the hip. These two tests evaluate hip stability and are the favored diagnostic exams for patients 3 months of age and younger. The Klisic and Galeazzi signs are often performed on patients older than 3 months of age to assess for decreased hip abduction and unequal thigh length.

9. d

Phimosis presents with foreskin that is not retractable over the tip of the penis. This condition is considered common in infant patients and is often resolved by 3 years of age. Hypospadias results in the opening of the urethra manifesting on the underside, rather than the tip, of the penis; epispadias similarly affects the urethra, causing it to open on the top or side of the penis. Chordee refers to curvature of the penis at the junction of head and shaft.

10. c

The suggested ibuprofen regimen for managing a fever in infants older than 6 months is 10 mg/kg every 6 hours; thus, a 90-mg dose of ibuprofen would be recommended for an infant weighing 9 kg. A recommended dose of 90 mg for an infant who weighs 7.5 kg would suggest that the dose is 12 mg/kg, which is not the case. If the suggested dose were 11 mg/kg, the nurse practitioner would recommend 90 mg for an infant who weighs approximately 8.18 kg. These dosing regimens would be appropriate for acetaminophen, however, because the recommended dose is 10–15 mg/kg. For a 10 kg patient taking 90 mg of ibuprofen, the recommended dosing ratio would have to be 9 mg/kg.

DISCUSSION

Child Health Supervision

Overview

The American Academy of Pediatrics' (AAP) *Bright Futures: Guidelines of Health Supervision of Infants, Children, and Adolescents* acts as a primary guide for supervision of child health and promotes optimal health development in children through preventive care.[1] To accomplish this goal, supervision of infant health includes screenings at regularly scheduled intervals, known as Well

Child Checks (WCCs), starting at 1 month of age.[2] In addition to measuring the child's growth and development, WCCs help detect and treat diseases early and prevent diseases through routine vaccinations, education, and anticipatory guidance.[3]

Definition

In child health supervision, the newborn period begins at birth and lasts up to the first month of life; infancy, on the other hand, is the period after birth through 11 months of age. Early childhood spans ages 1–4 years. Middle childhood spans from 5 to 10 years of age, and adolescence occurs thereafter until 21 years of age.[4]

Focus

Physical

Infant WCCs should include an assessment of the child's growth and development. The physical examination should include a measurement of weight, height, and head circumference.[5] Additionally, the child's gross and fine motor development should be assessed, as should social interaction.[6]

Cognitive

The nurse practitioner (NP) should assess the cognitive and sensorimotor development of children. The NP can make these assessments through direct observations, a thorough history, and observations from parents, teachers, and child care providers.[4]

Psychosocial

Psychosocial development of infants is marked by development of trust.[7] The infant's social development and parent-child interactions should also be assessed.[3]

Well Child Checks

Overview

WCCs should begin 1 month post-birth, followed by visits at 2, 4, 6, 9, and 12 months of age.[2,8] If the infant is discharged from the hospital prior to 48 hours, his or her first visit should be within 48 hours of discharge.[8] Many providers also choose to check weight gain and feeding at a 2 week visit.

Stage Appropriate Screening

WCCs use both subjective and objective data to assess a child's health. The WCC may include a physical exam; laboratory tests; health and developmental history; immunizations; lead, hearing, vision, and dental screenings; and health education.[9] Additionally, developmental screening can be assessed by the Ages and Stages Questionnaire (ASQ), which is the parents' assessment of their child's language, social, motor, and problem solving

skills. The Denver Developmental Screening Test, second edition (Denver II), can also be implemented to detect developmental delays or children at risk of development problems.[10] Management plans for the infant are determined by the results of screening.

The Physical Examination: Necessary Elements

Overview

A complete physical examination is recommended for all children and should be performed at regular intervals.[11] The examination should measure the infant's height and weight; head circumference should also be measured until the child is 3 years of age.[11] These measurements are recorded on approved growth charts for the specific child. The NP should also assess the infant's vital signs, including temperature, blood pressure, respiratory rate, and heart rates.[11]

Head control is expected in infants by 4 months of age, and no lag is expected when the infant is pulled to sitting at 6 months. A lag may indicate a neurodevelopmental concern such as palsy.[12] The infant's fontanels should also be assessed. The posterior fontanel usually closes within the first few months, and the anterior fontanel typically closes around 15–18 months. Early or late closure of fontanels may signal significant anomalies, such as hyperthyroidism, trisomy disorders, or microcephaly.[13] The nose should be assessed for nasal flaring, which may indicate difficulty breathing, or a flattened bridge, which may indicate an underlying congenital disorder such as fetal alcohol syndrome.[14] The NP should also examine the child's skin for lesions, rashes, or other abnormalities.[11,15]

A nose, mouth, and throat exam can help detect infections and common childhood abnormalities.[16] These abnormalities may be caused by too little or too much fluoride, sleeping with a bottle, or an unusual tooth eruption sequence. Fissures at the patient's lip corners may indicate vitamin deficiencies, and asymmetrically enlarged tonsils may suggest infection, as well as immunologic or anatomic anomalies.[17]

Voice abnormalities in infants may indicate underlying disorders. For instance, a shrill or high-pitched cry may indicate increased intracranial pressure.[18] In addition to assessing the infant's voice, the NP should perform a chest and lung exam, assessing for normal heart sounds and breathing. Mild pectus carinatum (pigeon chest) and pectus excavatum (sunken chest) are common findings in children, and gynecomastia and galactorrhea may present up to 3 months of age; if these presentations persist or exacerbate, however, the patient may have a genetic disorder.[5,17] An abdominal exam should likewise be performed. In most infants, the abdomen is prominent and the liver edge is palpable 1–2 cm below the right costal margin.[17] Diastasis recti, a disorder marked by the separation of the rectus abdominis muscle, is a common abnormal abdominal finding in infants; this condition typically resolves on its own and does not necessitate intervention.[12]

The genitals should be examined in infants of both genders. When dealing with female patients, the NP should assess for signs of labial adhesions and ensure that the vaginal opening is fully visible. When dealing with male patients, the NP should assess for abnormalities of the penis and testes. The testes typically descend by the age of 3 months, and many male infants present with a large scrotum. When examining the penis, the NP should assess for genitourinary abnormalities such as phimosis, where the foreskin is unable to fully retract, or hypospadias, where the urethra appears on the underside of the penis.[12,17]

Developmental dysplasia of the hip (DDH), a dislocation of the hip, is typically present at birth but may develop within the first year of life. DDH may be indicated by findings such as asymmetry of skin fold thickness and unequal leg length. DDH can be detected by the Ortolani maneuver, in which a palpable "clunk" is present upon reduction of the hip.[19,20] DDH can also be detected by the Galeazzi sign, which manifests an inequality in the height of the pediatric patient's knees while the patient lies down with his or her feet drawn in towards the buttocks.[21]

In normal infants, lymph nodes are not typically palpable.[22] Infants may present with enlargements in the inguinal and cervical nodes, which are normal variants that typically only last a short period of time.[12] Shotty nodes may indicate past infection in the infant, but do not typically indicate active infection unless they are warm, tender, and enlarged.[22] Palpable supraclavicular lymph nodes or nodes larger than 3 mm should warrant urgent referral for possible malignancy.[22]

Standardized Tests

According to the AAP, children should be screened for developmental disabilities during WCCs at 9 months, 18 months, and 24 or 30 months of age.[23] Several standardized tests may be used to assess the development of infants, including the Denver II, the Bayley Scales of Infant Development, the Bayley Infant Neurodevelopmental Screener, and the ASQ, among others.[17] The Newborn Behavioral Assessment Scale includes 27 behavioral responses and 20 reflex items to assess higher cortical function, including consolability and habituation.[24] The Modified Checklist for Autism in Toddlers should also be used in pediatric screening protocols.[12]

Reflexes and Motor Skills

The presence and strength of an infant's reflexes, such as the Moro reflex and tonic neck reflex, is important in assessing the infant's nervous system development and function. If an infant's reflex persists after the age at which the reflex normally disappears, this may be a sign of neurodevelopmental abnormalities.[12]

Cognitive Development

When evaluating the cognitive development of an infant, the NP should assess the infant's response to environment and voice. Visual acuity is measured by the blink reflex and pupil constriction. Hearing screening, using tests such as otoacoustic emissions and auditory brainstem response, is indicated for all infants.[25]

Sensorimotor development, as defined by Jean Piaget, should also be assessed. By these standards, infants should be able to adapt their reflexes to their environment and engage in simple problem-solving.[26]

Psychosocial Development

There is a range of temperaments in infants; some may adapt easily to situations and people, but others may have a more difficult time adapting and may react more intensely.[12] Infants typically develop a fear of strangers and a fear of separation from their parents at approximately 7–9 months of age.[12] Attachment is defined as an affective bond that develops over the course of the first year of life and will differentiate into other emotions later. Although breastfeeding promotes maternal sensitivity and attachment development, breastfeeding is not necessary for, and does not always result in, secure attachment. Insecure attachment results in infants with detachment issues, such as avoidance, anxiety, and disorganization.[4,17]

Nutrition/Feeding

There are many benefits to breastfeeding, as breast milk has the optimal combination of nutrients for the growth and development of infants.[8,27] In addition to breast milk, infants should also receive supplements to ensure an adequate intake of vitamin D.[28] According to the AAP, children should be breastfed exclusively until 6 months of age, at which time solid foods should begin to be introduced. Breastfeeding should continue until approximately 12 months of age. After 12 months of age, infants should be transitioned to whole milk with a limit of 24 ounces per day to avoid micro-gastrointestinal bleeding with resultant iron deficiency anemia. Excessive milk intake can also lead to poor nutrition from lack of food intake due to satiety from milk.[4,12] Weaning may be delayed if breastfeeding is mutually desired by both the mother and infant.[28]

Dental Health

The NP should assess the infant for tooth decay due to use of a baby bottle. Before the patient's teeth erupt, the infant's mouth should be cleaned by wiping with a soft cloth; this process will help to minimize the risk of tooth decay once primary dentition begins. Once the teeth erupt, the parents should be encouraged to clean their child's mouth twice daily with a soft brush. The infant's fluoride intake should also be monitored; if supplements are necessary, administration should begin at 6 months of age.[29] The AAP recommends that infants have their first dental visit by the time they reach 1 year of age.[30]

Sleep

Infants between the ages of 2 months and 1 year should sleep 16–18 hours per day, including two to three naps daily.[31] It is strongly recommended that parents or caregivers avoid sleeping with infants because bed-sharing can increase the risk of sudden infant death syndrome (SIDS).[8,32] SIDS can also be prevented by putting infants to sleep on their back, using a firm sleep surface, keeping soft objects out of the crib, offering a pacifier at naptime and bedtime, and breastfeeding.[33]

Injury Prevention: Special Consideration for Infants

Knowledge of developmental phases, awareness of external occurrences that may cause the infant harm, and constant supervision of the infant are ways to facilitate injury prevention. Because infants do not yet understand consequences, they are at an increased risk of unintentional injury, such as falls, burns, poisoning, choking, and drowning. Constant supervision and educating the infant (e.g., teaching the importance of approaching authority figures and staying away from strangers) are also ways to safeguard against potential harm.[8]

Developmental Warning Signs (see table 5.1)

Visual delays, such as retinopathy, infant cataracts, and strabismus, are developmental warning signs in infants.[4,12] Other developmental warning signs include an infant's failure to raise his or her head when lying on his or her stomach by 3 months of age, and the failure to manually play with toys by 6 months of age.

Fever in the Very Young Infant

Infants generally have higher temperatures than older children and adults because they have a greater surface-area-to-body-weight ratio and a higher metabolic rate.[34] An infant is considered to have a fever when the infant's rectal temperature is greater than 100.4 °F (38 °C). In newborns, however, fevers can be indicated by lower than normal temperatures because newborns are unable to regulate their body temperatures when they are very ill.

Fever in Early Infancy (the first 2 months of life)

Although almost any infection can cause fevers

in infants, fevers in this population are usually indicative of an upper respiratory illness or other type of viral infection. The degree of the fever does not always directly correlate with the severity of the illness.[35] Group B *Streptococcus* and Gram-negative enteric organisms are common causes of fevers in the first month of age, whereas *Streptococcus pneumoniae* and *Haemophilus influenzae* are more likely causes of fevers in the second month of age.[17]

Assess the Degree of Illness: Responses are Behavioral

Infants who are mildly ill often act relatively normal, appearing alert and active, feeding well, and smiling. Moderately ill infants, on the other hand, may be fussy or irritable. They may, however, eat normally, be consolable, and smile. Severely ill infants with temperatures of 104 °F (40 °C) or higher typically appear listless, cannot be consoled, and either feed poorly or do not feed at all. Hospital admission is recommended if the infant's fever is above 100.4 °F.[17] Diagnostic studies depend on the infant's age: Neonates should receive a full sepsis evaluation, whereas infants older than 28 days should undergo studies to determine the source of the fever. These studies may include lumbar punctures, urine and stool cultures, or complete blood counts, depending on the presentation. Additionally, radiographic studies may be indicated if the patient presents with signs of respiratory illness, such as coughing, wheezing, or coryza.[36] When no local site of infection can be clearly identified, the NP should consider the diagnosis of a urinary tract infection, pneumonia, or another type of infection.[17]

Management

Over-the-counter medications, such as acetaminophen, are recommended to manage fevers in infants as long as the source of fever is located and treated.[35] Ibuprofen should only be used in infants younger than 6 months of age when they are not responding to acetaminophen and they are being closely monitored in the hospital or undergoing a septic workup.[37] Alternating medications is not recommended because medication errors are common as a result of dosage and timing inaccuracies. Moreover, there is no evidence that a patient's temperature is better controlled by alternating medications.[8,35]

Table 5.1	Developmental Warning Signs During the Infant Stage
2 months	Doesn't respond to loud sounds
	Doesn't watch things as they move
	Doesn't smile at people
	Doesn't bring hands to mouth
	Can't hold head up when pushing up from stomach
4 months	Doesn't watch things as they move
	Doesn't smile at people
	Can't hold head steady
	Doesn't coo or make sounds
	Doesn't bring things to mouth
	Doesn't push down with legs when feet are on hard surface
	Has trouble moving one or both eyes in all directions
6 months	Doesn't try to get things in reach
	Doesn't show affection to caregivers
	Doesn't respond to sounds
	Has difficulty putting things in mouth
	Doesn't make vowel sounds
	Doesn't roll over in either direction
	Doesn't laugh/make squealing sounds
	Seems stiff with tight muscles
	Seems floppy like a rag doll
9 months	Doesn't bear weight on legs with support
	Doesn't sit with help
	Doesn't babble
	Doesn't play games back and forth
	Doesn't respond to name
	Doesn't seem to recognize familiar people
	Doesn't look where you point
	Doesn't transfer toys from one hand to the other
1 year	Doesn't crawl
	Can't stand when supported
	Doesn't search for things that she sees you hide
	Doesn't say single words
	Doesn't learn gestures (waving, shaking head)
	Doesn't point to things
	Loses skills he/she once had
18 months	Doesn't point to things to show others
	Can't walk
	Doesn't know what familiar things are used for
	Doesn't copy others
	Doesn't gain new words
	Doesn't have a vocabulary of 6 words or more
	Doesn't notice/care when caretaker leaves/returns
	Loses skills he/she once had

Note. Adapted with permission from Developmental milestones. CDC. http://www.cdc.gov/ncbddd/actearly/milestones/index.html. Published 2014. Accessed April 2015.

References

1. Hagan JF, Shaw JS, Duncan PM, eds. *Bright Futures: Guidelines for Health Supervision of Infants, Children, and Adolescents*. 3rd ed. Elk Grove Village, IL: American Academy of Pediatrics; 2008.

2. Well-child visits. MedlinePlus Web site. http://www.nlm.nih.gov/medlineplus/ency/article/001928.htm. Updated January 27, 2013. Accessed April 8, 2015.

3. Consolini DM. Health supervision of the well child. In: Porter RS, Kaplan JL, eds. The Merck Manual Online. http://www.merckmanuals.com/professional/pediatrics/health_supervision_of_the_well_child/health_supervision_of_the_well_child.html?qt=colson%20held%20and%20chapman&alt=sh. Updated April 2014. Accessed April 13, 2015.

4. Kliegman RM, Stanton BF, St. Geme JW III, Schor NF, Behrman RE. *Nelson Textbook of Pediatrics*. 19th ed. Philadelphia, PA: Elsevier Saunders; 2011.

5. Drutz JE. The pediatric physical examination: Chest and abdomen. In: Basow DS, ed. *UpToDate*. Waltham, MA: UpToDate; 2015. http://www.uptodate.com/contents/the-pediatric-physical-examination-chest-and-abdomen?source=search_result&search=pediatric+physical+examination&selectedTitle=3~150. Updated October 14, 2013. Accessed April 13, 2015.

6. Boyse K. Developmental milestones. University of Michigan Health System Web site. http://www.med.umich.edu/yourchild/topics/devmile.htm. Updated August 2013. Accessed April 13, 2015.

7. Crocetti E, Meeus WHJ, Ritchie RA, Meca A, Schwartz SJ. Adolescent identity: Is this the key to unraveling associations between family relationships and problem behaviors? In: Scheier LM, Hansen WB, eds. *Parenting and Teen Drug Use: The Most Recent Finding from Research, Prevention, and Treatment*. New York, NY: Oxford University Press; 2014: 92–109.

8. Recommendations for preventive pediatric health care. American Academy of Pediatrics Web site. http://www.aap.org/en-us/professional-resources/practice-support/Periodicity/Periodicity%20Schedule_FINAL.pdf. Published 2014. Accessed April 14, 2015.

9. Well child exams. Lake Cumberland District Health Department Web site. http://www.lcdhd.org/children/well_child_exams. Accessed April 14, 2015.

10. Ringwalt S. Developmental screening and assessment instruments with an emphasis on social and emotional development for young children ages birth through five. National Early Childhood Technical Assistance Center Web site. http://www.nectac.org/~pdfs/pubs/screening.pdf. Published May 2008. Accessed April 14, 2015.

11. Drutz JE. The pediatric physical examination: General principles and standard measurements. In: Basow DS, ed. *UpToDate*. Waltham, MA: UpToDate; 2015. http://www.uptodate.com/contents/the-pediatric-physical-examination-general-principles-and-standard-measurements. Updated March 2015. Accessed April 14, 2015.

12. Burns CE, Dunn AM, Brady MA, Starr NB, Blosser CG. *Pediatric Primary Care*. 5th ed. Philadelphia, PA: Elsevier Saunders; 2013.

13. Gallagher ER, Hing AV, Cunningham ML. Evaluating fontanels in the newborn skull. *Contemp Peds*. 2013; 30(11): 12. http://contemporarypediatrics.modernmedicine.com/contemporary-pediatrics/content/tags/cerebrospinal-fluid-dynamics/evaluating-fontanels-newborn-skull?page=full

14. Fuller RA. Newborn assessment. In: Sawyer SS, ed. *Pediatric Physical Examination & Health Assessment*. Sudbury, MA: Jones & Bartlett Learning; 2012: 103–142.

15. PEDS: Basic pediatric clerkship. University of Washington Department of Pediatrics Web site. https://www.washington.edu/medicine/pediatrics/docs/students/PEDS%20Clerkship%20Manual_Website_0614.pdf. Last updated May 2014. Accessed April 14, 2015.

16. Allen PJ. Nose, mouth, and throat. In: Duderstadt K, ed. *Pediatric Physical Examination: An Illustrated Handbook*. 2nd ed. St. Louis, MO: Elsevier Mosby; 2014: 178–197.

17. Barkley TW Jr. Infant health and issues. In *Pediatric Primary Care Nurse Practitioner: Certification Review/Clinical Update Continuing Education Course*. West Hollywood, CA: Barkley & Associates; 2015: 38–44.

18. Increased intracranial pressure. Nationwide Children's Hospital Web site. www.nationwidechildrens.org/Document/Get/40003. Updated January 2015. Accessed April 14, 2015.

19. Schwend RM, Shaw BA, Segal LS. Evaluation and treatment of developmental hip dysplasia in the newborn and infant. *Pediatr Clin North Am*. 2014; 61(6): 1095–1107. doi: 10.1016/j.pcl.2014.08.008

20. Tamai J, McCarthy JJ. Developmental dysplasia of the hip. In: Jaffe WL, ed. Medscape. http://emedicine.medscape.com/article/1248135-overview#showall. Updated March 31, 2014. Accessed April 14, 2015.

21. Storer SK, Skaggs DL. Developmental dysplasia of the hip. *Am Fam Physician*. 2006; 74(8): 1310–1316. http://www.aafp.org/afp/2006/1015/p1310.html

22. Drutz JE. The pediatric physical examination: Back, extremities, nervous system, skin, and lymph nodes. In: Basow DS, ed. *UpToDate*. Waltham, MA: UpToDate; 2015. http://www.uptodate.com/contents/the-pediatric-physical-examination-back-extremities-nervous-system-skin-and-lymph-nodes?source=search_result&search=pediatric+physical+examination&selectedTitle=5~150. Updated March 2015. Accessed April 14, 2015.

23. U.S. Department of Health and Human Services, Centers for Disease Control and Prevention. Developmental monitoring and screening. http://www.cdc.gov/ncbddd/childdevelopment/screening.html. Updated February 12, 2015. Accessed April 14, 2015.

24. Kotagal S. Neurological examination of the newborn. In: Basow DS, ed. *UpToDate*. Waltham, MA: UpToDate; 2015. http://www.uptodate.com/contents/neurologic-examination-of-the-newborn?source=search_result&search=neurological+examination+of+the+newborn&selectedTitle=1~150. Updated May 28, 2014. Accessed April 14, 2015.

25. Delaney AM. Newborn hearing screening. In: Meyers AD, ed. Medscape.. http://emedicine.medscape.com/article/836646-overview#showall. Updated September 11, 2014. Accessed April 14, 2015.

26. Cherry K. Sensorimotor stage of cognitive development. About Education Web site. http://psychology.about.com/od/piagetstheory/p/sensorimotor.htm. Accessed April 14, 2015.

27. Infant feeding and nutrition module. Oregon Health Authority Web site. https://public.health.oregon.gov/HealthyPeopleFamilies/wic/Documents/modules/infant-feeding-and-nutrition-staff.pdf. Updated April 2014. Accessed April 14, 2015.

28. American Academy of Pediatrics. Breastfeeding and the use of human milk. *Pediatrics*. 2012; 129(3): 600–603. doi: 10.1542/peds.2011-3553

29. Nowak AJ, Warren JJ. (2015). Preventive dental care and counseling for infants and young children. In: Basow DS, ed. *UpToDate*. Waltham, MA: UpToDate; 2015. http://www.uptodate.com/contents/preventive-dental-care-and-counseling-for-infants-and-young-children?source=search_result&search=Preventive+dental+care+and+counseling+for+infants+and+young+children&selectedTitle=1~150. Updated February 13, 2015. Accessed April 14, 2015.

30. Your child's age 1 dental visit. Simple Steps Web site. http://www.simplestepsdental.com/SS/ihtSSPrint/r.WSIHW000/st.31840/t.31887/pr.3/c.354252.html. Updated July 3, 2012. Accessed April 14, 2015.

31. U.S. Department of Health and Human Services, Centers for Disease Control and Prevention. How much sleep do I need? http://www.cdc.gov/sleep/about_sleep/how_much_sleep.htm. Updated July 1, 2013. Accessed April 14, 2015.

32. UNICEF UK Baby Friendly Initiative statement on bed sharing research. UNICEF Web site. http://www.unicef.org.uk/BabyFriendly/News-and-Research/News/UNICEF-UK-Baby-Friendly-Initiative-statement-on-new-bed-sharing-research. Published May 21, 2014. Accessed April 14, 2015.

33. American Academy of Pediatrics. SIDS and other sleep-related infant deaths: Expansion of recommendations for a safe infant sleeping environment. *Pediatrics*. 2011; 128(5): e1341–e1367. doi: 10.1542/peds.2011-2285

34. Ward MA. Fever in infants and children: Pathophysiology and management. In: Basow DS, ed. *UpToDate*. Waltham, MA: UpToDate; 2015. http://www.uptodate.com/contents/fever-in-infants-and-children-pathophysiology-and-management?source=search_result&search=Pathophysiology+and+management+of+fever+in+infants+and+children&selectedTitle=1~150. Updated December 15, 2014. Accessed April 14, 2015.

35. Sullivan JE, Farrar HC, Section on Clinical Pharmacology and Therapeutics, Committee on Drugs. Fever and antipyretic use in children. *Pediatrics*. 2011; 127(3): 580–587. doi: 10.1542/peds.2010-3852

36. Gould JM, Aronoff SC. Fever in the infant and toddler workup. In: Steele RW, ed. Medscape. http://emedicine.medscape.com/article/1834870-workup#showall. Updated January 30, 2014. Accessed April 14, 2015.

37. Hockenberry MJ, Wilson D. *Wong's Essentials of Pediatric Nursing*. 9th ed. St. Louis, MO: Elsevier; 2013.

Chapter 6
Toddler/Preschool Health and Issues

1. Johnny, age 3, is brought into the clinic by his parents, who state that he has been unable to perform certain skills that he used to be able to perform. They also say that his ability to use language has started to deteriorate, and he does not want to play with the other children at school. Which of the following conditions would be the most likely diagnoses?

   a. Autistic disorder

   b. Asperger's syndrome

   c. Rett's disorder

   d. Childhood disintegrative disorder

2. By what age would not knowing what to do with common objects be first considered a developmental delay?

   a. At 1 year

   b. At 2 years

   c. At 3 years

   d. At 4 years

3. Dan and Kara bring their toddler son, Ian, to your office because they are worried about his feeding habits. They explain that they still have to feed him because he is unable to use utensils—even a spoon—on his own. As the practitioner, you know that at what earliest age would Ian have to be for this issue to be a developmental concern?

   a. Twelve months old

   b. Fifteen months old

   c. Seventeen months old

   d. Twenty months old

4. Two 2 year olds are playing in a sandbox. They are both scooping and pouring sand, occasionally glancing over at each other but not interacting. How would the nurse practitioner best characterize this type of play?

   a. This behavior is abnormal, as by now they should want to play together.

   b. This behavior demonstrates parallel play, which is common in this age group.

   c. These children are participating in associative play, which is not expected in this age group.

   d. This is active play and is typical in this age group.

5. What is the average age by which toddlers achieve daytime control of bowel and bladder movements?

   a. By 18 months of age

   b. By 2 years of age

   c. By 2.5 years of age

   d. By 3 years of age

6. A 3-year-old male patient presents for a well-child checkup. While interviewing his parents, you learn that the patient's family comes from a working-class neighborhood in downtown Los Angeles. All of the following laboratory exams are especially indicated at this age except:

    a. Hemoglobin and hematocrit

    b. Vitamin D level

    c. Cholesterol

    d. Lead level

7. At what age does taking a blood pressure reading usually become a part of a child's physical examination?

    a. At 2 years

    b. At 3 years

    c. At 4 years

    d. At 5 years

8. Which of the following values most likely indicates the normal visual acuity of a 5-year-old child?

    a. Vision is 20/80

    b. Vision is 20/50

    c. Vision is 20/30

    d. Vision is 20/20

9. A concerned father says that his daughter recently turned 5 years old, and he has noticed she is beginning to stutter. The nurse practitioner tells the father that his daughter's condition is probably normal, but you will be watching with him to see if it persists or if she avoids speaking. As the nurse practitioner, you know that it is usually acceptable to wait before referring the son for his stuttering until how long?

    a. Three months

    b. Six months

    c. Nine months

    d. Twelve months

10. Leonard, a 4-year-old toddler, is brought to your office by his parents who have some concerns regarding his development. Which of the following factors should Leonard's parents be most concerned about?

    a. He has only eaten mashed potatoes for the previous 4 weeks.

    b. He has had a stutter for the previous 4 months.

    c. He struggles with nighttime bowel and bladder control.

    d. He has never acquired the motor skill of skipping.

RATIONALES

1. d

Based on the age of the patient and the recent decline in multiple areas of functioning, the most likely condition is childhood disintegrative disorder. This condition generally presents with a regression after at least 2 years of normal development. Autistic disorder, on the other hand, typically presents with impaired social interaction or language delay within the patient's first year. Asperger's syndrome does not typically result in language delays and would likely present with repetitive behaviors or interests. Lastly, Rett's disorder typically manifests after the first 5 months of the patient's life and results in neurodegenerative development. This condition has predominately been diagnosed in females; thus, it would not likely present in a male patient.

2. b

It would be considered a developmental warning sign for a toddler to not know what to do with common objects by the age of 2 years. At the age of 1 year, an infant is not yet expected to know what do with common objects. A child not being aware of his or her external environment could be considered a developmental warning sign at 3 years of age. Not listening or not speaking in sentences would be a developmental warning sign at 4 years.

3. d

The inability to use a spoon would not be considered a warning sign for developmental delay until 18 months of age or after; so, of the choices, 20 months would be the earliest age at which this would be considered a warning sign for Ian. Children are typically still using their hands to eat food at 12 months of age. A spoon could be introduced as early as 15 months of age, and the ability to use the spoon is often acquired by 17 months.

4. b

Two year olds most frequently exhibit parallel or onlooker play. Parallel play is characterized by children mimicking each other's behavior without actively engaging with one another. Preschoolers exhibit associative, dramatic, and interactive play.

5. b

Although toddlers may be physiologically and psychologically ready for toilet training at 18 months of age, they are, on average, able to control daytime bowel and bladder movements by 2 years of age. Since toilet training does not start at a specific age, some children may be ready to begin toilet training at 2.5 years; this age does not, however, represent the median age at which the child achieves daytime control. By 3 years of age, toddlers should be able to control nighttime bowel and bladder control, which usually lags behind daytime control by 1 year.

6. b

Vitamin D is frequently measured but there are no requirements for this test at this age. Children in inner city and impoverished environments are expected to be tested for anemia; thus, hemoglobin/hematocrit and lead poisoning (which is common in this population), in addition to cholesterol (if greater than the 95th percentile) tests, are usually warranted.

7. b

Blood pressure (BP) readings usually become part of a child's physical examination at 3 years of age. Although BP readings may be conducted before the age of 3 years, results are often difficult to isolate; as such, these readings are usually only considered in cases when the child shows signs of underlying renal or cardiovascular disease. BP readings should already be part of a child's physical examination by 4 or 5 years of age.

8. c

Normal visual acuity for a 5-year-old child is usually 20/30. A 5-year-old with a visual acuity of 20/80 or 20/50 is lower than the average visual acuity for this age and, in such cases, the child should be referred to an optometrist or ophthalmologist. Likewise, 20/20 vision is not expected at this stage of development.

9. b

The nurse practitioner should advise the father to bring in his daughter for an evaluation if her stuttering persists for more than 6 months or if she avoids speaking. Because stuttering normally resolves within anywhere from a few weeks to 6 months, bringing a child in for evaluation after 3 months does not allow enough time for the condition to resolve spontaneously. However, if the stuttering persists, waiting up to 9 months or longer may be detrimental to language development as therapy practices should be implemented prior to that point.

10. c

The fact that Leonard still struggles with nighttime bowel and bladder control gives most substantial grounds for concern. On average, daytime bowel and bladder control is acquired by 2 years of age, and nighttime control is acquired within the following year. Toilet training is often completed by 4 years of age. Food jags are common behaviors in toddlers. This behavior is taken on by toddlers to assert their independence, and may be relieved by continuing to offer new foods and encouraging kids to at least taste them. Stutters that present before 6 years of age are not of concern unless the stuttering persists for longer than 6 months or leads to the child avoiding speaking. Lastly, skipping is a motor skill that is generally acquired by age 5, so the fact that Leonard has never skipped is of little concern at this point in his life.

DISCUSSION

Definition

The toddler age is defined as 1 to 3 years of age, whereas the preschool age is considered to last from ages 4 to 5 years.[1]

Focus

Physical

The physical development of toddlers is assessed by measurements of the child's body. These measurements consist of the toddler's length, height, weight, and head circumference, which are taken at each checkup until the toddler is 2 years of age.[1,2]

Cognitive

According to Jean Piaget's theory of cognitive development, the preoperational thinking stage lasts from 2 to 7 years of age.[3] During this stage, children are typically egocentric in their thoughts and communications. One characteristic of childhood egocentrism is the concept of animism, in which the child believes that inanimate objects are alive and have feelings.[4] Moreover, children typically begin to engage in pretend play during the preoperational stage.[3] Around age 4 years, children enter the intuitive thinking substage, which lasts until approximately age 7 years. In this substage, children often learn by asking questions and display centration in their thinking.[5]

Psychosocial

Erik Erikson's theory of psychosocial development categorizes toddlers as entering the autonomy vs. shame and doubt stage, whereas preschoolers enter the initiative vs. guilt stage. During the autonomy vs. shame and doubt stage, toddlers commonly develop a greater sense of personal control which, in turn, promotes confidence.[6] The initiative vs. guilt stage, on the other hand, is usually marked by the child asserting power and control over the world via directing social interactions such as play.[6]

Well Child Checks

Overview

Well Child Checks (WCCs) measure a toddler's health by gathering subjective and objective data. A physical examination commonly measures anthropometrics, including the child's height, weight, and head circumference.[2]

Numerous tools are used in developmental screening, such as the Ages and Stages Questionnaire produced by the American Academy of Pediatrics (AAP) and the Denver Developmental Screening Test, second edition (Denver II). These tools are often used for developmental screening of children 6 years of age and under. Children should receive blood pressure assessments annually, starting at 3 years of age.[7] The AAP also recommends that additional screening for anemia should occur between 1 and 5 years of age.[8] To meet these recommendations, children may be screened for anemia via hematocrit testing. Furthermore, for children who live in high-risk areas such as large, urban cities, the Centers for Disease Control and Prevention (CDC)[9] recommend lead screening with questionnaires. Preschoolers should be screened for tuberculosis with a purified protein derivative test between the ages of 4 and 6 years if they are at risk for the disease. Finally, children should undergo cholesterol screenings at around 10 years of age to assess for cardiovascular risk factors.[10]

Management of toddlers should include the continuation and completion of the primary series of immunizations. The toddler's illnesses should be managed with appropriate supportive care or medications, and the nurse practitioner (NP) should also give health promotion strategies with anticipatory guidance. Moreover, the AAP recommends that the child's first dental screening should ideally occur after the first tooth eruption and no later than age 1.[11]

According to the recommended schedule for WCCs, toddlers should be screened at 12, 15, and 18 months of age. Beginning at 2 years of age, children should be screened annually.[12]

The Interview

Overview

When interviewing a toddler, the NP should be mindful that toddlers are often striving for autonomy. Tantrums are common in toddlers, and major fears emerge during this age as well. The NP should allow children to touch equipment, give choices when possible, and continue progression from a non-invasive exam to an invasive exam. Additionally, the child should be undressed for as little of the exam as possible in order to keep discomfort to a minimum.[1,13]

The Physical Examination: Necessary Elements

Overview

Measurement of the standard growth parameters is essential for assessing a child's normal development.[14] In a physical examination, a toddler's weight and length (i.e., height) should be measured at each visit up to 2 years of age, at which point these measurements should then be taken annually. Body mass index measures the proportion between the child's weight and height, and is the best clinical standard for defining obesity in children older than age 2 years.[15] Furthermore, head circumference is measured during each visit up to 2 years of age. The anterior fontanel usually closes between 12 and 18 months of age; delayed closure may indicate an underlying condition, such as hypothyroidism or Down syndrome.[1,13] Chest circumference, on the other hand, is usually measured in the examination of a newborn, but is not a typical part of subsequent routine examinations for toddlers.[14] A child's chest and head are typically equal until the age of 2 years, after which the chest size usually becomes larger than the head.[16]

In addition to these measurements, the toddler's vital signs should also be measured, including temperature, respiratory and heart rates, and blood pressure.[14] Typical dental development consists of the appearance of primary teeth at 6 months of age and permanent teeth at 6 years of age.[1,13] An eye exam should be performed at each WCC to assess for conditions, such as strabismus, which often appear shortly after birth.[1,13] In an ear examination, the child's tympanic membrane may appear red as a result of crying. Children should be assessed for neck masses. Shotty nodes are normal findings, as are nodes with 1–2 cm enlargement; both typically present post-infection.[17,18] Moreover, children should be assessed for periorbital edema, which is the presenting symptom in nearly all children with nephrotic syndrome.[19]

The NP should conduct a mouth and throat exam to assess for abnormalities. Dental abnormalities, such as cavities, may occur due to lack of fluoride; less commonly, too much fluoride can cause changes in the child's enamel.[20] Fissures at the lip corners may indicate a vitamin deficiency, and mouth breathing may be indicative of allergic rhinitis.[13] Furthermore, a nasal voice may be indicative of enlarged adenoids or tonsils, whereas a raspy voice may be indicative of laryngitis.[21]

Cardiac disorders may be indicated by increased respiratory rate at rest or during sleep, as well as eyelid or orbital edemas. If the child is squatting during play or sleeping in a knee-to-chest position, this may also indicate cardiac disorders.[22] The NP should perform a chest exam, and the point of maximal impulse (PMI) can usually be found near the fourth intercostal space in the midclavicular line; a displaced PMI may indicate a cardiac disorder.[23] Additionally, a lung exam should be performed to assess the pediatric patient's respiratory rate, diaphragm movement, and breath sounds.[24]

Prominent abdomens are often normal in toddlers, and palpation of the abdomen may be helpful in assessing whether or not the prominent abdomen is caused by an underlying complication.[25] A liver edge is palpable 1–2 cm beneath the right costal margin in most children. Labial adhesions are common in prepubertal females, and males may present with undescended testes or phimosis, a condition where the foreskin is too tight to be pulled back from the head of the penis.[26,27] Genu varum (bowed legs) and genu valgum (knock-knees) are both normal musculoskeletal variants in young children.[22] Genu varum, however, often resolves by age 2 years and warrants an orthopedic referral if it persists any longer; genu valgum typically resolves itself by age 7 years.[18] A turned-in foot may indicate femoral anteversion or tibial torsion.[18]

Developmental Monitoring

Motor Skills

The CDC outlines developmental milestones that indicate whether a toddler is developing normally.[28] At 2 years of age, the child should be able to walk up and down steps, run, kick a ball, and build a tower of four or more blocks. At 3 years of age, the child should be able to ride a tricycle and copy a circle. At age 4 years, children typically begin to hop and show the ability to draw a person with at least two body parts. Lastly, at 5 years of age, the child should be able to skip, as well as copy squares and other types of shapes.

Cognitive Development

According to Jean Piaget's theories of cognitive development, the preoperational period lasts from 2 to 7 years of age. During this stage, children display a tendency to understand their environment only through their own point of view, a tendency known as egocentrism. Moreover, children in this stage of development tend to demonstrate animism, which is the belief that inanimate objects are capable of feeling and thinking.[3]

Piaget's preoperational stage can be further divided into the preconceptual substage, which lasts from 2 to 4 years of age, and the intuitive substage, which lasts from 4 to 7 years of age. The preconceptual substage is characterized by the child's inability to understand the properties of classes used to identify objects. During the intuitive stage, on the other hand, children typically develop a more complete understanding of concepts.[29]

Visual acuity is often the best measurement to help determine if a child's vision is developing normally; visual acuity testing should be performed on all children older than 3 years of age. A toddler's visual acuity is about 20/30 and often continues to improve with age.[30] Furthermore, toddlers commonly begin to orient themselves with sound and language development at 2 years of age.[1] The recommended hearing test for children 3 years of age and older is play audiometry, which is similar to pure tone audiometry, except that the child performs specific play actions when he or she hears tones.[31]

By age 2 years, language development typically progresses to the point where the child has at least a 50-word vocabulary, talks constantly, and can follow simple instructions.[1,13,28] The child's vocabulary usually expands to include up to 900 words by 3 years of age, 1,500–1,600 words by 4 years of age, and more than 2,000 words by 5 years of age.[32] Moreover, at age 4 years, the child can understand phrases and simple analogies; by age 5 years, children use sentences regularly and know at least four colors. A tip in remembering meaningful word usage in sentences is recalling that children typically use two words in conjunction by 2 years of age, three words in conjunction by 3 years of age, four words in conjunction by 4 years of age, and five words in conjunction by 5 years of age.[18]

Psychosocial Development

According to Erik Erikson's stages of psychosocial development, the toddler years are characterized by the autonomy vs. shame and doubt stage, which lasts from 2 to 3 years of age. The autonomy versus shame and doubt stage is characterized by the child's development of a sense of independence by gaining personal control.[33] In order to curb aggression and encourage impulse control during this stage, discipline should be introduced. Furthermore, play is a major psychosocial medium during the autonomy vs. shame and doubt stage; toddlers often engage in onlooker and parallel play, and preschoolers often engage in associative, cooperative, dramatic, and physical play.[1,13]

Standardized Testing

Overview

The Bayley Scales of Infant and Toddler Development, third edition (BAYLEY-III), are the gold standard for recognizing and diagnosing developmental delays in infants and toddlers up to 42 months of age. The BAYLEY-III test measures a child's development with separate cognitive, language, motor, social-emotional, and adaptive functioning scales.[34] As mentioned earlier, the Denver II test may be used to screen a child's development up to 6 years of age. Additionally, the Ages and Stages Questionnaire is used to screen children from 4 months to 5 years of age.[35] The Modified Checklist for Autism in Toddlers is also used during this time, and is used to screen children and assess the risk of autism spectrum disorder.[13]

Nutrition/Feeding

As soon as parents begin introducing cow's milk, the bottle should be weaned to reduce the risk of tooth decay.[36] A sippy cup can even begin to be used around 10 months of age to reduce the time needed to wean from the bottle. The use of utensils should also be encouraged, and most toddlers are able to use forks and spoons by 18 months of age.[13] Concerning the toddler's diet, it is important to not force eating, to avoid simple sugar snacks and drinks, and to remember that food jags are common.[18]

Dental Health

According to the AAP, children should receive their first dental exam by 1 year of age.[37] Additionally, brushing is recommended for toddlers twice a day, including before bed.[38]

Sleep

Toddlers require 10–12 hours of sleep per night in addition to a daily afternoon nap.[39] During the toddler age, rituals and consistency at bedtime are necessary.[18] Nightmares, when they occur, generally start between 3 and 6 years of age; children at this age may also experience night terrors, which are episodes of extreme panic.[40] Most children outgrow night terrors as they grow older.[18]

Toilet Training

Toilet training does not start at a specific age, but depends on the toddler's physical and emotional readiness.[41] Usually, children are physiologically and psychologically ready for toilet training between 1.5 and 2.5 years of age. Daytime control of elimination is typically attained by 2 years of age. However, nighttime control often lags behind by approximately one year. Day and night control is typically achieved around 3–4 years of age.[13] Toilet training should not be started during stressful times, and children should be rewarded for all good efforts; a child should never be punished for incontinence.[41,42]

Developmental Warning Signs (see table 6.1)

Stuttering

Overview

Stuttering is defined as abnormal speech patterns marked by the presence of repetitions and pauses in speech, known as dysfluencies.[43] The precise cause of stuttering is unknown, but stuttering in young children is generally believed to be the result of developmental causes.[44] Stuttering is more common among males and has a high familial incidence.[45] The condition typically lasts anywhere from several weeks to 6 months but usually resolves without specialized care. Parents often need considerable reassurance that this is not uncommon and usually resolves spontaneously.[13]

Differential Diagnosis

Stuttering is diagnosed clinically by a speech language pathologist, who assesses factors such as the child's case history, stuttering behaviors, and speech and language abilities.[44] Furthermore, hearing and visual impairment should also be considered in the differential diagnosis.[18]

Management

The NP should recognize the initial presentation of stuttering and encourage the child's parents to be patient; however, health professionals recommend that children be referred if the stutter lasts longer than 6 months, if they are older than 6 years of age and stutter, or if they avoid speaking.[18,44] Stuttering may be treated with methods such as electronic

Table 6.1	Developmental Warning Signs During the Toddler Stage
2 years	Doesn't use 2 word phrases
	Doesn't know what to do with common things (i.e., brush, phone, fork)
	Doesn't copy actions and words
	Doesn't follow simple instruction
	Doesn't walk steadily
	Loses skills he/she once had
3 years	Falls down a lot or has trouble with stairs
	Drools or has very unclear speech
	Can't work simple toys (such as peg boards, simple puzzles, turning handle)
	Doesn't speak in sentences
	Doesn't understand simple instructions
	Doesn't play pretend or make believe
	Doesn't want to play with other children or with toys
	Doesn't make eye contact
	Loses skills he/she once had
4 years	Can't jump in place
	Has trouble scribbling
	Shows no interest in interactive games or make believe
	Ignores other children or doesn't respond to people outside of family
	Resists dressing, sleeping, using toilet
	Can't retell favorite story
	Doesn't follow 3 part commands
	Doesn't understand "same" and "different"
	Doesn't use "me" and "you" correctly
	Speaks unclearly
	Loses skills he/she once had
5 years	Doesn't show a wide range of emotions
	Shows extreme behavior
	Usually withdrawn, inactive
	Easily distracted
	Doesn't respond to people or responds superficially
	Can't tell what's real or make believe
	Doesn't play a variety of games
	Can't give first and last name
	Doesn't use plurals or tenses properly
	Doesn't talk about daily activities or experiences
	Doesn't draw pictures
	Can't brush teeth, wash and dry hands, or get undressed without help
	Loses skills he/she once had

Note. Adapted with permission from Developmental milestones. CDC. http://www.cdc.gov/ncbddd/actearly/milestones/index.html. Published 2014. Accessed April 2015.

devices, controlled fluency, and cognitive behavior therapy.[44,46]

Pervasive Development Disorders (PDD)

Overview

According to the fifth edition of the Diagnostic and Statistical Manual of Mental Disorders (DSM-5), pervasive development disorders (PDDs), also known as autism spectrum disorders, are a collection of disorders distinguished by impaired social interactions and altered reactions to environmental stimuli.[47] Individuals may avoid eye contact or not understand social cues. Repetitive movements and self-abusive behavior is also typical. Autism is the most common pervasive development disorder.[48] Autism is characterized by a marked impaired or abnormal social development, especially in terms of interaction; signs and symptoms may appear as early as infancy.[49] Moreover, autistic children often have a narrowly focused repertoire of interests and activities, and may exhibit language delay.

Unlike autism, Asperger's syndrome (AS) does not commonly present with any clinically significant delays in language acquisition; however, AS overlaps with high-functioning autism in its often severe and sustained impairments in social interaction.[50] Children with AS may exhibit obsessive compulsive tendencies, and may also develop narrow, repetitious patterns of interests, behavior, and activities.[51]

Rett's disorder (RTT) is a neurologic disorder that causes developmental reversals and occurs exclusively in females.[52] RTT is characterized by a clear and specific pattern of neurodegenerative developmental regression after a 5-month period of normal functioning and growth. After this period of normal development, there is commonly a lack of gain in developmental milestones, as well as loss of skills previously mastered, such as speech and hand skills. Typically, the first stage of the onset of RTT is a developmental arrest in which signs and symptoms, such as hypertonicity, become evident.[53] Delayed head growth is also a common finding and is often the first sign that a child has RTT. Stereotypic hand movements present in almost all patients with RTT, and scoliosis is common and typically increases with age.[54] Additional signs and symptoms may include central nervous system irritability, withdrawal symptoms, and seizures.

Childhood disintegrative disorder (CDD) begins with about two years of normal development, followed by significant regression in multiple areas of functioning. Although the cause of CDD is unknown, the condition may be caused by infections or neurological disorders due to brain insult in utero. Unlike RTT, CDD is overall more common in males, but is more severe in females.[18,55]

Presentation

Although signs and symptoms of PDDs vary depending on the specific disorder, the onset of developmental delay by the age of 3 years is common and is part of the diagnostic criteria.[1,13] Furthermore, the DSM-5 requires six total behaviors from three categories for a PDD diagnosis. These three categories are motor, language, and communication and social.[47] Classic autistic disorder usually appears during the child's first year and almost always manifests by 3 years of age.[56] Autism is characterized by speech and language delays; however, language often develops normally in children with Asperger's syndrome.[57] Autistic children with advanced speech may use speech abnormally and inappropriately. This is known as echolalia, characterized by repeating another person's words mechanically and meaninglessly.[58]

Management

Referral and early screening is of the utmost importance in the management of PDDs.[1,13] The NP may assess the child's behavior with diagnostics, such as the Autism Behavior Checklist, as well as first-stage screening tools, such as the Checklist for Autism in Toddlers and the Modified Checklist for Autism in Toddlers.[59] Treatment of PDDs is individualized, and children should be referred for community resources and family support.

References

1. Kliegman RM, Stanton BF, St. Geme JW III, Schor NF, Behrman RE, eds. *Nelson Textbook of Pediatrics*. Philadelphia, PA: Elsevier Saunders; 2011.

2. Growth charts: Taking your toddler's measurements. Baby Center web site. http://www.babycenter.com/0_growth-charts-taking-your-toddlers-measurements_10870.bc. Accessed April 10, 2015.

3. McLeod S. Preoperational stage. Simply Psychology web site. http://www.simplypsychology.org/preoperational.html. Published 2010. Accessed April 10, 2015.

4. Piaget's stages of cognitive development. In a Nutshell web site. http://www.telacommunications.com/nutshell/stages.htm. Accessed April 10, 2015.

5. Oswalt A. Early childhood cognitive development: Intuitive thought. Gulf Bend Center web site. http://www.gulfbend.org/poc/view_doc.php?type=doc&id=12759&cn=462. Accessed April 10, 2015.

6. Heffner CL. Chapter 3: Section 3: Erikson's stages of psychosocial development. AllPsych web site. http://allpsych.com/psychology101/social_development/#.VSfxCPnF_kU. Accessed April 10, 2015.

7. Riley M, Bluhm B. High blood pressure in children and adolescents. *Am Fam Physician*. 2010; 85(7): 693–700.

8. Dave H, Wayne AS. Childhood hematologic diseases. In: Rodgers GP, Young NS, eds. *The Bethesda Handbook of Clinical Hematology.* 3rd ed. Philadelphia, PA: Wolters Kluwer Health/Lippincott Williams & Wilkins; 2013: 121–136.

9. United States Department of Health and Human Services, Centers for Disease Control and Prevention. What do parents need to know to protect their children? http://www.cdc.gov/nceh/lead/acclpp/blood_lead_levels.htm. Last reviewed October 30, 2012. Last updated June 19, 2014. Accessed April 10, 2015.

10. Physicians recommend all children, ages 9-11, be screened for cholesterol. American Academy of Pediatrics web site. http://www.aap.org/en-us/about-the-aap/aap-press-room/ pages/Physicians-Recommend-all-Children,-Ages-9-11,-Be-Screened-for-Cholesterol.aspx. Published November 14, 2011. Accessed April 10, 2015.

11. Krol DM. Policy statement: Maintaining and improving the oral health of young children. *Pediatrics.* 2014; 134(6): 1224–1229. doi: 10.1542/peds.2014-2984

12. Well-child visits. A.D.A.M. Medical Encyclopedia. http://www.nlm.nih.gov/medlineplus/ency/article/001928.htm. Updated January 27, 2013. Accessed April 10, 2015.

13. Burns CE, Dunn AM, Brady MA, Starr NB, Blosser CG, eds. *Pediatric Primary Care.* 5th ed. Philadelphia, PA: Elsevier Saunders; 2013.

14. Drutz JE. The pediatric physical examination: General principles and standard measurements. In: Basow DS, ed. *UpToDate.* Waltham, MA: UpToDate; 2015. http://www.uptodate.com/contents/the-pediatric-physical-examination-general-principles-and-standard-measurements. Last updated August 13, 2013. Accessed April 10, 2015.

15. Phillips SM, Shulman RJ. Measurement of growth in children. In: Basow DS, ed. *UpToDate.* Waltham, MA: UpToDate; 2015. http://www.uptodate.com/contents/measurement-of-growth-in-children. Last updated February 10, 2014. Accessed April 10, 2015.

16. Increased head circumference. A.D.A.M. Medical Encyclopedia. http://www.nlm.nih.gov/medlineplus/ency/article/003305.htm. Updated May 10, 2013. Accessed April 10, 2015.

17. Drutz JE. The pediatric physical examination: HEENT. In: Basow DS, ed. *UpToDate.* Waltham, MA: UpToDate; 2015. http://www.uptodate.com/contents/the-pediatric-physical-examination-heent. Last updated September 25, 2014. Accessed April 10, 2015.

18. Barkley TW Jr. *Pediatric Primary Care Nurse Practitioner Certification Review/Clinical Update Continuing Education Course.* West Hollywood, CA: Barkley and Associates; 2015.

19. Lane JC. Pediatric nephrotic syndrome clinical presentation. In: Langman CB, ed. Medscape. http://emedicine.medscape.com/article/982920-clinical#showall. Updated October 27, 2014. Accessed April 10, 2015.

20. Fluoride in diet. A.D.A.M. Medical Encyclopedia. http://www.nlm.nih.gov/medlineplus/ency/article/002420.htm. Updated June 14, 2013. Accessed April 10, 2015.

21. Robin S. Laryngitis in toddlers. Global Post web site. http://everydaylife.globalpost.com/laryngitis-toddlers-9754.html. Accessed April 10, 2015.

22. Reuter-Rice K, Bolick B. *Pediatric Acute Care: A Guide for Interprofessional Practice.* Burlington, MA: Jones & Bartlett Learning; 2012.

23. Allen HD, Driscoll DJ, Shaddy RE, Feltes TF, eds. *Moss and Adams' Heart Disease in Infants, Children, and Adolescents: Including the Fetus and Young Adult.* 8th ed. Philadelphia, PA: Wolters Kluwer Health/Lippincott, Williams, & Wilkins; 2012.

24. Draper R. Paediatric examination. Patient web site. http://www.patient.co.uk/doctor/Paediatric-Examination.htm. Last reviewed June 13, 2014. Accessed April 10, 2015.

25. Hutson JM, Beasley SW. *The Surgical Examination of Children.* Berlin, Germany: Springer Science & Business Media; 2012.

26. Nepple KG, Cooper CS, Alagiri M. Labial adhesions. In: Zuckerman AL, ed. Medscape. http://emedicine.medscape.com/article/953412-overview#a0101. Updated July 14, 2014. Accessed April 11, 2015.

27. Phimosis and paraphimosis in children. Boston's Children Hospital web site. http://www.childrenshospital.org/health-topics/conditions/phimosis-and-paraphimosis. Accessed April 11, 2015.

28. United States Department of Health and Human Services, Centers for Disease Control and Prevention. Developmental milestones. http://www.cdc.gov/ncbddd/actearly/milestones. Last updated March 27, 2014. Accessed April 13, 2015.

29. The stages of cognitive development. Jean Piaget web site. http://piaget.weebly.com/stages-of-cognitive-development.html. Accessed April 13, 2015.

30. Coats DK. Visual development and vision assessment in infants and children. In: Basow DS, ed. *UpToDate.* Waltham, MA: UpToDate; 2015. http://www.uptodate.com/contents/visual-development-and-vision-assessment-in-infants-and-children. Last updated December 9, 2014. Accessed April 13, 2015.

31. Hearing assessments for young children. Australian Hearing web site. http://www.hearing.com.au/hearing-assessments-young-children. Published December 28, 2013. Accessed April 13, 2015.

32. Zundel I. Speech and language development from birth to age five. EduGuide web site. http://www.eduguide.org/article/speech-and-language-development-from-birth-to-age-five. Accessed April 13, 2015.

33. Erikson's stages of development. Learning Theories web site. http://www.learning-theories.com/eriksons-stages-of-development.html. Accessed April 13, 2015.

34. Weiss LG, Oakland T, Aylward GP, eds. *Bayley-III Clinical Use and Interpretation*. San Diego, CA: Academic Press; 2010.

35, LaRosa A. Developmental and behavioral screening tests in primary care. In: Basow DS, ed. *UpToDate*. Waltham, MA: UpToDate; 2015. http://www.uptodate.com/contents/developmental-and-behavioral-screening-tests-in-primary-care. Last updated September 2, 2014. Accessed April 13, 2015.

36. Weaning from the bottle. American Academy of Pediatrics web site. http://www.aap.org/en-us/about-the-aap/aap-press-room/aap-press-room-media-center/Pages/Weaning-from-the-Bottle.aspx. Accessed April 13, 2015.

37. Your child's age 1 dental visit. Palm Valley Pediatric Dentistry web site. http://www.palmvalleypediatricdentistry.com/index.php/about-us/item/76-your-child-s-age-1-dental-visit. Accessed April 13, 2015.

38. Caring for your toddler's teeth. Baby Centre web site. http://www.babycentre.co.uk/a539851/caring-for-your-toddlers-teeth. Last reviewed July 2012. Accessed April 13, 2015.

39. Toddler sleep: What to expect. Raising Children Network web site. http://raisingchildren.net.au/articles/toddlers_sleep_nutshell.html. Last updated February 15, 2012. Accessed April 13, 2015.

40. Cleveland Clinic Staff. Nightmares. Cleveland Clinic web site. http://my.clevelandclinic.org/disorders/sleep_disorders/hic_nightmares.aspx. Last reviewed May 17, 2013. Accessed April 13, 2015.

41. Wilson D. Health promotion of the toddler and family. In: Hockenberry MJ, Wilson D, eds. *Wong's Nursing Care of Infants and Children*. 9th ed. St. Louis, MO: Elsevier Mosby; 2011: 553–584.

42. Zweiback M. Rewards and potty training. Baby Center web site. http://www.babycenter.com/0_rewards-and-potty-training_65029.bc?page=1. Accessed April 13, 2015.

43. Stuttering. American Speech-Language-Hearing Association web site. http://www.asha.org/public/speech/disorders/stuttering.htm. Accessed April 13, 2015.

44. United States Department of Health and Human Services, National Institutes of Health (NIH), National Institute on Deafness and Other Communication Disorders. Stuttering. http://www.nidcd.nih.gov/health/voice/pages/stutter.aspx. Updated March 2010. Accessed April 13, 2015.

45. Carter J, Musher K. Etiology of speech and language disorders in children. In: Basow DS, ed. *UpToDate*. Waltham, MA: UpToDate; 2015. http://www.uptodate.com/contents/etiology-of-speech-and-language-disorders-in-children. Last updated April 1, 2015. Accessed April 13, 2015.

46. Mayo Clinic Staff. Stuttering. Mayo Clinic web site. http://www.mayoclinic.org/diseases-conditions/stuttering/basics/definition/CON-20032854. Updated August 20, 2014. Accessed April 13, 2015.

47. American Psychiatric Association. *Diagnostic and statistical manual of mental disorders: DSM-5*. Washington, D.C: American Psychiatric Association; 2013.

48. American Psychiatric Association. Autism spectrum disorder. American Psychiatric Association web site. http://www.dsm5.org/Documents/Autism%20Spectrum%20Disorder%20Fact%20Sheet.pdf. Published 2013. Accessed April 13, 2015.

49. United States Department of Health and Human Services, NIH, National Institute of Neurologic Disorders and Stroke (NINDS). Autism fact sheet. http://www.ninds.nih.gov/disorders/autism/detail_autism.htm. Last updated November 6, 2014. Accessed April 13, 2015.

50. Brasic JR. Asperger syndrome. In: Pataki C, ed. Medscape. http://emedicine.medscape.com/article/912296-overview. Updated March 26, 2014. Accessed April 13, 2015.

51. United States Department of Health and Human Services, NIH, NINDS. Asperger syndrome fact sheet. http://www.ninds.nih.gov/disorders/asperger/detail_asperger.htm. Last updated November 6, 2014. Accessed April 13, 2015.

52. Rett syndrome. Penn State Hershey web site. http://pennstatehershey.adam.com/content.aspx?productId=117&pid=1&gid=001536. Reviewed November 12, 2012. Accessed April 13, 2015.

53. Bernstein BE, Glaze DG. Rett syndrome. In: Pataki C, ed. Medscape. http://emedicine.medscape.com/article/916377-overview. Updated January 5, 2015. Accessed April 13, 2015.

54. Schultz RJ, Glaze DG. Rett syndrome. In: Basow DS, ed. *UpToDate*. Waltham, MA: UpToDate; 2015. http://www.uptodate.com/contents/rett-syndrome. Last updated October 22, 2013. Accessed April 13, 2015.

55. Childhood disintegrative disorder. Autism Program at Yale web site. http://medicine.yale.edu/childstudy/autism/information/cdd.aspx. Accessed April 13, 2015.

56. Autism spectrum disorders (ASD). In: Porter RS, Kaplan JL, eds. The Merck Manual Online. http://www.merckmanuals.com/professional/pediatrics/learning_and_developmental_disorders/autism_spectrum_disorders_asd.html. Last reviewed March 2013. Accessed April 13, 2015.

57. Chiu S, Hagerman RJ. Pervasive developmental disorder. In: Pataki C, ed. Medscape. http://emedicine.medscape.com/article/914683-overview. Updated December 12, 2013. Accessed April 13, 2015.

58. Heffner GJ. Echolalia – repetitive speech. Synapse web site. http://www.autism-help.org/communication-echolalia-autism.htm. Accessed April 13, 2015.

59. Bridgemohan C. Autism spectrum disorder: Screening tools. In: Basow DS, ed. *UpToDate*. Waltham, MA: UpToDate; 2015. http://www.uptodate.com/contents/autism-spectrum-disorder-screening-tools. Last updated April 9, 2014. Accessed April 13, 2015.

Chapter 7
School Age Health and Issues

1. Jack, age 12, is diagnosed with attention deficit hyperactivity disorder (ADHD). Which of the following is most strongly recommended regarding Jack's medication regimen?

   a. There should be a drug holiday at nighttime during the week.

   b. There should be a drug holiday on the weekends.

   c. There should be a drug holiday during holiday breaks from school.

   d. There should be no drug holiday in the course of treatment.

2. Jerome, an 11-year-old, wakes up every morning at 6 a.m. At what time should he go to bed in order to get the minimum recommended amount of sleep for his age?

   a. 8 p.m.

   b. 9 p.m.

   c. 10 p.m.

   d. 11 p.m.

3. A 7-year-old child arrives at your practice with a radial fracture and bruising around the lower arm. When asked how he received the fracture, the child says he fell while riding his bike earlier that day. Suspecting abuse, you decide to undertake a more thorough examination. All of the following signs would increase your concern of child abuse <u>except</u>:

   a. The child appears shy with a limited vocabulary.

   b. Closer examination of the lower arm reveals thin, finger-like bruises.

   c. You learn that the child exhibits poor academic performance.

   d. You note that the child has 'fallen off his bike' before and presented with a slight concussion.

4. According to Erik Erikson, the industry vs. inferiority stage occurs during school age. Which of the following would Piaget expect for appropriate cognitive development during this stage?

   a. Being active, energetic, and curious

   b. Magical thinking

   c. Understanding the concept of space

   d. Seeking rewards and approval

5. Which of the following is <u>not</u> a developmental warning sign in younger school age children?

   a. Lack of social interaction

   b. Not paying attention in class

   c. Worrying about the opinions of peers

   d. Dropping in test score performance

6. Between what ages should typical pediatric patients first receive a purified protein derivative test for tuberculosis?

    a. Two to 4 years

    b. Four to 6 years

    c. Six to 8 years

    d. Eight to 10 years

7. Which of the following is thought to be a predisposing psychosocial factor for attention deficit hyperactivity disorder?

    a. Family history of alcoholism

    b. Near-death experience from perinatal asphyxia

    c. Depression

    d. Current lack of friends

8. A parent wants to know when the best time is to give the medication being prescribed for attention deficit hyperactivity disorder. Your instructions are based on your knowledge that the earliest onset of action after the ingestion of methylphenidate in children is usually:

    a. 15 minutes

    b. 30 minutes

    c. 45 minutes

    d. 90 minutes

9. What are the last permanent teeth to fully erupt during development?

    a. Bicuspids

    b. Molars

    c. Incisors

    d. Canines

10. All of the following are school age fears the nurse practitioner should expect when interviewing a child <u>except</u>:

    a. Pain

    b. Death

    c. Isolation

    d. Loss of control

RATIONALES

1. d

It is recommended that children do not take drug holidays from their attention deficit hyperactivity disorder (ADHD) medication. Although some parents and practitioners of patients with ADHD encourage drug holidays on nights, weekends, and school breaks, this is typically based on the belief that continuous medication use will lead to dependency or significant adverse effects, for which there is no evidence.

2. c

School age children are recommended to get at least 8 hours of sleep, with a maximum of 11 hours of sleep per night; therefore, a child who wakes up at 6 a.m. should go to sleep at 10 p.m. to receive the minimum recommended amount of sleep. If he goes to bed at 8 p.m. or 9 p.m., the child would receive 10 and 9 hours of sleep, respectively; while designating the recommended amount of sleep, these answer choices do not refer to the minimum recommended amount of sleep. On the other hand, going to bed at 11 p.m. would only give him 7 hours of sleep, which would be the proper amount of sleep for an adult because adults require 7–8 hours of sleep; this amount of sleep, however, is not sufficient for a school age child.

3. c

Although notable changes in school performance and attendance may indicate possible child abuse, poor academic performance in itself is not sufficient to justify the suspicion of child abuse. Along with the vague and incompatible history ascribed to the injury, all of the other signs strongly indicate abuse. A limited vocabulary and a lack of self-esteem may indicate developmental delays, which may be a result of child abuse. Fractures and bruises in various stages of healing may indicate a delay in seeking care. Soft tissue markings in the shape of a hand, object, or weapon, as well as cigarette burns, may indicate non-accidental trauma or a human source of injury.

4. c

Piaget felt that concrete operational thinking— including understanding the concept of space— marked cognitive development during school age years. Erik Erikson's industry versus inferiority stage, which occurs during school age, is marked by a child becoming active, energetic, and curious. Magical thinking is a preschool trait and should not be dominant during this stage. Although children generally seek rewards and approval, this is not a specific tenet of Piaget's concrete operational thinking stage.

5. c

Putting increased emphasis on the opinions of peers is not a warning sign in school age children; rather, it shows normal psychosocial development because the child is now interested in his or her peers and capable of behaving in a peer environment. Developmental warning signs in younger school age children include poor adjustment to school (e.g., not paying attention in class), failure to work to ability (e.g., dropping in test scores), and either a lack of social interaction or experiencing peer problems. Older school age children may manifest similar signs, such as an inability to make or keep friends, poor school performance, or a disinterest in any extracurricular academic activity.

6. b

The purified protein derivative (PPD) test for tuberculosis (TB) is recommended to be administered only once to pediatric patients between 4 and 6 years of age prior to enrolling in school. This minimizes the chance that any children infected with TB will pass it on to their classmates. Although administration of the PPD test was once recommended for all pediatric patients, recent recommendations have suggested applying the PPD test only to populations at a heightened risk for TB, such as children who were born—or have traveled— outside of the United States, or children who have been exposed to individuals with TB. A range of 2–4 years of age is younger than the recommended age at which a child should receive the PPD test. Likewise, children over 6 years of age will not require the PPD test as a matter of course unless certain risk factors are present, such as low socioeconomic status or residence in an area where TB is prevalent.

7. a

A family history of alcoholism is a predisposing psychosocial factor that may lead to attention deficit hyperactivity disorder (ADHD) in children. Perinatal asphyxia is a medical condition that results from an inadequate intake of oxygen that occurs at birth. Although this factor may predispose a child towards ADHD, perinatal asphyxia is a biological, not psychosocial, influence. Depression is a predisposing psychosocial factor for adolescents with eating disorders. Depression may occur simultaneously with ADHD, but it is not a predisposing factor for ADHD. Lastly, a lack of friends is not considered a common psychosocial influence on ADHD, but it may indicate impaired psychosocial development and may occur as a result of ADHD.

8. b

Behavior changes can be identified in children with attention deficit hyperactivity disorder within approximately 30 minutes after ingestion of central nervous system (CNS) stimulants such as methylphenidate. This is important because the goal is for the drug to be in effect by the time the child is interacting with others at school. CNS stimulants commonly do not produce noticeable behavior changes as early as 15 minutes after ingestion, and these drugs typically show effects before 45 or 90 minutes.

9. b

Molars are the last set of permanent teeth to fully erupt; the first molars will come in around 6 years of age, the third molars will typically erupt somewhere between 17 and 21 years of age. Incisors will erupt between 6 and 8 years of age, with the lower central incisors usually developing first. The canines will erupt between 10 and 12 years of age, as will the bicuspids, or premolars.

10. c

Of the choices, it is not necessarily expected that a nurse practitioner (NP) should consider fear of isolation when interviewing a child. Although school age children may have specific fears of the dark or fears of parental separation, there does not tend to be a generalized fear of isolation. The NP should be mindful when interviewing a child that school age children are likely to fear pain, loss of control over personal circumstances or environment, and death.

DISCUSSION

Definition

School age is defined as 6 to 12 years of age.[1]

Focus

Physical

According to Freud's stages of psychosexual development, the latency stage lasts from ages 6 to 12. This stage is marked by repression of sexual urges, as children play mostly with peers of the same sex.[2]

Cognitive

According to Jean Piaget's stages of cognitive development, school age children enter the concrete thinking stage at approximately age 7. During this stage, which lasts until about 11 years of age, children become more organized and rational in their thinking. They become better at conservation tasks and understanding the quantity of something may remain constant even if its appearance changes.[3]

Psychosocial

According to Erik Erikson's stages of psychosocial development, children ages 6 to 12 go through the industry vs. inferiority stage. Children in this stage show a desire to please adults and become capable of performing more complex tasks.[4]

Well Child Checks

Overview

School age children should receive a Well Child Check (WCC) annually.[5] These check-ups measure a child's health by collecting both objective and subjective data. Subjective data in a WCC includes assessing the child for elimination disorders, such as constipation and enuresis, and observing developmental behaviors, such as daily activities and family relationships. Subjective data also includes risk factors and behaviors, such as the use of alcohol, tobacco, and caffeine.[1] Objective data can be gathered from the physical examination.

Immunizations are an important part of a WCC and one of the most successful ways of preventing diseases in children.[5,6] A second dose of the measles, mumps, rubella vaccine is recommended between the ages of 4 and 6 years prior to school entry. Children aged 11 and 12 years should receive a tetanus, diphtheria, pertussis vaccine; human papillomavirus vaccine; and meningococcal conjugate vaccine.[6] A school age child's WCC should also include a discussion of illness management with medications and health promotion strategies. If necessary, the NP should give anticipatory guidance. It is also recommended that pediatric patients receive a dental assessment and cleanings every 6 months.[7]

The Interview

Overview

Measures that can help the nurse practitioner (NP) maximize an interview with a pediatric patient include the use of diagrams, with visual diagrams commonly yielding best results.[1] As previously mentioned, school age children go through the industry vs. inferiority stage; hence, it is important for the NP to remember that children of this age group typically want to be brave. Older school age children should be expected to be more modest than younger children and experience fears related to pain, loss of control, and death.[1]

The Physical Examination: Necessary Elements

Overview

Children should receive a physical examination during each visit. The exam should proceed from head to foot and focus on whether or not the child is reaching normal developmental milestones.[8,9] The child's height and weight should be plotted on standard growth charts.[8] During the school age period, the child's rapid physical growth and development can be expected to level off. The average weight increase of school age children is 5–7 lb per year, and the average height increase is 2–3 inches per year. The average 10-year-old child is 70 lb and 52–56 inches tall; females typically reach peak height velocity at ages 11 and 12 years of age, prior to menarche.[1] It is also important to note the child's body mass index (BMI) in order to diagnose and prevent obesity.[9] Children with a BMI at the 80th percentile are at risk for becoming overweight; obesity is indicated by a BMI over the 95th percentile.[10]

The school age child's vital signs should be measured at each visit; as children get older, pulse and respiration rate decrease and blood pressure increases.[11] Further developments that characterize school age include the eruption of permanent teeth, visual acuity approaching 20/20, and the beginning of breast development in females. Tanner staging can be used to identify precocious puberty, which is puberty in females younger than 8 years of age and boys younger than 9 years of age.[12]

Recommended laboratory screenings in a WCC include a purified protein derivative (PPD) test for tuberculosis; some states require that the test be administered to all children between 4 and 6 years of age prior to school entry. PPD tests should be given annually to children with any of the following risk factors: low socioeconomic status, residence in areas where tuberculosis is prevalent, exposure to tuberculosis, or immigrant status.[1]

According to the American Academy of Pediatrics' (AAP) Bright Futures guidelines, hematocrit assessment is recommended annually during school age because it can be used to detect anemias before the child becomes symptomatic.[13,14]

Lastly, scoliosis is most likely to be identified early by school screening. School screening typically involves use of the Adam's Forward Bend Test or instruments such as a scoliometer. If scoliosis is indicated, radiography may be used in a clinical setting to further assess the degree of curvature.[1,15]

Developmental Monitoring

Motor Skills

School age children's motor skills typically become well developed, with a corresponding increase in muscle strength. Hand dominance can be expected to appear by 5 years of age.[16]

Cognitive Development

According to Erikson's industry vs. inferiority stage, school age children begin to develop a sense of pride in their accomplishments.[17] School age children also go through Piaget's concrete operational thinking stage, during which they develop logical thought and acquire new knowledge.[3]

The language of school age children becomes fluid and descriptive. Also, thought processes expand so that children of this age become capable of reversibility, can grasp the concept of conservation, and can classify objects based upon one characteristic. School age children also begin applying concepts of time and money, develop an understanding of the concept of space, become capable of deductive reasoning, and master the concept of cause and effect.[1]

Psychosocial Development

The psychosocial development of school age children expands markedly to include the outside world. Children during this age often feel competent in abilities such as learning and decision-making. School age children also work to develop self-esteem, which is the belief that they are accepted and valued by those who are important to them.[18]

Typically, school age children socialize through playing with others, such as through organized sports, as they become capable of fully interacting and cooperating in a peer environment and become interested in peer groups and clubs. In late school age, peers usually become extremely important, which can lead children to feel pressure to do what they think their peers are doing.[19]

School age children demonstrate responsibility by being proactive to meet needs and become capable of fulfilling household and school responsibilities (e.g., caring for a pet).[20]

Developmental Discussion/Guidance

Consistency is critical when disciplining school age children. Adults should act as role models and should emphasize natural and logical consequences. Parents should expect lying and should confront their children in a positive way when disciplining them.[21] Moreover, children should be assigned regular duties and chores.[20] As children develop language skills, their parents should be encouraged to listen and respond. Parents should reinforce honesty and respect their child's need for privacy. Lastly, the AAP recommends that children should be limited to less than 2 hours per day of screen time, which includes television programming, internet activity, video games, and all other digital media.[22]

Nutrition/Feeding

A school age child's diet should conform to the current food recommendations under the MyPlate guidelines. Foods that are high in calories and low in nutrients should be minimized. Also, weight is expected to increase at a steady pace according to height, although height velocity normally decreases prior to prepubertal growth spurts.[23]

Dental Health

School age children should learn to floss and should be encouraged to brush their teeth after meals and before bed. Children should receive a dental cleaning every 6 months, and sealants should be placed on the child's premolars and molars as soon as they come in.[24]

Injury Prevention

To help prevent injuries and other health consequences, communicate with school age children regarding tobacco, drugs, alcohol abuse, and the use of safety devices, such as helmets and seatbelts.[25]

Sexuality

Females should be prepared for menstruation, and males should be prepared for hormonal and bodily changes. Because school age children tend to display an increased curiosity towards sex, communication about sexually transmitted infections should be established, especially regarding HIV and AIDS. Moreover, it is vital for parents to give accurate information about sexual intercourse to ensure the child develops healthy sexuality.[26]

Sleep

According to the National Sleep Foundation, school age children should sleep approximately 10–11 hours per night.[27] The occurrence of nightmares typically peaks during preschool age and decreases during school age.[28]

Developmental Warning Signs

For younger children of school age, developmental warning signs include behaviors that interfere with social interaction and school performance.[29] Frequent illnesses that require a child to stay home from school may indicate a chronic condition.[30] In older school age children, warning signs may include reversion to shy or passive roles.[31] Additional developmental warning signs in older school age children include destructive behavior as a means of self-expression, a lack of interest in any extra academic activity, and poor school performance that leaves the child feeling "left behind."[1]

Obesity

Overview

Obesity is a condition in which a person's body has excess fat because of an imbalance between caloric intake and expenditure.[32] Obesity is determined primarily by a patient's BMI. The BMI does not directly measure body fat, however. It may overestimate adiposity in a child with increased muscle mass, or underestimate adiposity in a child with reduced muscle mass. Pediatric patients are considered overweight when their BMI is at or greater than the 85th percentile.[33] Patients are considered obese when their BMI is at, or greater than, the 95th percentile for their age and gender.[10] Increasing BMI is also a problem. A patient whose BMI is below the 85th percentile but is increasing more than three to four units per year and begins to cross percentile lines is at risk of becoming overweight.[33]

Usually, obesity is caused by a combination of genetic, physiologic, and environmental factors.[1] Environmental factors responsible for almost all cases of obesity include an inactive or sedentary lifestyle combined with a high caloric intake that is greater than the patient's needs.[10] As a result, the patient's body stores unused calories as fat.[34] Certain unhealthy eating habits contribute to weight gain, such as high-fat or high-carbohydrate diets, or the use of food for comfort or control.[1] Obesity can also sometimes be caused by genetic disorders such as Prader-Willi syndrome, or by physical disorders of decreased energy expenditure.[35] Preliminary evidence suggests that viruses and toxins also contribute to childhood obesity. Other environmental factors (e.g., sugar-sweetened beverages, television use, video game use) have been associated with childhood obesity.[36]

Differential Diagnosis

Differential diagnoses of obesity include endocrine diseases and genetic conditions.[1] Certain people with mesomorphic body states may have elevated BMIs as a result of increased muscle mass, rather than fat.[37] Certain types of medications, such as antipsychotics, are also known to produce obesity as a side effect.[1]

Workup

The goal of the evaluation is to identify treatable causes of the patient's obesity and any comorbidities.[33] The NP should begin by taking the patient's history. In order to distinguish between obesity due to overfeeding and obesity due to genetic causes, the age of onset of overweight status should be determined. The patient's eating patterns should also be assessed. The NP should note who feeds the child, what the child eats, and how frequently the child eats.[33] An activity history should also be taken. The NP should note the amount and type of the child's play time, physical exercise, after school activities, and screen time.[36] Medications should also be reviewed, especially weight-promoting medications.[33] A psychosocial history should be taken to assess for depression, school problems, or tobacco use. An overweight parent increases the likelihood of an overweight child becoming an overweight adult. For this reason, a family history is also important.[33]

In addition to taking the patient history, obese patients may undergo other diagnostic studies to rule out physical causes and determine potential complications. The NP should review the patient's body systems to probe for evidence of comorbidities or underlying etiologies, such as type 2 diabetes mellitus, sleep apnea, polycystic ovary syndrome, or vitamin D deficiency.[33]

Management

The safest way for obese patients to lose weight is through a combination of healthy eating and an active lifestyle.[34] The goal for preventative treatment in younger children is to stabilize weight through nutritional planning and increased activity; this will result in compensation through linear growth.[38,39] Patients with a higher degree of obesity may require gradual weight loss. Structured diets are not recommended, but the NP should focus on establishing healthy eating behaviors in the pediatric patient.[33]

Patients should also reduce sedentary activities and minimize screen time. Both the patient and the family should increase levels of physical activity. Young children can increase outdoor play time. Older children may want to participate in structured physical activities.[38,39]

In addition to anticipatory guidance, the NP should treat underlying physical causes and refer the patient for counseling if psychosocial issues are contributing to obesity.[1,40]

Child Abuse and Neglect

Overview

Child abuse is an umbrella term used to describe acts of omission or commission, including emotional, physical, and sexual acts, that pose a clear risk to the development and health of the child.[41] Of these types of acts, the most common type of child abuse is neglect.[42]

Child abuse is believed to occur relatively frequently.[42] A 2011 study estimated that approximately four children die daily in the United States due to child abuse, and the actual number is probably higher due to underreporting.[43] Many abusers are parents. Child abuse amongst Native Americans and African Americans reaches twice the national average of reported incidence.[1] Child abusers may display various personality traits, but these characteristics can generally be traced back to "a breakdown of impulse control."[44] Often, child abusers are former victims themselves and have psychiatric, cognitive, and emotional impairments.[1]

Presentation

When a child presents with injuries, the NP should obtain a detailed history to determine the underlying cause.[45] Obtaining the patient's history is particularly important because adults may bring injured children to the emergency room with explanations that are vague, strange, or incompatible with the injuries.[42] Injuries indicative of child abuse may include soft tissue markings with an outline of an object, weapon, cigarette burn, or hand.[44] Delay in seeking care is suspicious of abuse and may result in bruises and fractures in various stages of healing.[1]

In addition to assessing the child's physical signs and symptoms, the NP should evaluate whether the child's physical and developmental needs are being met. Children with developmental delays have historically had increased rates of abuse and neglect.[1,46] Because unusual parent-child interaction is characteristic of child abuse, the NP should carefully note interactions between the child and members of the child's family.[45]

Differential Diagnosis

Because accidental injuries often occur during childhood, the NP should obtain a history and conduct a physical examination to determine the cause of the child's injuries.[46] Differential diagnoses may include homeopathic or cultural practices. The NP should also consider underlying diseases such as coagulation disorders.[47]

Workup

Diagnostic studies and laboratory tests for an abused child are determined by the child's history and physical examination findings.[48] A coagulation profile is recommended for children who present with bruising and should include a complete blood count, platelet count, prothrombin time, and partial thromboplastin time.[45,49] Serum calcium, alkaline phosphatase, and phosphorus levels may be measured if bone disease is suspected.[45]

During the physical examination, the NP should rule out other conditions that may cause similar symptoms. For example, osteogenesis imperfecta may present with findings similar to those of abused children.[42] A local radiological evaluation is recommended for children who demonstrate bony tenderness or limited range of motion on examination. A skeletal survey is recommended for children with soft tissue findings who are either nonverbal or incapable of giving a clear history.[1] Computed tomography (CT) and magnetic resonance imaging scans are used to detect intracranial injuries; CT scans may also be useful in detecting abdominal trauma.[45,49] Ultrasonography is useful if visceral injuries are suspected.[1] A home assessment may also be requested by the NP, with social services or other local authorities evaluating whether the patient's home is a dangerous environment or not.

Management

In cases of child abuse, care should be aimed at ensuring the child's safety and addressing urgent medical needs. Parents or caregivers may require some type of counseling or intervention as well.[42,44] NPs are required to report suspected child abuse in all 50 states.[50]

Attention Deficit Hyperactivity Disorder (ADHD)

Overview

Attention deficit hyperactivity disorder (ADHD) is a chronic neurodevelopmental disorder that most commonly manifests in school age children.[51] The onset of ADHD is usually no later than 7 years of age, and the peak age of diagnosis is between 8 and 10 years of age.[52,53] Although it is generally acknowledged that ADHD is more common in boys than in girls, the estimated prevalence of ADHD varies depending on the diagnostic criteria and the populations studied.[54] Moreover, ADHD is often overdiagnosed, as some signs and symptoms overlap with other conditions, such as anxiety, depression, and learning disabilities.[53,55]

Patients with ADHD are often overactive and unable to focus or control their behavior.[56] Because of these behavioral inhibitions, the child's developing knowledge of how to self-regulate behaviors is disrupted, and behaviors that are appropriate only for young children continue into school age and adolescence. These behaviors may include inattention, distractibility, impulsivity, and hyperactivity.[55]

The pathology of ADHD is unclear, and there is no single cause responsible for the condition.[52,53] Genetics may play a role in the development of ADHD; there is a noted frequency of the condition among family members.[54] Prenatal exposure to tobacco, alcohol, or cocaine is also a risk factor.[53] Perinatal factors of ADHD include prematurity, prolonged labor, perinatal asphyxia, and signs of fetal distress. Postnatal factors include cerebral palsy, epilepsy, and central nervous system (CNS) trauma or infections.[1]

Table 7.1	Clinical Manifestations of Core Signs/Symptoms of ADHD	
Inattention	**Impulsivity**	**Hyperactivity**
Makes careless mistakes	Difficulties awaiting one's turn	Fidgetiness
Fails to pay attention to detail	Frequently blurts out answers	Difficulty remaining seated
Easily distracted	Interrupts or intrudes on others	Difficulty playing quietly
Difficulty concentrating long enough to complete task		Subjective feelings of restlessness
Difficulty following instructions		Difficulty with social relations
Difficulty organizing tasks and activities		Low frustration tolerance

In addition to these risk factors, environmental influences such as lead are also thought to play a role in the development of the condition.[57] ADHD may also be caused by psychosocial influences, such as disorganized or chaotic environments, child abuse or neglect, a family history of alcoholism, hysterical or sociopathic behaviors, and developmental learning disorders.[1]

Presentation

The fifth edition of the Diagnostic and Statistical Manual of Mental Disorders (DSM-5) classifies the symptoms of ADHD into two categories for diagnosis: (a) inattention, and (b) hyperactivity and impulsivity.[58] To confirm a diagnosis of ADHD in children, at least six symptoms from either category or a combination of both categories must be present.[58] These symptoms must present for at least 6 months to a degree that is inconsistent with normal development and functioning, and must interfere with the child's functioning in at least two settings, such as home and school.[52] Most children are diagnosed with a combination of both types of ADHD.[57]

Comorbid psychiatric disorders are common in children with ADHD.[54] These disorders include learning disabilities, anxiety, depression, oppositional defiant disorder, and conduct disorder.[59]

Differential Diagnosis

Differential diagnoses of ADHD include sensory impairment, age-appropriate activities, and situational anxiety.[1] Other disorders that should be ruled out include bipolar affective disorders, depression, and sleep disorders, among others.[52] It is important to accurately identify other possible causes of the child's signs and symptoms to avoid overdiagnosis of ADHD and provide accurate treatment.[53]

Workup

Diagnosis is usually made on the basis of the child's pattern of symptoms rather than any one test; the NP should determine whether these symptoms occur in several settings or only in one place.[56,57] Additional factors that should be considered in the child's medical evaluation include family history and the child's prenatal and perinatal history.[60] A variety of standardized tests and questionnaires may be used to assess the child's symptoms, including the Conners' Parent and Teacher Rating Scale, the Achenbach Child Behavior Checklist, and the Vanderbilt Assessment Tool.[61,62,63]

Management

Management of ADHD is multi-modal. The condition is best treated with a combination of medication and behavioral therapy.[64] Treating a child with ADHD likewise requires cooperation between the NP and the child's parents.[56]

Stimulants are the most commonly used medications for ADHD management and are considered to be highly effective.[52,56] CNS stimulants increase the availability of neurotransmitters to strengthen focus and attention.[1] The most widely used stimulant preparations for ADHD management are methylphenidate and amphetamines. Methylphenidate remains relatively consistent across its various brands, which include Ritalin, Concerta, Metadate, and Focalin; amphetamines, on the other hand, come in a variety of formulations, such as lisdexamfetamine (Vyvanse), dextroamphetamine (Dexedrine), and amphetamine/dextroamphetamine (Adderall, Adderall XR).[53,65]

The prescribing principle of ADHD medications is to start low and titrate up slowly.[1] The NP should titrate up at weekly intervals and receive feedback from teachers and parents in order to assess effectiveness. The usual dose of medications is 0.3–0.7 mg/kg, starting with 5–10 mg in the morning. If medications are not effective, the NP should increase dosage in increments of 2.5–5 mg per week until an effective level is reached. Changes in behavior can typically be identified within 30–90 minutes of ingestion.[66]

Short-acting preparations of stimulants are often the initial treatment for children younger than 6 years of age; however, these medications often require re-dosing multiple times per day.[67,68] Long-acting preparations generally last 10–12 hours and are recommended for children who require a duration of action longer than 4 hours.[67]

Because medications can affect children differently, the NP may need to try multiple stimulants, switching between methylphenidate and amphetamines if necessary, before finding the most effective medication with the least side effects.[64] The NP should also avoid evening doses to minimize insomnia.[1]

Pharmacologic treatment of ADHD is contraindicated in children with conditions such as heart disease, hypertension, or glaucoma.[69] Psychiatric contraindications include marked anxiety and increased risk for suicide.[1] Children with comorbid depression should undergo psychiatric evaluation and be assessed by subsequent primary care providers for potential multi-drug interactions. Common side effects of ADHD medications include stomach aches, headaches, anorexia, weight loss, tachycardia, tics, and sleep disturbances. There may also be a temporary decrease in the child's rate of growth and development, although the results of studies on this are not consistent.[53]

Besides medications, children with ADHD benefit from non-pharmacologic measures such as behavior treatment, parent education, and support.[64] In order to assess the patient's symptoms and need for medication, drug holidays may be implemented on occasions such as school breaks or summer vacations.[68]

References

1. Barkley TW Jr. *Pediatric Primary Care Nurse Practitioner Certification Review/Clinical Update Continuing Education Course*. West Hollywood, CA: Barkley and Associates; 2015.

2. Heffner CL. Freud's stages of psychosexual development. AllPsych Web site. http://allpsych.com/psychology101/sexual_development.html. Last updated August 21, 2014. Accessed April 27, 2015.

3. McLeod S. Concrete operational stage. Simply Psychology Web site. http://www.simplypsychology.org/concrete-operational.html. Published 2010. Accessed April 27, 2015.

4. McLeod S. Erik Erikson. Simply Psychology Web site. http://www.simplypsychology.org/Erik-Erikson.html. Published 2008. Updated 2015. Accessed April 27, 2015.

5. American Academy of Pediatrics. Well-child care: A checkup for success. Healthy Children Web site. http://www.healthychildren.org/English/family-life/health-management/pages/Well-Child-Care-A-Check-Up-for-Success.aspx. Last updated August 11, 2014. Accessed April 27, 2015.

6. Drutz JE. Standard immunizations for children and adolescents. In: Basow DS, ed. *UpToDate*. Waltham, MA: UpToDate; 2015. http://www.uptodate.com/contents/standard-immunizations-for-children-and-adolescents. Last updated April 15, 2015. Accessed April 27, 2015.

7. Your child's first dental visit. Cleveland Clinic Children's Web site. https://my.clevelandclinic.org/childrens-hospital/health-info/ages-stages/toddler/hic-your-childs-first-dental-visit. Last reviewed November 23, 2012. Accessed April 27, 2015.

8. Drutz JE. The pediatric physical examination: General principles and standard measurements. In: Basow DS, ed. *UpToDate*. Waltham, MA: UpToDate; 2015. http://www.uptodate.com/contents/the-pediatric-physical-examination-general-principles-and-standard-measurements. Last updated August 13, 2013. Accessed April 27, 2015.

9. Well-child visits. A.D.A.M. Medical Encyclopedia. http://www.nlm.nih.gov/medlineplus/ency/article/001928.htm. Updated January 27, 2013. Accessed April 27, 2015.

10. Klish WJ. Definition; epidemiology; and etiology of obesity in children and adolescents. In: Basow DS, ed. *UpToDate*. Waltham, MA: UpToDate; 2015. http://www.uptodate.com/contents/definition-epidemiology-and-etiology-of-obesity-in-children-and-adolescents. Last updated April 13, 2015. Accessed April 27, 2015.

11. Normal vital signs. School of Health Professions, University of Missouri Health System Web site. https://shp.missouri.edu/pt/pdf/emergency.pdf. Accessed April 27, 2015.

12. Kaplowitz PB. Precocious puberty: Overview. In: Kemp S, ed. Medscape. http://emedicine.medscape.com/article/924002-overview. Updated October 14, 2014. Accessed April 27, 2015.

13. Consolini DM. Health supervision of the well child. In: Porter RS, Kaplan JL, eds. The Merck Manual Online. http://www.merckmanuals.com/professional/pediatrics/health_supervision_of_the_well_child/health_supervision_of_the_well_child.html. Last reviewed April 2014. Accessed April 27, 2015.

14. Minnesota Department of Health, Minnesota Department of Human Services. Child and teen checkups (C&TC) fact sheet. http://www.health.state.mn.us/divs/fh/mch/ctc/factsheets/hgbhct.pdf. Published April 12, 2010. Accessed April 27, 2015.

15. Chowanska J, Kotwicki T, Rosadzinski K, Sliwinski Z. School screening for scoliosis: Can surface topography replace examination with scoliometer? *Scoliosis*. 2012; 7(1): 9. doi: 10.1186/1748-7161-7-9.

16. Brooks A. Physical development in babies and children. Kidspot.com.au Web site. http://www.kidspot.com.au/Development-Development-Physical-development-in-babies-and-children+5367+553+article.htm. Published April 9, 2011. Accessed April 27, 2015.

17. Heffner CL. Erikson's stages of psychosocial development. AllPsych Web site. http://allpsych.com/psychology101/social_development.html. Last updated August 21, 2014. Accessed April 27, 2015.

18. DeBord K. Self-esteem in children. NC State University College of Agriculture and Life Sciences Web site. http://www.ces.ncsu.edu/depts/fcs/pdfs/fcsw_506.pdf. Accessed April 27, 2015.

19. Barker J. Teens and peer pressure. WebMD Web site. http://www.webmd.com/parenting/teenabuse-cough-medicine-9/peer-pressure. Reviewed September 12, 2011. Accessed April 27, 2015.

20. Davis SE, Needlman R. Chores for school aged children. Raising Children Web site. http://raisingchildren.net.au/articles/chores_for_school aged_children.html/context/476. Last updated April 30, 2014. Accessed April 27, 2015.

21. Lehman J. How to deal with lying in children and teens. Empowering Parents Web site. http://www.empoweringparents.com/How-to-Deal-with-Lying-in-Children-and-Teens.php. Accessed April 27, 2015.

22. American Academy of Pediatrics. Managing media: We need a plan. American Academy of Pediatrics Web site. http://www.aap.org/en-us/about-the-aap/aap-press-room/pages/Managing-Media-We-Need-a-Plan.aspx. Published October 28, 2013. Accessed April 27, 2015.

23. Boom JA. Normal growth patterns in infants and prepubertal children. In: Basow DS, ed. *UpToDate*. Waltham, MA: UpToDate; 2015. http://www.uptodate.com/contents/normal-growth-patterns-in-infants-and-prepubertal-children. Last updated April 13, 2015. Accessed April 27, 2015.

24. Drescher S. Dental health: Sealants. WebMD Web site. http://www.webmd.com/oral-health/guide/dental-sealants. Reviewed April 14, 2013. Accessed April 27, 2015.

25. American Academy of Child and Adolescent Psychiatry. Facts for families: Teens: Alcohol and other drugs. American Academy of Child and Adolescent Psychiatry Web site. http://www.aacap.org/App_Themes/AACAP/docs/facts_for_families/03_teens_alcohol_and_other_drugs.pdf. Published July 2013. Accessed April 27, 2015.

26. Mayo Clinic Staff. Sex education: Talking to your teen about sex. Mayo Clinic Web site. http://www.mayoclinic.org/sex-education/art-20044034. Updated July 23, 2014. Accessed April 27, 2015.

27. Children and sleep. National Sleep Foundation Web site. http://www.sleepfoundation.org/article/sleep-topics/children-and-sleep. Accessed April 27, 2015.

28. Lyness D. Nightmares. KidsHealth Web site. http://kidshealth.org/parent/general/sleep/nightmare.html#. Reviewed July 2013. Accessed April 27, 2015.

29. Harris W. Behavioural and developmental paediatrics. In: Harris W. *Examination Paediatrics*. 4th ed. Chatswood, NSW, Australia: Elsevier Churchill Livingstone; 2011: 25–66.

30. Boyse K, Boujaoude L, Laundy J. Children with chronic conditions. University of Michigan Health System Web site. http://www.med.umich.edu/yourchild/topics/chronic.htm. Updated November 2012. Accessed April 27, 2015.

31. Hyson MC, Van Trieste K. Shyness: How to help the shy child and teenager. Child Development Institute Web site. http://childdevelopmentinfo.com/child-psychology/anxiety_disorders_in_children/shy_child. Accessed April 27, 2015.

32. United States Department of Health and Human Services, Centers for Disease Control and Prevention. Childhood obesity facts. http://www.cdc.gov/healthyyouth/obesity/facts.htm. Last updated April 24, 2015. Accessed April 27, 2015.

33. Klish WJ. Clinical evaluation of the obese child and adolescent. In: Basow DS, ed. *UpToDate*. Waltham, MA: UpToDate; 2015. http://www.uptodate.com/contents/clinical-evaluation-of-the-obese-child-and-adolescent?source=search_result&search=clinical+evaluation+of+the+obese+child+and+adolescent&selectedTitle=1~150. Last updated October 9, 2014. Accessed May 11, 2015.

34. Obesity. A.D.A.M. Medical Encyclopedia. http://www.nlm.nih.gov/medlineplus/ency/article/007297.htm. Updated August 17, 2014. Accessed April 27, 2015.

35. Mayo Clinic Staff. Obesity. Mayo Clinic Web site. http://www.mayoclinic.com/health/obesity/DS00314. Updated May 13, 2014. Accessed April 27, 2015.

36. Klish WJ. Definition; epidemiology; and etiology of obesity in children and adolescents. In: Basow DS, ed. *UpToDate*. Waltham, MA: UpToDate; 2015. http://www.uptodate.com/contents/definition-epidemiology-and-etiology-of-obesity-in-children-and-adolescents?source=search_result&search=epidemiology+and+etiology+of+obesity+in+children&selectedTitle=1~150. Last updated April 13, 2015. Accessed May 11, 2015.

37. Hamdy O, Uwaifo GI, Oral EA. Obesity. In: Khardori R, ed. Medscape. http://emedicine.medscape.com/article/123702-overview. Updated February 27, 2015. Accessed April 27, 2015.

38. Skelton JA. Management of childhood obesity in the primary care setting. In: Basow DS, ed. *UpToDate*. Waltham, MA: UpToDate; 2015. http://www.uptodate.com/contents/management-of-childhood-obesity-in-the-primary-care-setting?source=search_result&search=management+of+childhood+obesity+in+primary+care+setting&selectedTitle=1~150. Last updated April 13, 2015. Accessed May 11, 2015.

39. Mayo Clinic Staff. Childhood obesity. Mayo Clinic Web site. http://www.mayoclinic.org/diseases-conditions/childhood-obesity/basics/definition/con-20027428. Accessed May 11, 2015.

40. Schwarz SM. Obesity in children. In: Bhatia J, ed. Medscape. http://emedicine.medscape.com/article/985333-overview. Updated February 27, 2015. Accessed May 11, 2015.

41. Child abuse. A.D.A.M. Medical Encyclopedia. http://www.nlm.nih.gov/medlineplus/childabuse.html. Accessed April 27, 2015.

42. Child abuse – physical. A.D.A.M. Medical Encyclopedia. http://www.nlm.nih.gov/medlineplus/ency/article/001552.htm. Updated November 20, 2014. Accessed April 27, 2015.

43. Mayo Clinic Staff. Child abuse facts and resources. Mayo Clinic Web site. http://www.mayoclinic.org/departments-centers/childrens-center/child-family-advocacy-center/child-abuse-facts-resources. Accessed April 27, 2015.

44. Pekarsky AR. Overview of child maltreatment (child abuse). In: Porter RS, Kaplan JL, eds. The Merck Manual Online. http://www.merckmanuals.com/professional/pediatrics/child_maltreatment/overview_of_child_maltreatment.html?qt=child%20abuse&alt=sh. Last reviewed June 2014. Accessed April 27, 2015.

45. Boos SC, Endom EE. Physical abuse in children: Diagnostic evaluation and management. In: Basow DS, ed. UpToDate. Waltham, MA: UpToDate; 2015. http://www.uptodate.com/contents/physical-abuse-in-children-diagnostic-evaluation-and-management. Last updated July 16, 2014. Accessed April 27, 2015.

46. Giardino AP, Giardino ER, Moles RL. Physical child abuse. In: Pataki C, ed. Medscape. http://emedicine.medscape.com/article/915664-overview. Updated June 30, 2014. Accessed April 27, 2015.

47. Segal M. The differential diagnosis of child abuse. SimulConsult Web site. http://www.simulconsult.com/resources/abuse.html. Accessed April 27, 2015.

48. Moles RL, Asnes AG. Has this child been abused?: Exploring uncertainty in the diagnosis of maltreatment. Pediatr Clin North Am. 2014; 61(5): 1023–1036. doi: 10.1016/j.pcl.2014.06.009

49. Magana J, Kaufhold M. Child abuse. In: Bechtel KA, ed. Medscape. http://emedicine.medscape.com/article/800657-overview. Updated January 22, 2014. Accessed April 27, 2015.

50. United States Department of Health and Human Services, Administration for Children and Families, Children's Bureau, Child Welfare Information Gateway. Reporting child abuse and neglect. https://www.childwelfare.gov/responding/reporting.cfm. Accessed April 27, 2015.

51. Attention deficit/hyperactivity disorder. American Speech-Language-Hearing Association Web site. http://www.asha.org/public/speech/disorders/adhd. Accessed April 27, 2015.

52. Soreff S. Attention deficit hyperactivity disorder. In: Dunayevich E, ed. Medscape. http://emedicine.medscape.com/article/289350-overview. Updated April 13, 2015. Accessed April 27, 2015.

53. Sulkes SB. Attention-deficit/hyperactivity disorder (ADHD, ADD). In: Porter RS, Kaplan JL, eds. The Merck Manual Online. http://www.merckmanuals.com/professional/pediatrics/learning-and-developmental-disorders/attention-deficit-hyperactivity-disorder-adhd-add. Last reviewed March 2013. Accessed April 27, 2015.

54. Krull KR. Attention deficit hyperactivity disorder in children and adolescents: Epidemiology and pathogenesis. In: Basow DS, ed. UpToDate. Waltham, MA: UpToDate; 2015. http://www.uptodate.com/contents/attention-deficit-hyperactivity-disorder-in-children-and-adolescents-epidemiology-and-pathogenesis. Last updated March 27, 2015. Accessed April 27, 2015.

55. United States Department of Health and Human Services, Centers for Disease Control and Prevention. Attention-deficit/hyperactivity disorder (ADHD): Symptoms and diagnosis. http://www.cdc.gov/ncbddd/adhd/diagnosis.html. Last updated September 29, 2014. Last reviewed March 18, 2015. Accessed April 27, 2015.

56. Attention deficit hyperactivity disorder. A.D.A.M. Medical Encyclopedia. http://www.nlm.nih.gov/medlineplus/ency/article/001551.htm. Updated February 24, 2014. Accessed April 27, 2015.

57. United States Department of Health and Human Services, National Institutes of Health, National Institute of Mental Health. Attention deficit hyperactivity disorder (ADHD). http://www.nimh.nih.gov/health/topics/attention-deficit-hyperactivity-disorder-adhd/index.shtml. Accessed April 27, 2015.

58. American Psychiatric Association. DSM-5 Attention deficit/hyperactivity disorder fact sheet. American Psychiatric Association DSM-5 Development Web site. http://www.dsm5.org/documents/adhd%20fact%20sheet.pdf. Published 2013. Accessed April 27, 2015.

59. Wilkes MA, Cobb SM, Spratt EG. Pediatric attention deficit hyperactivity disorder: Differential diagnoses. In: Pataki C, ed. Medscape. http://emedicine.medscape.com/article/912633-differential. Updated December 29, 2014. Accessed April 27, 2015.

60. Krull KR. Attention deficit hyperactivity disorder in children and adolescents: Clinical features and evaluation. In: Basow DS, ed. UpToDate. Waltham, MA: UpToDate; 2015. http://www.uptodate.com/contents/attention-deficit-hyperactivity-disorder-in-children-and-adolescents-clinical-features-and-evaluation. Last updated March 12, 2015. Accessed April 27, 2015.

61. Wilkes MA, Cobb SM, Spratt EG. Pediatric attention deficit hyperactivity disorder: Workup. In: Pataki C, ed. Medscape. http://emedicine.medscape.com/article/912633-workup#aw2aab6b5b3. Updated December 29, 2014. Accessed April 27, 2015.

62. Perlstein D. ADHD testing. In: Shiel WC Jr, ed. eMedicineHealth. http://www.emedicinehealth.com/adhd_testing/article_em.htm. Reviewed November 17, 2014. Accessed April 27, 2015.

63. Bhandari S. ADHD tests. WebMD Web site. http://www.webmd.com/add-adhd/guide/adhd-tests-making-assessment?page=2. Reviewed January 20, 2015. Accessed April 27, 2015.

64. United States Department of Health and Human Services, Centers for Disease Control and Prevention. Attention deficit/hyperactivity disorder: Treatment. http://www.cdc.gov/ncbddd/adhd/treatment.html. Last updated April 1, 2015. Accessed April 27, 2015.

65. Wilkes MA, Cobb SM, Spratt EG. Pediatric attention deficit hyperactivity disorder: Medication. In: Pataki C, ed. Medscape. http://emedicine.medscape.com/article/912633-medication#showall. Updated December 29, 2014. Accessed April 27, 2015.

66. Sub-Committee on Attention-Deficit/Hyperactivity Disorder Steering Committee on Quality Improvement Management. ADHD: clinical practice guideline for the diagnosis, evaluation, and treatment of attention-deficit/hyperactivity disorder in children and adolescents: Implementing the key action statements—an algorithm and explanation for process of care for the evaluation, diagnosis, treatment, and monitoring of ADHD in children and adolescents. *Pediatrics.* 2011; 128:1007–1022.

67. Krull KR. Attention deficit hyperactivity disorder in children and adolescents: Treatment with medications. In: Basow DS, ed. *UpToDate*. Waltham, MA: UpToDate; 2015. http://www.uptodate.com/contents/attention-deficit-hyperactivity-disorder-in-children-and-adolescents-treatment-with-medications. Last updated April 15, 2015. Accessed April 27, 2015.

68. O'Brien JM, Christner JG, Biermann B, et al. Guidelines for clinical care: Attention-deficit hyperactivity disorder. University of Michigan Faculty Group Practice Web site. http://www.med.umich.edu/1info/FHP/practiceguides/adhd/adhd.pdf. Published August 2015. Last updated April 2013. Accessed April 27, 2015.

69. Chayer RP. Basic principles in the pharmacologic management of ADHD. Children's Hospital of Wisconsin Web site. http://www.chw.org/~/media/Files/Medical%20Professionals/Medical%20Care%20Guidelines/ADHD.pdf. Approved March 2013. Accessed April 27, 2015.

Chapter 8
Adolescent Health and Issues

QUESTIONS

1. During a physical exam on a 17-year-old female, you note a sore throat, parotid gland enlargement, and dental erosion. You begin to suspect a possible eating disorder. Which of the following findings would most strongly indicate bulimia nervosa in this patient?

    a. Amenorrhea

    b. Russell's sign

    c. Lanugo

    d. Thinning hair

2. Key immunizations to offer during adolescence include all the following <u>except</u>:

    a. Meningococcal

    b. Measles, mumps, and rubella

    c. Tetanus, diphtheria, and attenuated pertussis

    d. Human papillomavirus

3. As a nurse practitioner, you know that the eating disorder mortality rate is about 10% but that a complication from the eating disorder, and not the eating disorder itself, is frequently listed as the cause of death. Which cause of death is most likely to be listed as the cause of an individual who dies from an eating disorder?

    a. Asphyxia

    b. Organ failure

    c. Anemia

    d. Dehydration

4. A Tanner sexual maturity rating of 3 in a male indicates which of the following?

    a. A penis that is adult in shape and appearance with adult pattern pubic hair

    b. A rough, red scrotum with sparse, fine pubic hair

    c. An elongated penis with darker, curlier pubic hair

    d. Development of glans and rugae on the penis and curly, sparse pubic hair

5. Which type of diet practiced by adolescents warrants the closest monitoring by parents?

    a. Vegetarian

    b. High-protein

    c. Lactose-free

    d. Pescetarian

6. When implementing the Guidelines for Adolescent Preventive Services in a Well Child Check with a 16-year-old female, which piece of information would you be most likely to share with her parent?

    a. She mentions that she is depressed and wonders if life is worth living.

    b. She had unprotected sex with her boyfriend last month and is late for her period.

    c. She has three best girlfriends and they have all started experimenting with marijuana.

    d. She thinks her mother's new boyfriend is "creepy."

7. The acronym SAFETEENS provides a checklist of preventive care topics for nurse practitioners. Going by this checklist, which of the following is not a significant concern in preventive care?

a. Sexual abstinence

b. Suicide

c. School performance

d. Involvement in hobbies

8. After which Tanner stage do males usually begin spermarche or nocturnal emissions?

a. Stage 1

b. Stage 2

c. Stage 3

d. Stage 4

9. Which of the following are two psychosocial developments that are associated primarily with adolescence?

a. Sense of identity and narcissism

b. Narcissism and desire to please adult figures

c. Sense of identity and development of self-esteem

d. Development of self-esteem and desire to please adult figures

10. Which test or exam should be performed at every female adolescent Well Child Check regardless of personal or family medical history?

a. Scoliosis assessment

b. Blood pressure

c. Liver function tests

d. A pelvic exam

RATIONALES

1. b

Russell's sign, characterized by bruises on the knuckles that result from self-induced vomiting, is often an indicator of bulimia. Amenorrhea can indicate either anorexia nervosa or bulimia nervosa. Thinning hair is commonly a sign of anorexia nervosa. Lanugo is more typical of anorexia than bulimia.

2. b

The Centers for Disease Control and Prevention recommend that children 12–15 months old receive the measles, mumps, and rubella vaccination. No booster shot is necessary during adolescence. Children 15–18 months old should receive a diphtheria, tetanus, and pertussis vaccination, and then a booster vaccination should be given to children 11–12 years old. The meningococcal conjugate vaccine and human papillomavirus vaccine should also be administered to children 11–12 years old.

3. b

Organ failure is the most common cause of death in eating disorders, producing as a result of severe malnutrition; cardiac complications, such as arrhythmias and loss of muscle are common, but eating disorders may also result in liver damage and multi-organ failure. Suicide is also a common cause of death in individuals with an eating disorder. Although eating disorders may result in anemia and dehydration, patients are not likely to die from anemia or dehydration. Although asphyxia may result due to improper vomiting, it is rarely the cause of death.

4. c

An elongated penis is a 3 on the Tanner stage of genital development, and darker, curlier pubic hair is also a 3 on the Tanner stage of pubic hair development; the combined average of these scores indicates a sexual maturity rating of 3. A rough, red scrotum and sparse, fine pubic hair are associated with a 2 under each category. Development of glans, rugae, and pubic hair that is adult in character but not volume is associated with a 4 for each category. A penis that is adult in shape and appearance is associated with a 5 in genital development; whereas adult pattern pubic hair is associated with a 5 in pubic hair development.

5. a

Parents should most closely monitor vegetarian diets in adolescents because vegetarian diets may not provide all nutritional requirements. Alternative sources of protein, fatty acids, calcium, zinc, iron, and vitamins B12 and D may need to be incorporated into the diet. Pescetarian diets may not require the level of strict monitoring that is required with vegetarian diets because fish provide a steady source of protein and fatty acids. High-protein diets can be especially helpful in teenage athletes because strength and endurance training requires extra protein. A lactose-free diet may require calcium-intake monitoring, but otherwise the diet would not require extensive parental monitoring.

6. a

Confidentiality should be assured when implementing the Guidelines for Adolescent Preventive Services, but a nurse practitioner is expected to disclose confidentiality when there is concern about a patient hurting herself or someone else. While recreational drug use and a possible pregnancy may require advisement or medical attention, the nurse practitioner does not need to alert the patient's parent. The patient's relationship with her mom's boyfriend should be explored carefully but does not require divulgence at this stage.

7. d

Although SAFETEENS may cover exercise concerns, involvement in hobbies is not a typical concern of preventive care covered under the auspices of SAFETEENS. SAFETEENS is an acronym for Sexuality, Accidents, Firearms/Violence, Emotions, Toxins, Environment, Exercise, Nutrition, and Shots. Sexual abstinence falls under the Sexuality heading. Suicide falls under Emotions, and school performance is included in Environment.

8. c

Spermarche begins shortly after Tanner stage 3 of genital development. Spermarche or nocturnal emissions do not yet begin at Tanner stages 1 and 2, which are distinguished by the initial development and enlargement of the testes, scrotum, and penis. Tanner stage 4 occurs after spermarche or nocturnal emissions begin.

9. a

The two main psychosocial developments during adolescence are sense of identity and narcissism. Unlike pathological narcissism, adolescent narcissism typically focuses on internal reflection and development of a personal identity. Development of self-esteem and the desire to please adult figures usually also occur but are not as strongly definitive. The period of psychosocial development within younger adolescence is characterized by parent and child conflict, which may become resolved during older adolescence.

10. b

The blood pressure of adolescent females should be measured at every Well Child Check. Scoliosis should be assessed at every visit until 2 years after the patient has reached her peak height velocity. Pelvic exams should be performed if clinically warranted, such as if the patient is sexually active or experiences irregular menses. Liver function tests should be performed if the patient has a history of drug use.

DISCUSSION

Definition

Adolescence is considered the bridge from school age to adulthood, ranging from 12 to 20 years of age. The three transitional periods of adolescence are called early adolescence, from 12 to 14 years of age; middle adolescence, from 15 to 17 years of age; and late adolescence, from 18 to 20 years of age.[1]

Focus

Physical

Adolescence is often marked by the onset of difficult changes. Rapid changes in the reproductive, skeletal, muscular, and cardiovascular systems, along with the development of secondary sexual characteristics, occur. Peak height velocity (PHV), or the period where maximum rate of growth occurs, also happens during adolescence.[2]

Cognitive

Adolescents begin to develop logical thinking during this stage of growth. They develop the ability to understand abstract ideas, such as the ability to comprehend higher-level math concepts, and to establish moral philosophies, including rights and privileges.[3]

Psychosocial

Adolescents typically begin to search for a sense of identity and may demonstrate narcissism during this stage.[3]

Well Child Checks

Overview

The framework for Well Child Checks (WCCs) comes from the Guidelines for Adolescent Preventive Services by the American Medical Association. WCCs measure the growth and development of adolescents through stage appropriate screenings. These screenings involve collecting subjective and objective data and creating a management plan for the patient.[4]

Subjective data often include the adolescent's school performance and attendance. Relationships with family and friends are also taken into account, as well as hobbies and work interests. The patient should also be evaluated on how he or she manages or copes with stress and anger. Any history of, or any present inclination, to commit self-inflicted injury or injury to others should be noted.[5] Inquiries should be made into the adolescent's sexual activities, reproductive and gender issues, and any worries or stressors that he or she may have. The nurse practitioner (NP) should also speak to the parents or caregiver and hear their perspectives on the adolescent's communication and relationship with the family. Strengths and weaknesses, as well as any particular attitudes or behaviors, should be discussed. The NP should also inquire about disciplinary practices within the household and how the adolescent responds to those disciplinary measures.

Objective data includes information obtained via a physical examination and laboratory tests. The physical examination may involve observing the interaction between the parent or caregiver and the adolescent.[5] The NP should evaluate whether or not the parent or caregiver is supportive of the adolescent and allows the adolescent to answer questions. The physical examination may include determining blood pressure readings; body mass index (BMI); scoliosis screenings up until 2 years after PHV is attained; Tanner staging; a clinical breast exam and pelvic exam for females; and instructing male and female patients in self-exams of the breasts and testes, respectively. Laboratory tests may include a hematocrit test to assess for risk of anemia. A liver function test may be ordered if the patient has a history of drug use. A cholesterol screening is indicated at least once between 17 and 21 years of age. Cervical cytology (i.e., Pap smear) is routine for female patients after age 21. Testing for sexually transmitted diseases or infections may be required for patients of all genders who are sexually active or who have a history of sexual abuse.[5]

A management plan should be drafted to reflect both existing concerns and findings of the WCC. This often involves immunizations and a completion of vaccine series, such as the meningococcal vaccine; the vaccine for tetanus, diphtheria, and pertussis (Tdap); and the human papillomavirus (HPV) vaccine. If illness is identified, the plan should include a medication regimen aimed at management and treatment. The plan should incorporate health promotion strategies with anticipatory guidance, including recommendations for a dental assessment and cleaning every 6 months.[4]

The Interview

Overview

The interview with the patient and parents or caregivers is an important component of the WCC process to facilitate understanding about their health care. The NP may need to structure part of the interview alone and should be alert for cues that the adolescent does not want to discuss certain issues in front of parents. The NP should encourage expression of feelings and concerns, while being aware that the adolescent is identity-seeking, attempting to establish independence, and may be rebellious. Adolescents are often inflexible and are refining their sex role and sexuality.

Several methods can assist in obtaining the adolescent's history. The HEADSS format, which stands for Home environment, Employment and education, Activities, Drugs, Social, and Sexuality, is a psychosocial interview for adolescents.[6] The PACES format emphasizes the importance of Parents/peers; Accident, alcohol, and/or drugs; Cigarettes; Emotional issues; and School and/or sexuality. SAFETEENS, another commonly used format, typically directs the conversation by the following topics: Sexuality, Accident and/or abuse, Firearms and homicide, Emotions (e.g., suicide/depression), Toxins (e.g., tobacco, alcohol, and others), Environment (e.g., school, home, and friends), Exercise, Nutrition, and Shots (e.g., immunization status and school performance).[7]

The Physical Examination: Necessary Elements

Overview

The adolescent stage is marked by the rapid, dramatic development of secondary sexual characteristics. Vision and hearing screening, along with an assessment of the patient's vitals, should be performed on each visit. The physical examination of adolescents should proceed from head to foot.

Tanner Staging (see figures 8.1–8.3)

Tanner staging is used to rate sexual maturity in adolescents. An adolescent's sexual maturity rating (SMR) is obtained by taking the average of the Tanner stages from the appropriate charts for that adolescent's gender.[8] Precocious puberty is indicated by the onset of puberty before age 8 in girls and before age 9 in boys.

The three charts for the Tanner staging of an adolescent are secondary sexual characteristic development for boys, breast development for girls, and pubic hair development for both genders. Each of these charts has five stages.

The first stage for the secondary sexual characteristic development in boys is marked by the development of preadolescent testes, scrotum, and penis. The second stage is marked by enlargement of the scrotum and testes, with the scrotum roughening and reddening. The third stage is characterized by penis elongation; it is soon after this stage that spermarche typically occurs. Rugae appear and glans develop in the fourth stage while the penis enlarges in breadth. The fifth and final stage is marked by adult shape and appearance.[9]

The first stage for the breast development chart is characterized by preadolescent breasts. Stage 2 is characterized by the breasts budding with areolar enlargement. Stage 3 is marked by breast enlargement but without separate nipple contour. The areola and nipple then project as a secondary mound in the fourth stage, whereas the fifth stage is marked by adult breast appearance with receding areolas and retracting nipples.[9] Menarche typically starts in between stages 3 and 4.

On the Tanner scale regarding pubic hair development, the first stage is characterized by a preadolescent, bare appearance. Sparse, pale, fine hair begins to develop in stage 2, with stage 3 seeing an increased amount of darker, curlier hair. The hair begins to look adult in character in stage 4, but is still not as voluminous. Stage 5 is marked by an adult appearance.

Developmental Monitoring

Physical Development

An adolescent's pubertal growth spurt will account for about 20% of final adult height; it is during this spurt that PHV is typically reached.[10] Musculoskeletal development during this phase commonly results in adolescents progressing from a "long and gangly" frame to adult appearance.

Cognitive Development

Erik Erikson's identity vs. role confusion stage of cognitive development is illustrated during adolescence.[11] During this stage, adolescents assume the roles they are to fill as an adult and attempt to find their sexual and occupational identities.[12] Jean Piaget's formal operational stage of abstract thinking is also observed during adolescence. During this stage, adolescents demonstrate an expansion in abstract thinking and creativity, begin to enjoy intellectual stimulation and challenge, and start to employ humor and critical thinking on a routine basis.[13]

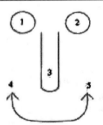

Figure 8.1. Boys: Secondary Sexual Characteristic Development

1) Preadolescent testes, scrotum, penis
2) Enlargement of scrotum and testes; scrotum roughens and reddens
3) Penis elongates
4) Penis enlarges in breadth and development of glans; rugae appear
5) Adult shape and appearance

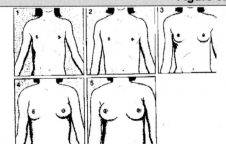

Figure 8.2. Girls: Breast Development

1) Preadolescent breasts
2) Breast buds with areolar enlargement
3) Breast enlargement without separate nipple contour
4) Areola and nipple project as secondary mound
5) Adult breast: areola recedes, nipple retracts

Figure 8.3. Pubic Hair: For Males and Females
1) Preadolescent
2) Sparse, pale, fine
3) Darker, increased amount, curlier
4) Adult in character but not as voluminous
5) Adult pattern

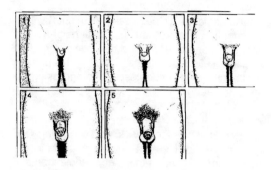
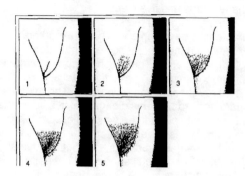

Psychosocial Development

Different phases of psychosocial development present at different ages in adolescence. Younger adolescence is typically characterized by an increase in parent and child conflict. The child tries to establish a sense of independence and identity and is very influenced by his or her peers. Anger and histrionics are commonly displayed.

Older adolescence is marked by a decrease in emotional lability, usually resulting in a decrease in conflict between parent and child. Although older adolescents are still attempting to develop independence and their own sense of identity, a re-establishment of rapport with parents is often sought. Older adolescents are more likely to have increased self-esteem and confidence than younger adolescents. Furthermore, an increased interest in sex is quite common.

Developmental Discussion/Guidance

Although peer groups become increasingly influential during adolescence, it is the parents who remain the primary influence for guidance. As such, it is of paramount importance that parents and other adults serve as good examples for children. As adolescents grow older and begin to reach young adulthood, it is optimal for parents to begin to treat the children as adults. Honesty in communication should be reinforced, and the adolescent's privacy should be respected. Discipline should begin to incorporate negotiation between parent and child, and should reflect flexibility with trivial matters. The monitoring of television and internet activity should be maintained throughout adolescence.

Nutrition/Feeding

Because adolescents are still physically developing, there are more nutritional requirements for this age group than for adults. High-calorie, low-nutrient food must be minimized, and the regular consumption of balanced meals should be encouraged. Vegetarian or vegan diets, as well as other specific diets that omit certain food groups, should be discussed between parents and adolescents and should be closely monitored to ensure nutritional needs are met.[14]

Eating Disorders

Overview

Eating disorders are chronic disturbances in eating patterns accompanied by a distorted body image. Peak incidence for eating disorders is typically between 14 and 18 years of age. Overall mortality is as high as 10% and is related to both suicide and health consequences, namely organ failure, that arise from the disorders, and may also include severe electrolyte imbalances, such as potassium.

Anorexia nervosa is characterized by eating disturbances such as food restriction and avoidance of eating in public, as well as weight loss and persistent behavior that prevents weight gain.[15] Amenorrhea usually ensues from anorexia. Bulimia nervosa, on the other hand, is characterized by episodic binging and purging.[15] The cause of bulimia is not clearly defined, but it is believed to arise from familial issues, social pressure, low self-esteem, and a desire for control.

Presentation

Presentations of anorexia nervosa may include weight loss, anemia, amenorrhea, constipation, jaundice, cold body temperature, lanugo, and brittle bones, hair, and nails. Presentations of bulimia nervosa may include worn tooth enamel, chronic sore throat, dehydration, swollen salivary glands, and intestinal distress.[16] Bruised and abraded knuckles, known as Russell's sign, may indicate anorexia or bulimia.

Differential Diagnosis

Differential diagnoses for eating disorders include pregnancy, depression, substance abuse, and organic diseases resulting in weight loss, among others.[4]

Workup

Vital signs should be assessed for any patients assumed to be anorexic or bulimic. The level of malnutrition, if any, should also be determined. A patient is considered to be mildly malnourished if he or she weighs less than 20% below their ideal body weight (IDW). A weight 20% to 30% below IDW would indicate moderate malnutrition, whereas a weight that is 30% or more below the IDW would indicate severe malnutrition. Additional diagnostic tests may be necessary to rule out any organic diseases resulting in weight loss, such as cancer or esophageal motility disorders.[17]

Management

An interdisciplinary approach is generally employed in the management of eating disorders in adolescents, aimed at addressing both the psychological underpinnings of the disorder and the physiologic changes resulting from malnutrition. Courses of treatment in adolescents may focus on behavior modification and psychotherapy. In severe cases, adolescents may require hospitalization.[16]

Dental Health

Dental health includes brushing after meals and before bed, having a dental cleaning every 6 months, and flossing.[4]

Sexuality

As adolescents' interest and knowledge in sexuality begins to expand, it is important for them to receive accurate information about sex and sexual maturity. Patients should be prepared for the bodily changes that often come with spermarche and menarche, such as nocturnal emissions and menstruation. Curiosity or conflict with one's gender and sexual identity may present, as adolescents are attempting to develop their sense of identity in various contexts. Adolescents should also receive thorough education in disease and pregnancy prevention measures.[18]

Preventative Health Issues

Preventative health issues for adolescents include mental health care for depression or suicide. Adolescents should be observed for signs indicative of depression, such as behavior changes, self-harm, or sudden weight loss. Treatment for depression centers on psychotherapy, with medications, such as selective serotonin reuptake inhibitors and sometimes tricyclic antidepressants, are prescribed when necessary.[19] Special care must be taken to assess the child for proclivities to violence.

Developmental Warning Signs

Changes in personality, school performance, friendships, or sleeping and eating patterns are often considered to be developmental warning signs.[19] Other signs may include difficulty accepting failure, talk of suicide, and withdrawal from friends or family.

Figures

Figure 8.1. Boys: Secondary sexual characteristic development. Barkley TW Jr. Adolescent health and issues. In: Barkley TW Jr, ed. *Family Nurse Practitioner Certification Review/ Clinical Update Continuing Education Course.* West Hollywood, CA: Barkley and Associates; 2015: 63–71.

Figure 8.2. Girls: Breast development. Barkley TW Jr. Adolescent health and issues. In: Barkley TW Jr, ed. *Family Nurse Practitioner Certification Review/Clinical Update Continuing Education Course.* West Hollywood, CA: Barkley and Associates; 2015: 63–71.

Figure 8.3. Pubic hair: For males and females. Barkley TW Jr. Adolescent health and issues. In: Barkley TW Jr, ed. *Family Nurse Practitioner Certification Review/Clinical Update Continuing Education Course.* West Hollywood, CA: Barkley and Associates; 2015: 63–71.

References

1. Hagan JF, Shaw JS, Duncan PM, eds. *Bright Futures: Guidelines for Health Supervision of Infants, Children, and Adolescents.* 3rd ed. Elk Grove Village, IL: American Academy of Pediatrics; 2008.

2. The growing child: Adolescent (13 to 18 years). Lucille Packard Children's Hospital Stanford web site. http://www.lpch.org/DiseaseHealthInfo/HealthLibrary/growth/adsct138.html. Accessed April 13, 2015.

3. Adolescent development. A.D.A.M. Medical Encyclopedia. http://www.nlm.nih.gov/medlineplus/ency/article/002003.htm. Updated January 27, 2013. Accessed April 13, 2015.

4. Barkley TW Jr. Adolescent health and issues. In: Barkley TW Jr, ed. *Family Nurse Practitioner Certification Review/Clinical Update Continuing Education Course.* West Hollywood, CA: Barkley and Associates; 2015: 63–71.

5. Sloane PD, Slatt LM, Ebell MH, Jacques LB, Smith MA, eds. *Essentials of Family Medicine.* 6th ed. Philadelphia, PA: Wolters Kluwer Health/Lippincott Williams & Wilkins; 2011.

6. Bradford S, Rickwood D. Psychosocial assessments for young people: A systematic review examining acceptability, disclosure and engagement, and predictive utility. *Adolesc Health Med Ther.* 2012; 3: 111–125. doi: 10.2147/AHMT.S38442

7. Loretz L. *Primary Care Tools for Clinicians: A Compendium of Forms, Questionnaires, and Rating Scales for Everyday Practice.* St. Louis, MO: Elsevier Mosby; 2005.

8. Biro FM, Chan Y-M. Normal puberty. In: Basow DS, ed. *UpToDate.* Waltham, MA: UpToDate; 2015. http://www.uptodate.com/contents/normal-puberty. Last updated March 27, 2015. Accessed April 13, 2015.

9. Ethington MD, Gallagher MR, Wilson D. Health promotion of the adolescent and family. In: Hockenberry MJ, Wilson D, eds. *Wong's Nursing Care of Infants and Children.* 10th ed. St. Louis, MO: Elsevier Mosby; 2015: 651–686.

10. Neinstein LS. Puberty to Normal growth and development (A1). USC web site. https://www.usc.edu/student-affairs/Health_Center/adolhealth/content/a1.html. Accessed April 13, 2015.

11. McLeod SA. Erik Erikson. Simply Psychology web site. http://www.simplypsychology.org/Erik-Erikson.html. Published 2008. Updated 2013. Accessed April 13, 2015.

12. Block M. Identity versus role confusion. In: Goldstein S, Naglieri A, eds. *Encyclopedia of Child Behavior and Development.* New York , NY: Springer; 2011: 785–786.

13. Colyar MR. *Assessment of the School-Age Child and Adolescent.* Philadelphia, PA: F. A. Davis Company; 2011.

14. Demory-Luce D, Motil KJ. Adolescent eating habits. In: Basow DS, ed. *UpToDate.* Waltham, MA: UpToDate; 2015. http://www.uptodate.com/contents/adolescent-eating-habits. Last updated September 25, 2014. Accessed April 14, 2015.

15. Forman SF. Eating disorders: Overview of epidemiology, diagnosis, and course illness. In: Basow DS, ed. *UpToDate.* Waltham, MA: UpToDate; 2015. http://www.uptodate.com/contents/eating-disorders-overview-of-epidemiology-diagnosis-and-course-of-illness. Last updated January 24, 2015. Accessed April 14, 2015.

16. U. S. Department of Health and Human Services, National Institutes of Health, National Institute of Mental Health. Eating disorders: About more than food. http://www.nimh.nih.gov/health/publications/eating-disorders/index.shtml. Revised 2014. Accessed April 14, 2015.

17. Bernstein BE. Anorexia nervosa differential diagnosis. In: Pataki C, ed. Medscape. http://emedicine.medscape.com/article/912187-differential. Updated December 14, 2014. Accessed April 14, 2015.

18. Benson PAS. Patient information: Adolescent sexuality (Beyond the Basics). In: Basow DS, ed. *UpToDate.* Waltham, MA: UpToDate; 2015. http://www.uptodate.com/contents/adolescent-sexuality-beyond-the-basics. Last updated July 7, 2014. Accessed April 14, 2015.

19. Mayo Clinic Staff. Mental illness in children: Know the signs. http://www.mayoclinic.com/health/mental-illness-in-children/MY01915. Updated February 11, 2015. Accessed April 14, 2015.

Chapter 9
Cardiovascular Disorders

QUESTIONS

1. A mother brings her 1-year-old to your practice, claiming that the child has had a fever for 6 days. She thought it was a simple illness at first, but she has noticed recent swelling in the hands and feet. An examination shows that the child has inflammation in the lips and oral cavity, as well as redness in both eyes without exudate. To rule out Kawasaki disease, which test would best help to isolate the child's most likely condition?

    a. Hemoglobin and hematocrit level

    b. Erythrocyte sedimentation rate

    c. White blood cell count

    d. Blood urea nitrogen

2. Which of the following types of congenital heart defects is most likely to present with right-to-left shunting?

    a. Transposition of the great vessels

    b. Coarctation of the aorta

    c. Tetralogy of Fallot

    d. Pulmonary stenosis

3. Which of the following diagnostics is least likely to indicate a diagnosis of rheumatic fever?

    a. Electrocardiogram

    b. Aldosterone level

    c. Echocardiogram

    d. Throat culture

4. How would you best auscultate to confirm a venous hum?

    a. Have the patient lay supine; auscultate the left upper sternal border.

    b. Have the patient stand; auscultate between the left lower sternal border and the apex.

    c. Have the patient sit up; auscultate the right upper sternal border.

    d. Have the patient turn his or her head; auscultate the apex.

5. What feature best distinguishes the characteristic murmur of patent ductus arteriosus?

    a. A holosystolic thrill at the left lower sternal border

    b. A "machinery" noise at the left upper sternal border

    c. An ejection murmur with radiation to the left interscapular area

    d. A click at the left upper sternal border that decreases with inspiration and increases with expiration

6. Which of these heart sounds would most strongly indicate a cardiac disorder in a pediatric patient?

    a. S1

    b. S2

    c. S3

    d. S4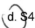

7. Which of the following types of heart murmurs is <u>not</u> typically considered an innocent heart murmur?

   a. Continuous humming murmur

   b. Radiating murmur

   c. Murmur that may vary with position changes

   d. Musical systolic murmur

8. During auscultation of a newborn, a grade IV murmur is heard with a holosystolic thrill at the left lower sternal border. You suspect a congenital heart defect and order an x-ray. What findings would be most consistent with a suspected diagnosis of ventricular septal defect?

   a. A normal chest x-ray

   b. Cardiomegaly with rib notching

   c. Boot-shaped heart

   d. Cardiomegaly with increased pulmonary vascular markings

9. What finding is <u>not</u> a classic characteristic of a 3-month-old with congenital heart disease and signs of heart failure?

   a. Failure to thrive

   b. Irritability

   c. Rales upon lung auscultation

   d. Frequent vomiting with feeding

10. Which of the following patients, all of whom have a known history of congenital heart disease, is <u>least</u> likely to require prophylactic antibiotics prior to a dental procedure?

   a. A patient with a heart transplant

   b. A patient with a ventricular septal defect with a patch repair

   c. A patient with a previous history of endocarditis

   d. A patient with a partially repaired cyanotic heart defect

RATIONALES

1. b

An erythrocyte sedimentation rate test can help to rule out a diagnosis of Kawasaki disease, which, although rare, most commonly manifests in children younger than 2 years of age and typically produces a fever that lasts at least 5 or more days. Kawasaki disease also often causes changes in the extremities, such as erythema, edema, and desquamation. Other common presentations include inflammatory changes in the lips and oral cavity, bilateral conjunctivitis without exudate, and cervical lymphadenopathy. Patients with the cardinal signs should have a pediatric cardiac referral to evaluate for latent adverse outcomes associated with Kawasaki disease. Hemoglobin and hematocrit levels are more confirmatory for anemia, whereas a blood urea nitrogen test may help to identify abnormalities in the kidneys. White blood cell count may be elevated in patients with Kawasaki disease, but this finding is not confirmatory.

2. c

Cyanotic cardiac defects, such as tetralogy of Fallot, are congenital heart defects that typically present with right-to-left shunting. Both pulmonary stenosis and a large ventricular septal defect are commonly seen with tetralogy of Fallot; however, pulmonary stenosis on its own is considered an obstructive lesion, whereas ventricular septal defect is typically considered an acyanotic cardiac defect (i.e., left-to-right shunting). Coarctation of the aorta is commonly considered an obstructive lesion.

3. b

Plasma aldosterone levels are least likely to provide an indication of rheumatic fever, as the condition does not typically produce altered plasma aldosterone levels. Plasma aldosterone levels may be ordered when hypertension is present in order to rule out aldosteronism. Throat culture is a key diagnostic for rheumatic fever when used to confirm prior streptococcal infection; other common diagnostics include a rapid strep assay and a strep antibody titer. An echocardiogram may reveal cardiomegaly in patients with rheumatic fever, whereas an electrocardiogram may show a prolonged PR interval.

4. c

A venous hum is typically considered benign and is best auscultated at the right upper sternal border just below the clavicle while the patient is sitting upright during diastole. Asking the patient to either lay supine or turn his or her head may eliminate the venous hum. Still's murmur, rather than a venous hum, is best auscultated between the left lower sternal border and the apex.

5. b

Patent ductus arteriosus is commonly characterized by a grade II to IV/VI holosystolic murmur at the left upper sternal border (LUSB) with a distinguishing "machinery" noise. Pulmonic stenosis is also typically auscultated at the LUSB, but is more often characterized by an ejection click that increases in intensity with expiration and decreases with inspiration. A holosystolic thrill at the lower left sternal border would commonly indicate ventricular septal defect. Coarctation of the aorta is commonly characterized by an ejection murmur that radiates to the left interscapular area.

6. d

The S4 heart sound is best heard at the apex and is almost always considered to be pathological. S4, characterized by a cadence similar to "Ten-ne-ssee," is produced by stiff ventricular walls, which cause increased resistance to inflow within the ventricle. The S1 and S2 heart sounds are normal and associated with the opening and closing of the atrioventricular and semilunar valves, respectively. The S3 heart sound may be considered an indicator of heart failure in older patients but is usually considered normal in children.

7. b

A radiating murmur is not typically associated with an innocent heart murmur, as this type of murmur may be indicative of an obstructive defect. Congenital innocent heart murmurs may be indicated by a continuous humming murmur (i.e., venous hum), a murmur that may vary with position changes, or a musical systolic murmur (commonly called a Still's murmur).

8. d

Ventricular septal defect commonly presents with a grade II to V/VI systolic ejection murmur with holosystolic thrill in the left lower sternal border, as well as a chest x-ray that shows cardiomegaly with increased pulmonary vascular markings. Rib notching due to collateral circulation is a distinguishing feature of coarctation of the aorta, which also commonly presents with cardiomegaly. A heart that appears normal on x-rays may appear with aortic and pulmonic stenosis, though congestive heart failure may be visible if the aortic stenosis is severe. A boot-shaped heart is a characteristic x-ray finding of tetralogy of Fallot.

9. d

While infants with congestive heart failure (CHF) may have some feeding intolerance, vomiting is not commonly considered a cardinal sign of CHF. Irritability and restlessness are common in infants with CHF. Rales typically derive from pulmonary congestion; as the congestion progresses, there is often leaking into the alveoli and interstitium of the lung from increased intracardiac pressure. Failure to thrive is one of the common hallmarks for CHF; feeding becomes exhaustive as coordination of sucking, swallowing, and breathing taxes the ill infant.

10. a

A heart transplant patient does not typically require prophylactic antibiotics prior to dental work unless they have developed valvular disease post-transplant. Any patch repair for a cardiac defect, a partially repaired cyanotic congenital heart defect, or a previous incidence of endocarditis would indicate a need for antibiotics prior to dental procedures to prevent infective endocarditis. Premedication with a penicillin, such as amoxicillin, is recommended 30–60 minutes prior to the procedure.

DISCUSSION

Cardiovascular

Overview

The cardiovascular system consists of the heart, vessels, and blood. The purpose of the system is to transport blood throughout the body. Components of the cardiovascular system, in the order of blood flow, include the following: the superior and inferior vena cava; right atrium; tricuspid valve; right ventricle; pulmonic valve; pulmonary artery; lungs; pulmonary veins; left atrium; mitral valve; left ventricle; aortic valve; and the aorta. From the aorta, blood is pumped to the rest of the body.[1,2]

Nurse practitioners (NPs) commonly use four different heart sounds to determine the anatomic and physiologic state of the heart. One heart sound is the S1, which is produced by mitral and/or tricuspid atrioventricular valve closure. The S2 heart sound is produced by aortic and pulmonic, or semilunar, valve closure. Systole occurs in the period between the S1 and S2 sounds, whereas diastole occurs in the period between the S2 and S1 sounds. The S3 heart sound is known as the "Ken-tuck-y" gallop. It is heard during the rapid entry of blood from the atrium to the ventricle; on the left side, it is best heard at the apex, whereas a right ventricular S3 sound is best audible at the left lower sternal border (LLSB). Lastly, the S4 heart sound is the "Ten-ne-ssee" sound. The S4 sound occurs when active atrial contraction leads to late ventricular filling; like the S3, the S4 sound is best heard at the apex in the left ventricle and at the LLSB in the right ventricle.[1,3]

There are five main auscultatory areas of the cardiovascular system. The aortic area is the right upper sternal border (RUSB). The pulmonic area is the left upper sternal border (LUSB). The mitral area is located in the fifth intercostal space at the apex. Erb's point is located in the third intercostal space at the left sternal border. The ventricular septal defect (VSD) or tricuspid area is the fourth intercostal space at the LLSB.[1]

Congenital Heart Diseases/Defects

Overview

Congenital heart diseases and defects are cardiovascular malformations resulting from abnormal structural development in the first trimester. The etiology of these conditions is multifactorial and often includes chromosomal abnormalities and adverse environmental conditions.[1] Congenital heart disease occurs in 6–13 per 1,000 births.[4] VSDs comprise up to 30% of all congenital heart defects.[5] Congenital heart defects include acyanotic lesions (left to right shunting), cyanotic lesions (right to left shunting), and obstructive lesions.[4]

Presentation

Infants with cardiovascular defects may present with feeding intolerance, sweating during feeding, or poor growth.[4] Older children may also present with poor growth, as well as repeated infections or activity intolerance.[6]

Acyanotic Defects (left to right shunting)

Overview

Acyanotic defects occur when a shunt causes blood to flow from the left side to the right side of the heart. This condition is due to a structural defect of the heart, such as a hole in the interventricular septum. There are three types of acyanotic defects: atrial septal defect (ASD), VSD, and patent ductus arteriosus (PDA).[7]

Presentation

ASD typically presents with a murmur. The murmur is characterized as a grade II/VI to III/VI systolic ejection, which is heard best at the LUSB. VSD usually presents with a grade II/VI to V/VI regurgitant systolic murmur, and a systolic thrill may be palpated at the LLSB. PDA often presents with a grade II to IV/VI continuous murmur at the LUSB that produces a characteristic machinery sound.[8]

Workup

Electrocardiograms (ECGs), x-rays, and echocardiograms are often used to diagnose acyanotic defects. X-rays commonly show the same results—cardiomegaly and increased pulmonary vascular markings—for all three acyanotic defects. With ASD, an ECG typically shows right ventricular hypertrophy (RVH), whereas left ventricular hypertrophy (LVH) would indicate a VSD. An ECG would typically show an LVH progressing to biventricular hypertrophy in cases of PDA, as well as in cases of large VSD.[8] Final diagnosis of these types of lesions is best done through consultation and evaluation with a pediatric cardiologist.

Cyanotic Defects (right to left shunting)

Overview

Cyanotic heart defects, characterized by right to left shunting, are structural defects of the heart that cause deoxygenated blood to bypass the lungs and enter the systemic circulation. Cyanotic defects can also cause a mixing of oxygenated and unoxygenated blood, which then enters the systemic circulation.[9]

Two major cyanotic defects are transposition of the great arteries and tetralogy of Fallot. Transposition of the great arteries can be either dextrotransposition of the great arteries or levotransposition of the great arteries. Tetralogy of Fallot consists of the following defects: large VSD, pulmonary stenosis, an overriding aorta, and RVH.[8]

Presentation

Transposition of the great arteries and tetralogy of Fallot both commonly present with a murmur. VSD usually occurs alongside transposition of the great arteries. Therefore, a loud, harsh systolic murmur characteristic of VSD is often present.[10,11] In tetralogy of Fallot, the murmur is characterized by a loud systolic ejection click at the middle and upper left sternal border.[12]

Workup

Both transposition of the great arteries and

tetralogy of Fallot can be diagnosed with an ECG and x-rays. However, an echocardiogram will likely also be done to more definitively visualize all structures within the heart. Radiographs of transposition of the great arteries show an "egg on a string" heart with cardiomegaly and increased pulmonary vascular markings.[13] An ECG shows a right axis deviation and RVH.[13] Abnormal origins of great arteries from the ventricles can be identified on an echocardiogram.[8] Radiographs of tetralogy of Fallot will show decreased or increased heart size, decreased pulmonary vascularity, and a boot-shaped heart.[8] Large VSD and an overriding aorta can usually be seen in an ECG of patients with tetralogy of Fallot.[12] Echocardiograms typically show right atrial enlargement and RVH.[12]

Obstructive Lesions

Overview

Obstructive cardiac lesions involve the narrowing of the pathways or major vessels where blood flows in the heart, which increases blood pressure (BP). Aortic stenosis, pulmonic stenosis, and coarctation of the aorta are three types of obstructive cardiac lesions.[6]

Presentation

Aortic stenosis, pulmonic stenosis, and coarctation of the aorta all commonly present with a murmur. Aortic stenosis is characterized by a grade II/VI to IV/VI systolic ejection murmur at the second right or left intercostal space.[8] A thrill at the RUSB is also commonly present.[14] Pulmonic stenosis is characterized by a grade II/VI to V/VI systolic murmur with ejection click that is loudest at the LUSB.[8] The intensity of the click commonly decreases with inspiration and increases with expiration. A left parasternal systolic thrill can be felt at the 2nd intercostal space.[15] Coarctation of the aorta is characterized by a systolic thrill that can be felt in the suprasternal notch.[8] A grade II/VI to III/VI systolic ejection murmur may be heard in the left interscapular area.[8,16] Additionally, with coarctation of the aorta, the provider may note diminished pulses in the lower extremities.[8] Diminished growth may be noted if the coarctation is not critical.

Workup

Aortic stenosis is primarily diagnosed through an echocardiogram, although x-rays and an ECG can also be beneficial.[14] An echocardiogram shows prominent thickening of the septum and abnormal mitral valve motions.[8] Radiographs are typically normal but may show a dilated ascending aorta or cardiomegaly.[8,14] An ECG is also likely to be normal, but mild LVH may be detected.[8]

Pulmonic stenosis is diagnosed through an ECG and x-rays, but an echocardiogram is typically used to confirm the diagnosis.[17] In mild cases, an ECG will be normal. In moderate cases, the ECG will show right axis deviation or RVH.[8] Radiographs typically show a normal heart size but occasionally may show dilated pulmonary arteries.[8,17] An echocardiogram can confirm the diagnosis by showing decreased motion of the pulmonary valve leaflets and poststenotic dilation of the main pulmonary artery segment.[8]

Coarctation of the aorta may show cardiomegaly on x-rays, but some patients may have normal x-rays.[8] X-rays may also show increased pulmonary venous congestion.[18] An ECG may also be normal, but some patients may show LVH.[18] An echocardiogram will show the localized area of coarctation by demonstrating increased velocities and turbulence.[18] With coarctation of the aorta, BP in lower extremities will usually be lower than in upper extremities.[1]

Common Genetic Syndromes and Associated Cardiac Defects

Overview

Numerous genetic syndromes, such as DiGeorge syndrome, trisomies, Marfan syndrome, and Turner syndrome, typically present with cardiac defects.[19] For instance, DiGeorge syndrome is associated with conotruncal defects, such as interrupted aortic arch, truncus arteriosus, and tetralogy of Fallot. These defects often cause cyanotic heart disease in newborns.[20] Marfan syndrome is associated with aortic root disease, which can lead to aneurysmal dilation, aortic regurgitation, and dissection. Mitral valve prolapse is also common.[21] Turner syndrome is associated with coarctation of the aorta and aortic valve abnormalities, primarily bicuspid aortic valve.[22] Trisomy 18 (i.e., Edward's syndrome) is characterized by acyanotic heart defects (e.g., VSD, ASD, PDA).[23] Approximately half of all patients with Trisomy 21 (i.e., Down syndrome) have congenital heart disease. Complete atrioventricular septal defects and VSD are the two most common primary lesions.[24]

Presentation

Assessment for cardiovascular disorders should begin with a careful history and physical examination. A family history of hereditary diseases or congenital heart defects is significant and suggests further evaluation. The neonatal history should include a history of frequent respiratory infections, color changes, cyanosis, tachypnea during sleep, feeding problems, diaphoresis, abnormal heart sounds, edema, clubbing, and congestive heart failure. The physical examination should include inspection, palpation, and auscultation.[8]

Workup

Referral to a pediatric cardiologist is the standard of care for patients with significant cardiac defects.

Additionally, the NP should ensure optimal primary care and provide anticipatory guidance.[1]

Innocent Murmurs (Functional, Benign, or Physiologic)

Overview

Innocent murmurs, which occur in more than 50% of all children, are heart murmurs mostly due to physiological conditions (e.g., extra blood flow), not structural defects of the heart.[25,26] Innocent murmurs are most common in children 3 to 7 years old. The murmur can be easily heard because of the child's thin chest and may become louder when the child is scared or febrile. The murmur may vary with position, often presenting with greater intensity in the sitting position compared to the standing position. Typically, innocent murmurs do not radiate to the neck or back.[27] Most innocent murmurs are grade I/VI or grade II/VI.[28]

Presentation

The most common innocent murmur is the Still's murmur.[28] This type of murmur is musical, systolic, and heard best between LLSB and the apex due to vibrations of the left outflow tract.[28,29] The murmur is often more difficult to hear when patients are sitting or lying on their stomach.[27]

A venous hum is a continuous murmur at the RUSB that can be heard as blood flows into the jugular veins.[27] This presentation is heard best in the sitting position and commonly disappears in the supine position or when the child's head is turned.[28]

Hypertension

Overview

Hypertension is a persistent elevation of BP that is greater than or equal to the 95th percentile for age and sex. In children, secondary hypertension, frequently from renal parenchymal disease or renovascular disease, is more common than primary hypertension.[30]

Presentation

Patients with hypertension are typically asymptomatic.[31] Signs and symptoms of hypertensive emergencies may include headaches, visual problems, dizziness, respiratory distress, irritability, and nosebleeds. Cardiovascular complaints of heart failure, such as chest pain, palpitations, cough, and shortness of breath, are also consistent with a hypertensive emergency.[32]

Workup

Hypertension is diagnosed after the child has three elevated BP readings over the course of at least three doctor's visits.[31] Once hypertension is confirmed, several laboratory tests are used in conjunction with other diagnostic criteria to determine the cause of hypertension. X-rays are used to check the posteroanterior and lateral chest for an enlarged heart or other significant markings.[33] A plasma aldosterone level is often used to rule out aldosteronism.[32] Urinalysis, basic metabolic panel, and complete blood count (CBC) are also helpful in determining the etiology.[31,32] An echocardiogram can be used to detect LVH.[32]

Treatment

Management of patients with primary hypertension can be conducted by the primary care providers. Patients with secondary hypertension typically require a referral to a cardiologist or nephrologist. BP goals for these patients should be based on etiology. Most children with primary and secondary hypertension will require antihypertensive medications and lifestyle modifications.[30]

Rheumatic Fever/Heart Disease

Overview

Rheumatic fever is a post-infectious inflammatory disease that can negatively impact the heart, joints, and central nervous system. Rheumatic fever follows an upper respiratory tract infection that derives from a group "A" streptococcal infection and is most common in ages 6 to 15 years.[1,34] Rheumatic heart disease may develop years after one or more episodes of rheumatic fever.[35]

Presentation

Common signs and symptoms of rheumatic fever include abdominal pain, fever, and joint pain and swelling. Patients may experience arthritis in the knees, elbows, ankles, and wrists. A ring-shaped rash may also appear on the trunk and upper part of the arms or legs. Sydenham chorea, which is a neurologic disorder characterized by muscle weakness, may also present.[36] Children with rheumatic heart disease may experience the same symptoms of rheumatic fever, but do not typically experience symptoms from heart damage.[37]

Workup

Rheumatic fever is diagnosed by using the Jones criteria. A diagnosis necessitates one required criteria and either two major criteria or one major criteria and two minor criteria.[38] The required criteria is evidence of an antecedent Strep infection.[38] Major criteria include carditis, polyarthritis, chorea, erythema marginatum, and subcutaneous nodules. Minor criteria include arthralgia without objective inflammation, fever higher than 102.2 °F (39 °C), elevated levels of acute phase reactants (e.g., erythrocyte sedimentation rate [ESR] and C-reactive protein), and a prolonged PR interval.[1,38]

In diagnosing rheumatic heart disease, the NP should check for signs of a recent Strep infection. Indications of rheumatic fever, such as joint pain and inflammation, should also be noted. A chest x-ray and echocardiogram are beneficial in assessing the size of the heart and the presence of any excess fluid.[37]

Treatment

Rheumatic fever is primarily treated by antibiotics and antiinflammatory agents. Antibiotics, primarily penicillin, are used to eradicate the group A beta-hemolytic streptococcus carriage.[36,39] Antiinflammatory agents are used in treating arthritis.[39] Bed rest is recommended if acute carditis is present.[1]

Patients with rheumatic heart disease are typically prescribed penicillin for many years to prevent the recurrence of rheumatic fever. If the patient has a severe valve leak, surgery is required to either repair or replace the valve.[37]

Kawasaki Disease

Overview

Kawasaki disease is an acute febrile vasculitic syndrome that involves inflammation of the blood vessels.[40] This condition often causes cardiac complications in children by damaging the coronary arteries that supply oxygen to the heart.[41] Kawasaki disease is most prevalent in children of Asian ethnicities.[42]

Presentation

Kawasaki disease has three stages: the acute, subacute, and convalescent phases. Prior to the onset of fever, patients may be irritable or vomit. The acute phase is characterized by fever lasting 7 to 14 days. Other findings include nonexudative bilateral conjunctivitis, anterior uveitis, perianal erythema, and lymphadenopathy.[40]

The subacute phase begins once fever abates and lasts until about week four. Findings include desquamation of the digits, thrombocytosis, and development of coronary aneurysms. Risk of sudden death is highest during the subacute phase.[40] The convalescent phase is characterized by the resolution of clinical signs of illness. Patients typically enter this phase within 3 months of presentation.[40]

Workup

Diagnosis of Kawasaki disease requires presentation of fever and four of the following criteria: bilateral bulbar conjunctival injection, oral mucous membrane changes, peripheral extremity changes, polymorphous rash, and cervical lymphadenopathy.[43]

Acute-phase reactants (i.e., erythrocyte sedimentation rate, C-reactive protein levels, alpha1-antitrypsin levels) are typically elevated at the start of the illness.[36,44] A CBC will often show mild anemia.[44] ECG changes indicative of Kawasaki disease include prolonged PR or QT intervals.[44] An echocardiogram should be conducted periodically throughout the phases of the illness to evaluate for coronary artery aneurysms.[40]

Treatment

Immediate referral to a pediatric cardiologist is recommended. Inpatient therapy should be initiated with a high dose of aspirin and a single infusion of intravenous immune globulin. Once fever has been absent for 48 hours, a low dose of aspirin should be administered daily for its antiplatelet effect. Aspirin therapy should be continued until laboratory markers indicate an absence of acute inflammation. The NP should discontinue aspirin therapy in collaboration with a cardiologist.[42,45]

References

1. Barkley TW Jr. Cardiovascular issues and disorders. In: Barkley TW Jr, ed. *Pediatric Primary Care Nurse Practitioner*. West Hollywood, CA: Barkley & Associates, Inc.; 2015: 72–81.

2. Cardiovascular. A.D.A.M. Medical Encyclopedia. http://www.nlm.nih.gov/medlineplus/ency/article/002310.htm. Updated January 21, 2013. Accessed April 14, 2015.

3. Mangla A. Heart sounds. In: Lang RA, ed. Medscape. http://emedicine.medscape.com/article/1894036-overview#showall. Updated April 24, 2014. Accessed June 2, 2015.

4. Altman CA. Congenital heart disease (CHD) in the newborn: Presentation and screening for critical CHD. In: Basow DS, ed. *UpToDate*. Waltham, MA: UpToDate; 2015. http://www.uptodate.com/contents/congenital-heart-disease-chd-in-the-newborn-presentation-and-screening-for-critical-chd. Last updated February 4, 2015. Accessed April 14, 2015.

5. Ashraf A. Ventricular septal defects. University of Texas Medical Branch Web site. http://www.utmb.edu/pedi_ed/core/cardiology/page_06.htm. Accessed June 2, 2008.

6. Singh RK, Singh TP. Etiology and diagnosis of heart failure in infants and children. In: Basow DS, ed. *UpToDate*. Waltham, MA: UpToDate; 2015. http://www.uptodate.com/contents/etiology-and-diagnosis-of-heart-failure-in-infants-and-children. Last updated May 28, 2014. Accessed April 14, 2015.

7. Webb GD, Smallhorn JF, Therrien J, Redington AN. Congenital heart disease. In: Zipes DP, Libby P, Bonow RO, eds. *Braunwald's Heart Disease: A Textbook of Cardiovascular Medicine*. 9th ed. Philadelphia, PA: Elsevier Saunders; 2011: 1411–1467.

8. Lott JW. Cardiovascular system. In: Kenner C, Lott JW, eds. *Comprehensive Neonatal Nursing Care*. 5th ed. New York, NY: Springer Publishing Company; 2014: 152–188.

9. Cyanotic heart disease. A.D.A.M. Medical Encyclopedia. http://www.nlm.nih.gov/medlineplus/ency/article/001104.htm. Updated November 5, 2013. Accessed April 14, 2015.

10. Bernstein D. Cyanotic congenital heart disease: Evaluation of the critically ill neonate with cyanosis and respiratory distress. In: Kliegman RM, Behrman RE, Jenson HB, Stanton BF, eds. *Nelson Textbook of Pediatrics.* 19th ed. Philadelphia, PA: Elsevier Saunders; 2011: 1572.

11. Fulton DR, Kane DA. L-transposition of the great arteries. In: Basow DS, ed. *UpToDate.* Waltham, MA: UpToDate; 2015. http://www.uptodate.com/contents/l-transposition-of-the-great-arteries?source=search_result&search=L-transposition+of+the+great+arteries&selectedTitle=1~6. Last updated September 26, 2014. Accessed June 2, 2015.

12. Doyle T, Kavanaugh-McHugh A. Pathophysiology, clinical features, and diagnosis of tetralogy of Fallot. In: Basow DS, ed. *UpToDate.* Waltham, MA: UpToDate; 2015. http://www.uptodate.com/contents/pathophysiology-clinical-features-and-diagnosis-of-tetralogy-of-fallot?source=search_result&search=pathophysiology%2C+clinical+features%2C+and+diagnosis+of+tetralogy+of+fallot&selectedTitle=1~115. Last updated May 6, 2015. Accessed June 2, 2015.

13. Geggel RL. Diagnosis and initial management of cyanotic heart disease in the newborn. In: Basow DS, ed. *UpToDate.* Waltham, MA: UpToDate; 2015. http://www.uptodate.com/contents/diagnosis-and-initial-management-of-cyanotic-heart-disease-in-the-newborn. Last updated June 17, 2014. Accessed April 14, 2015.

14. Brown DW. Valvar aortic stenosis in children. In: Basow DS, ed. *UpToDate.* Waltham, MA: UpToDate; 2015. http://www.uptodate.com/contents/valvar-aortic-stenosis-in-children. Last updated March 31, 2015. Accessed April 14, 2015.

15. Armstrong GP. Pulmonic stenosis. In: Porter RS, Kaplan JL, eds. Merck Manual Professional Version. http://www.merckmanuals.com/professional/cardiovascular-disorders/valvular-disorders/pulmonic-stenosis. Last reviewed July 2014. Accessed April 14, 2015.

16. Frank JE, Jacobe KM. Evaluation and management of heart murmurs in children. *Am Fam Physician.* 2011; 84(7): 793–800. http://www.aafp.org/afp/2011/1001/p793.html

17. Peng LF, Perry S. Pulmonic stenosis (PS) in neonates, infants, and children. In: Basow DS, ed. *UpToDate.* Waltham, MA: UpToDate; 2015. http://www.uptodate.com/contents/pulmonic-stenosis-ps-in-neonates-infants-and-children?source=search_result&search=pulmonic+stenosis+in+neonates&selectedTitle=1~52. Last updated July 22, 2014. Accessed June 2, 2015.

18. Agarwala BN, Bacha E, Cao QL, Hijazi ZM. Clinical manifestations and diagnosis of coarctation of the aorta. In: Basow DS, ed. *UpToDate.* Waltham, MA: UpToDate; 2015. http://www.uptodate.com/contents/clinical-manifestations-and-diagnosis-of-coarctation-of-the-aorta?source=search_result&search=clinical+manifestations+and+diagnosis+of+coarctation+of+the+aorta&selectedTitle=1~124. Last accessed February 9, 2015. Accessed June 2, 2015.

19. Wiesmann-Günzler S. Congenital syndromes with malformations of the heart. Corience Web site. http://www.corience.org/about-heart-defects/syndromes. Last updated March 13, 2014. Accessed April 14, 2015.

20. Seroogy CM. DiGeorge (22q11.2 deletion) syndrome: Clinical features and diagnosis. In: Basow DS, ed. *UpToDate.* Waltham, MA: UpToDate; 2015. http://www.uptodate.com/contents/digeorge-22q11-2-deletion-syndrome-clinical-features-and-diagnosis?source=search_result&search=digeorge+syndrome+clinical+features&selectedTitle=1~66. Last updated April 29, 2015. Accessed June 2, 2015.

21. Wright MJ, Connolly HM. Genetics, clinical features, and diagnosis of Marfan syndrome and related disorders. In: Basow DS, ed. *UpToDate.* Waltham, MA: UpToDate; 2015. http://www.uptodate.com/contents/genetics-clinical-features-and-diagnosis-of-marfan-syndrome-and-related-disorders?source=search_result&search=genetics%2C+clinical+features%2C+and+diagnosis+of+marfan+syndrome&selectedTitle=1~150. Last updated March 18, 2015. Accessed June 2, 2015.

22. Saenger P. Clinical manifestations and diagnosis of Turner syndrome (gonadal dysgenesis). In: Basow DS, ed. *UpToDate.* Waltham, MA: UpToDate; 2015. http://www.uptodate.com/contents/clinical-manifestations-and-diagnosis-of-turner-syndrome-gonadal-dysgenesis?source=search_result&search=clinical+manifestations+and+diagnosis+of+turner+syndrome&selectedTitle=1~144. Last updated September 17, 2014. Accessed June 2, 2015.

23. Chan H. Trisomy 18 clinical presentation. In: Rohena LO, ed. Medscape. http://emedicine.medscape.com/article/943463-clinical. Updated August 27, 2014. Accessed June 2, 2015.

24. Ostermaier KK. Down syndrome: Clinical features and diagnosis. In: Basow DS, ed. *UpToDate.* Waltham, MA: UpToDate; 2015. http://www.uptodate.com/contents/down-syndrome-clinical-features-and-diagnosis?source=search_result&search=down+syndrome%3A+clinical+features+and+diagnosis&selectedTitle=1~150. Last updated April 28, 2015. Accessed June 2, 2015.

25. Innocent heart murmur. Congenital & Children's Heart Centre Web site. http://www.childrensheartcentre.com/selectedheartconditions/innocentmurmur.html. Accessed June 2, 2015.

26. U.S. Department of Health and Human Services, National Institute of Health (NIH), National Heart, Lung, and Blood Institute. What causes heart murmurs? National Heart, Lung, and Blood Institute Web site. http://www.nhlbi.nih.gov/health/health-topics/topics/heartmurmur/causes. Updated September 20, 2012. Accessed June 2, 2015.

27. Punnoose AR, Burke AE, Golub RM. Innocent (harmless) heart murmurs in children. *JAMA*. 2012; 308(3): 305. doi: 10.1001/jama.2012.6223

28. McConnell ME, Adkins SB III, Hannon DW. Heart murmurs in pediatric patients: When do you refer? *Am Fam Physician*. 1999; 60(2): 558–564. http://www.aafp.org/afp/1999/0801/p558.html

29. Gersh BJ. Auscultation of cardiac murmurs. In: Basow DS, ed. *UpToDate*. Waltham, MA: UpToDate; 2015. http://www.uptodate.com/contents/auscultation-of-cardiac-murmurs. Last updated April 23, 2014 Accessed April 14, 2015.

30. Riley M, Bluhm B. High blood pressure in children and adolescents. *Am Fam Physician*. 2012; 85(7): 693–700. http://www.aafp.org/afp/2012/0401/p693.html

31. Mayo Clinic Staff. High blood pressure. Mayo Clinic Web site. http://www.mayoclinic.org/diseases-conditions/high-blood-pressure-in-children/basics/symptoms/con-20033799. Updated December 18, 2012. Accessed June 2, 2015.

32. Mattoo TK. Evaluation of hypertension in children and adolescents. In: Basow DS, ed. *UpToDate*. Waltham, MA: UpToDate; 2015. http://www.uptodate.com/contents/evaluation-of-hypertension-in-children-and-adolescents?source=search_result&search=evaluation+of+hypertension+in+children+and+adolescents&selectedTitle=1~150. Last updated January 21, 2014. Accessed June 2, 2015.

33. Berger S. Pediatric primary pulmonary hypertension. In: Bye MR, ed. Medscape. http://emedicine.medscape.com/article/1004828-overview. Updated December 31, 2013. Accessed June 2, 2015.

34. Gibofsky A, Zabriskie JB. Clinical manifestations and diagnosis of acute rheumatic fever. In: Basow DS, ed. *UpToDate*. Waltham, MA: UpToDate; 2015. http://www.uptodate.com/contents/clinical-manifestations-and-diagnosis-of-acute-rheumatic-fever?source=search_result&search=clinical+manifestations+and+diagnosis+of+acute+rheumatic+fever&selectedTitle=1~110. Last updated October 4, 2013. Accessed June 2, 2015.

35. Mayosi B. Natural history, screening, and management of rheumatic heart disease. In: Basow DS, ed. *UpToDate*. Waltham, MA: UpToDate; 2015. http://www.uptodate.com/contents/natural-history-screening-and-management-of-rheumatic-heart-disease?source=search_result&search=natural+history%2C+screening%2C+and+management+of+rheumatic+heart+disease&selectedTitle=1~85. Last updated January 8, 2014. Accessed June 2, 2015.

36. Rheumatic fever. A.D.A.M. Medical Encyclopedia. http://www.nlm.nih.gov/medlineplus/ency/article/003940.htm. Updated May 11, 2014. Accessed April 14, 2015.

37. Rheumatic heart disease diagnosis. UCSF Benioff Children's Hospital San Francisco Web site. http://www.ucsfbenioffchildrens.org/conditions/rheumatic_heart_disease/diagnosis.html. Accessed June 2, 2015.

38. Jones criteria for diagnosis of rheumatic fever. Medscape. http://reference.medscape.com/calculator/jones-criteria-diagnosis-rheumatic. Accessed June 2, 2015.

39. Gibofsky A, Zabriskie JB. Treatment and prevention of acute rheumatic fever. In: Basow DS, ed. *UpToDate*. Waltham, MA: UpToDate; 2015. http://www.uptodate.com/contents/treatment-and-prevention-of-acute-rheumatic-fever?source=search_result&search=treatment+and+prevention+of+acute+rheumatic+fever&selectedTitle=1~110. Last updated October 7, 2013. Accessed June 2, 2015.

40. Scheinfeld NS. Kawasaki disease. In: Steele RW, ed. Medscape. http://emedicine.medscape.com/article/965367-overview. Updated January 12, 2015. Accessed April 14, 2015.

41. Kawasaki disease. American Heart Association Web site. http://www.heart.org/HEARTORG/Conditions/More/CardiovascularConditionsofChildhood/Kawasaki-Disease_UCM_308777_Article.jsp. Last reviewed March 22, 2013. Accessed April 14, 2015.

42. Porth CM. Disorders of cardiac function. In: Porth CM, ed. *Essentials of Pathophysiology: Concepts of Altered Health States*. 3rd ed. Philadelphia, PA: Wolters Kluwer Health/Lippincott Williams & Wilkins; 2011: 447–485.

43. Sundel R. Kawasaki disease: Clinical features and diagnosis. In: Basow DS, ed. *UpToDate*. Waltham, MA: UpToDate; 2015. http://www.uptodate.com/contents/kawasaki-disease-clinical-features-and-diagnosis?source=search_result&search=kawasaki+disease+clinical+features+and+diagnosis&selectedTitle=1~150. Last updated May 5, 2015. Accessed June 2, 3015.

44. Horeczko T, Inaba AS. Cardiac disorders. In: Marx JA, Hockberger RS, Walls RM, eds. *Rosen's Emergency Medicine: Concepts and Clinical Practice*. 8th ed. Philadelphia, PA: Elsevier Saunders; 2014: 2139–2167.

45. Sundel R. Kawasaki disease: Initial treatment and prognosis. In: Basow DS, ed. *UpToDate*. Waltham, MA: UpToDate; 2015. http://www.uptodate.com/contents/kawasaki-disease-initial-treatment-and-prognosis?source=search_result&search=kawasaki+disease+in+pediatrics&selectedTitle=2~150. Last updated November 18, 2014. Accessed June 2, 2015.

Chapter 10

Gastrointestinal Disorders

QUESTIONS

1. You are evaluating a 4-month-old, whose mother says, "She's been vomiting and doesn't seem to be taking any milk or fluids. She's also been sleeping a lot more than usual." You note that the patient's fontanel is slightly sunken, and that her skin is cool to the touch and has poor turgor. These findings are least likely to be an initial indication of which condition?

   a. Intussusception

   b. Gastroenteritis

   c. Pyloric stenosis

   d. Hirschsprung's disease

2. Which test would provide the most definitive diagnosis of neuroblastoma?

   a. Physical exam

   b. Low levels of urine catecholamines

   c. Abdominal computed tomography scan

   d. Surgical biopsy

3. A mother brings her 18-month-old daughter to your practice with complaints of watery diarrhea. The mother says that she has noticed her child "has not looked too well." She also says that her daughter has been refusing to eat and has been unable to keep her food down. The mother also reports hearing loud rumbling noises coming from the child's stomach. Based on these findings, which finding would you most expect to see in this patient during your exam?

   a. Enlarged abdominal mass

   b. Visible peristaltic waves

   c. Abdominal distention

   d. Positive psoas sign

4. Vitamin deficiency resulting from malabsorption is most likely to present with:

   a. Vomiting

   b. Chronic diarrhea

   c. Fatigue

   d. Thin stools

5. A 6-month-old male is brought to your clinic with complaints of vomiting. His mother says that her son was fine, but then "he just got really irritable and started crying, and then just started throwing up green barf." The mother says that she noticed her son has not been as energetic as usual, and that there was "jelly-like poop" when changing his diaper. Based on these findings, which gastrointestinal disorder would you most likely suspect?

a. Gastroenteritis

b. Hirschsprung's disease

c. Pyloric stenosis

d. Intussusception

6. How and where does the obturator sign present in pediatric patients with appendicitis?

a. Sharp pain in the right lower quadrant of the abdomen

b. Pain with internal rotation of the right hip

c. Pain with extension of the right hip

d. Tenderness one-third the distance from the anterior superior iliac spine to the umbilicus

7. You are teaching the parents of an 8-month-old infant with gastroesophageal reflux disease. Which of the following actions should you advise the parents to perform immediately after meals specifically to decrease reflux activity?

a. Position the infant in a semi-supine position

b. Assist the newborn to burp after meals

c. Elevate the newborn's head

d. Administer a histamine 2-receptor antagonist

8. Incidence of viral gastroenteritis in pediatric patients usually peaks during which season?

a. Spring

b. Summer

c. Autumn

d. Winter

9. Management of symptoms in infants with gastroesophageal reflux disease is more likely to include which of these in non-severe cases?

a. Thickening of feedings

b. Histamine 2-receptor antagonist

c. A diet that either reduces or eliminates protein

d. Switching to hydrolyzed or amino acid-based formula

10. Which test can be used to diagnose either Hirschsprung's disease or intussusception?

a. Barium enema

b. Rectal biopsy

c. Ultrasound

d. Colon biopsy

RATIONALES

1. c

Decreased skin turgor and a slightly sunken fontanel are signs of dehydration; however, pyloric stenosis is least likely to result in an infant who remains hungry after vomiting. Dehydration and poor feeding may accompany Hirschsprung's disease, intussusception, pyloric stenosis, and gastroenteritis.

2. d

A surgical biopsy is the most definitive diagnosis for neuroblastoma. Elevated urinary catecholamine levels, rather than low urinary catecholamine levels, may be used to diagnose neuroblastoma. Imaging studies, such as a computerized tomography scan and physical exams, may strongly suggest the presence of this condition, but are unable to confirm a diagnosis.

3. c

Abdominal distention is an expected finding of gastroenteritis, which often produces watery diarrhea, hyperactive bowel sounds, non-bilious vomiting, and anorexia in infants. An enlarged abdominal mass, on the other hand, may be a sign of neuroblastoma, but this condition is accompanied by profuse sweating and tachycardia. Although gastroenteritis may present with peristaltic rushes, peristaltic waves are more likely a sign of pyloric stenosis. A positive psoas sign indicates appendicitis, not gastroenteritis.

4. c

Fatigue is most likely to be associated with vitamin deficiency due to malabsorption because it may be a sign of anemia resulting from malabsorption of vitamin B12, folate, and iron. Vomiting and chronic diarrhea are also symptoms of malabsorption, but are not directly caused by vitamin deficiency. Thin stools usually are not indications of an abnormal condition, but may result from irritable bowel syndrome.

5. d

Intussusception is a medical emergency that presents with sudden onset of bilious vomiting, progressive lethargy, and acute colicky pain, which may be indicated in infants by crying. A "currant-jelly" stool is a hallmark symptom of the latter stages of the condition as the intestine sheds its mucosa. Hirschsprung's disease also presents in infancy with pain and bilious vomiting, but may produce bloody diarrhea. Pyloric stenosis is associated with non-bilious, projectile vomiting, as opposed to bilious vomiting. Gastroenteritis, which also may present with vomiting, would produce watery diarrhea rather than a "currant-jelly" stool.

6. b

The obturator sign presents as pain with internal rotation of the right hip, as the inflamed appendix comes into contact with the obturator internus muscle. Although psoas sign also produces through action on the right thigh, it produces through extension of the thigh rather than rotation. Appendicitis presents with tenderness at McBurney's point, which is found one-third of the distance from the anterior superior iliac spine to the umbilicus. Sharp stomach pain that originates around the navel and shifts to the right lower quadrant after several hours may indicate a perforation, which is much more common in pediatrics due to age-related communication barriers.

7. c

Parents of infants with gastroesophageal reflux disease (GERD) should be advised to elevate the infant's head after feeding to decrease reflux activity. Parents should also be told that burping should be performed frequently during the infant's feeding session, not after. Positioning the infant in a semi-supine position is not advised because it would increase reflux, rather than decrease it. Histamine 2-receptor antagonists should be reserved only for severe or complicated cases, because symptoms of GERD typically resolve in infants without medical intervention.

8. d

Incidence of viral gastroenteritis in pediatric patients usually peaks during the winter. Viral causes of gastroenteritis include the norovirus and the rotavirus, which is particularly more active during the winter, from November to February.

9. a

Management of symptoms in infants with non-severe gastroesophageal reflux disease (GERD) is more likely to include small, frequent feeds that are thickened with cereal. Conservative management with optimization of positioning, feeding, and nutrition is often sufficient to manage healthy and thriving infants with symptoms due to physiological GERD. Severe cases of GERD, rather than non-severe cases, may require pharmacologic intervention with histamine 2-receptor antagonists, with proton pump inhibitors (PPIs) co-administered to block gastric acid secretion caused by histamine or other PPIs, but the administration of these drugs may lead to malabsorption of B12. Because an allergy to cow's milk protein may mimic symptoms of GERD, formula-fed infants with persistent vomiting may benefit from a 2–4 week trial of a hydrolyzed or amino acid-based formula. Although some breast-fed infants with symptoms may benefit from a maternal diet excluding all dairy and egg, a diet that either reduces or eliminates protein is more often used to manage symptoms associated with pediatric viral hepatitis than GERD.

10. a

A barium enema is a diagnostic for both Hirschsprung's disease and intussusception. Rectal and colon biopsies are only useful for diagnosis of Hirschsprung's disease. Ultrasounds, on the other hand, are useful in the diagnosis of intussusception but not for Hirschsprung's disease.

DISCUSSION

Gastroenteritis

Overview

Gastroenteritis is a broad term applied to a syndrome of acute vomiting, nausea, and diarrhea that stems from acute irritation and inflammation of the gastric mucosa. Although gastroenteritis has many causes, the condition is most commonly caused by viruses, which are particularly active in the months of winter.[1] Gastroenteritis may also be caused by bacterial or parasitic infections which

Table 10.1	Signs and Symptoms of Dehydration		
Variable	Mild (3%–5%)	Moderate (6%–9%)	Severe (≥ 10%)
Blood Pressure	Normal	Normal	Normal, decreased
Pulse/Heart Rate	Normal	Increased	Severe, decreased
CAP Refill	WNL	WNL	Prolonged (> 3 seconds)
Skin Turgor	Normal	Decreased	Decreased
Fontanel	Normal	Sunken (slightly)	Sunken
Urine	Slightly decreased	< 1 ml/kg/hour	< 1 ml/kg/hour

Used with permission from Barkley TW Jr. *Pediatric Primary Care Nurse Practitioner Certification Review/Clinical Update Continuing Education Course*. West Hollywood, CA: Barkley and Associates; 2015.

can be transmitted by food, water, dirty surfaces, or contact with infected persons.[2] Moreover, inorganic food content and emotional stress may lead to gastroenteritis.[3]

The majority of viral gastroenteritis cases are due to rotavirus and norovirus. Astrovirus and adenoviruses are also common viral causes of the condition.[4] The three leading causes of bacterial diarrhea are bacteria in the *Salmonella*, *Campylobacter*, and *Shigella* genera.[5] Although *Salmonella* bacteria do not tend to produce distinctive symptoms, *Campylobacter* bacteria often cause malodorous stool, whereas *Shigella* bacteria can be distinguished by fever spikes, bloody stools, and febrile seizures. *Escherichia coli* bacteria, another common cause of bacterial gastroenteritis, may produce loose stools.[3]

Presentation

Characteristic findings include abdominal distention, nausea and vomiting, cramping abdominal pain, and diarrhea.[6] Patients may also present with a fever, hyperactive bowel sounds, and anorexia.

Diarrhea and vomiting may lead to dehydration.[2] Dehydration can appear in mild, moderate, or severe forms. These forms can be classified by assessing the patient's signs and symptoms according to table 10.1.[3]

Workup

In most cases, gastroenteritis is diagnosed clinically. No diagnostic tests are indicated for gastroenteritis unless the patient's symptoms persist for more than 72 hours, bloody stool is present, or the patient has a fever.[3] A complete blood count (CBC) can be performed to help determine a possible bacterial etiology, whereas a blood urea nitrogen test can be performed to note dehydration.[7] A stool culture can be used to determine the specific bacterial etiology after 72 hours.[4]

Treatment

The mainstay of supportive care focuses on drinking fluids to maintain hydration.[2,8] Infants should continue to be breastfed or formula fed.

Older children can gradually resume a regular diet once rehydrated. The BRAT diet, which consists of bananas, rice, applesauce, and toast, is often recommended because these foods are well tolerated by most people and are easy to digest.[9] However, virtually any food or drink that a child would normally partake in is acceptable to maintain hydration and avoid electrolyte imbalance.

Children with gastroenteritis should be excluded from daycare, particularly if their condition is caused by rotavirus, *E. coli*, or *Shigella spp.* In bacterial cases caused by *E. coli* and *Shigella spp.*, two negative stool cultures collected consecutively at least 24 hours apart are required prior to the child's return to daycare.[3,10]

In-patient pediatric patients should be treated by oral rehydration therapy at 50–100 ml/hr to remedy their fluid deficit.[11] Antidiarrheal medications are not recommended because it may prolong symptoms.[2,3]

Gastroesophageal Reflux Disease (GERD)

Overview

Gastroesophageal reflux disease (GERD) is a condition where gastric contents pass from the stomach into the esophagus due to incompetence of the lower esophageal sphincter.[12] GERD frequently presents in premature infants and infants with low birth weight but typically resolves by 18 months of age.[13]

The three classes of GERD are physiological, functional, and pathological.[3] Physiological GERD is characterized by infrequent, episodic vomiting. Functional GERD, on the other hand, presents with painless, effortless vomiting with no physical sequelae. Pathological GERD presents with frequent vomiting with alteration in physical functioning, which may include failure to thrive (FTT) or aspiration pneumonia.

Presentation

The most common and prominent symptom of GERD is heartburn, which may be accompanied by other findings such as acid regurgitation and dysphagia.[14] Heartburn usually occurs after eating, or when the patient is bending over or lying supine. Conditions that cause issues with the ear or teeth, such as otitis media and dental erosion, may result from abnormal reflux.[15] Vomiting and irritability are common symptoms of GERD in infants, whereas coughing and wheezing may appear in infants and adults alike.[12] Patients may also experience additional signs and symptoms affecting the throat such as pharyngitis, choking, and painful belching. Weight loss, abdominal pain, and stool pattern changes may also present.[3]

Workup

Most cases of GERD are made clinically.[16] However, when a patient's signs and symptoms are longstanding or do not improve with conservative management, an endoscopy may be helpful.[12] Additional studies that may be considered include ambulatory 24-hour pH monitoring,[15] a CBC, and urinalysis. When the diagnosis is not clear, an abdominal ultrasonography can help to rule out pyloric stenosis.[3]

Treatment

Infant cases of GERD can usually be treated with dietary and behavioral modifications, but more severe cases may require a referral to a gastrointestinal specialist.[17] Infant GERD patients should receive small, frequent feedings and should be burped frequently during feedings. The pediatric patient's head should be elevated for 60 minutes after feeding.[18] Breastfeeding should continue, and formula changes should be avoided. For pediatric patients who require thickened formula in GERD management, one tablespoon of rice cereal may be added per ounce of formula.[3,17]

When dietary and behavioral modifications do not provide relief, pharmacological measures may be instituted. Treatment should begin with over-the-counter antacids to control heartburn.[19] Other medications that may be ordered to treat GERD include histamine H2-receptor antagonists, such as ranitidine (Zantac) and famotidine (Pepcid AC). If histamine H2-receptor antagonists prove ineffective, proton pump inhibitors such as omeprazole (Prilosec) may be ordered to inhibit gastric acid secretion produced by acetylcholine, histamine, or gastrin.[19]

Pyloric Stenosis

Overview

Pyloric stenosis is a rare obstruction disorder in which the stomach is unable to empty into the small intestine because of the thickening of the circular muscles of the pylorus.[20] The cause of pyloric stenosis is unclear, although the condition may involve genetic or familial predisposition as well as environmental factors.[21] Males are more often affected than females, and the condition is more common in Caucasians. Pyloric stenosis most often affects children younger than 6 months of age.[20]

Presentation

Pyloric stenosis typically presents in children between 3 weeks and 4 months of age.[3] Projectile non-bilious vomiting occurs after eating. Afterward, the patient remains apparently hungry.[22] A palpable olive-shaped mass may be observed in the right side of the patient's abdomen. As the condition progresses, the patient may become dehydrated and either loses weight or fails to gain weight.[23] The appearance of peristaltic waves in the patient's abdomen is also a sign of pyloric stenosis.[24]

Workup

Pyloric stenosis is diagnosed by an abdominal ultrasound that shows increased thickness and elongation of the pylorus.[23] An upper gastrointestinal imaging (GI) test can be useful when an ultrasound or other imaging tests are not conclusive.[22] An upper GI study commonly shows delayed gastric emptying and a "string sign," a thin strip of contrast material in the lumen which indicates the narrowing of the pyloric channel.[23]

Treatment

Patients usually need a surgical procedure known as a pyloromyotomy, which opens the thickened area of the pylorus and allows food to pass through.[24] Surgery typically relieves all of the patient's symptoms. Within a few hours post-surgery, the patient can often tolerate small, frequent feedings.[20]

Intussusception

Overview

Intussusception is a disorder in which one part of the intestine experiences an acute inversion into an adjacent segment of the intestine. This process, known as telescoping, often blocks food or fluids.[14] Most cases of intussusception occur prior to 2 years of age, and the condition is more common in males.[3] Intussusception commonly occurs in children who are otherwise healthy. Although the cause of intussusception is unknown, the condition is associated with viral triggers such as adenovirus.[25] Patients with celiac disease and cystic fibrosis also have an increased incidence of intussusception.[3]

Presentation

Acute colicky pain, usually accompanied by vomiting, is often the first sign of intussusception.[26] This vomiting is initially non-bilious but becomes bilious when the patient's intestine becomes obstructed.[27] Progressive lethargy is also a common symptom and in some cases may be the patient's sole presenting symptom.[27] As intussusception progresses, a palpable, sausage-shaped mass may develop in the right side of the patient's abdomen.[25] The patient's stool may be mixed with blood and mucus, which gives the appearance of currant jelly.[25] Patients may present with progressive abdominal distention and tenderness, which may indicate intestinal perforation.[3]

Workup

An ultrasonography is the preferred diagnostic test to detect intussusception.[25] If the ultrasonography is not clear, a radiograph of the patient's abdomen should be considered to exclude intussusception, but should not be relied upon to confirm a diagnosis.[25,27] A barium enema is both diagnostic and therapeutic because it can reduce the telescoped segments of the patient's intestine. However, barium enemas have fallen out of favor as a diagnostic, as the barium may enter a clinically unsuspected perforation and produce peritonitis.[26]

Treatment

When a diagnosis of intussusception is confirmed, the patient should be treated with a non-operative reduction, if possible.[25] Enemas are the primary non-operative treatments.[25] If these treatments are not successful, the patient will require emergent surgery because intussusception is fatal if not treated urgently.[3,28]

Hirschsprung's Disease (Aganglionic Megacolon)

Overview

Hirschsprung's disease, or aganglionic megacolon, is a developmental disorder in which functional bowel obstruction is caused by improper muscle movement in the bowel and the absence of ganglion cells in the distal colon.[29] Although the cause of Hirschsprung's disease is unknown, the disease sometimes occurs in families or develops spontaneously from genetic mutations.[3,30] If untreated, enterocolitis, an inflammation of the colon with potentially fatal results, may develop in patients. Hirschsprung's disease is rare, more common in boys than girls, and may present both in infancy and in older children.[29]

Presentation

Infants with Hirschsprung's disease frequently fail to pass meconium shortly after birth.[31] Newborns and infants may also present with abdominal distention, bilious vomiting, FTT, jaundice, and infrequent and explosive bowel movements.[32] Older children often present with abdominal distention, constipation, and malnutrition.[32]

Workup

A rectal biopsy, which confirms an absence of ganglion cells, is the standard for diagnosing Hirschsprung's disease.[29,33] A barium enema and abdominal x-ray may also be helpful, but an abdominal x-ray is only suggestive of the disease and a barium enema is less sensitive.[29]

Treatment

Patients should be referred to a gastroenterologist for management and surgery.[29] Surgical treatment of Hirschsprung's disease typically involves a one-stage procedure focused on resecting the aganglionic portion of the colon.[31,33]

Appendicitis

Overview

Appendicitis is an acute inflammation of the vermiform appendix.[34] Typically, appendicitis is precipitated by obstruction of the appendix by fecalith, foreign bodies, or neoplasms.[35] If the condition remains untreated, perforation and gangrene may develop within 36 hours. Appendicitis affects approximately 10% of the general population and most commonly occurs in males 10–30 years of age.[3]

Presentation

Appendicitis typically begins with vague, colicky umbilical pain, which shifts to the right lower quadrant of the abdomen within several hours. The pain often worsens, localizes with coughing, and is followed by nausea, vomiting, fever, and anorexia.[36] Nausea accompanied by one to two episodes of vomiting is characteristic of appendicitis, but more vomiting may suggest another diagnosis.[3] Diarrhea is a less common finding.[34]

Although more difficult to elicit in children than adults, the psoas sign, the obturator sign, McBurney's point tenderness, and Rovsing's sign each have a high specificity for appendicitis.[37] Psoas sign is pain with right thigh extension. Obturator sign occurs when the right thigh is rotated internally. McBurney's point can be found by tracing a line from the anterior superior iliac spine to the umbilicus, then finding a point at one-third of the line starting from the iliac spine; tenderness at this point commonly indicates appendicitis. Lastly, Rovsing's sign, also known as indirect tenderness, is pain in the right lower quadrant upon palpation of the left lower quadrant.[37]

Workup

A diagnosis of appendicitis can be made clinically in patients who present with the classic signs and symptoms of anorexia, periumbilical pain, migration of pain to the right lower quadrant, fever, and vomiting.[36] Along with a history and physical exam, a possible elevated erythrocyte sedimentation rate and an elevated white blood cell count between 10,000 and 20,000 cells/µL will further support a diagnosis of appendicitis.[3] An ultrasound or computed tomography (CT) are diagnostic.[37]

Treatment

An appendectomy is the only curative treatment for appendicitis.[34] The prognosis is very good in patients experiencing the early stages of the condition.[38] The prognosis for advanced appendicitis is also good, but special attention must be given to postoperative care to reduce wound infection and other possible complications.[38]

Malabsorption

Overview

Malabsorption is a state where the intestine is unable to fully absorb essential nutrients and electrolytes.[39] Celiac disease and cystic fibrosis can cause malabsorption, as can infection, inflammation, and other conditions that may result in damage to the intestine.[40]

Presentation

Severe, chronic diarrhea is the most common finding of malabsorption.[41] Bulky, foul stool (i.e., steatorrhea) occurs in patients who excrete more than 7 grams of fat per day.[42] Other common signs and symptoms may include FTT, vomiting, abdominal pain, and a protuberant abdomen. Patients with vitamin deficiencies may also present with pallor, fatigue, hair and dermatological abnormalities, cheilosis, and peripheral neuropathy.[3]

Workup

Although a diagnosis of malabsorption is often apparent based on the patient's clinical presentation, this diagnosis may be further established by iron and folate tests.[39,41] Other diagnostic tests for malabsorption include a stool assessment for ova and parasites, liver function tests, and tests to assess serum calcium, phosphorus, alkaline phosphatase, and total protein levels.[3]

Further diagnostic tests can be done to determine the etiology. Differential diagnoses of malabsorption include conditions such as FTT, cystic fibrosis, immune deficiency, hepatic disease, inflammatory bowel disease, chronic diarrhea, and celiac disease.[3]

Treatment

Patients should be referred to a gastroenterologist for treatment. Treatment should be aimed at correcting nutritional deficiencies and managing causative diseases.[41] Dietary modifications are useful, particularly in treating diarrhea due to malabsorption.[43] The appropriate dietary treatment depends on the patient's underlying condition. For example, patients with celiac disease should avoid wheat, oat, rye, and barley. Cystic fibrosis patients should be treated with pancreatic enzyme replacement and fat soluble vitamins.[3]

Neuroblastoma

Overview

Neuroblastoma is a malignant tumor that arises from the neural tissue. Most cases of neuroblastoma are in the adrenal gland or abdomen and can expand to the bone marrow, lymph nodes, skin, liver, and orbits of the eyes.[44] Neuroblastoma is the most common cancer in infants and most always occurs in children younger than 5 years of age.[45]

Presentation

Signs and symptoms vary depending on the location of the tumor and the extent of metastasis.[46] Children with localized disease are typically asymptomatic, but systemic manifestations appear in children with disseminated neuroblastoma.[47] The most common findings are an abdominal mass, abdominal pain, and discomfort.[41] Other common findings include FTT, general malaise, and bone pain.[47]

Workup

After referring to a pediatric oncologist, neuroblastoma may be diagnosed by a surgical biopsy and elevated urinary catecholamine levels. An abdominal CT scan may also be used as a diagnostic study.[3] Once neuroblastoma is diagnosed, staging of the disease is determined by the patient's age, the location of the tumor, and the extent of tumor spread.[44]

Treatment

The NP should refer the patient to a pediatric oncologist for treatment. Surgery is used to treat low-stage neuroblastoma. More advanced stages are treated with multiple-agent chemotherapy and surgery.[47]

Hepatitis

Overview

Hepatitis is an inflammation of the liver that results in liver dysfunction.[48] Manifestation of symptoms can range anywhere from mild and self-limiting to profound and life-threatening. Hepatitis may be caused by a variety of viral subtypes; in pediatric patients, the most common subtypes are A, B, and C.[49]

The hepatitis A virus is an enteral virus transmitted via the oral-fecal route. The mortality rate of this condition is very low, and almost all patients recover completely.[50] Common sources of the hepatitis A virus are contaminated water and food, particularly shellfish.[51] Symptoms of hepatitis A typically manifest 2–6 weeks after infection, but patients' blood and stool are infectious 2 weeks before symptoms appear and 1 week after the onset of clinical illness.[52] Because many patients are asymptomatic, infections frequently go unnoticed or unreported.[52]

The hepatitis B virus is found in blood and all body fluids. The virus has an incubation period of 30–180 days.[54] Hepatitis B may be transmitted perinatally or via blood or sexual activity.[55] Hepatitis

Table 10.2	Hepatitis Serology
Virus	**Serology**
Active hepatitis A	Anti-HAV, IgM
Recovered hepatitis A	Anti-HAV, IgG
Active hepatitis B	HBsAg, HBeAg, Anti-HBc, IgM
Chronic hepatitis B	HBsAg, Anti-HBc, Anti-Hbe, IgM, IgG
Recovered hepatitis B	Anti-HBc, Anti-HBsAg
Acute hepatitis C	Anti-HCV, HCV RNA
Chronic hepatitis C	Anti-HCV, HCV RNA

Barkley TW Jr. *Pediatric Primary Care Nurse Practitioner Certification Review/Clinical Update Continuing Education Course.* West Hollywood, CA: Barkley and Associates; 2015.

A and B share similar clinical features, but onset tends to be more insidious in cases of hepatitis B. Although the risk of fulminant hepatitis B is less than 1%, the mortality rate is high when it does occur.[56,57]

Hepatitis C is traditionally associated with blood transfusions; however, in the United States, donated blood is now screened for the disease.[58] The virus is most commonly transmitted through intravenous drug use.[59] Hepatitis C may also be transmitted through sexual intercourse with an infected person, but the risk of sexual transmission is lower than that of intravenous drug use transmission.[60] The incubation period of hepatitis C is variable and ranges from 4 to 12 weeks.[59]

Presentation

Hepatitis presents with different signs and symptoms in its pre-icteric and icteric states. Signs and symptoms of the pre-icteric phase include malaise, anorexia, fever, nausea, and vomiting.[59] The icteric phase, characterized by jaundice, also features weight loss, itching, right upper quadrant abdominal pain, mild splenomegaly, clay-colored stool, and dark urine.[61]

Workup

Depending on the type of hepatitis, diagnostics may include a CBC, urinalysis, and serology tests. Both alanine aminotransferase (ALT) and aspartate aminotransferase (AST) levels increase prior to the onset of jaundice and decrease after jaundice presents. If ALT and AST levels indicate acute viral hepatitis, a prothrombin time test may be used, with slightly elevated results further indicating the disease. Urinalysis may reveal bilirubinuria and proteinuria, with urinary bilirubin typically preceding jaundice.[62]

Once the likelihood of hepatitis has been established, serology is the primary means of isolating the particular strain. Patients with acute hepatitis A will present with immunoglobulin M (IgM) hepatitis A antibodies (anti-HAV), whereas the presence of immunoglobulin G (IgG) anti-HAV will indicate a patient who has recovered from hepatitis A. Acute hepatitis B is indicated by hepatitis B virus surface antigen (HBsAg), hepatitis B e antigen (HBeAg), antibodies to the hepatitis B c antigen (anti-HBc), and IgM. If IgG and antibodies to HBeAg present alongside HBsAg, the patient has chronic hepatitis B; if anti-HBc and antibodies to HBsAg are present, the patient has likely recovered from hepatitis B. Both acute and chronic cases of hepatitis C will show hepatitis C antibodies (anti-HCV) and hepatitis C virus RNA. A patient who has recovered from hepatitis C will typically show anti-HCV but no hepatitis C virus RNA.[62]

Treatment

As there is no established antiviral therapy for hepatitis, management is generally supportive. Patients should be encouraged to rest during the active phase of the condition.[59] The NP should encourage fluid intake to prevent electrolyte or fluid imbalances, with the goal of increasing the patient's fluids to 3,000–4,000 ml per day. Vitamin K is recommended for patients with a prolonged prothrombin time longer than 15 seconds.[3] Patients with hepatitis should avoid excessive protein, alcohol, and medications detoxified by the liver.[61]

Vaccines exist for hepatitis A and hepatitis B. The hepatitis A vaccine should be administered at 1 year of age, and hepatitis A immune globulin is recommended as a short-term protection for those exposed to the virus. Once a pediatric patient recovers from hepatitis A, the vaccine is typically not necessary, as anti-HAV remains in the patient's system for life.[52] Hepatitis B vaccine should be administered within 12 hours of birth, with follow-up doses at 1 and 6 months of age. Patients who have not received the hepatitis B vaccine may receive it as prophylaxis within 24 hours of exposure to the virus; however, there is little benefit to administering the vaccine to someone who has already developed hepatitis B.[63]

References

1. Mayo Clinic Staff. Viral gastroenteritis (stomach flu). Mayo Clinic web site. http://www.mayoclinic.org/diseases-conditions/viral-gastroenteritis/basics/risk-factors/con-20019350. Updated December 2, 2014. Accessed April 15, 2015.

2. Cleveland Clinic Foundation. Diseases and conditions: Gastroenteritis. Cleveland Clinic web site. http://my.clevelandclinic.org/disorders/gastroenteritis/hic_gastroenteritis.aspx. Last reviewed April 4, 2012. Accessed April 15, 2015.

3. Barkley TW Jr. *Pediatric Primary Care Nurse Practitioner Certification Review/Clinical Update Continuing Education Course.* West Hollywood, CA: Barkley and Associates; 2015.

4. Boyce TG. Overview of gastroenteritis. In: Porter RS, Kaplan JL, eds. The Merck Manual Online. http://www.merckmanuals.com/professional/gastrointestinal_disorders/gastroenteritis/overview_of_gastroenteritis.html?qt=gastroenteritis&alt=sh. Last reviewed July 2014. Accessed April 15, 2015.

5. Bonheur JL, Arya M, Tarner MA. Bacterial gastroenteritis. In: Anand BS, ed. Medscape. http://emedicine.medscape.com/article/176400-overview#showall. Updated October 2, 2014. Accessed April 15, 2015.

6. Mayo Clinic Staff. Gastroenteritis: First aid. Mayo Clinic web site. http://www.mayoclinic.com/health/first-aid-gastroenteritis/FA00030. Updated February 7, 2015. Accessed April 15, 2015.

7. Patient information: Viral gastroenteritis (the basics). In: Basow DS, ed. *UpToDate*. Waltham, MA: UpToDate; 2015. http://www.uptodate.com/contents/viral-gastroenteritis-the-basics. Accessed April 15, 2015.

8. Gastroenteritis. WedMD web site. http://www.webmd.com/digestive-disorders/gastroenteritis. Reviewed April 25, 2014. Accessed April 15, 2015.

9. Stöppler MC. The BRAT diet. In: Doerr S, ed. MedicineNet. http://www.medicinenet.com/the_brat_diet/article.htm. Reviewed February 18, 2015. Accessed April 15, 2015.

10. Minnesota Department of Health. Specific disease exclusion guidelines for childcare and preschool. http://www.health.state.mn.us/divs/idepc/dtopics/foodborne/exclusions.html. Accessed April 15, 2015.

11. Prescilla RP. Pediatric gastroenteritis. In: Steele RW, ed. Medscape. http://emedicine.medscape.com/article/964131-overview#showall. Updated September 29, 2014. Accessed April 15, 2015.

12. DiMarino MC. Gastroesophageal reflux disease (GERD). In: Porter RS, Kaplan JL, eds. The Merck Manual Online. http://www.merckmanuals.com/professional/gastrointestinal_disorders/esophageal_and_swallowing_disorders/gastroesophageal_reflux_disease_gerd.html?qt=gastroesophageal%20reflux%20disease&alt=sh. Last reviewed May 2014. Accessed April 15, 2015.

13. Schwarz SM. Pediatric gastroesophageal reflux. In: Cuffari C, ed. Medscape. http://emedicine.medscape.com/article/930029-overview#aw2aab6b2b5. Updated April 26, 2014. Accessed April 23, 2015.

14. Mayo Clinic Staff. Intussusception. Mayo Clinic web site. http://www.mayoclinic.com/health/intussusception/DS00798. Updated December 14, 2012. Accessed April 15, 2015.

15. Patti MG. Gastroesophageal reflux disease. In: Katz J, ed. Medscape. http://emedicine.medscape.com/article/176595-overview. Updated April 16, 2014. Accessed April 15, 2015.

16. Kahrilas PJ. Clinical manifestations and diagnosis of gastroesophageal reflux in adults. In: Basow DS, ed. *UpToDate*. Waltham, MA: UpToDate; 2015. http://www.uptodate.com/contents/clinical-manifestations-and-diagnosis-of-gastroesophageal-reflux-in-adults. Last updated March 11, 2015. Accessed April 15, 2015.

17. Lightdale JR. Gastroesophageal reflux: Management guidance for the pediatrician. *Pediatrics*. 2013; 131(5): e1684–e1695. doi: 10.1542/peds.2013-0421

18. Schwarz SM. Pediatric gastroesophageal reflux treatment & management. In: Cuffari C, ed. Medscape. http://emedicine.medscape.com/article/930029-treatment#aw2aab6b6b2. Updated April 26, 2014. Accessed April 23, 2015.

19. Mayo Clinic Staff. GERD. Mayo Clinic web site. http://www.mayoclinic.org/diseases-conditions/gerd/basics/treatment/con-20025201. Updated July 31, 2014. Accessed April 16, 2015.

20. Pyloric stenosis. A.D.A.M. Medical Encyclopedia. http://www.nlm.nih.gov/medlineplus/ency/article/000970.htm. Updated August 22, 2013. Accessed April 16, 2015.

21. Olivé AP, Endom EE. Infantile hypertrophic pyloric stenosis. In: Basow DS, ed. *UpToDate*. Waltham, MA: UpToDate; 2015. http://www.uptodate.com/contents/infantile-hypertrophic-pyloric-stenosis. Last updated April 10, 2015. Accessed April 16, 2015.

22. Singh J. Pediatric pyloric stenosis. In: Bechtel KA, ed. Medscape. http://emedicine.medscape.com/article/803489-overview. Updated October 9, 2014. Accessed April 16, 2015.

23. Cochran WJ. Hypertrophic pyloric stenosis. In: Porter RS, Kaplan JL, eds. The Merck Manual Online. http://www.merckmanuals.com/professional/pediatrics/gastrointestinal_disorders_in_infants/hypertrophic_pyloric_stenosis.html?qt=pyloric%20stenosis&alt=sh. Last reviewed October 2014. Accessed April 16, 2015.

24. Mayo Clinic Staff. Pyloric stenosis. Mayo Clinic web site. http://www.mayoclinic.com/health/pyloric-stenosis/DS00815/DSECTION=tests-and-diagnosis. Updated November 16, 2012. Accessed April 16, 2015.

25. Kitagawa S, Miqdady M. Intussusception in children. In: Basow DS, ed. *UpToDate*. Waltham, MA: UpToDate; 2015. http://www.uptodate.com/contents/intussusception-in-children. Last reviewed April 6, 2015. Accessed April 16, 2015.

26. Cochran WJ. Intussusception. In: Porter RS, Kaplan JL, eds. The Merck Manual Online. http://www.merckmanuals.com/professional/pediatrics/gastrointestinal_disorders_in_infants/intussusception.html?qt=intussusception&alt=sh. Last reviewed October 2014. Accessed April 16, 2015.

27. Blanco F. Intussusception. In: Cuffari C, ed. Medscape. http://emedicine.medscape.com/article/930708-overview. Updated April 22, 2014. Accessed April 16, 2015.

28. Intussusception – children. A.D.A.M. Medical Encyclopedia. http://www.nlm.nih.gov/medlineplus/ency/article/000958.htm. Updated May 14, 2014. Accessed April 16, 2015.

29. Wesson DE. Congenital aganglionic megacolon (Hirschsprung disease). In: Basow DS, ed. *UpToDate*. Waltham, MA: UpToDate; 2015. http://www.uptodate.com/contents/congenital-aganglionic-megacolon-hirschsprung-disease. Last updated January 29, 2015. Accessed April 16, 2015.

30. Mayo Clinic Staff. Hirschsprung's disease. Mayo Clinic web site. http://www.mayoclinic.com/health/hirschsprungs-disease/DS00825/DSECTION=causes. Updated March 28, 2013. Accessed April 16, 2015.

31. Cochran WJ. Hirschsprung disease. In: Porter RS, Kaplan JL, eds. The Merck Manual Online. http://www.merckmanuals.com/professional/pediatrics/congenital_gastrointestinal_anomalies/hirschsprung_disease.html?qt=megacolon&alt=sh. Last reviewed March 2013. Accessed April 16, 2015.

32. Hirschsprung's disease. A.D.A.M. Medical Encyclopedia. http://www.nlm.nih.gov/medlineplus/ency/article/001140.htm. Updated December 4, 2013. Accessed April 16, 2015.

33. Wagner JP. Hirschsprung disease. In: Katz J, ed. Medscape. http://emedicine.medscape.com/article/178493-overview. Updated May 30, 2014. Accessed April 16, 2015.

34. Craig S. Appendicitis. In: Brenner BE, ed. Medscape. http://emedicine.medscape.com/article/773895-overview#showall. Updated July 21, 2014. Accessed April 16, 2015.

35. Appendicitis. A.D.A.M. Medical Encyclopedia. http://www.ncbi.nlm.nih.gov/pubmedhealth/PMH0001302. Accessed April 16, 2015.

36. Ansari P. Appendicitis. In: Porter RS, Kaplan JL, eds. The Merck Manual Online. http://www.merckmanuals.com/professional/gastrointestinal_disorders/acute_abdomen_and_surgical_gastroenterology/appendicitis.html. Last reviewed June 2014. Accessed April 16, 2015.

37. Wesson DE. Acute appendicitis in children: Clinical manifestations and diagnosis. In: Basow DS, ed. *UpToDate*. Waltham, MA: UpToDate; 2015. http://www.uptodate.com/contents/acute-appendicitis-in-children-clinical-manifestations-and-diagnosis. Last updated December 4, 2014. Accessed April 16, 2015.

38. Wesson DE. Acute appendicitis in children: Management. In: Basow DS, ed. *UpToDate*. Waltham, MA: UpToDate; 2015. http://www.uptodate.com/contents/acute-appendicitis-in-children-management?source=search_result&search=appendicitis+in+children&selectedTitle=2~150. Last updated February 6, 2015. Accessed April 24, 2015.

39. Ruiz AR Jr. Malabsorption syndromes. In: Porter RS, Kaplan JL, eds. The Merck Manual Online. http://www.merckmanuals.com/professional/gastrointestinal_disorders/malabsorption_syndromes/overview_of_malabsorption.html?qt=malabsorption&alt=sh. Last reviewed May 2014. Accessed April 16, 2015.

40. Kerr M. Malabsorption syndrome. Healthline web site. http://www.healthline.com/health/malabsorption. Published June 14, 2012. Accessed April 16, 2015.

41. Goebel SU. Malabsorption. In: Katz J, ed. Medscape. http://emedicine.medscape.com/article/180785-clinical#showall. Updated December 16, 2014. Accessed April 16, 2015.

42. Malabsorption. A.D.A.M. Medical Encyclopedia. http://www.nlm.nih.gov/medlineplus/ency/article/000299.htm. Updated August 10, 2012. Accessed April 16, 2015.

43. Mason JB, Milovic V. Overview of the treatment of malabsorption. In: Basow DS, ed. *UpToDate*. Waltham, MA: UpToDate; 2015. http://www.uptodate.com/contents/overview-of-the-treatment-of-malabsorption. Last updated April 14, 2014. Accessed April 16, 2015.

44. Neuroblastoma. A.D.A.M. Medical Encyclopedia. http://www.nlm.nih.gov/medlineplus/ency/article/001408.htm. Updated October 30, 2013. Accessed April 16, 2015.

45. United States Department of Health and Human Services, National Institutes of Health, National Cancer Institute. Neuroblastoma treatment. http://www.cancer.gov/cancertopics/pdq/treatment/neuroblastoma/HealthProfessional/page1. Updated December 15, 2014. Accessed April 16, 2015.

46. Shohet JM, Nuchtern JG. Clinical presentation, diagnosis, and staging evaluation of neuroblastoma. In: Basow DS, ed. *UpToDate*. Waltham, MA: UpToDate; 2015. http://www.uptodate.com/contents/clinical-presentation-diagnosis-and-staging-evaluation-of-neuroblastoma. Last updated December 30, 2013. Accessed April 17, 2015.

47. Joyner BD. Neuroblastoma. In: Kopell BH, ed. Medscape. http://emedicine.medscape.com/article/439263-overview#showall. Updated March 27, 2015. Accessed April 17, 2015.

48. Rutherford AE. Overview of hepatitis. In: Porter RS, Kaplan JL, eds. The Merck Manual Online. http://www.merckmanuals.com/professional/hepatic_and_biliary_disorders/hepatitis/overview_of_hepatitis.html?qt=hepatitis&alt=sh. Last reviewed February 2014. Accessed April 17, 2015.

49. Ben Joseph EP. Hepatitis. KidsHealth web site. http://kidshealth.org/teen/sexual_health/stds/hepatitis.html#. Reviewed February 2014. Accessed April 17, 2015.

50. United States Department of Health and Human Services, Centers for Disease Control and Prevention. Hepatitis A FAQs for the public. http://www.cdc.gov/hepatitis/A/aFAQ.htm#overview. Last updated March 6, 2015. Accessed April 17, 2015.

51. Bennett NJ, Domachowske J. Pediatric hepatitis A. In: Steele RW, ed. Medscape. http://emedicine.medscape.com/article/964575-overview#showall. Updated March 3, 2014. Accessed April 17, 2015.

52. United States Department of Health and Human Services, Centers for Disease Control and Prevention. Hepatitis A information for health professionals. http://www.cdc.gov/hepatitis/HAV/. Updated April 14, 2014. Accessed April 24, 2015.

53. Hepatitis A. A.D.A.M. Medical Encyclopedia. http://www.nlm.nih.gov/medlineplus/ency/article/000278.htm. Updated October 13, 2013. Accessed April 17, 2015.

54. World Health Organization. Hepatitis B. World Health Organization web site. http://www.who.int/mediacentre/factsheets/fs204/en. Updated March 2015. Accessed April 17, 2015.

55. United States Department of Health and Human Services, Centers for Disease Control and Prevention. Hepatitis B FAQs for the public. http://www.cdc.gov/hepatitis/b/bFAQ.htm#overview. Last updated March 6, 2015. Accessed April 17, 2015.

56. Rapti IN, Hadziyannis SJ. Chronic hepatitis B infection: Treatment of special populations: HBV prophylaxis following liver transplantation. http://www.medscape.org/viewarticle/743845_6. Updated June 8, 2011. Accessed April 17, 2015.

57. Government of Canada, Canadian Centre for Occupational Health and Safety. Hepatitis B. http://www.ccohs.ca/oshanswers/diseases/hepatitis_b.html. Last updated August 28 ,2013. Accessed April 17, 2015.

58. United States Department of Health and Human Services, Centers for Disease Control and Prevention. Hepatitis C information for the public. http://www.cdc.gov/hepatitis/C/index.htm. Updated May 6, 2013. Accessed April 24, 2015.

59. United States Department of Health and Human Services, Centers for Disease Control and Prevention. The ABCs of hepatitis. http://www.cdc.gov/hepatitis/resources/professionals/pdfs/abctable.pdf. Updated 2014. Accessed April 17, 2015.

60. World Health Organization. Hepatitis C. World Health Organization web site. http://www.who.int/mediacentre/factsheets/fs164/en. Updated April 2014. Accessed April 17, 2015.

61. Hepatitis C. A.D.A.M. Medical Encyclopedia. http://www.nlm.nih.gov/medlineplus/ency/article/000284.htm. Updated October 13, 2013. Accessed April 18, 2015.

62. Rutherford AE. Acute viral hepatitis. In: Porter RS, Kaplan JL, eds. The Merck Manual Online Web site. http://www.merckmanuals.com/professional/hepatic-and-biliary-disorders/hepatitis/acute-viral-hepatitis. Last reviewed February 2014. Accessed April 24, 2015.

63. United States Department of Health and Human Services, Centers for Disease Control and Prevention. Hepatitis B FAQs for health professionals. http://www.cdc.gov/hepatitis/HBV/HBVfaq.htm. Last updated March 6, 2015. Accessed April 18, 2015.

Chapter 11

Dermatological Disorders

QUESTIONS

1. You are examining Ryan, a 17-year-old male, and note inflamed papules on his face and upper trunk. He admits to using steroids in order to keep up with his teammates in baseball; these steroids appear to have exacerbated the symptoms. Of the following, which dermatological disorder is the most likely diagnosis?

   a. Acne

   b. Psoriasis

   c. Atopic dermatitis

   d. Pityriasis rosea

2. Which of these dermatological disorders is most commonly associated with elevated serum immunoglobulin E (IgE) levels?

   a. Atopic dermatitis

   b. Acne

   c. Pityriasis rosea

   d. Varicella zoster virus

3. Which of these treatments is primarily recommended for management of tinea capitis?

   a. Oral acyclovir

   b. Aluminum subacetate solution

   c. Neem shampoo

   d. Griseofulvin

4. The most common findings of impetigo include all of the following choices except:

   a. Pain

   b. Pruritic rash

   c. Honey-crusting lesions

   d. Regional lymphadenopathy

5. A 5-month-old infant's parent describes him as being recently irritable and constantly rubbing at his skin. Your examination reveals red-brown vesiculopapular lesions on his soles. Which drug would be the best choice to manage the most likely condition?

   a. Lindane lotion (Kwell)

   b. Calamine with topical diphenhydramine (Ivarest)

   c. Permethrin (Nix) 5% rinse

   d. Griseofulvin (Grifulvin V)

6. An infant presents to the clinic with an angry red diaper rash with satellite lesions. A potassium hydroxide preparation used to examine the lesion is negative. Your treatment would consist of which of these methods?

   a. Hydrocortisone 1% cream

   b. Zinc oxide ointment

   c. Acyclovir 5% cream

   d. Nystatin 100,000 units/gram

7. A 14-year-old patient presents to your clinic with complaints of stiff joints and pain that starts in her shoulders before traveling down her arms. She reports that, following a recent nature hike, she found a tick on her leg. Within a few days, a lesion that "looks like a bull's eye" had developed at the tick site. She also tells you that she has been experiencing severe headaches, and that her heart occasionally "races like a drum." Which stage of the most likely diagnosis is the patient experiencing?

   a. Stage 1

   b. Stage 2

   c. Stage 3

   d. Stage 4

8. Of the following, which viral infection most commonly presents with Koplik spots?

   a. Rubeola

   b. Roseola infantum

   c. Rubella

   d. Lyme disease

9. A 5-year-old patient is brought to your clinic with extensive second-degree burns. The burns cover the entirety of the back of his head but do not extend any further than that. Approximately how much of his body has been burned?

   a. Approximately 6%

   b. Approximately 7%

   c. Approximately 9%

   d. Approximately 10%

10. While assessing a patient during a physical, you find a small elevated area on her lower back. The area is a firm lesion of approximately 1.5 cm; it feels smooth to the touch, is not filled with fluid, and does not appear to extend below the epidermis. This morphology best describes which type of lesion?

   a. Wheal

   b. Tumor

   c. Cyst

   d. Nodule

RATIONALES

1. a

Because the patient presents with papules and cysts on his face and upper trunk and has a history of steroid use, he is most likely experiencing acne. Psoriasis typically presents as lesions with red, sharply defined plaques with silvery scales, not comedones or pustules, and commonly occurs due to genetic predisposition, not steroid use. Atopic dermatitis often involves dry scaly skin rather than comedones or papules, and commonly presents with intense pruritus along the face, neck, trunk, wrists, hands, and antecubital and popliteal folds. Lastly, although pityriasis rosea also typically manifests on the upper trunk, it usually manifests as a pruritic rash, not comedones and cysts, and is often treated with, not exacerbated by, steroids.

2. a

Atopic dermatitis commonly presents with elevated serum immunoglobulin E (IgE) and eosinophilia. Allergic rhinitis, asthma, and parasitic diseases are also typically associated with elevated IgE, but pityriasis rosea, acne, or varicella zoster virus are not.

3. d

Primary treatment for tinea capitis often utilizes griseofulvin, given in doses of 20 mg/kg/day for 6 weeks. Oral acyclovir is a common primary treatment for the varicella zoster virus, not tinea capitis. Aluminum subacetate solution often treats both tinea manuum and pedis. Neem shampoo is a common treatment for scabies.

4. b

Pruritic rash is not a standard sign or symptom of impetigo, and is more commonly associated with pityriasis rosea. Honey-crusting lesions are a classic symptom of impetigo, and the bacterial infection of the skin often produces pain and regional lymphadenopathy.

5. c

Permethrin (Nix) 5% rinse is a common primary treatment for scabies, which is indicated by the infant's irritability, itching, and red-brown vesiculopapular lesions on his soles. Lindane lotion is also a common treatment of choice for scabies; however, as the patient in the scenario is younger than 6 months old, it should be avoided, as lindane is often neurotoxic to this population and can cause seizures or death. As scabies is easily spread among family members, it is important to treat the household in order to reduce the incidence of reacquisition and retreatment. Calamine with a topical antihistamine, such as diphenhydramine, may relieve the patient's pruritus, but it will not typically affect the mites that cause scabies. Griseofulvin is meant to remedy fungal, not parasitic, skin infections.

6. a

Irritant diaper dermatitis presenting with satellite lesions is typically treated with 1% hydrocortisone cream in order to reduce inflammation. Nystatin may be called for if secondary *Candida albicans* infection is suspected; however, as the patient's potassium hydroxide preparation turned up negative for the fungus, this medication is not necessarily indicated. Zinc oxide ointment functions as a barrier emollient and is typically recommended for more mild cases of irritant diaper dermatitis. Acyclovir cream is commonly reserved for viral lesions stemming from the herpes simplex virus or other viral skin infections.

7. b

Headache, stiff joints, migratory pains, and cardiac irregularities all typically characterize Stage 2 of Lyme disease, as would aseptic meningitis, Bell's palsy, and peripheral neuropathy. Although muscle and joint pain may present in Stage 1, this stage is more commonly characterized by flu-like symptoms, fatigue, and erythema migrans. Stage 3 is also often characterized by pain, stiffness, and swelling in the joints, but these symptoms would typically evolve into clear manifestations of arthritis, usually presenting in the knees. Furthermore, other symptoms such as acrodermatitis chronicum atrophicans, characterized by bluish-red discoloring of the distal extremity with edema, or subacute encephalopathy may produce in Stage 3. There is no Stage 4 for Lyme disease.

8. a

Rubeola (measles) commonly presents with Koplik spots, which are small, white, granular spots surrounded by red rings found inside the oro-pharynx. Small, pink, and flat to raised bumps often appear in roseola infantum (Sixth disease), rather than white spots. Rubella typically presents with a fine, erythematous maculopapular rash that first manifests on the face before spreading to the trunk and extremities. Lyme disease is characterized by erythema migrans in a distinctive "bulls-eye" pattern, not Koplik spots.

9. b

For a 5-year-old child, the back of the head is commonly considered 7% of the surface area of the skin. The surface area of a child's head, thighs, and legs changes during early development, and thus has varying values based on age. The back of the head would typically be considered 10% of total skin surface area in a newborn, 9% in a 1-year-old, and 6% in a 10-year-old.

10. d

Nodules are classified as elevated, firm lesions that extend beyond 1 cm. Although tumors are also firm and elevated, they commonly take on the appearance of lumps, which are masses of indefinite size, rather than lesions, which are more circumscribed. A wheal typically appears both above the surface of the skin and extends below the epidermis; many times, it is a sign of an allergic reaction. A cyst is often filled with either air, fluid, or semi-solid material, such as in the case of a pilonidal cyst.

DISCUSSION

Burns

Overview

Burns are traumatic injuries to the skin and underlying tissues caused by exposure to or contact with thermal or non-thermal sources.

Burn injuries can be thermal, chemical, electrical, or radiological.[1,2]

Burn injuries are categorized as first-degree, second-degree, third-degree, and fourth-degree burns. Healing time depends on the depth and size of the burn area, care given, and a timely treatment.

Presentation

Superficial or first-degree burns are burns that affect only the epidermis. Typically, the site of injury is dry and red, with later development of moisture. These injuries are painful and include severe sunburns and burns caused by scalding hot water.[3]

Partial-thickness or second-degree burns extend beyond the epidermis. These burns may be described as superficial or deep, and may present with a variety of findings, such as moist wounds, blisters, and pain, among others.[3,4]

Full-thickness or third-degree burns extend beyond the dermis to the underlying subcutaneous tissues. Third-degree burns result in eschar, leaving a dry, hard, leathery surface. The site may be black, pearly, or red and waxy. As with partial-thickness burns, the skin appears flat and dehydrated, and may be peeled with ease. The patient feels no pain due to destruction of pain sensors.[3,4]

Fourth-degree burns are full-thickness burns affecting the deeper tissues. These types of burns involve total destruction of the skin, subcutaneous tissue, tendons, muscle, and/or bone, and the damaged areas are typically black and charred in appearance.[2,3,4]

Workup (see figures 11.1–11.2 and table 11.1)

Burns to certain parts of the body warrant special consideration.[5] Burns to the eyes should be immediately assessed by an ophthalmologist. Burns to the face may be accompanied by inhalation injury and facial edema, which may affect the airway. Burns to the genitalia and surrounding region (i.e., the perineum) require immediate hospitalization.

Assessing the extent of a burn injury, which is expressed as a percentage of the total body surface area (TBSA), is necessary to determine severity, estimate fluid resuscitation requirements, and assess whether or not the patient should be transported to emergency care. The TBSA is calculated by using either the "Rule of Nines" or the Lund and Browder Chart. Inhalation injuries can increase the TBSA estimate.

The "Rule of Nines" is an estimation of TBSA measured in multiples of 9, but is calculated differently for pediatric patients than in adult patients.[6] In pediatrics, a larger percentage is assigned to the surface area of the head, whereas the legs are assigned a smaller percentage. For example, the TBSA of an infant's head ranges from 18% to 20% and the legs range from 13% to 14% for each leg— half the percentage is attributed to the anterior and posterior surface areas. For adults, the head and neck are 9%, and each leg equals 18% of TBSA.[7]

The Lund and Browder chart is the preferred method in most burn units, as it correlates TBSA with age-related proportions, while also further subdividing the areas of the body and taking the patient's age and TBSA into account.[8]

Treatment

As the first 6 hours following a burn injury are critical, children with severe burns should be transported to the emergency department as soon as possible. For all burns, patients should be assessed for the ABCs—airway, breathing, and circulation— and for signs that warrant prophylactic intubation (e.g., singed nares or eyebrows, soot and/or black mucous in nares or mouth).[5] In minor burns, all burnt clothing should be removed, and the burn should be immersed in cool, not iced, water for 30 minutes to prevent further damage and reduce pain. Once this is done, a clean wrap should be applied to the wound. The burn should not be covered with lotion, butter, or other products.

According to guidelines established by the American College of Surgeons, pediatric patients with severe and major burns should be referred to a burn center for treatment and recovery.[11] This includes patients with partial-thickness burns covering more than 10% of the TBSA, burns that involve areas especially prone to damage (e.g., face, hands, feet, genitalia, perineum, major joints), full-thickness burns, electrical or chemical burns, inhalation injury, burn injuries in patients with preexisting conditions that may complicate management, and burns with concomitant trauma where the burn poses the highest risk of mortality. Pediatric patients should also be referred to a burn center if the hospital lacks qualified personnel or equipment for the care of children, or if the patient requires special social, emotional, or rehabilitative intervention.[11]

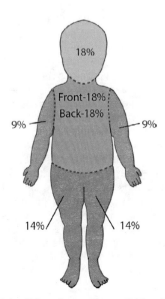

Figure 11.1. Rule of Nines diagram for a pediatric patient

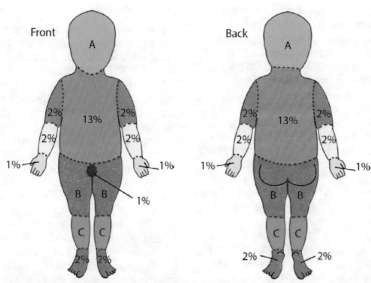

Figure 11.2. Lund and Browder diagram for pediatric patients

Table 11.1	Relative Percentage of Body Surface Area for Lund and Browder Chart			
Area	Age 0	1 year	5 years	10 years
A=1/2 of head	10%	9%	7%	6%
B=1/2 of one thigh	3%	3%	4%	5%
C=1/2 of one leg	2%	3%	3%	3%

Used with permission from Barkley TW Jr. *Adult-Gerontology Primary Care Nurse Practitioner Certification Review/Clinical Update Continuing Education Course*. West Hollywood, CA: Barkley and Associates; 2015.

Evaluation of Skin Disorders

Overview

The systematic approach to evaluating skin disorders consists of identifying the morphology, configuration, and distribution of lesions. A macule is a flat discoloration on the surface of the skin.[12] A patch is a flat discoloration that appears as a collection of multiple, tiny pigment changes. Papules are elevated, firm skin lesions smaller than 1 cm in diameter. A nodule is an elevated, firm lesion greater than 1 cm in diameter.[13] A tumor is a firm, elevated mass of tissue. Wheals, which are caused by either a contact or systemic allergic reaction, are raised above the skin surface and extend slightly below the epidermis.[14] Plaques are scaly, elevated lesions, which are classically associated with psoriasis. Vesicles are lesions smaller than 1 cm that are filled with serous fluid; bullae are serous fluid-filled vesicles greater than 1 cm in diameter.[15] A pustule is a small pus-filled lesion smaller than 1 cm in diameter, whereas an abscess is a pus-filled lesion greater than 1 cm in diameter.[16] Lastly, cysts are large, raised lesions filled with serous fluid, blood, and/or pus.[17]

Presentation

Skin lesions are grouped into two categories: primary and secondary. Primary lesions are lesions that develop on previously unaltered skin as a result of disease, trauma, or insult. Secondary lesions result from changes over time to primary lesions or may develop as a consequence of insult to the lesion (e.g., infection, scratching, etc.).[18] Furthermore, solitary or discrete lesions present as individual or distinct lesions that remain separate. Grouped lesions form a linear cluster, whereas confluent lesions run together.[18] Linear lesions may resemble scratches, streaks, lines, or stripes. Annular lesions present in a circular pattern, beginning in the center and spreading to the periphery. In some patients, annular lesions may merge to form polycyclic lesions.[19] Usually, lesions develop on the face, trunk, upper extremities, groin, feet, axilla, and dermatomal regions.

Acne

Overview

Acne vulgaris is a common skin disorder characterized by the formation of comedones, papules, pustules, and cysts. The onset is both more common and more severe in males.[20] Although

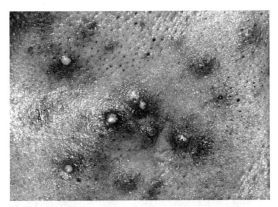

Figure 11.3. Acne

exact causes of acne are unknown, androgens play a role in genetically predisposed individuals.[21] Acne is also exacerbated by the use of steroids and anticonvulsants.[22]

Presentation (see figure 11.3)

Patients with acne present with comedones on the face and upper trunk. Comedones can be either open or closed.[23] Open comedones, also known as blackheads, are openings in the skin capped with blackened skin debris. Closed comedones, also known as whiteheads, are obstructed openings capped with white skin debris. Depending on the severity of acne, papules, pustules, nodules, cysts, or a combination of the four may also present. More severe acne lesions may result in atrophic (i.e., depressed) or hypertrophic scars.[24] In adolescents, acne may be exacerbated by hormonal fluctuations related to menses.[25]

Workup

The diagnosis of acne is based on clinical appearance.[26]

Treatment

Patients with acne should first be encouraged to wash their face several times per day. Non-pharmacologic management of acne focuses on avoidance of topical, oil-based products and use of oil-free mild soaps, cleansers, and moisturizers. Pharmacologic management options include salicylic acid preparations and topical antibiotics such as erythromycin and clindamycin.[27] For patients with mild acne, topical treatment with benzoyl peroxide (2.5%–10%) is first recommended. If not effective, others agents may be considered, such as retinoic acid (0.025%–0.1%) cream or gel. Retinoic acid should be prescribed with caution in females, as it is classified as a Pregnancy Category C drug.[28] Topical tretinoin is also highly effective in the treatment of acne.[29]

Moderate and severe pustular acne often requires topical treatments with systemic antibiotics, such as doxycycline (Vibramycin), erythromycin (Erythrocin), or minocycline (Minocin).[30] Patients with severe acne that does not respond to antibiotics should be referred to a dermatologist.

Fungal Infections

Overview

The various types of fungal infections are distinguished by the causal species of fungi and the location of affected areas of the body. Fungal infections are classified based on location on the body.[31]

Many fungal infections in pediatric patients are caused by dermatophytes, including tinea capitis, located on the scalp; tinea corporis, or ringworm (usually the legs, arms, and trunk), tinea cruris (groin), tinea pedis (feet), and tinea versicolor (trunk and legs).[32,33] Tinea pedis may be accompanied by tinea manuum (surfaces of the palms).[34]

Presentation

Some fungal infections, such as tinea capitis, may be asymptomatic at first; eventually, however, tinea capitis presents with papules, pruritus, and detachment of hair from the scalp. Pruritus is common, but may be more severe in tinea cruris and tinea pedis.[35] Tinea corporis is characterized by erythematous rings.[36] Tinea versicolor is distinguished by the appearance of solitary areas of hypopigmented or hyperpigmented macules.[34,37]

Workup

The diagnosis of fungal infections is determined via a clinical examination.[38] A potassium hydroxide (KOH) microscopy may also be necessary; on a KOH preparation, fungal infections are distinguished by a "spaghetti and meatballs" pattern.[39,40]

Treatment

Tinea capitis is treated with antifungal shampoo, but may require systemic management. The traditional choice for systemic treatment is griseofulvin (Gris-PEG), 20–25 mg/kg/day for approximately six weeks. Newer therapeutic options with shorter courses of treatment include oral terbinafine, itraconazole, and fluconazole.[41]

Like most other fungal infections, tinea corporis responds well to topical antifungals, including miconazole 2% and ketoconazole 2%.[42] Griseofulvin may be ordered for severe cases. Terbinafine cream is effective in more than 80% of all cases when prescribed twice a day for 7 days.[43]

The treatment regimen for tinea manuum and tinea pedis depends on the stage of infection. In the macerated stage of infection, aluminum subacetate solution is used for 20 minutes twice a day.[44] The dry, scaly stage is treated with topical antifungals.

The standard treatment for tinea versicolor is selenium sulfide for 5–15 minutes daily over 7 days.

Itraconazole, given at 200 mg every day by mouth, may serve as an alternative treatment in patients 3 years of age or older.[40]

Varicella Zoster Virus (Chickenpox)

Overview

Varicella zoster is an acute, contagious disease caused by primary infection of the varicella zoster virus, transmitted through direct contact with lesions.[45] Patients are contagious 48 hours before the outbreak of the disease, with contagion persisting until lesions have crusted over.[46] Varicella zoster is most common in children between 5 and 10 years of age.[47]

Presentation (see figure 11.4)

Varicella zoster is characterized by the outbreak of erythematous macules and subsequent development of papules.[48] In most cases, vesicles initially appear on the trunk before developing on the scalp and face, accompanied by intense pruritus, low-grade fever, and generalized lymphadenopathy.[48]

Workup

Typically, a clinical examination is sufficient to diagnose varicella zoster.[49] Lab tests may be required in cases with immunocompromised patients or atypical lesions.[49]

Treatment

Varicella zoster may be prevented with varicella vaccine; the initial dose is administered to infants at 12–15 months of age, followed by a second dose at 4–6 years of age.[50] The standard treatment for varicella zoster is oral acyclovir, 20 mg/kg every 6 hours for 5 days, not to exceed 800 mg; this dosage may need to be adjusted based on age, weight, and immunocompetence.[51] Supportive treatment may include antihistamine and calamine (Caladryl) for pruritus, as well as acetaminophen for fever.[52,53] Aspirin should be avoided, however, as children given acetylsalicylic acid during cases of varicella zoster may develop Reye's syndrome.

Molluscum Contagiosum

Overview

Molluscum contagiosum is a benign viral skin infection, causing small pearly or flesh-colored papules that may disappear within 6–12 months without treatment.[54]

Presentation (see figure 11.5)

Patients with molluscum contagiosum present with pruritus and very small, firm, pink or flesh-colored discrete papules.[55] Lesions develop on the face, axillae, antecubital fossa, trunk, and extremities. Although not easily treated, these lesions frequently disappear over the course of a few months.[56,57,58]

Workup

The diagnosis of molluscum contagiosum can be determined based on clinical presentation.[59]

Treatment

Because molluscum contagiosum is self-limiting, treatment may not be necessary. Curettage is a useful treatment but should not be used on sensitive areas due to risk of scarring.[12]

Molluscum contagiosum is treated with agents such as tretinoin, salicylic acid, liquid nitrogen, trichloroacetic acid, podofilox, silver nitrate, or electrocautery.[60,61] Cantharidin 0.7% may be applied to individual lesions and covered with clear tape.[62] Cantharidin should, however, be avoided on facial lesions since it may cause blistering within 24 hours.

Scratching and touching lesions should be avoided to prevent further spread.[63]

Atopic Dermatitis (Eczema)

Overview

Atopic dermatitis, also known as eczema, is a chronic skin condition characterized by intense pruritus, as well as plaques with a typical pattern of distribution and periods of remission and exacerbation. In infants and young children, plaques commonly appear on facial and extensor surfaces.

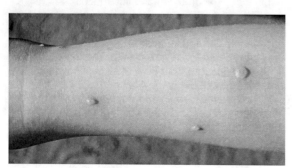

Figure 11.4. Chickenpox

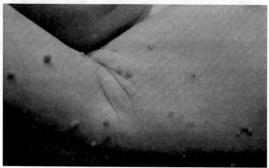

Figure 11.5. Molluscum contagiosum

This condition is particularly sensitive to low humidity and often worsens in the winter.[64]

Presentation (see figure 11.6)

Patients with atopic dermatitis have plaques that may appear along the face, neck, trunk, wrists, and/or antecubital and popliteal folds.[65] These patches are often inflamed or scabbed and exhibit diffuse erythema and scaling, followed by dry, leathery lichenification. Acute flare-ups show red, shiny, or thickened patches.[66]

Workup

The patient's personal or family history of asthma, allergic rhinitis, atopic dermatitis, and predisposition to skin infections should be considered during the diagnostic evaluation. Laboratory tests may reveal eosinophilia and elevated serum immunoglobulin E levels.[67] A radioallergosorbent (RAST) test or allergy tests may be used to determine the causative allergen.[44]

Treatment

Treatment of eczema focuses on managing dry skin. Patients should blot themselves dry after every bath or shower prior to applying medication or moisturizing cream to the area.[68]

Topical steroids, such as hydrocortisone cream, fluocinonide cream 0.05%, desonide, and triamcinolone 0.1%, among others, may be thinly applied 2–4 times daily and should only be used for exacerbations.[69,70] Systemic steroids such as prednisone should only be used in extremely severe cases. For acute weeping lesions that are moist, either saline, aluminum subacetate solution, or colloidal oatmeal baths (e.g., Aveeno) are beneficial. Ultraviolet therapy may also see use, and immune modulators may be used in immunocompetent patients over the age of 2 years with severe atopic dermatitis.[71]

Allergic Contact Dermatitis

Overview

Allergic contact dermatitis is a condition characterized by inflammation that results from direct skin contact with chemicals or allergens.[72]

Presentation

A variety of findings, including redness, pruritus, and scabbing, among others, are seen in patients with allergic contact dermatitis. The acute phase is characterized by small vesicles and oozing, encrusted lesions. The chronic phase involves scaling, erythema, and thickened, lichenified skin.[71] Affected areas may appear inflamed and swollen.

Workup

Diagnosis of allergic contact dermatitis is made by clinical evaluation and, sometimes, by patch testing.[73]

Treatment

Management depends on the severity of findings and the offending agent. Supportive treatment consists of compresses applied locally. Patients should avoid scrubbing the affected area with soap and water. High potency topical steroids applied locally are considered first-line treatment for localized allergic contact dermatitis.[74] If severe, management may incorporate prednisone, 60 mg daily on a 14-day tapered course for older children and adolescents. Younger children should be dosed based on weight.[75] Antihistamines may also be used.

Irritant (Diaper) Dermatitis

Overview

Diaper dermatitis is a common skin irritation of the genital-perianal region in infants, caused by exposure to chemical irritants or prolonged contact with urine or feces. This exposure can lead to infection by bacteria or *Candida albicans*.[76] Irritant

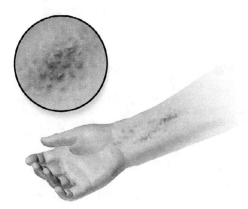

Figure 11.6. Allergic contact dermatitis

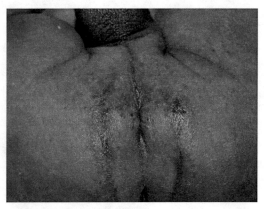

Figure 11.7. Irritant diaper dermatitis

dermatitis occurs at some time in 95% of all infants, with the incidence peaking at 9–12 months.[77]

Presentation (see figure 11.7)

A fiery red rash with papules, vesicles, crusts, and ulcerations is common in cases of irritant diaper dermatitis.[78]

Workup

The diagnosis for irritant diaper dermatitis is made clinically, with a focus on ruling out other conditions. A KOH test may be used to confirm the presence of a *Candida* infection.[78]

Treatment

In mild cases, barrier emollients improve skin condition.[79] When erythema and papules are present, 1% hydrocortisone is recommended to reduce skin inflammation.[80] Burow's (Domeboro) compresses may be used to relieve severe erythema and vesicles.[77]

Cases with secondary bacterial or fungal infection require topical antibiotics or antifungal cream, respectively.[42] The NP should also educate parents about preventive measures, such as allowing the diaper area to be open to air several times daily.[77]

Psoriasis

Overview

Psoriasis is a benign hyperproliferative inflammatory skin disease that affects the protective function of the epidermis. The disorder may be either acute or chronic, and may be associated with more serious diseases. The development of psoriasis is dependent upon a genetic predisposition affecting approximately 2%–3% percent of the population, although environmental and immunologic factors may play a role.[81,82]

In most cases of psoriasis, normal maturation of the skin cells cannot take place, keratinization is faulty, the epidermis is thickened, and immature nucleated cells are seen on the stratum corneum (i.e., the horny layer).[83]

Presentation

Some patients may present with no more than pruritus, whereas others experience red, sharply defined plaques with silvery scales.[84] Lesions commonly develop on the scalp, elbows, knees, palms, soles, and nails.[85] Fine pitting of the nails and separation of the nail plate from the bed are additional findings commonly noted in psoriasis.[86] Pink or red lines may be seen in the intergluteal fold. Auspitz sign is another common finding, consisting of pinpoint bleeding spots that appear when scales are removed.[87]

Workup

Psoriasis can be clinically diagnosed through a physical exam and medical history. In rare cases, skin biopsy may be used to determine the exact type of psoriasis.[88]

Treatment

Common management options for psoriasis include topicals for the scalp, such as coal tar or salicylic acid shampoo and medium potency topical steroid oil.[89] Coal tar shampoo is not approved for use in patients under 2 years of age. Topical steroids may be applied to affected regions twice a day for 2 weeks.[90] Following treatment with steroids, management of psoriasis is usually resumed with calcipotriene (Dovonex).[91] Alternatively, the treatment may be continued with either betamethasone dipropionate 0.05% (Diprolene AF) or triamcinolone acetonide 0.5% (Aristocort). Moisturizers may be used for supportive treatment. Ultraviolet B phototherapy may be combined with topical or systemic agents to increase efficacy of treatment, especially if more than 30% of the body surface is involved.[92]

Pityriasis Rosea

Overview

Pityriasis rosea is a mild, acute self-limiting inflammatory disorder, lasting 3–8 weeks. According to current theories, this disorder is viral in origin, although the causes remain unknown.[93] Pityriasis rosea is more common in the spring and fall seasons, presents more often in females than in males, and has an age-related onset. Patients with pityriasis rosea often have a history of recent upper respiratory infections.[94]

Presentation

A "herald patch" is commonly seen as the initial finding of pityriasis rosea.[95] This patch is usually 2–10 cm in diameter and is macular, oval, and fawn-colored with a crinkled appearance and collarette scale. A mild pruritic rash follows within 1–2 weeks of onset, often developing in a "Christmas tree pattern" that runs along the trunk and proximal extremities.[96]

Workup

A diagnosis of pityriasis rosea is made by considering the clinical distribution and appearance of the patient's lesions. A serologic test for syphilis should also be performed if the patient's lesions are small in number, perfectly-shaped, not pruritic, or located on the palmar or plantar surfaces.[52]

Treatment

Cases of pityriasis rosea with pruritus may require hydroxyzine hydrochloride (Atarax), topical antipruritic lotions, or oral antihistamines.[97] Medium-strength topical steroids (e.g., triamcinolone 0.1%), cool compresses, and baths—either with or without colloidal oatmeal—may also be used for pruritus.[98]

Daily sunlight exposure is also known to hasten the healing process. Another option is ultraviolet B treatment, which is most effective when administered daily over the course of 1 week.[99]

Impetigo

Overview

Impetigo is a bacterial infection of the skin caused by gram-positive streptococcal or staphylococcal (e.g., *Staphylococcus aureus*) organisms. This disorder predominantly affects the face but can occur anywhere on the body.[52,100] Impetigo occurs most often in the summer and is highly contagious and autoinoculable.

Presentation

Impetigo is characterized by thin-walled vesicles that can easily rupture and honey-crusting lesions.[101] Satellite lesions commonly spread to remote areas of the skin. Other findings include inflammation, pain, swelling, warmth, systemic infection, fever, chills, malaise, and anorexia, among others.[52]

Workup

Impetigo is diagnosed through a clinical exam. In some cases, a culture test may be called for to confirm the causative organism.[102]

Treatment

Systemic treatment of impetigo should be directed at the offending organism. Minor infections may be treated with topical antimicrobials (e.g., bacitracin, mupirocin, etc.).[103] Depending on the offending organism, the NP should consider prescribing oral beta-lactamase resistant antibiotics (e.g., dicloxacillin, cephalexin, erythromycin, clindamycin).[104] In cases of severe cellulitis, intravenous agents (e.g., nafcillin, vancomycin, and doxycycline) may be ordered in an acute care facility.[105] Burow's (Domeboro) solution should be applied to clean lesions.[106] Lastly, a patient with impetigo should abstain from school and other community events until the completion of 48 hours of treatment.

Scabies

Overview

Scabies is a highly contagious skin infestation caused by a parasitic mite that burrows into the stratum corneum. The outbreak of the infestation is usually preceded by an incubation period of 4–6 weeks. Scabies spreads through direct skin-to-skin contact, but can also be transmitted indirectly through contact with an infected patient's personal items.[96]

Presentation

Clinical findings of scabies in infants include linear or curved burrows, intense itching, and irritability. Infants with scabies may present with red-brown vesiculopapular lesions on the head, neck, palms, or soles.[107] Red papules on the umbilicus, abdomen, or skin folds frequently present in older children. Regional adenopathy may be observed in some cases.

Workup

To confirm a diagnosis, skin scrapings are examined for mites, ova, or feces.[34]

Treatment

For patients older than 2 months of age, permethrin (Nix) 5% rinse is the standard management option for scabies. Permethrin should be left on overnight for 8–12 hours upon the first treatment, and then repeated in 1 week.[108] Ivermectin may also be used to treat scabies, but is contraindicated in certain patients (e.g., pregnant/lactating mothers, children under 15 kg). Lindane lotion (Kwell) may be used with caution in children over 6 months of age.[109]

Antihistamines may be used for pruritus. Because a scabies rash may persist, it is recommended that washable items be washed in hot water and dried.[110]

Lyme Disease

Overview

Lyme disease, the most common vector-borne disease in the United States, is caused by the spirochete bacterium *Borrelia burgdorferi*. The majority of cases are concentrated in the Northeast and Upper Midwest regions, and less commonly on the Pacific West Coast; incidence peaks during the summer months.[111]

Deer ticks (*Ixodes scapularis*) are the source of transmission for Lyme disease. After latching onto a host, ticks carrying the pathogen typically take 36–48 hours to transmit the bacteria via feeding.[112,113]

Presentation (see figure 11.8)

Clinical manifestation of Lyme disease occurs in three stages. The first stage is characterized by erythema migrans, a rash that is the hallmark sign of Lyme disease.[114] The rash begins as a flat or slightly raised annular, erythematous lesion that gradually grows to assume a characteristic "bulls eye" shape. An erythema migrans lesion usually appears 1 week after the host has been infected. Although most tick bites occur in areas of tight clothing, they can present anywhere on the body.

About 50% of all patients present with non-specific, virus-like findings during the first stage, including fever, fatigue, headache, neck pain,

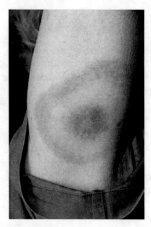

Figure 11.8. Lyme disease

arthralgia, and myalgia.[115] Asymptomatic cases during the first stage are rare. Erythema migrans and associated symptoms generally resolve within 3–4 weeks.

Findings and complications associated with the second and third stages include headache, stiff and painful joints, migratory and periarticular pain, Bell's palsy, peripheral neuropathy, acrodermatitis chronicum atrophicans (bluish-red discoloration of the distal extremity with edema), aseptic meningitis, and subacute encephalopathy.[116]

Workup

A clinical diagnosis of Lyme disease should take into account whether the patient was exposed to a tick habitat within the last 30 days.

Initial diagnosis of Lyme disease involves ELISA screening for *B. burgdorferi* antibodies. A Western blot assay is then used to confirm the diagnosis.[117] A complete blood count may also be ordered to check for elevated erythrocyte sedimentation rate.

Treatment

In cases of infection confined to the skin, patients younger than 7 years of age should be given either amoxicillin or cefuroxime axetil. Patients older than age 7 should be prescribed doxycycline.[68] Patients with second or third stage Lyme disease may need to be referred to an infectious disease specialist.

Rubeola

Overview

Rubeola, commonly known as ordinary measles, is an acute viral disease that is transmitted through inhalation of infective droplets and person-to-person contact. Although rubeola usually causes a mild illness, it may produce serious complications. Rubeola is a leading cause of death in young pediatric patients globally, and is more prevalent in non-vaccinated populations.[118]

Because of strict vaccination and prevention measures, rubeola was previously declared to be eliminated in the United States. However, the disease is highly contagious, can be imported, and may spread in unvaccinated communities.[49] In most cases, infected individuals are contagious about four days prior to and four days following the onset of rash.[119]

Complications can be life-threatening, including pneumonia, encephalitis, and pericarditis, among others.[120]

Presentation

Characteristic findings of rubeola include high-grade fever, maculopapular rash, and/or signs and symptoms similar to a respiratory illness.

Rubeola infections generally occur in four stages, beginning with an incubation period that lasts from 7 to 21 days. The incubation stage is followed by a prodromal stage, exanthema, and recovery.[119,121]

Initial findings during the prodromal stage, which can last from 2 to 10 days, commonly include a high fever, malaise, and anorexia. Within 2 days, additional findings may include coryza (i.e., rhinitis and sore throat); a productive, persistent cough; and conjunctivitis, which may be accompanied by photophobia, discharge or lacrimation, and swelling. In severe cases, patients may develop generalized lymphadenopathy and splenomegaly.[120,121,122]

A characteristic finding is Koplik's spots, 1–3 mm elevations that manifest as granular spots surrounded by red rings with an erythematous base. These spots may be white, gray, or blue in color, and are found on the buccal mucosa, opposite the first and second upper molars, but may spread to the hard and soft palate.[121]

The exanthema stage typically manifests a few days after the appearance of fever, and begins with a deep red, irregular maculopapular rash on the face, consisting of small papules the size of a pinhead. After originating around the hairline, the rash typically spreads to the face and neck, the trunk, and then to the extremities. This stage may be accompanied by additional findings, such as respiratory complications and hyperpigmentation in fair-skinned patients. The rash begins to fade after a couple days and resolves within a week.[118,120]

During the recovery period, a cough may persist for up to 2 weeks. Patients diagnosed with rubeola develop an immunity to the virus after recovery.

Workup

A clinical diagnosis of rubeola is determined from the presence of a rash lasting 3 or more days, high fever, and either cough or coryza.[119]

If required, diagnostic labs may be useful. Thrombocytopenia is a common finding, and a white blood cell count may show leukopenia. Other diagnostic findings include serologic assays showing rubeola antibodies, or a polymerase chain reaction that shows measles virus RNA.[120,121]

Treatment

Rubeola resolves within 2–3 weeks, and mainly requires supportive treatment. However, the patient may need to be hospitalized if complications manifest.

Vaccination is indicated in young pediatric patients, as severe complications are more commonly seen in children younger than age 5.[118] In the United States, the two combination vaccines approved for use are the measles-mumps-rubella (MMR) and measles-mumps-rubella-varicella (MMRV) vaccines. The MMR vaccine is administered to infants younger than age 1, and the MMRV vaccine is administered to children between 12 months and 12 years of age. Although the MMR and MMRV vaccines rarely cause fever and febrile seizures, neither vaccine has been linked to cases of hearing deficits or autism.[119]

Rubella

Overview

Rubella, also known as German measles or 3-day measles, is a contagious disease that causes a mild illness and characteristic rash. Transmission of the rubella virus occurs through contact with an infected patient's fluids (e.g., coughing, sneezing).

Although rubella manifests as an acute illness in pediatric patients and adults, the disease can cause birth defects or fetal death in pregnant women if the virus is transmitted through the placenta. The effects of infection on the fetus are most severe in the early weeks of gestation, particularly within the first 12 weeks. Additionally, infants infected in utero may be born with congenital rubella syndrome (CRS), which can lead to congenital heart disease, developmental delays, and hearing impairment.[123]

The incidence of rubella is virtually non-existent in the Unites States due to strict prevention measures, which include early vaccination programs and surveillance; however, there is a chance for cases to be imported from international travel or other countries that do not implement strict measures to control the disease.[124]

Presentation

Patients who are pregnant and have a history of inadequate immunization or show signs of infection are referred for further management.

The incubation period for rubella lasts 14–21 days after transmission.[125]

Characteristic findings of rubella include low-grade fever and a fine, erythematous, non-pruritic maculopapular rash that is red to light pink in color. The rash begins on the face, then rapidly spreads to the extremities and trunk. The rash fades rapidly and is gone within 3 days.[120,123]

About one to five days prior to onset of rash, patients may develop signs and symptoms that include malaise, joint pain or general body aches, and lymphadenopathy. A reddish maculopapular eruption on the soft palate (i.e., the Forchheimer sign) may also develop. Signs and symptoms generally last no more than 3 days and are seen in only about half of all rubella cases.[123,125] Less common complications of rubella include postinfectious encephalopathy, thrombocytopenia, vascular damage, duodenal stenosis, and mild hepatitis.[120]

Workup

An enzyme immunoassay (EIA) is the most common method used to detect rubella-specific immunoglobulin M (IgM) antibodies. Adolescents who may be pregnant or are considering pregnancy should be tested for antibodies following exposure.[120]

Diagnostic testing also includes an analysis of the patients' nasal, throat, urine, and blood specimens.[124]

Treatment

Vaccination against rubella requires 2 doses: The first dose is administered to infants between 12 and 15 months of age, and the second dose is administered to children between the ages of 4 and 6 years.[123]

Infants born with CRS are considered to be infectious until 1 year of age. To prevent spreading the virus, it is important to restrict contact with others. Surveillance of CRS should be implemented in cases involving suspected or confirmed rubella infection in the fetus.[124]

Erythema Infectiosum (Fifth Disease)

Overview

Erythema infectiosum, also known as fifth disease, is a mild contagious disease caused by human parvovirus B19, which is usually benign and peaks in incidence in the spring. The virus is mainly seen in children between 5 and 14 years of age, but can affect adults as well.[68,126] Erythema infectiosum can be transmitted through respiratory secretions, blood transfusions, and blood-derived products, and has an incubation period that typically lasts for 4–14 days. Adolescents who are pregnant and infected with erythema infectiosum may also transmit the virus to the fetus.[127]

Presentation (see figure 11.9)

Initial findings during the prodromal stage are usually non-specific and vary according to each patient. Headache, fever, and sore throat may manifest, as well as malaise, pruritus on the palms and soles, coryza, and arthralgias.[127,128] After the initial findings subside, a characteristic facial exanthema manifests with a sudden onset, producing the appearance of fiery red, flushed cheeks (i.e., "slapped cheek" appearance).[120] The facial exanthema fades within 2–4 days and is followed by onset of a lacy, erythematous maculopapular rash that spreads to the upper arms, legs, trunk, and dorsum of the hands and feet. On average, the rash lasts one-and-a-half weeks, but may persist up to 40 days.[67]

Workup

Diagnosis of erythema infectiosum in pediatrics can be determined through clinical observation. If further confirmation is necessary, a diagnostic analysis of the patient's blood may be performed to detect parvovirus B19 antibodies.[129] Diagnostic testing is commonly required if infection is suspected in pregnant adolescents.[128]

Treatment

Erythema infectiosum is a self-limiting disease that usually does not require treatment in children.[128]

Roseola Infantum (Sixth Disease)

Overview

Roseola infantum, often referred to as sixth disease, is a mild contagious disease caused by human herpesvirus type 6 (HHV-6) that occurs in infants between 6 months and 2 years of age. Roseola infantum is a major cause of febrile seizures in infants, and the incidence is rare in children older than 4 years of age.[68]

Presentation (see figure 11.10)

Roseola infantum is characterized by a high fever that is followed by a distinctive maculopapular rash. The initial high fever onsets abruptly and can last from 3 to 8 days. During this time, infants are susceptible to febrile seizures. Additional findings may include inflammation of the tympanic membrane and cold-like signs and symptoms. After the fever resolves, a rash initially manifests on the trunk

and then spreads to the extremities, characterized by papules that are small, pink, flat, or slightly raised.[68,130]

Workup

Diagnosis is determined through clinical observation, with a particular focus on the presentation of the rash.[131] A lab diagnostic is rarely required, but blood antibody titers and viral cultures may be performed to confirm a diagnosis, if necessary.[130]

Treatment

Roseola infantum resolves on its own. Management is mainly supportive, as there is no cure. Antipyretics may be used for fever reduction.[131,132]

Coxsackie Virus (Hand, Foot, and Mouth Disease)

Overview

The coxsackie virus is an RNA enterovirus that resides in the digestive tract. There are several strains of the coxsackie virus, but the one most commonly seen in pediatric patients younger than age 10 is hand, foot, and mouth disease (HFMD).[133,134]

Pediatric patients with HFMD are most contagious within the first week of infection, and transmission occurs through contact with the infected patient's fluids (e.g., oral and respiratory secretions, vesicle fluid) or the fecal-oral route.[135] Viral coxsackie infections are rare in adults, but women are more susceptible to infection during pregnancy.[136] Transmission of infection from the pregnant mother to the fetus is extremely rare, but neonates are highly susceptible to infection.[137] In rare cases, referral is necessary for complications.[133,135]

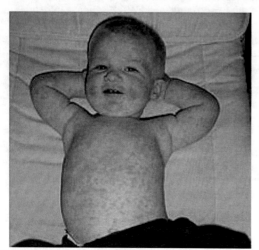

Figure 11.9. Fifth disease

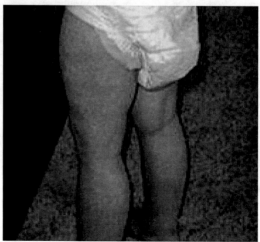

Figure 11.10. Sixth disease

Presentation

Findings of HFMD include soreness in the mouth or throat, loss of appetite or refusal to eat, and malaise. A low-grade fever is also present, lasting 24–48 hours.[138]

The most characteristic features of HFMD are oral enanthema or exanthema. Oral sores initially appear as erythematous macules that progress to vesicles surrounded by an erythematous halo, which characteristically appear on the tongue and buccal mucosa but may manifest anywhere in the mouth or throat.[138] Skin rashes manifest on the palms of the hands, soles of the feet, buttocks, legs, and arms, and present with similar appearance to oral sores.[135,139]

Workup

Diagnosis of HFMD is determined through clinical observation of the patient's findings, with special focus on the characteristic oral sores and exanthema. Labs and diagnostics are usually unnecessary.[136]

Treatment

Treatment of HFMD is supportive, as HFMD typically resolves within a week. Management consists of antipyretics (e.g., acetaminophen) for fever reduction and mouthwash for mouth sores and pain.[135]

Figures

Figure 11.1. Rule of Nines diagram for a pediatric patient. Barkley & Associates, Inc. Published 2015.

Figure 11.2. Lund and Browder diagram for pediatric patients. Barkley & Associates, Inc. Published 2015.

Figure 11.3. Acne vulgaris. In: Cavallini J. Phototake. Reproduced with permission.

Figure 11.4. Chickenpox. In: Ager-Wick R. http://commons.wikimedia.org/wiki/File:Bem_chicken-pox_vannkopper_20140318.jpg. Reproduced with permission.

Figure 11.5. Molluscum contagiosum. In Herk E. http://commons.wikimedia.org/wiki/File:Mollusca1klein.jpg. Reproduced with permission.

Figure 11.6. Allergic contact dermatitis. In: Blausen.com staff. *Blausen gallery 2014*. Wikiversity Journal of Medicine. DOI:10.15347/wjm/2014.010. ISSN 20018762. Reproduced with permission.

Figure 11.7. Diaper dermatitis. http://commons.wikimedia.org/wiki/File:Irritant_diaper_dermatitis.jpg. Reproduced with permission.

Figure 11.8. Lyme disease. In: J. Gathany. http://upload.wikimedia.org/wikipedia/commons/0/01/Erythema_migrans_-_erythematous_rash_in_Lyme_disease_-_PHIL_9875.jpg. Copyright by CDC. Reproduced with permission.

Figure 11.9. Fifth disease. In: Kerr A. http://commons.wikimedia.org/wiki/File:Fifth_disease.jpg. Reproduced with permission.

Figure 11.10. Sixth disease. In: Davis A. http://commons.wikimedia.org/wiki/File:Roseola_on_a_21-month-old_girl.jpg. Reproduced with permission.

References

1. Burn Classification. The University of New Mexico Hospitals Web site. http://hospitals.unm.edu/burn/classification.shtml. Accessed April 23, 2015.

2. Huether SE, McCance KL, eds. *Understanding Pathophysiology*. 5th ed. St. Louis, MO: Elsevier Mosby; 2012.

3. Deshaies L. Burns. In: Cooper C, ed. *Fundamentals of Hand Therapy: Clinical Reasoning and Treatment Guidelines for Common Diagnoses of the Upper Extremity*. 2nd ed. Philadelphia: Elsevier; 2014: 479–490.4.

4. Rice PL Jr, Orgill DP. Classification of burns. In: Basow DS, ed. *UpToDate*. Waltham, MA: UpToDate; 2015. http://www.uptodate.com/contents/classification-of-burns?detectedLanguage=en&source=search_result&search=burns&selectedTitle=2~150&provider=noProvider. Updated January 16, 2014. Accessed April 23, 2015.

5. County of Los Angeles Department of Health Services, Emergency Medical Services Agency, Disaster Services. Burn resource manual. http://file.lacounty.gov/dhs/cms1_206654.pdf. Published June 2010. Accessed April 24, 2015.

6. Sharma RK, Parashar A. Special considerations in paediatric burn patients. *Indian J Plast Surg*. 2010; 43(Suppl): S43–S50.

7. United States Department of Health and Human Services, Office of the Assistant Secretary for Preparedness and Response, National Library of Medicine. Burn triage and treatment – thermal injuries. Chemical Hazards Emergency Medical Management Web site. http://chemm.nlm.nih.gov/burns.htm. Updated June 25, 2011. Accessed April 24, 2015.

8. Hinkle JL, Cheever KH. *Brunner & Suddarth's Textbook of Medical-Surgical Nursing*. 13th ed. Philadelphia, PA: Wolters Kluwer Health/Lippincott Williams & Wilkins; 2014.

9. LeMone P, Burke K, Levett-Jones T, et al. *Medical-Surgical Nursing: Critical Thinking for Person-Centered Care*. 2nd ed. Frenchs Forest, NSW, Australia: Pearson Australia; 2014.

10. Trauma/burn clinical guidelines: A quick guide for the management of trauma/burn disasters for emergency department personnel. Yale New Haven Health Web site. http://yalenewhavenhealth.org/emergency/PDFs/TraumaBurn_ClinicalGuidelines_Final.pdf. Updated August 2013. Accessed April 27, 2015.

11. Burn center referral criteria. American Burn Association Web site. http://www.ameriburn.org/BurnCenterReferralCriteria.pdf. Accessed April 27, 2015.

12. Usatine, RP. Anesthesia. In: Usatine RP, Pfenninger JL, Stulberg DL, Small R, eds. *Dermatologic and Cosmetic Procedures in Office Practice*. Philadelphia, PA: Elsevier Saunders; 2012: 20–29.

13. Wolff K, Johnson RA, Saavedra AP. *Fitzpatrick's Color Atlas and Synopsis of Clinical Dermatology*. 7th ed. New York, NY: McGraw-Hill Education; 2013.

14. Tully A, Studdiford JS. *USMLE Images for the Boards: A Comprehensive Image-Based Review*. Philadelphia, PA: Elsevier Saunders; 2013.

15. Rhoads J, Petersen SW. *Advanced Health Assessment and Diagnostic Reasoning*. 2nd ed. Burlington, MA: Jones & Bartlett Learning; 2013.

16. Bristow I, Turner R. Dermatological assessment. In: Yates B, ed. *Merriman's Assessment of the Lower Limb*. 3rd ed. Philadelphia, PA: Elsevier Churchill Livingstone; 2012: 164–200.

17. Derrer DT. Cysts, lumps, bumps, and your skin. WebMD Web site. http://www.webmd.com/skin-problems-and-treatments/guide/cysts-lumps-bumps?page=5. Updated September 21, 2014. Accessed April 27, 2015.

18. Williams G, Katcher M. Primary care dermatology: Nomenclature of skin lesions. The University of Wisconsin Department of Pediatrics Web site. http://www.pediatrics.wisc.edu/education/derm/. Accessed April 27, 2015.

19. Sharma A, Lambert PJ, Maghari A, Lambert WC. Arcuate, annular, and polycyclic inflammatory and infectious lesions. *Clin Dermatol*. 2011; 29(2): 140–150.

20. Greydanus DE. The acnes: Acne vulgaris, acne rosacea, and acne excoriée. In: Tareen RS, Greydanus DE, Jafferany M, Patel DR, Merrick J, eds. *Pediatric Psychodermatology: A Manual of Child and Adolescent Psychocutaneous Disorders*. Boston, MA: Walter de Gruyter; 2013: 163–192.

21. Cole GW. Acne. In: Stöppler MC, ed. eMedicine Health. http://www.emedicinehealth.com/acne/page2_em.htm. Updated November 7, 2014. Accessed April 27, 2015.

22. Sylvia LM. Drug allergy, pseudoallergy, and cutaneous diseases. In: Tisdale JE, Miller DA, eds. *Drug-Induced Diseases: Prevention, Detection, and Management*. 2nd ed. Bethesda, MD: American Society of Health-System Pharmacists; 2010: 51–97.

23. Zouboulis CC, Abdel-Naser MB. Acne and its variants. In: Krieg T, Bickes DR, Miyachi Y, eds. *Therapy of Skin Diseases: A Worldwide Perspective on Therapeutic Approaches and Their Molecular Basis*. New York, NY: Springer; 2010: 359–375.

24. Fabbrocini G, Annunziata MC, D'Arco V, et al. Acne scars: Pathogenesis, classification and treatment. *Dermatol Res Pract*. 2010; 2010: 893080. http://www.ncbi.nlm.nih.gov/pmc/articles/PMC2958495/# Accessed May 1, 2015.

25. Bowers ES. How your period affects acne. WebMD Web site. http://www.webmd.com/skin-problems-and-treatments/acne/features/period. Updated April 11, 2011. Accessed May 1, 2015.

26. Bauer KA, Schlosser B, Mirowski GW. Acne vulgaris and steroid acne. In: Fife RS, Schrager SB, eds. *The APC Handbook of Women's Health*. Philadelphia, PA: ACP Press; 2009: 337–346.

27. Graber E. Treatment of acne vulgaris. In: Basow DS, ed. *UpToDate*. Waltham, MA: UpToDate; 2015. http://www.uptodate.com/contents/treatment-of-acne-vulgaris?detectedLanguage=en&source=search_result&search=acne+treatment&selectedTitle=1~150&provider=noProvider. Updated February 18, 2015. Accessed May 1, 2015.

28. Herrier RN. Dermatotherapy and drug-induced skin disorders. In: Alldredge BK, Corelli RL, Ernst ME, et al, eds. *Koda-Kimble and Young's Applied Therapeutics: The Clinical Use of Drugs*. 10th ed. Philadelphia, PA: Wolters Kluwer Health/Lippincott Williams & Wilkins; 2013: 925–946.

29. Kober MM, Bowe WP, Shalita AR. Topical therapies for acne. In: Zeichner JA, ed. *Acneiform Eruptions in Dermatology: A Differential Diagnosis*. New York, NY: Springer; 2014: 19–26.

30. Titus S, Hodge J. Diagnosis and treatment of acne. *Am Fam Physician*. 2012; 86(8): 734–740. http://www.aafp.org/afp/2004/0501/p2123.html. Accessed May 1, 2015.

31. Richardson MD, Warnock DW. *Fungal Infection: Diagnosis and Management*. 4th ed. Hoboken, NJ: Wiley-Blackwell; 2012.

32. Van der Vlugt TM. Regional dermatitis. In: Amieva-Wang NE, Shandro J, Fassl B, Sohoni A, eds. *A Practical Guide to Pediatric Emergency Medicine: Caring for Children in the Emergency Department*. New York, NY: Cambridge University Press; 2011: 147–150.

33. Robbins CM, Elewski BE. Tinea pedis. In: Elston DM, ed. Medscape. http://emedicine.medscape.com/article/1091684-overview. Updated December 10, 2014. Accessed May 4, 2015.

34. Cafardi JA. *The Manual of Dermatology*. New York, NY: Springer; 2012.

35. McKinney ES, James SR, Murray SS, Nelson K, Ashwill JW. *Maternal-Child Nursing*. 4th ed. Philadelphia, PA: Elsevier Saunders; 2012.

36. Lescher JL Jr. Tinea corporis. In: Elston DM, ed. Medscape. http://emedicine.medscape.com/article/1091473-overview. Updated July 21, 2014. Accessed May 4, 2015.

37. Craft N, Fox LP, Goldsmith LA, Papier A, Birnbaum R, Mercurio MG. *VisualDx: Essential Adult Dermatology*. Philadelphia, PA: Wolters Kluwer Health/Lippincott Williams & Wilkins; 2011.

38. Burkhart CG, Burkhart CN. Tinea versicolor workup. In: Elston DM, ed. Medscape. http://emedicine.medscape.com/article/1091575-workup. Updated July 21, 2014. Accessed May 4, 2015.

39. Dourmishev LA. Pediatric tinea versicolor workup. In: Elston DM, ed. Medscape. http://emedicine.medscape.com/article/911138-workup. Updated November 4, 2014. Accessed May 4, 2015.

40. Rakel RE, Rakel DP. *Textbook of Family Medicine*. 9th ed. Philadelphia, PA: Elsevier Saunders; 2015.

41. Michaels BD, Del Rosso JQ. Tinea capitis in infants: Recognition, evaluation, and management suggestions. *J Clin Aesthet Dermatol*. 2012; 5(2): 49–59.

42. McQueen L, Lio P. Pediatric dermatologic conditions. In: Aghababian RV, ed. *Essentials of Emergency Medicine*. 2nd ed. Sudbury, MA: Jones & Bartlett Learning; 2011: 551–561.

43. Phillips RM, Rosen T. Topical antifungal agents. In: Wolverton SE, ed. *Comprehensive Dermatologic Drug Therapy*. 3rd ed. Philadelphia, PA: Elsevier Saunders; 2013: 460–472.

44. Berger TG. Dermatologic disorders. In: Papadakis MA, McPhee SJ, Rabow MW, eds. *Current Medical Diagnosis & Treatment*. 53rd ed. New York, NY: McGraw-Hill; 2014: 90–158.

45. Weber DJ, Rutala WA. Prevention and control of varicella-zoster virus in hospitals. In: Basow DS, ed. *UpToDate*. Waltham, MA: UpToDate; 2015. http://www.uptodate.com/contents/prevention-and-control-of-varicella-zoster-virus-in-hospitals. Updated September 20, 2013. Accessed May 5, 2015.

46. Albrecht MA. Clinical features of varicella-zoster virus infection: Chickenpox. In: Basow DS, ed. *UpToDate*. Waltham, MA: UpToDate; 2015. http://www.uptodate.com/contents/clinical-features-of-varicella-zoster-virus-infection-chickenpox?source=search_result&search=chickenpox&selectedTitle=1~150. Updated June 30, 2014. Accessed May 5, 2015.

47. Mersch J. Chickenpox. In: Stöppler MC, ed. eMedicineHealth. http://www.emedicinehealth.com/chickenpox/article_em.htm. Reviewed June 18, 2015. Accessed June 19, 2015.

48. Papadopoulos J, Janniger CK, and Schwartz RA. Chickenpox clinical presentation. In: Elston DM, ed. Medscape. http://emedicine.medscape.com/article/1131785-clinical. Updated February 10, 2015. Accessed May 5, 2015.

49. Albrecht M. Diagnosis of varicella-zoster virus infection. In: Basow DS, ed. *UpToDate*. Waltham, MA: UpToDate; 2015. http://www.uptodate.com/contents/diagnosis-of-varicella-zoster-virus-infection. Updated October 8, 2013. Accessed May 5, 2015.

50. United States Department of Health and Human Services, Centers for Disease Control and Prevention. Chickenpox VIS. http://www.cdc.gov/vaccines/hcp/vis/vis-statements/varicella.html. Updated June 18, 2013. Accessed May 5, 2015.

51. Acyclovir (oral route, intravenous route). Mayo Clinic Web site. http://www.mayoclinic.org/drugs-supplements/acyclovir-oral-route-intravenous-route/proper-use/drg-20068393. Updated April 1, 2015. Accessed May 5, 2015.

52. Marks JG Jr, Miller JJ. *Lookingbill and Marks' Principles of Dermatology*. 5th ed. Philadelphia, PA: Elsevier Saunders; 2013.

53. United States Department of Health and Human Services, Centers for Disease Control and Prevention. Chickenpox (varicella): Prevention & treatment. http://www.cdc.gov/chickenpox/about/prevention-treatment.html. Updated November 16, 2011. Accessed May 5, 2015.

54. United States Department of Health and Human Services, Centers for Disease Control and Prevention. Molluscum (molluscum contagiosum). http://www.cdc.gov/ncidod/dvrd/molluscum/faq/everyone.htm#whatis. Updated January 13, 2011. Accessed May 5, 2015.

55. Saavedra A, Rosmarin D. Tropical dermatology. In: Magill AJ, Ryan ET, Hill D, Solomon T, eds. *Hunter's Tropical Medicine and Emerging Infectious Diseases*. 9th ed. Philadelphia: Elsevier Saunders; 2012: 68–76.

56. Eckert LO, Lentz GM. Infections of the lower and upper genital tracts: Vulva, vagina, cervix, toxic shock syndrome, endometritis, and salpingitis. In: Lentz GM, Lobo RA, Gershenson DM, Katz VL, eds. *Comprehensive Gynecology*. 6th ed. Philadelphia, PA: Elsevier Mosby; 2012: 519–560.

57. Isaacs, SN. Patient information: Molluscum contagiosum (beyond the basics). In: Basow DS, ed. *UpToDate*. Waltham, MA: UpToDate; 2015. http://www.uptodate.com/contents/molluscum-contagiosum-beyond-the-basics. Updated October 17, 2013. Accessed May 5, 2015.

58. Warrell DA. Molluscum contagiosum. In: Warrell DA, Cox TM, Firth JD, Török E, eds. *Oxford Textbook of Medicine: Infection*. Oxford, UK: Oxford University Press; 2012: 264–266.

59. Brice SL. Viral diseases of the skin. In: Bope ET, Kellerman RD, eds. *Conn's Current Therapy 2013*. 65th ed. Philadelphia, PA: Elsevier Saunders; 2013: 288–293.

60. Medically prescribed treatments for molluscum contagiosum. Natural Molluscum Web site. http://www.naturalmolluscum.com/treatments. Accessed May 5, 2015.

61. Bhatia AC. Molluscum contagiosum treatment & management. In: Elston DM, ed. http://emedicine.medscape.com/article/910570-treatment#aw2aab6b6b2. Updated November 4, 2014. Accessed May 5, 2015.

62. Mathes EFD, Frieden IJ. Treatment of molluscum contagiosum with cantharidin: A practical approach. *Pediatr Ann*. 2010; 39(3): 124–128.

63. Berk DR. Tutorial: Dermatologic medications and dermatologic diagnostics. In: Amieva-Wang NE, Shandro J, Sohoni A, Fassl B, eds. *A Practical Guide to Pediatric Emergency Medicine: Caring for Children in the Emergency Department*. New York: Cambridge University Press; 2011: 176-183.

64. United States Department of Health and Human Services, National Institutes of Health, National Institute of Arthritis and Musculoskeletal and Skin Diseases. Handout on health: Atopic dermatitis (a type of eczema). http://www.niams.nih.gov/health_info/atopic_dermatitis/#d. Published May 2013. Accessed May 6, 2015.

65. Weston WL, Howe W. Epidemiology, clinical manifestations, and diagnosis of atopic dermatitis (eczema). In: Basow DS, ed. *UpToDate*. Waltham, MA: UpToDate; 2015. http://www.uptodate.com/contents/epidemiology-clinical-manifestations-and-diagnosis-of-atopic-dermatitis-eczema?source=search_result&search=atopic+dermatitis&selectedTitle= 2~150. Updated April 29, 2015. Accessed May 6, 2015.

66. Honig PJ, Castelo-Soccio L, Yan AC. Dermatologic urgencies and emergencies. In: Fleisher GR, Ludwig S, eds. *Textbook of Pediatric Emergency Medicine*. Philadelphia, PA: Lippincott Williams & Wilkins; 2010: 730–757.

67. Nagaraju K. *Manual of Pediatric Allergy*. London and New Dehli: JP Medical; 2014.

68. Barkley TW Jr. *Family Nurse Practitioner Certification Review / Clinical Update Continuing Education Course*. West Hollywood, CA: Barkley and Associates; 2015.

69. Topical corticosteroids. National Eczema Association Web site. http://nationaleczema.org/eczema/treatment/topical-corticosteroids/. Accessed May 6, 2015.

70. Basics of topical corticosteroids. National Eczema Association Web site. http://nationaleczema.org/eczema/treatment/topical-corticosteroids/basics-of-topical-corticosteroids/. Accessed May 6, 2015.

71. Winland-Brown JE, Porter BO, Allen S. Skin problems. In: Dunphy LM, Winland-Brown JE, Porter BO, Thomas DJ, eds. *Primary Care: The Art and Science of Advanced Practice Nursing*. 3rd ed. Philadelphia, PA: F. A. Davis Company; 2011: 145–244.

72. Ratini M. Contact dermatitis: Facts about skin rashes. WebMD web site. http://www.webmd.com/skin-problems-and-treatments/contact-dermatitis?page=2. Accessed May 6, 2015.

73. Hogan DJ. Allergic contact dermatitis. In: James WD, ed. Medscape. http://emedicine.medscape.com/article/1049216-overview. Updated April 23, 2015. Accessed May 6, 2015.

74. Usatine RP, Riojas M. Diagnosis and management of contact dermatitis. *Am Fam Physician*. 2010; 82(3): 249–255.

75. Singh AK, Loscalzo J. *The Brigham Intensive Review of Internal Medicine*. 2nd ed. New York, NY: Oxford University Press; 2014.

76. Horii KA, Prossick TA. Overview of diaper dermatitis in infants and children. In: Basow DS, ed. *UpToDate*. Waltham, MA: UpToDate; 2015. http://www.uptodate.com/contents/overview-of-diaper-dermatitis-in-infants-and-children?source=search_result&search=irritant+diaper+dermatitis&selectedTitle=1~150. Updated July 9, 2013. Accessed May 7, 2015.

77. Findlay JS. Dermatologic conditions. In: Silbert-Flagg J, Sloand E, eds. *Pediatric Nurse Practitioner Certification Review Guide*. 5th ed. Sudbury, MA: Jones and Bartlett Publishing; 2011: 153–192.

78. Cadeliña R. Diaper rash: Clinical considerations and evaluation. The University of British Columbia Web site. http://learnpediatrics.com/body-systems/neonate/diaper-rash-clinical-considerations-and-evaluation/. Updated February 9, 2011. Accessed May 7, 2015.

79. Dib R, Kazzi AA. Diaper rash treatment & management. In: Bachur RG, ed. Medscape. http://emedicine.medscape.com/article/801222-treatment. Updated September 16, 2014. Accessed May 7, 2015.

80. Schalock PC. Topical therapy. In: Schalock PC, Hsu JTS, Arndt KA. *Lippincott's Primary Care Dermatology*. Philadelphia: Lippincott Williams & Wilkins; 2011: 12–19.

81. Meffert J. Psoriasis. In: James WD, ed. Medscape. http://emedicine.medscape.com/article/1943419-overview#showall . Updated January 22, 2015. Accessed May 8, 2015.

82. Cane EM. Psoriasis condition. Psoriasis Free Life Web site. http://www.psoriasisfreelife.net/psoriasis-condition.html. Published 2012. Accessed May 8, 2015.

83. White L, Duncan G, Baumle W. *Medical-Surgical Nursing: An Integrated Approach*. 3rd ed. Clifton Park, NY: Cengage Learning; 2013.

84. Schalock PC. Psoriasis. In: Porter RS, Kaplan JL, eds. The Merck Manual Online. http://www.merck-manuals.com/professional/dermatologic-disorders/psoriasis-and-scaling-diseases/psoriasis. Updated November 2014. Accessed May 8, 2015.

85. Ko HC, Jwa SW, Song M, Kim MB, Kwon KS. Clinical course of guttate psoriasis: Long-term follow-up study. *J Dermatol*. 2010; 37(10): 894–899.

86. Tidy C. Psoriatic nail disease. Patient.co.uk Web site. http://www.patient.co.uk/doctor/psoriatic-nail-disease. Updated November 20, 2012. Accessed May 8, 2015.

87. Knee NW, Blair G. Psoriasis. In: Buttaro TM, Trybulski J, Bailey PP, Sandberg-Cook J, eds. *Primary Care: A Collaborative Practice*. 4th ed. St. Louis, MO: Elsevier Mosby; 2013: 62–63.

88. Psoriasis: Tests and diagnosis. Mayo Clinic Web site. http://www.mayoclinic.org/diseases-conditions/psoriasis/basics/tests-diagnosis/con-20030838. Published April 11, 2014. Accessed May 5, 2015.

89. Topical treatment for psoriasis. National Psoriasis Foundation Web site. https://www.psoriasis.org/document.doc?id=164. Published September, 2013. Accessed May 11, 2015.

90. Kupetsky EA, Keller M. Psoriasis vulgaris: An evidence-based guide for primary care. *J Am Board Fam Med*. 2013; 26(6): 787–801.

91. Mild psoriasis: Non-steroidal prescription topical treatments. National Psoriasis Foundation Web site. https://www.psoriasis.org/about-psoriasis/treatments/topicals/non-steroid. Accessed May 11, 2015.

92. Phototherapy. National Psoriasis Foundation Web site. https://www.psoriasis.org/phototherapy. Accessed May 11, 2015.

93. Gruskin KD. Rash-maculopapular. In: Fleisher GR, Ludwig S, eds. *Textbook of Pediatric Emergency Medicine*. 6th ed. Philadelphia, PA: Wolters Kluwer Health/Lippincott Williams & Wilkins; 2010: 509–520.

94. Fletcher ST, Chaney SE. Dermatological disorders. In: Miller SK, ed. *Adult Nurse Practitioner Certification Review Guide*. 5th ed. Burlington, MA: Jones & Bartlett; 2012: 29–44.

95. Tidy C. Pityriasis rosea. Patient.co.uk Web site. http://www.patient.co.uk/doctor/pityriasis-rosea. Updated February 8, 2013. Accessed May 11, 2015.

96. Goldstein AO, Goldstein BG. Pityriasis rosea. In: Basow DS, ed. *UpToDate*. Waltham, MA: UpToDate; 2015. http://www.uptodate.com/contents/pityriasis-rosea?source=search_result&search=pityriasis+rosea&selectedTitle=1~18. Updated November 25, 2014. Accessed May 11, 2015.

97. Pityriasis rosea – Treatment. National Health Service Web site. http://www.nhs.uk/Conditions/pityriasis-rosea/Pages/Treatment.aspx. Updated March 23, 2015. Accessed May 14, 2015.

98. Perman MJ, Lucky AW, Marino BS. Dermatology. In: Marino BS, Fine KS, eds. *Blueprint Pediatrics*. 6th ed. Philadelphia, PA: Wolters Kluwer Health/Lippincott Williams & Wilkins; 2013: 74–85.

99. Pityriasis rosea. MedlinePlus Web site. http://www.nlm.nih.gov/medlineplus/ency/article/000871.htm. Updated October 14, 2012. Accessed May 14, 2015.

100. Baddour LM. Impetigo. In: Basow DS, ed. *UpToDate*. Waltham, MA: UpToDate; 2015. http://www.uptodate.com/contents/impetigo?source=search_result&search= impetigo&selectedTitle=1~62. Updated February 26, 2015. Accessed May 14, 2015.

101. Lewis LS. Impetigo. In: Steele RW, ed. Medscape. http://emedicine.medscape.com/article/965254-overview. Updated September 10, 2014. Accessed May 15, 2015.

102. Santiago TMG, Cardona JMO. Cutaneous disorders in the intensive care unit. In: Sánchez NP, ed. *Atlas of Dermatology in Internal Medicine*. New York, NY: Springer; 2011: 129–142.

103. Woo TM. Drugs used in treating infectious diseases. In: Woo TM, Wynne AL, eds. *Pharmacotherapeutics for Nurse Practitioner Prescribers*. 3rd ed. Philadelphia, PA: F. A. Davis Company; 2011: 741–868.

104. Gutierrez K. Infectious diseases. In: Bernstein D, Shelov S. *Pediatrics for Medical Students*. 3rd ed. Philadelphia, PA: Wolters Kluwer Health/Lippincott Williams & Wilkins; 2012: 160–223.

105. Kyle T, Carman S. *Essentials of Pediatric Nursing*. 2nd ed. Philadelphia, PA: Lippincott Williams & Wilkins; 2013.

106. Bose SK. Skin diseases. In: Srivastava RN, Kabra SK, eds. *Pediatrics: A Concise Text*. New Delhi, India: Elsevier India; 2011: 263–268.

107. Albakri L, Goldman RD. Permethrin for scabies in children. *Can Fam Physician*. 2010; 56(10): 1005–1006.

108. McCord S. Health problems of middle childhood. In: Hockenberry MJ, Wilson D, eds. *Wong's Nursing Care of Infants and Children Multimedia Enhanced Version*. 9th ed. St. Louis, MO: Elsevier Mosby; 2011: 684–737.

109. Workowski KA, Berman S. Sexually transmitted diseases treatment guidelines. *MMWR Morb Mortal Wkly Rep*. 2010; 59(RR-12): 1–110. http://origin.glb.cdc.gov/mmwr/pdf/rr/rr5912.pdf.

110. Beard CB. Epidemiology of Lyme disease. In: Basow DS, ed. *UpToDate*. Waltham, MA: UpToDate; 2015. http://www.uptodate.com/contents/epidemiology-of-lyme-disease?source=search_result&search=lyme+disease&selectedTitle=6~150. Accessed May 26, 2015.

111. United States Department of Health and Human Services, Centers for Disease Control and Prevention. Lifecycle of blacklegged ticks. Retrieved from http://www.cdc.gov/lyme/transmission/blacklegged.html. Updated November 15, 2011. Accessed May 26, 2015.

112. Misinformation about Lyme disease. American Lyme Disease Foundation Web site. http://aldf.com/lyme-disease/. Updated February 21, 2015. Accessed May 26, 2015.

113. Meyerhoff JO, Steele RW, Zaidman GW. Lyme disease clinical presentation. In: Diamond HS, ed. Medscape. http://emedicine.medscape.com/article/330178-clinical. Updated January 22, 2015. Accessed May 26, 2015.

114. Shapiro ED. Lyme disease: Clinical manifestations in children. In: Basow DS, ed. *UpToDate*. Waltham, MA: UpToDate; 2015. http://www.uptodate.com/contents/lyme-disease-clinical-manifestations-in-children?source=search_result&search=lyme+disease+children&selectedTitle=4~150#H3. Updated January 30, 2014. Accessed May 26, 2015.

115. Philip SS. Spirochetal infections. In: Papadakis MA, Mcphee SJ, Rabow MJ, eds. *Current Medical Diagnosis & Treatment*. 53rd ed. New York, NY: McGraw-Hill Education; 2014: 1417–1435.

116. Hu, L. Diagnosis of Lyme disease. In: Basow DS, ed. *UpToDate*. Waltham, MA: UpToDate; 2015. http://www.uptodate.com/contents/diagnosis-of-lyme-disease?source=search_result&search=lyme+disease&selectedTitle=3~150#H9. Updated March 20, 2015. Accessed May 26, 2015.

117. Measles. World Health Organization Web site. http://www.who.int/mediacentre/factsheets/fs286/en/. Updated February, 2015. Accessed May 26, 2015.

118. Fiebelkorn AP, Goodson JL. Measles (rubeola). In: Brunette GW, ed. *CDC Health Information for International Travel 2014: The Yellow Book*. New York, NY: Oxford University Press; 2013: 249–253.

119. Roig IL, Shandera WX. Viral and Rickettsial infection. In: Papadakis MA, McPhee SJ, Rabow MW, eds. *Current Medical Diagnosis & Treatment*. 53rd ed. New York, NY: McGraw-Hill Education; 2014: 1305–1370.

120. Barinaga JL, Skolnik PR. Clinical presentation and diagnosis of measles. In: Basow DS, ed. *UpToDate*. Waltham, MA: UpToDate; 2015. http://www.uptodate.com/contents/clinical-manifestations-and-diagnosis-of-measles. Updated February 12, 2015. Accessed May 26, 2015.

121. Pillitteri A. *Maternal & Child Health Nursing: Care of the Childbearing & Childrearing Family*. 7th ed. Philadelphia, PA: Wolters Kluwer Health/Lippincott Williams & Wilkins; 2013.

122. United States Department of Health and Human Services, Centers for Disease Control and Prevention. Rubella (German measles, three-day measles). http://www.cdc.gov/rubella/about/index.html. Updated December 17, 2014. Accessed May 26, 2015.

123. McLean H, Redd S, Abernathy E, Icenogle J, Wallace G. Congenital rubella syndrome. In: Roush SW, McIntyre L, Baldy LM, eds. *Centers for Disease Control and Prevention, Manual for the Surveillance of Vaccine-Preventable Diseases*. 5th ed. Atlanta, GA: Centers for Disease Control and Prevention; 2012. http://www.cdc.gov/vaccines/pubs/surv-manual/chpt15-crs.pdf. Accessed May 26, 2015.

124. Ezike E, Ang JY. Pediatric rubella clinical presentation. In: Steele RW, ed. Medscape. http://emedicine.medscape.com/article/968523-clinical#showall. Updated December 18, 2014. Accessed May 26, 2015.

125. Dijkmans AC, de Jong EP, Dijkmans BA, et al. Parvovirus B19 in pregnancy: prenatal diagnosis and management of fetal complications. *Curr Opin Obstet Gynecol*. 2012; 24(2): 95–101. doi: 10.1097/GCO.0b013e3283505a9d

126. Zellman GL. (2014). Erythema infectiosum. In: Elston DM, ed. Medscape. http://emedicine.medscape.com/article/1132078-overview#showall. Updated September 15, 2014. Accessed May 26, 2015.

127. Jordan JA. Clinical manifestations and pathogenesis of human parvovirus B19 infection. In: Basow DS, ed. *UpToDate*. Waltham, MA: UpToDate; 2015. http://www.uptodate.com/contents/clinical-manifestations-and-pathogenesis-of-human-parvovirus-b19-infection?source=search_result&search=erythema+infectiosum&selectedTitle=1~30. Updated December 15, 2014. Accessed May 26, 2015.

128. Pagana KD. *Mosby's Manual of Diagnostic and Laboratory Tests*. 5th ed. Philadelphia, PA: Elsevier Mosby; 2014.

129. Porth C. *Essentials of Pathophysiology: Concepts of Altered Health States*. 3rd ed. Philadelphia, PA: Wolters Kluwer Health/Lippincott Williams & Wilkins; 2011.

130. Tremblay C, Brady MT. Human herpesvirus 6 infection in children: Clinical manifestations; diagnosis; and treatment. In: Basow DS, ed. *UpToDate*. Waltham, MA: UpToDate; 2015. http://www.uptodate.com/contents/human-herpesvirus-6-infection-in-children-clinical-manifestations-diagnosis-and-treatment?source=search_result&search=roseola+infantum+children&selectedTitle=2~150#H11. Updated January 7, 2015. Accessed May 26, 2015.

131. Gorman CR. Roseola infantum: Treatment & management. In: James WD, ed. Medscape. http://emedicine.medscape.com/article/1133023-treatment#showall. Updated October 13, 2014. Accessed May 26, 2015.

132. Davis CP. Coxsackie virus. In: Shiel WC Jr, ed. eMedicine Health. http://www.medicinenet.com/coxsackie_virus/article.htm. Updated July 11, 2014. Accessed May 26, 2015.

133. United States Department of Health and Human Services, Centers for Disease Control and Prevention. About hand, foot, and mouth disease (HFMD). http://www.cdc.gov/hand-foot-mouth/about/index.html. Updated July 7, 2014. Accessed May 26, 2015.

134. Romero JR. Hand, foot, and mouth disease and herpangina: An overview. In: Basow DS, ed. *UpToDate*. Waltham, MA: UpToDate; 2015. http://www.uptodate.com/contents/hand-foot-and-mouth-disease-and-herpangina-an-overview?source=-search_result&search=coxsackievirus&selectedTitle=2~70#H456270554. Updated December 2, 2014. Accessed May 26, 2015.

135. Hand-foot-mouth disease. A.D.A.M. Medical Encyclopedia Web site. http://www.nlm.nih.gov/medlineplus/ency/article/000965.htm. Updated August 18, 2013. Accessed May 26, 2015.

136. Modlin JF. Clinical manifestations and diagnosis of enterovirus and parechovirus infections. In: Basow DS, ed. *UpToDate*. Waltham, MA: UpToDate; 2015. http://www.uptodate.com/contents/clinical-manifestations-and-diagnosis-of-enterovirus-and-parecho-virus-infections?source=search_result&search=coxsackievirus&selectedTitle=1~70#H5882578. Updated October 7, 2014. Accessed May 26, 2015.

137. Nervi SJ, Schwartz RA, Kapila R. Hand-foot-and-mouth disease. In: Bronze MS, ed. Medscape. http://emedicine.medscape.com/article/218402-overview#-showall. Updated June 10, 2014. Accessed May 26, 2015.

138. Balentine JR. Encephalitis and meningitis. In: Shiel WC Jr, ed. eMedicine Health. http://www.medicinenet.com/encephalitis_and_meningitis/article.htm. Updated February 10, 2015. Accessed May 26, 2015.

Chapter 12
Eye, Ear, Nose, and Throat Disorders

QUESTIONS

1. A 2-year-old is brought to your clinic presenting with red, irritated eyes. The mother says the symptoms manifested after they had visited a public swimming pool the day prior. Upon examination, you see no discharge. The child does not indicate any pain, only an itching sensation. You tell the mother that the condition is self-limiting, and you proceed with a normal saline flush on the patient's eyes. Which is the most likely diagnosis?

   a. Bacterial conjunctivitis

   b. Hordeolum

   c. Chemical conjunctivitis

   d. Viral conjunctivitis

2. Which of the following is most likely to be caused by *Chlamydia trachomatis*?

   a. Pharyngitis

   b. Croup

   c. Infectious mononucleosis

   d. Epiglottitis

3. Which of the following statements is most true regarding sinusitis in young children?

   a. Sinusitis occurs in children beginning at 6 years of age or older.

   b. Sinusitis is distinguished from acute otitis media by its typical pathogens.

   c. Radiological studies are the most common method of confirming a diagnosis.

   d. The paranasal sinuses are the most commonly affected sinuses.

4. A patient reports to your clinic with intense fatigue and a fever. Suspecting infectious mononucleosis, you begin a physical exam. Which of the following signs is not consistent with the common presentation of this condition?

   a. White exudate on the tonsils

   b. Generalized lymphadenopathy

   c. Discolored nasal discharge

   d. Petechial rash

5. Of the following, which eye disorder is characterized by an abrupt or sudden onset with painful swelling on the lid margin?

   a. Hordeolum

   b. Strabismus

   c. Conjunctivitis

   d. Chalazion

6. All of the following are viral causes of pharyngitis and tonsillitis except:

   a. Mumps virus

   b. Respiratory syncytial virus

   c. Influenza A and B

   d. Epstein-Barr virus

7. Which of the following conditions does not have a bacterial etiology?

   a. Epiglottitis

   b. Infectious mononucleosis

   c. Acute otitis media

   d. Conjunctivitis

8. Which of the following pathogens is most commonly responsible for epiglottitis?

    a. *Neisseria gonorrhoeae*

    b. *Streptococcus pneumoniae*

    c. *Moraxella catarrhalis*

    d. *Haemophilus influenzae*

9. Which of the following best distinguishes epiglottitis from croup?

    a. Epiglottitis presents with fever, whereas croup does not.

    b. Epiglottitis targets children between 3 months and 6 years of age, whereas croup usually presents in children 6–10 years of age.

    c. An x-ray for epiglottitis will show a thumb sign, whereas an x-ray for croup will show a steeple sign.

    d. Epiglottitis is entirely bacterial in nature, whereas croup is entirely viral.

10. Of the following, which form of conjunctivitis most often presents with watery discharge?

    a. Bacterial

    b. Viral

    c. Gonococcal

    d. Allergic

RATIONALES

1. c

Because the patient was treated with a normal saline flush and no discharge was present at the site, the most likely diagnosis is chemical conjunctivitis. Bacterial conjunctivitis, as well as viral conjunctivitis, can be self-limiting as well; however, purulent discharge accompanies bacterial conjunctivitis, and watery discharge typically accompanies viral conjunctivitis. The child's findings do not indicate a hordeolum, which presents with an abscess and is typically accompanied by pain, edema, and abrupt onset of symptoms.

2. a

Of the four choices, pharyngitis, or tonsillitis, is most likely caused by *Chlamydia trachomatis*. Common pathogens for epiglottitis include *Streptococci, Pneumococci*, and *Haemophilus influenzae*, but not *C. trachomatis*. Croup and infectious mononucleosis are both primarily caused by viral infections, rather than bacterial infections. Croup is mostly caused by parainfluenza, whereas infectious mononucleosis is caused by the Epstein-Barr virus.

3. d

In young children, the two sinuses most commonly affected by sinusitis are two of the paranasal sinuses: the maxillary and ethmoid sinuses. Sinusitis can occur in children younger than 6 years of age because the ethmoid and maxillary sinuses are present at birth. Sinusitis cannot be distinguished from acute otitis media (AOM) by its typical pathogens, as sinusitis shares the same typical pathogens with AOM, such as *Streptococcus pneumoniae, Haemophilus influenzae*, and *Moraxella catarrhalis*. Radiological studies are not commonly used to confirm a diagnosis in uncomplicated presentations of sinusitis, which is often diagnosed on clinical presentation. When imaging is required, CT scans are favored over standard x-rays, as a CT scan is more sensitive and equal in price.

4. c

Discolored nasal discharge is a presentation of sinusitis, not infectious mononucleosis. A petechial or maculopapular rash, white exudate on the tonsils, and generalized lymphadenopathy are all physical findings of infectious mononucleosis.

5. a

Of the choices, hordeolum is the only eye disorder that presents abruptly with painful swelling. Symptoms associated with strabismus, conjunctivitis, and cataracts develop over time. Strabismus is an ocular misalignment and does not normally cause painful swelling. Conjunctivitis has various types according to etiology; some types, such as allergic and bacterial conjunctivitis, can appear abruptly, but swelling is not typically painful with conjunctivitis as it is with hordeolum. Lastly, chalazia are typically not painful and usually occur inside the eyelid, rather than on the lid margin.

6. a

Although the mumps virus belongs to the same family as parainfluenza, which can produce pharyngitis and tonsillitis, it produces neither condition; the virus affects the salivary glands, genitals, and nervous system, rather than the throat and pharynx. The respiratory syncytial virus, Epstein-Barr virus, and influenza A and B are all viral causes of pharyngitis and tonsillitis.

7. b

Infectious mononucleosis is caused by the Epstein-Barr virus; thus, it does not have a bacterial etiology. Epiglottitis can be caused by a bacterial infection, with the most common pathogens being *Haemophilus influenzae* and members of the *Streptococci* and *Pneumococci* genera. *Streptococcus pneumoniae* and *H. influenzae* are the pathogens most commonly responsible for acute otitis media. Chlamydial and gonococcal pathogens can cause conjunctivitis.

8. d

Epiglottitis is most often caused by *Haemophilus influenzae* infection; as such, the number of cases has dropped in recent years due to widespread implementation of the *H. influenza* type B vaccine. *Moraxella catarrhalis* can be a bacterial cause of epiglottitis; however, the pathogen is more commonly associated with sinusitis. *Neisseria gonorrhoeae* is more likely to cause pharyngitis. *Streptococcus pneumoniae* does not typically produce epiglottitis but may produce conjunctivitis and sinusitis.

9. c

X-rays may be used to distinguish epiglottitis from croup; the former condition manifests as a thumb sign, whereas the latter condition manifests as a steeple sign upon x-ray. Both conditions can present with fever, and although patients with croup are typically afebrile, there are some manifestations of the condition, such as laryngotracheitis, that tend to produce fever. Epiglottitis produces high-grade fever in over half of all cases. Although croup is most commonly a viral infection, it may also be caused by bacteria, which results in bacterial tracheitis. Further, epiglottitis may be caused by bacterial or viral etiologies. Epiglottitis most often affects children 6–10 years of age, whereas croup affects children between 3 months and 6 years of age.

10. b

Of the choices, viral conjunctivitis most often presents with watery discharge. Bacterial conjunctivitis, along with gonococcal conjunctivitis, can present with purulent, not watery, discharge. With allergic conjunctivitis, patients may experience increased tearing, but the discharge is stringy, not watery.

DISCUSSION

Hordeolum (Stye)

Overview

Hordeolum, or stye, is a common type of staphylococcal abscess that presents on the upper or lower eyelid.[1]

Presentation

Styes typically have an abrupt onset with localized pain and edema. The eyelid is often extremely tender, and the amount of pain is usually proportional to the amount of edema.[2]

Workup

Differential diagnoses for a stye include conjunctivitis, chalazion, blepharitis, or dacryocystitis.[3] Before diagnosing a stye, the health care practitioner should closely examine the pediatric patient's general health to ensure that no other health conditions are complicating the diagnosis.[4] Generally, a diagnosis can be made by examining the patient's eyelid.

Treatment

Styes can be managed with warm compresses and antibiotics, such as topical bacitracin or erythromycin ophthalmic ointment. For severe cases, the nurse practitioner (NP) may refer the pediatric patient to an ophthalmologist for possible incision and drainage.[5]

Chalazion

Overview

A chalazion is a granulomatous nodule that slowly develops, blocks the oil gland in the eyelid, and causes swelling. This condition develops from an infection or retention cyst of the meibomian gland.[3]

Chalazia are more common in adults but may occur in children as well.[6] Sometimes chalazia appear due to an internal hordeolum that does not drain or resolve.[3] Unlike styes, chalazia are usually painless.

Presentation

Although often asymptomatic, signs and symptoms of a chalazion may include red conjunctiva, eyelid swelling, light sensitivity, itching, visual distortion, and increased tearing. If the chalazion pushes against the eye, the patient may also experience blurred vision due to pressure exerted on the cornea.[7]

Workup

Chalazia may be quite small and initially confused with styes. Other eye conditions may resemble a chalazion, including conjunctivitis, blepharitis, or dacryocystitis.[3] In order to diagnose a stye, the health care practitioner should closely examine the pediatric patient's eyelid, noting the lid structure, skin texture, and eyelash appearance. A patient history should also be conducted.[8]

Treatment

Chalazia can be treated with a warm compress.[3] A pediatric patient with a persistent chalazion should be referred to an ophthalmologist for possible surgical removal.

Conjunctivitis

Overview

Conjunctivitis (i.e., pink eye) is the most common eye disorder. Conjunctivitis is an inflammation of the conjunctiva. It may result from a variety of causes, such as allergies, chemical irritation, or bacterial or viral infection.[9]

Presentation

Signs and symptoms of conjunctivitis include inflammation, redness, irritation, itching, burning, increased tears, blurred vision, eyelid swelling, foreign body sensation, and discharge. The type of discharge that presents can often aid in distinguishing between variants of conjunctivitis. Both bacterial and gonococcal conjunctivitis may present with purulent discharge, but the discharge is typically more copious in cases of gonococcal infection. Watery discharge may indicate viral conjunctivitis, whereas stringy discharge and increased tearing may indicate allergic conjunctivitis.[10]

Workup

Because conjunctivitis has a variety of causes, a health care practitioner must identify the etiology in order to appropriately treat the condition. Viral conjunctivitis is often diagnosed based on clinical features alone. Severe cases may warrant culture and smear. Gram stains help to identify bacterial characteristics, whereas Giemsa stains help identify chlamydial bodies.[11,12] Bacterial cultures on blood and chocolate agar, along with a Gram stain and polymerase chain reaction assay, are indicated in neonatal cases.[13]

Treatment

As previously indicated, the proper identification of etiology of conjunctivitis is vital for appropriate management. See table 12.1 for treatment considerations for each type of conjunctivitis infection.

Cataracts

Overview

Cataracts are an abnormal, uniform, progressive opacity of the eye. Children with this condition most likely have comorbidities such as Down syndrome, diabetes mellitus, Marfan syndrome, or atopic dermatitis.[14] Cataracts may be congenital as a result of prolonged steroid use, trauma, undernutrition, or radiation.[15]

Presentation

Cataracts are painless, and pediatric patients typically present with decreased visual acuity; cloudy, blurred, dim vision; white reflex; poor visual fixation; and photophobia.[16]

Workup

In order to diagnose an infant or child with cataracts, the NP must consider the patient's medical history and ascertain if the patient has any systemic diseases that may cause cataracts. Laboratory and diagnostic tests may be unnecessary. If cataracts are indicated, the health care practitioner should refer the pediatric patient to an ophthalmologist.[15]

Treatment

Some cataracts that occur in infants do not need to be removed because the pediatric patient's vision will eventually develop normally. However, cataracts that continue to interfere with a child's vision must be surgically removed by an ophthalmologist.[17]

Strabismus

Overview

Strabismus is an ocular misalignment that results from uncoordinated ocular muscles. If strabismus is acquired after 6 months of age, the condition is usually related to underlying problems such as cerebral palsy, Down syndrome, hydrocephalus, or brain tumors.[16]

Presentation

Signs and symptoms of strabismus may include squinting; decreased visual acuity; head tilt; face-turning; inward deviation of the eyes (i.e., esotropia); outward deviation of the eyes (i.e., exotropia); upward deviation of the eyes (i.e., hypertropia); downward deviation of the eyes (i.e., hypotropia); and an unequal Hirschberg papillary light reflex.[18]

Table 12.1	Treatment Considerations for Conjunctivitis	
Type	**Discharge**	**Treatment Considerations**
Bacterial	Purulent; thick; white, yellow, or green; mostly at lid margins and corners of eyes[14]	1) Erythromycin ophthalmic ointment 2) Bacitracin ointment 3) Sulfacetamide ointment 4) Bacitracin-polymyxin B ointment[14]
Gonococcal (ophthalmic emergency)	Purulent; profuse exudate; swollen eyelids[15]	1) Hospitalization 2) Ceftriaxone, 25–50 mg/kg IV or IM, or 3) Cefotaxime, 100 mg/kg IV or IM (preferred if hyperbilirubinemia is present) 4) Frequent saline irrigation[15]
Chlamydial	Mild swelling of eyelids with mucopurulent, watery discharge; marked swelling of eyelids with thick, red conjunctivae[16]	1) Oral erythromycin, 50 mg/kg/day for 14 days, or 2) Oral azithromycin, 20 mg/kg/day for 3 days[16]
Allergic	Bilateral redness; itchy; may have morning crusting[14]	1) Topical antihistamines with mast cell stabilizers 2) Topical antihistamine/vasoconstrictors 3) Refer to allergist/ophthalmologist in refractory cases[17]
Viral	Watery; may have morning crusting; occasional scants of mucous throughout the day; burning, sandy feeling in one eye[14]	1) Symptomatic: 2) Nonantibiotic lubricating agents 3) Topical antihistamine/decongestants[14]

Used with permission from Barkley TW Jr. Eyes, ears, nose, and throat issues and disorders. In: *Pediatric Primary Care Nurse Practitioner Certification Review/Clinical Update Continuing Education Course*. West Hollywood, CA: Barkley and Associates; 2015: 109–124.

Workup

If a pediatric patient presents with strabismus, an NP should conduct a thorough examination of the eyes. Indications for referral to an ophthalmologist include strabismus that is fixed or continuous at 6 months of age or later; hypertropia or hypotropia; or signs that an underlying condition is the cause of strabismus.[19]

Treatment

Treatment for strabismus may include contact lenses, eyeglasses, or eye exercises. Patching may be required if amblyopia is also present. In some cases, surgical alignment of the eyes may be necessary.[19]

Otitis Externa (Swimmer's Ear)

Overview

Otitis externa is an inflammation of the external auditory canal or auricle. Though this condition is usually caused by a bacterial infection, the origin may also be viral or fungal. This condition occurs in all age groups, though children's narrow ear canals put them at increased risk. Recent water exposure is another risk factor because the retained water prevents not only drying, but removal of cerumen from the ear. Other causes of otitis externa include mechanical trauma, a foreign body in the ear, or excess cerumen.[20,21]

Presentation

Signs and symptoms of otitis externa include otalgia, pruritus, and purulent discharge.[20] Ear canal erythema, edema, purulent exudate, or pain upon manipulation of the auricle may also occur.

Workup

Diagnosis is based on a history and physical exam. Cultures should be obtained only in severe or recalcitrant cases of otitis externa.[22]

Treatment

In treating otitis externa, NSAIDs or corticosteroid ear drops may be administered to remedy inflammation. For otitis externa limited to the ear canal and not extending to adjacent tissues, topical antibiotics—or antifungals, if warranted—are the standard of care. In severe cases of malignant otitis externa, hospitalization is required; intravenous antibiotics are commonly administered, and surgery may be indicated. It is recommended that the patient keep the ear dry for 7-10 days, substitute showers for baths, and refrain from using earplugs or hearing aids until healed.[21]

Acute Otitis Media (AOM)

Overview

Acute otitis media (AOM) is a bacterial infection of the middle ear.[23] Although AOM may occur at any age, it is most prevalent in infants and young children. Between 60%–80% of all infants experience AOM in their first year, with 80%–90% experiencing it in their first 3 years. Risk factors include family history, lack of breastfeeding, exposure to tobacco smoke and air pollution, and pacifier use. Though viral infection is possible, AOM is more commonly caused by the bacteria *Streptococcus pneumoniae*, *Haemophilus influenzae*, or *Moraxella catarrhalis*.[24]

Presentation

Signs and symptoms of AOM include decreased hearing, otalgia, fever, aural pressure, vertigo, and nausea or vomiting. Other physical findings may include an erythematous and edematous tympanic membrane, purulent exudate from the ear, and the appearance of a bulging tympanic membrane. Impaired mobility of the tympanic membrane is another common indicator for AOM.[24]

Workup

In order to test for AOM, an NP should conduct a physical exam and diagnostic tests. A pneumatic otoscopy or a tympanometry test should be conducted to assess the status of the tympanic membrane; these measures will also help to confirm AOM and differentiate it from otitis media with effusion.[23]

Treatment

Pediatric patients may be administered acetaminophen to manage the pain associated with AOM. Benzocaine otic drops can be used for pain relief if the tympanic membrane has not perforated. These drops should only be used for 24–48 hours, as the pain should be decreased by then, and prolonged use can mask progressing symptoms. Otherwise, healthy children with the disorder should be observed. If the condition persists, amoxicillin can be administered orally at 80–90 mg/kg/day, twice daily. Cephalosporins may be administered to children with a delayed response penicillin allergy, whereas macrolides and lincosamides may be administered to children with an immediate responding penicillin allergy.[25]

AOM may be prevented by the *H. influenzae* type B and pneumococcal conjugate vaccines, as well as by annual flu vaccinations. Parents should also ensure that their children are not exposed to second-hand smoke, as there is an association between increased AOM and smoke exposure.[26]

Otitis Media with Effusion (OME)/Serous Otitis Media

Overview

Otitis media with effusion (OME), or serous otitis media, is the buildup of fluid in the middle ears without infection. The fluid may build up as a result of allergies or respiratory infection. Although this condition can occur at any age, it is most common in children younger than 3 years of age due to their increased incidence of upper respiratory tract infections. Additionally, eustachian tubes are smaller and more horizontally aligned in children than in adults, making drainage more difficult. OME is most prevalent during the winter.[27]

Presentation

Unlike AOM, OME is mostly asymptomatic, although children may experience mild hearing loss, a popping sensation when pressure is altered, or a feeling of fullness in the ear.[28]

Workup

When a pediatric patient presents with symptoms of OME, a health care practitioner should conduct a physical exam. OME will typically present with opacity, impaired mobility of the tympanic membrane, bubbles, or an air fluid level. Furthermore, acute signs or symptoms should be absent, as these symptoms would more traditionally indicate AOM.[28] For prolonged cases of OME, especially in young children developing language abilities, audiometry to check for hearing loss would be indicated for lack of resolution after about four to six weeks.[29]

Treatment

Pediatric patients with OME should be monitored for 3 months. If fluid has not resolved by 3 months, pneumoeustacian tubes will typically be inserted to allow the fluid to drain, optimize normal hearing, and consequently improve verbal acquisition skills. Pediatric patients with OME should be re-evaluated 6 months after the first evaluation.[30]

Hearing Loss

Overview

Hearing loss is any degree of impairment in the ability to perceive sound, and may be conductive, sensorineural, or central.[31,32] Conductive hearing loss is characterized by the decreased ability to conduct sound from the external ear to inner ear. The most common causes of conductive hearing loss are cerumen impaction and middle ear fluid. Sensorineural hearing loss is characterized by problems of the inner ear, usually occurring at the cochlea, eighth cranial nerve, internal auditory canal, or the brain. Central hearing loss is the misperception of auditory information due to flaws in the central auditory nervous system or auditory nerve.[32]

Presentation

Pediatric patients with hearing loss should undergo both the Weber test and Rinne test (see table 12.1). The Weber test assesses if a pediatric patient hears sound equally in both ears and not laterally, whereas the Rinne test evaluates whether the patient's air conduction (AC) of sound is greater than bone conduction (BC) of sound.[33] The Weber test indicates conductive hearing loss if sound lateralizes to the affected ear; if the sound lateralizes to the unaffected ear, sensorineural hearing loss is indicated instead. A Rinne test presents normal results in the affected ear in cases of sensorineural hearing loss; in conductive hearing loss, however, the results of the Rinne test are abnormal in the affected ear, indicating that AC may be less than BC. [33]

Workup

An NP can administer a variety of diagnostic tests and labs to determine if hearing loss is present and possibly even determine the etiology. An otoscopic exam can be conducted to evaluate mobility of the tympanic membrane. Diminished mobility may indicate fluid or a mass in the middle ear cavity. Increased mobility may indicate ossicular chain disruption. Audiometric testing determines the softest decibel threshold a patient can hear. The test can be performed in an office but may fail to detect mild hearing loss. A complete neurological exam should be conducted to test for neurologic deficits. If a neurologic condition is suspected, a computerized tomography (CT) scan of the temporal bone and internal auditory meatus should be obtained. Finally, serum blood tests and tests for congenital infection should be obtained as warranted.[33]

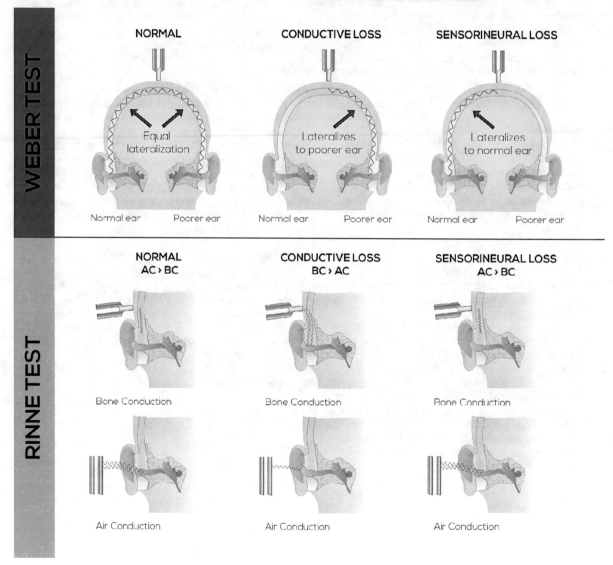

Figure 12.1. Weber and Rinne hearing loss tests.

Treatment

Treatment for hearing loss depends on etiology. Some causes of hearing loss are surgically correctable, such as hearing loss due to benign growths or malignant tumors. Amplification devices, such as hearing aids, are helpful for many people. Patients may benefit from hearing aids that either selectively amplify high frequencies or perform simple amplification. In those cases where traditional hearing aids are ineffective, bone conduction hearing aids and cochlear implants may be used. Children with permanent hearing loss should be managed by a multidisciplinary team of experts.[34]

Common Cold

Overview

The common cold occurs in the upper respiratory tract and is characterized as a self-limiting viral infection. Rhinoviruses are responsible for up to 50% of all colds in adults and children. Respiratory syncytial, influenza, parainfluenza, and adenoviruses are other common causes of colds in preschool children.[35]

Presentation

Symptoms of a common cold may include headache, rhinorrhea, sore throat, coughing, sneezing, and fever.[36]

Workup

To diagnose a common cold, a health care practitioner must conduct a physical exam focusing on the eyes, ears, nose, and throat, as well as determine the recent history of the patient. Based on physical exam findings, the health care practitioner can rule out other possible infections or illnesses that have similar symptoms to the common cold, such as influenza or sinusitis. [35]

Treatment

Treatment of the common cold is generally limited to supportive care. The NP should advise patients to rest and stay hydrated. Nasal saline drops and a humidifier can also provide some relief. Antibiotics should not be prescribed, and patients should be educated that time will alleviate the symptoms.[37]

Epistaxis (Nosebleed)

Overview

Epistaxis, commonly known as a nosebleed, involves bleeding from the inside of the nose.[38]

Presentation

Nosebleeds usually occur in one nostril.[38] Nosebleeds can result in an upset stomach due to drainage from the back of the throat into the stomach.

Workup

Nosebleeds are diagnosed by observation or evaluation of the pediatric patient's symptoms. Nosebleeds are typically caused from dryness, nose-picking, upper respiratory infections, or sinus complications. Frequent or prolonged nosebleeds may require an evaluation for a bleeding disorder.[38]

Treatment

In order to manage a nosebleed, the pediatric patient must sit upright, and the patient or parent must apply pressure for 10 minutes at Kiesselbach's triangle, which is the anterior inferior aspect of the nasal septum—the end of the bony ridge.[39] Ice should also be applied.[16] When compression is unsuccessful, cautery, matrix sealant, fibrin glue, or nasal packing may be used.

Pharyngitis/Tonsillitis

Overview

Pharyngitis is inflammation of the pharynx, whereas tonsillitis is inflammation of the tonsils. Pharyngitis and tonsillitis can occur at the same time or separately. Viruses such as respiratory syncytial virus, influenza A or B, or Epstein Barr virus are among the main causes of pharyngitis and tonsillitis. These conditions can also be caused by bacteria such as group A β-hemolytic *Streptococci* (GABHS), *Neisseria gonorrhoeae*, *Mycoplasma*, *Chlamydia trachomatis*, and *Corynebacterium*.[40]

Presentation

Pediatric patients with either condition typically present with the following symptoms: erythematous pharynx, dysphagia and cough, malaise, rhinorrhea, anterior cervical adenopathy, painful throat, and exudate. Fever may or may not be present.[41]

Workup

Diagnosing pharyngitis or tonsillitis does not typically require any routine testing. Numerous studies have shown that clinical judgment is not effective in determining if a sore throat is streptococcal pharyngitis or not. Consequently, a rapid strep test should be obtained. If the test is negative, a throat culture should be obtained and the patient should be treated appropriately.

Treatment

Treating pharyngitis or tonsillitis often requires supportive care measures, such as hydration, warm salt water gargles, and antipyretics. If a bacterial infection is present, antibiotics should be prescribed.[42] Penicillin VK, 250 mg orally, 3 times daily, for 10 days is the treatment of choice; however, this treatment tastes terrible, often making it a challenge to obtain compliance from pediatric patients. Amoxicillin, 45 mg/kg/day, is an acceptable alternative to prevent rheumatic complications of streptococcal A infection. For patients who are allergic to penicillin, erythromycin at 250 mg, 4 times daily, for 10 days is also commonly prescribed.[41]

Epiglottitis

Overview

Epiglottitis is a sudden and severe swelling of the epiglottis. The majority of pediatric cases are caused by *H. influenzae* type b, although *Streptococci* and *Staphylococcus aureus* may cause epiglottitis as well.[43]

Presentation

Pediatric patients with epiglottitis often present with a sudden onset of high fever, drooling, dysphagia, a restless and fearful state, and rapidly progressive signs of respiratory distress. Patients often prefer to sit, hyperextending their necks in an attempt to open the obstructed airway.[43]

Workup

Lab tests for epiglottitis include blood and tracheal cultures to determine the causative organism. A radiograph of the neck often shows a thumb-shaped patch, or "thumb sign."[44]

Treatment

Epiglottitis requires immediate hospitalization. Keeping the child calm is very important, and preparation for emergent intubation must be expedited in order to avoid cardiopulmonary arrest.[43,45] Intravenous third-generation cephalosporins should be started while waiting for culture verification of the offending pathogen.[46]

Croup

Overview

Croup is a parainfluenza viral infection of the larynx. The severity of this illness can range from mild to severe.[47] Croup affects males more often than females, with a peak incidence in pediatric patients occurring between the ages of 3 months and 6 years. Additionally, cases of croup are more common in the fall and winter.[48]

Presentation

Signs and symptoms of croup include a recent upper respiratory infection, a bark-like cough, a low-grade fever, dyspnea, and, in severe cases, stridor. Cyanosis may present late and is often indicative of impending respiratory failure.[49]

Workup

Croup is often diagnosed clinically, based on the physical examination and history of the patient. A pulse oximetry reading may be obtained to determine the child's oxygenation status, and x-rays may be obtained to differentiate croup from epiglottitis. However, neither of these measures confirms a diagnosis of croup.[50]

Treatment

The severity of croup must first be determined before treatment can begin. Corticosteroids or epinephrine may be used to reduce inflammation, though corticosteroids, such as dexamethasone, are preferred for more long-lasting effects.[49] Severe cases of croup require hospitalization and may require intubation.[51,52]

Infectious Mononucleosis

Overview

Infectious mononucleosis (mono) is an acute infectious disease that is caused by the Epstein-Barr virus and usually occurs in children older than the age of 10 years. Mono is transmitted via saliva and usually lasts about one month. The condition is usually self-limiting, but malaise and fatigue may endure for several months.[53]

Presentation

Fever, sore throat, swollen lymph nodes, and extreme fatigue are the typical presenting signs and symptoms of mono. A physical exam may reveal white tonsillar exudate and a maculopapular or petechial rash. Splenomegaly or hepatosplenomegaly, as well as jaundice, may also occur.[54]

Workup

Mono is often diagnosed clinically, based upon a physical examination that confirms the presence of the signs and symptoms listed above.[54] Lab tests should also be conducted to look for lymphocytic leukocytosis, neutropenia, an early rise in immunoglobulin M, and a permanent rise in immunoglobulin G. A positive heterophil antibody test or monospot test will also help to confirm a diagnosis.[53,55]

Treatment

Mono can be managed with supportive care, including NSAIDs and warm saline gargles.[56] Patients with strep throat should be prescribed penicillin or erythromycin instead of amoxicillin or ampicillin because amoxicillin and ampicillin often cause a rash in mono patients. In order to avoid splenic rupture, contact sports should be avoided for 3 weeks to several months, even in cases where splenomegaly is not clinically detectable.[57]

Sinusitis (Rhinosinusitis)

Overview

Sinusitis, also known as rhinosinusitis, occurs when one or more of the sinuses that drain into the nose become inflamed. The maxillary and ethmoid sinuses are the most commonly affected sinuses in patients with sinusitis. Sinusitis is most often caused by viral infections, such as the common cold.[58]

Presentation

Signs and symptoms of sinusitis include pain and pressure over the cheek, headache, and halitosis. Sinusitis also commonly presents with purulent postnasal drip and cough, usually occurring during the day and sometimes exacerbated at night. Additionally, patients may experience a dull, throbbing pain that worsens when the patient's head is in a dependent position.[59]

Workup

Diagnosis of sinusitis is often determined according to clinical presentation, especially when symptoms have lasted longer than 7–10 days. In some patients, the NP may need to order a CT scan to confirm the diagnosis.[59]

Treatment

Antibiotic therapy should be provided for children with a severe onset or worsening condition; amoxicillin with or without clavulanate is the typical first-line treatment.[60] For uncomplicated sinusitis with mild symptoms, pediatric patients should be treated as outpatients. Decongestants and antihistamines are not useful for acute sinusitis, but may be helpful for chronic sinusitis. The pain associated with sinusitis can be managed with acetaminophen. To reduce mucosal drying, nighttime humidification and supportive care can be used. In cases of chronic, refractory, or recurrent sinusitis, the patient should be referred to an otolaryngologist.[60]

Figures

Figure 12.1. Weber and Rinne hearing loss tests. Barkley & Associates, Inc. Published 2015.

References

1. Mayo Clinic Staff. Stye: definition. Mayo Clinic Web site. http://www.mayoclinic.com/health/sty/DS00257. Updated June 13, 2012. Accessed April 19, 2015.

2. Mayo Clinic Staff Sty: symptoms. Mayo Clinic Web site. http://www.mayoclinic.org/diseases-conditions/sty/basics/symptoms/con-20022698. Updated June 13, 2012. Accessed April 19, 2015.

3. Ghosh C, Ghosh T. Eyelid lesions. In: Basow DS, ed. *UpToDate*. Waltham, MA: UpToDate; 2015. http://www.uptodate.com/contents/eyelid-lesions. Last updated September 27, 2013. Accessed April 19, 2015.

4. Testing & diagnosis for stye (hordeolum) in children. Boston Children's Hospital Web site. http://www.childrenshospital.org/conditions-and-treatments/conditions/s/stye-hordeolum/testing-and-diagnosis. Accessed April 19, 2015.

5. Lindsley K, Nichols JJ, Dickersin K. Interventions for acute internal hordeolum. *Cochrane Database Syst Rev.* 2013; 4. doi: 10.1002/14651858.CD007742.pub3

6. Deschênes J, Fansler JL, Plouznikoff A. Chalazion. In: Roy H Sr, ed. Medscape. http://emedicine.medscape.com/article/1212709-overview#showall. Updated October 31, 2014. Accessed April 19, 2015.

7. Deschênes J, Fansler JL, Plouznikoff A. Chalazion clinical presentation. In: Roy H Sr, ed. Medscape. http://emedicine.medscape.com/article/1212709-clinical#-showall. Updated October 31, 2014. Accessed April 19, 2015.

8. Chalazion. American Optometric Association Web site. http://www.aoa.org/patients-and-public/eye-and-vision-problems/glossary-of-eye-and-vision-conditions/chalazion?sso=y. Accessed April 19, 2015.

9. Azari AA, Barney NP. Conjunctivitis: A systematic review of diagnosis and treatment. *JAMA.* 2013; 310(16): 1721–1729. doi: 10.1001/jama.2013.280318

10. Conjunctivitis (pink eye). Centers for Disease Control and Prevention Web site. http://www.cdc.gov/conjunctivitis/about/symptoms.html. Last reviewed January 9, 2014. Accessed April 19, 2015.

11. Scott IU, Luu K. Viral conjunctivitis workup. In: Roy H Sr, ed. Medscape. http://emedicine.medscape.com/article/1191370-workup#showall. Updated May 2, 2014. Accessed April 19, 2015.

12. Yeung KK, Weissman BA, De Shazer ME. Bacterial conjunctivitis workup. In: Roy H Sr, ed. Medscape. http://emedicine.medscape.com/article/1191730-workup#showall. Updated March 27, 2014. Accessed April 19, 2015.

13. McCourt EA, Enzenauer RW, Jatla KK, Zhao F. Neonatal conjunctivitis workup. In: Roy H Sr, ed. Medscape. http://emedicine.medscape.com/article/1192190-workup#showall. Updated February 20, 2014. Accessed April 19, 2015.

14. McCreery KM. Cataract in children. In: Basow DS, ed. *UpToDate*. Waltham, MA: UpToDate; 2015. www.uptodate.com/contents/cataract-in-children. Last updated March 4, 2015. Accessed April 19, 2015.

15. Colby K. Cataract. In: Porter RS, Kaplan JL, eds. The Merck Manual Online. http://www.merckmanuals.com/professional/eye_disorders/cataract/cataract.html. Last reviewed July 2014. Accessed April 19, 2015.

16. Barkley TW Jr. Eyes, ears, nose, and throat issues and disorders. In: *Pediatric Primary Care Nurse Practitioner Certification Review/Clinical Update Continuing Education Course*. West Hollywood, CA: Barkley and Associates; 2015: 109–124.

17. Bashour M, Menassa J, Cerontis CC. Congenital cataract treatment & management: Surgical care. In: Roy H Sr, ed. Medscape. http://emedicine.medscape.com/article/1210837-treatment#a1128. Updated March 5, 2014. Accessed April 19, 2015.

18. Strabismus. A.D.A.M. Medical Encyclopedia. http://www.nlm.nih.gov/medlineplus/ency/article/001004.htm. Updated September 2, 2014. Accessed April 19, 2015.

19. Fecarotta C, Huang WW. Strabismus. In: Porter RS, Kaplan JL, eds. The Merck Manual Online. http://www.merckmanuals.com/professional/pediatrics/eye_defects_and_conditions_in_children/strabismus.html?qt=Strabismus&alt=sh#v7540269. Last reviewed December 2012. Accessed April 19, 2015.

20. Waitzman AA. Otitis externa. In: Elluru RG, ed. Medscape. http://emedicine.medscape.com/article/994550-overview#showall. Updated December 29, 2014. Accessed April 19, 2015.

21. McCarthy AA. Otitis externa. Surgical Center of South Jersey Web site. http://www.scasouthjersey.com/apps/healthgate/article.aspx?chunkiid=100689. Last reviewed August 2014. Accessed April 19, 2015.

22. Goguen LA. External otitis: Pathogenesis, clinical features, and diagnosis. In: Basow DS, ed. *UpToDate*. Waltham, MA: UpToDate; 2015. http://www.uptodate.com/contents/external-otitis-pathogenesis-clinical-features-and-diagnosis. Last updated September 19, 2014. Accessed April 19, 2015.

23. Wald ER. Acute otitis media in children: Diagnosis. In: Basow DS, ed. *UpToDate*. Waltham, MA: UpToDate; 2015. http://www.uptodate.com/contents/acute-otitis-media-in-children-diagnosis. Last updated October 21, 2014. Accessed April 19, 2015.

24. Klein JO, Pelton S. Acute otitis media in children: Epidemiology, microbiology, clinical manifestations, and complications. In: Basow DS, ed. *UpToDate*. Waltham, MA: UpToDate; 2015. http://www.uptodate.com/contents/acute-otitis-media-in-children-epidemiology-microbiology-clinical-manifestations-and-complications. Last reviewed November 11, 2014. Accessed April 19, 2015.

25. Klein JO, Pelton S. Acute otitis media in children: Treatment. In: Basow DS, ed. *UpToDate*. Waltham, MA: UpToDate; 2015. http://www.uptodate.com/contents/acute-otitis-media-in-children-treatment. Last updated January 31, 2014. Accessed April 19, 2015.

26. Vaccine recommendations of the ACIP. Centers for Disease Control and Prevention Web site. http://www.cdc.gov/vaccines/hcp/acip-recs/index.html. Last reviewed July 16, 2013. Last updated March 30, 2015. Accessed April 19, 2015.

27. Otitis media with effusion. Penn State Hershey Web site. http://pennstatehershey.adam.com/content.aspx?productId=117&pid=1&gid=007010. Reviewed August 30, 2014. Accessed April 19, 2015.

28. Klein JO, Pelton S. Otitis media with effusion (serous otitis media) in children: Clinical features and diagnosis. In: Basow DS, ed. *UpToDate*. Waltham, MA: UpToDate; 2015. http://www.uptodate.com/contents/otitis-media-with-effusion-serous-otitis-media-in-children-clinical-features-and-diagnosis. Last updated May 28, 2013. Accessed April 19, 2015.

29. Higgins TS Jr. Otitis media with effusion. In: Meyers AD, ed. Medscape. http://emedicine.medscape.com/article/858990-overview. Updated February 20, 2015. Accessed April 19, 2015.

30. Lieberthal AS, Carrol AE, Chonmaitree T, et al. The diagnosis and management of acute otitis media. *Pediatrics*. 2013; 131(3): e964–e999. doi: 10.1542/peds.2012-3488

31. Hearing loss. A.D.A.M. Medical Encyclopedia. http://www.nlm.nih.gov/medlineplus/ency/article/003044.htm. Updated May 18, 2014. Accessed April 19, 2015.

32. Smith RJH, Gooi A. Hearing impairment in children: Etiology. In: Basow DS, ed. *UpToDate*. Waltham, MA: UpToDate; 2015. http://www.uptodate.com/contents/hearing-impairment-in-children-etiology. Last updated March 25, 2014. Accessed April 19, 2015.

33. Smith RJH, Gooi A. Hearing impairment in children: Evaluation. In: Basow DS, ed. *UpToDate*. Waltham, MA: UpToDate; 2015. http://www.uptodate.com/contents/hearing-impairment-in-children-evaluation. Last updated January 14, 2015. Accessed April 19, 2015.

34. Smith RJH, Gooi A. Hearing impairment in children: Treatment. In: Basow DS, ed. *UpToDate*. Waltham, MA: UpToDate; 2015. http://www.uptodate.com/contents/hearing-impairment-in-children-treatment. Last updated January 20, 2015. Accessed April 19, 2015.

35. Pappas DE, Hendley JO. The common cold in children: Clinical features and diagnosis. In: Basow DS, ed. *UpToDate*. Waltham, MA: UpToDate; 2015. http://www.uptodate.com/contents/the-common-cold-in-children-clinical-features-and-diagnosis. Last updated January 15, 2014. Accessed April 19, 2015.

36. Mayo Clinic Staff. Common cold. Mayo Clinic Web site. http://www.mayoclinic.org/diseases-conditions/common-cold/basics/symptoms/con-20019062. Updated April 17, 2013. Accessed April 19, 2015.

37. Pappas DE, Hendley JO. The common cold in children: Treatment and prevention. In: Basow DS, ed. *UpToDate*. Waltham, MA: UpToDate; 2015. http://www.uptodate.com/contents/the-common-cold-in-children-treatment-and-prevention. Last updated January 20, 2015. Accessed April 19, 2015.

38. Mayo Clinic Staff. Nosebleeds. Mayo Clinic Web site. http://www.mayoclinic.org/symptoms/nosebleeds/basics/definition/sym-20050914. Updated August 10, 2012. Accessed April 19, 2015.

39. Messner AH. Management of epistaxis in children. In: Basow DS, ed. *UpToDate*. Waltham, MA: UpToDate; 2015. http://www.uptodate.com/contents/management-of-epistaxis-in-children. Last updated September 10, 2014. Accessed April 19, 2015.

40. Pharyngitis and tonsillitis. Cincinnati's Children Hospital Web site. http://www.cincinnatichildrens.org/health/p/pharyngitis-tonsillitis. Last updated September 2013. Accessed April 19, 2015.

41. Drutz JE. Sore throat in children and adolescents: Symptomatic treatment. In: Basow DS, ed. *UpToDate*. Waltham, MA: UptoDate; 2015. http://www.uptodate.com/contents/sore-throat-in-children-and-adolescents-symptomatic-treatment. Last updated January 6, 2014. Accessed April 19, 2015.

42. Shah UK, Conrad DE, Grindle CR. Tonsillitis and pharyngitis organism–specific therapy. In: Bronze MS, ed. Medscape. http://emedicine.medscape.com/article/2011872-overview. Updated August 16, 2013. Accessed April 19, 2015.

43. Woods CR. Epiglottitis (supraglottitis): Clinical features and diagnosis. In: Basow DS, ed. *UpToDate*. Waltham, MA: UpToDate; 2015. http://www.uptodate.com/contents/epiglottitis-supraglottitis-clinical-features-and-diagnosis. Last updated October 2, 2013. Accessed April 19, 2015.

44. Abdallah C. Acute epiglottitis: Trends, diagnosis and management. *Saudi J Anaesth*. 2012; 6(3): 279–281. doi: 10.4103/1658-354X.101222

45. Epiglottitis. A.D.A.M. Medical Encyclopedia. http://www.nlm.nih.gov/medlineplus/ency/article/000605.htm. Updated February 25, 2014. Accessed April 19, 2015.

46. Gompf SG. Epiglottitis medication. In: Dyne PL, ed. Medscape. http://emedicine.medscape.com/article/763612-medication#2. Updated August 8, 2014. Accessed April 19, 2015.

47. Holmes A. Croup: What it is and how to treat it. *US Pharmacist*. 2013; 38(7): 47–50. http://www.medscape.com/viewarticle/809211

48. Woods CR. Croup: Clinical features, evaluation, and diagnosis. In: Basow DS, ed. *UpToDate*. Waltham, MA: UpToDate; 2015. http://www.uptodate.com/contents/croup-clinical-features-evaluation-and-diagnosis. Last updated February 18, 2015. Accessed April 19, 2015.

49. Defendi GL, Muñiz A, Molodow RE. Croup clinical presentation. In: Steele RW, ed. Medscape. http://emedicine.medscape.com/article/962972-clinical#showall. Updated April 15, 2014. Accessed April 19, 2015.

50. Perlstein D. Croup diagnosis. In: Davis CP, ed. eMedicineHealth. http://www.emedicinehealth.com/croup/page5_em.htm#croup_diagnosis. Reviewed June 20, 2014. Accessed April 19, 2015.

51. Perlstein D. Croup treatment. In: Davis CP, ed. eMedicineHealth. http://www.emedicinehealth.com/croup/page7_em.htm#croup_treatment. Reviewed June 20, 2014. Accessed April 19, 2015.

52. Mayo Clinic Staff. Croup. Mayo Clinic Web site. http://www.mayoclinic.org/diseases-conditions/croup/basics/treatment/con-20014673. Updated January 30, 2013. Accessed April 19, 2015.

53. Epstein-Barr virus and infectious mononucleosis. Centers for Disease Control and Prevention Web site. http://www.cdc.gov/epstein-barr/index.html. Last updated January 7, 2014. Accessed April 19, 2015.

54. Infectious mononucleosis symptoms & causes. Boston Children's Hospital Web site. http://www.childrenshospital.org/conditions-and-treatments/conditions/i/infectious-mononucleosis/symptoms-and-causes. Accessed April 19, 2015.

55. Mono test. Lab Tests Online Web site. http://labtestsonline.org/understanding/analytes/mono/tab/test. Last reviewed January 8, 2013. Accessed April 19, 2015.

56. Snellman L, Anderson G, Godfrey A, et al. Diagnosis and treatment of respiratory illness in children and adults. Institute for Clinical Systems Improvement Web site. https://www.icsi.org/_asset/1wp8x2/RespIllness.pdf. Published 2013. Accessed April 19, 2015.

57. Stöppler MC. Infectious mononucleosis. In: Shiel WC Jr. eMedicineHealth. http://www.medicinenet.com/infectious_mononucleosis/page5.htm#what_is_the_usual_course_and_treatment_of_mono. Reviewed February 3, 2015. Accessed April 19, 2015.

58. Ramadan H. Pediatric sinusitis. American Rhinologic Society Web site. http://care.american-rhinologic.org/pediatric_sinusitis. Revised February 17, 2015. Accessed April 19, 2015.

59. U.S. Department of Health and Human Services, National Institutes of Health, National Institute of Allergy and Infectious Diseases. Sinusitis. http://www.niaid.nih.gov/topics/sinusitis/Pages/Index.aspx. Last reviewed March 9, 2011. Last updated April 3, 2012. Accessed April 19, 2015.

60. Wald ER, Applegate KE, Bordley C, et al. Clinical practice guideline for the diagnosis and management of acute bacterial sinusitis in children aged 1 to 18 years. *Pediatrics*. 2013; 132(1): e262–e280. doi: 10.1542/peds.2013–1071

Chapter 13

Respiratory Disorders

QUESTIONS

1. In general, how frequently would a typical pediatric patient with mild persistent asthma use a rescue inhaler?

    a. Less than 2 days per week

    b. Several times per day

    c. More than 2 days per week

    d. Once per day

2. Which of the following regimens would best constitute Step 3 in the stepwise management of a patient with asthma, according to national recommendations?

    a. Preferred low-dose inhaled corticosteroid (ICS)

    b. Cromolyn or montelukast as required

    c. Preferred medium-dose ICS with considered oral systemic corticosteroid short course

    d. Preferred short-acting B2-agonist as required

3. In considering the need to refer a child to a specialist for cystic fibrosis, all of the following statements from the mother would typically support the decision except:

    a. "My child's stool is often bulky and foul smelling with an oily residue."

    b. "My child doesn't seem to be growing. Am I not breastfeeding her enough?"

    c. "My child always seems to be coughing and has a running nose that won't quit."

    d. "My child wets his diaper six times a day and nearly soaks it through each time."

4. A premature infant should typically be given palivizumab (Synagis) for the prevention of respiratory syncytial virus bronchiolitis if gestation is less than:

    a. 29 weeks

    b. 33 weeks

    c. 35 weeks

    d. 40 weeks

5. The practitioner would expect which of the following laboratory tests to be least useful in a workup for cystic fibrosis?

    a. Pilocarpine iontophoresis sweat test

    b. Pulmonary function tests

    c. White blood cell count

    d. Sputum culture

6. What is the most common etiology of pneumonia in children 1–3 years old?

    a. *Streptococcus pneumoniae*

    b. *Mycoplasma*

    c. Group B Streptococcus

    d. *Haemophilus influenzae*

7. A 7-year-old presents with symptoms indicative of asthma. His mother states that he typically experiences symptoms once per day. His mother adds that the symptoms also keep him out of some of the more active past times of his peers and cause him to wake 2–3 nights per week. How should you classify the patient's asthma?

   a. Intermittent

   b. Persistent mild

   c. Persistent moderate

   d. Persistent severe

8. Which of the following pathogens responsible for pneumonia does not typically demonstrate lobar consolidation as a radiographic characteristic?

   a. *Streptococcus pneumoniae*

   b. *Haemophilus influenzae*

   c. *Pneumocystis jiroveci*

   d. *Klebsiella pneumoniae*

9. Which two laboratory findings best characterizes the findings of restrictive disease in pulmonary function test results?

   a. Reduced airflow rates and lung volumes within normal range or larger

   b. Primarily reduced volumes and, to some extent, reduced expiratory flow rates

   c. Normal volumes and reduced expiratory flow rates

   d. Primarily reduced airflow rates and, to some extent, increased lung volumes

10. You are assessing for egophony in a young patient with suspected pneumonia. You ask the patient to produce a long "E" sound. What sound should you anticipate to auscultate when the patient has lung consolidation?

    a. A long "A," or "ay," sound

    b. A short "A," or "ah," sound

    c. A long "E," or "ee," sound

    d. A short "E," or "eh," sound

RATIONALES

1. c

Patients with mild persistent asthma commonly tend to use a rescue inhaler for symptom control more than 2 days per week. Use of a rescue inhaler less than 2 days per week, on the other hand, more often indicates intermittent asthma. Daily use of a rescue inhaler is typically indicated for moderate persistent asthma but not for lesser degrees of severity. Using a rescue inhaler several times per day is mostly seen in cases of severe persistent asthma.

2. c

Step 3 in managing a patient with moderate to severe asthma would commonly involve administering a medium-dose inhaled corticosteroid (ICS) and considering a short course of oral systemic corticosteroids. A low-dose ICS is often the preferred course in Step 2 of asthma management, with cromolyn and montelukast suggested as alternatives. Lastly, short-acting B2-agonists are the common preferred course in Step 1 of managing a patient with asthma.

3. d

Urinary frequency and polyuria are not signs and symptoms typically associated with cystic fibrosis. In infants and young children, cystic fibrosis is more likely to present with steatorrhea, or greasy, foul-smelling stool produced as a result of non-absorption of dietary fats. Other common signs and symptoms of cystic fibrosis may include failure to thrive, chronic cough, and rhinorrhea.

4. a

A premature infant born under 29 weeks gestation should be given palivizumab as prophylaxis for potential respiratory syncytial virus (RSV) infection. A premature infant born under 32 weeks gestation would qualify for prophylaxis if he or she required oxygenation for the first 28 days after birth, but not commonly on the basis of gestation. Earlier standards for RSV prophylaxis had qualifiers for children born at 32–35 weeks gestation, but these standards have since been modified. There is no common requirement for RSV prophylaxis in children born under 40 weeks gestation.

5. c

A white blood cell count is not a common diagnostic for cystic fibrosis. The pilocarpine iontophoresis sweat test is often considered the hallmark diagnostic for cystic fibrosis, with elevated salt levels serving as a bedrock for diagnosis. Pulmonary function tests see use to determine the possibility of airway obstruction, but may not be as reliable in patients under the age of 5. Sputum culture may likewise see use to find the presence of confirmatory pathogens for cystic fibrosis such as *Pseudomonas aeruginosa*.

6. a

The most common bacterial etiology for pediatric pneumonia in children 1–3 years old is by *Streptococcus pneumoniae*. The preferred outpatient oral antibiotic treatment for community-acquired pneumonia in this age group is amoxicillin, 90 mg/kg/day, dosed twice a day. The most common source of pediatric pneumonia is viral, which does not typically need any treatment other than supportive care.

7. c

A patient between the ages of 5 and 11 years who presents with daily asthma symptoms, some limitation of activity, and nighttime awakening more than once per week should be classified as experiencing persistent moderate asthma. Intermittent asthma typically presents with no limitation of activity, symptoms less than 2 days per week, and nighttime awakenings less than 2 nights per month. Mild persistent asthma commonly presents with minor activity limitation, as well as symptoms more than 2 days per week, but not daily and nighttime awakenings more than 3–4 times per month. Severe persistent asthma presents with nighttime awakenings more than once per week, but also presents with asthma symptoms throughout the day and extreme activity limitation.

8. c

Radiographic characteristics of pneumonia stemming from *Pneumocystis jiroveci* commonly include diffuse interstitial, alveolar, apical, or upper lobe infiltrates, but not lobar consolidation. Lobar consolidation is, however, a common shared radiographic characteristic of pneumonia stemming from *Haemophilus influenzae*, *Streptococcus pneumoniae*, and *Klebsiella pneumoniae*.

9. b

Restrictive disease in pulmonary function test results is primarily characterized by reduced volumes and, to some extent, expiratory flow rates. Primarily, reduced airflow rates and expiratory flow rates accompanied by lung volumes within the normal range or larger are, to some extent, more indicative of obstructive disease, not restrictive disease.

10. a

The technique to check for egophony requires listening to the lungs with a stethoscope as the patient says the letter "E"; when lung consolidation is present, the sound will typically be transmitted as the long "A," or "ay," sound. When the lungs are normal, the long "E," or "ee," sound can commonly be heard through the stethoscope. Short "A" ("ah") and short "E" ("eh") sounds are not typical findings of this technique, regardless of the state of the lungs. This assessment can be performed in conjunction with percussion to validate findings by assessment of resonance versus dullness for consolidation.

DISCUSSION

Respiratory Assessment

Overview

A respiratory assessment evaluates the type and location of a patient's breath sounds and consists of four components: inspection, palpation, percussion, and auscultation.[1] The nurse practitioner (NP) should inspect the thorax, vertebral column, and chest wall. The palpation component consists of palpating the trachea for mobility and any deviation from the midline. The lymph nodes of the head and neck should also be palpated. Percussion can be used to determine if the regions of the chest are hyper-resonant, dull, or flat. The NP should auscultate each lobe of both lungs, and should be able to recognize any abnormal breath sounds on either inspiration or expiration.[2] Egophony, which is a change in timbre from "E" to "A" that can be heard while auscultating, indicates lung consolidation and compression.[3] In cases of respiratory complications and if indicated, pulmonary function tests should also be included in a respiratory assessment if the patient is older than 5 years of age and is cooperative.[4]

Presentation

When a respiratory assessment detects abnormalities that derive from recurring respiratory complications, the patient's pulmonary condition can be classified as an obstructive or restrictive disease. Obstructive diseases are characterized by reduced airflow rates and lung volumes either within the normal range or higher. These findings are typical of conditions such as asthma, chronic bronchitis, and cystic fibrosis. Restrictive diseases, such as pneumonia, are characterized by reduced expiratory flow rates and volumes.[5]

Bronchiolitis

Overview

Bronchiolitis is a viral illness that affects the lower respiratory tract and produces inflammation, which then leads to blockage of the small respiratory airways. Most cases of bronchiolitis are caused by the respiratory syncytial virus (RSV) or the parainfluenza 3 virus.[6] Bronchiolitis usually affects children younger than 2 years of age and often occurs in epidemics.[6] Although bronchiolitis may occur at any age, severe symptoms of the condition usually appear only in young infants.[7]

Presentation

Bronchiolitis usually begins with a mild upper respiratory infection lasting for several days. After a few days, the patient presents with a moderate fever and signs of respiratory distress, (e.g., a wheezy or hacking cough, retractions, tachypnea).[6,8] More severe cases may present with additional signs of distress, such as cyanosis and nasal flaring.[7] Restlessness and changes in mental status may also accompany respiratory distress.[3] The patient's liver and spleen may be palpable due to hyperinflated lungs.[9]

Workup

A diagnosis of bronchiolitis is confirmed by a number of factors, such as seasonal occurrence, the patient's age, presentation, and physical examination findings.[7] A chest x-ray, usually reserved for if the patient exhibits severe symptoms or has a pre-existing condition, typically shows hyperinflated lungs and may show scattered areas of consolidation.[3,6] Other diagnostic tests that may be done include a nasal fluid culture, which helps to determine the causative virus, and arterial blood gas analysis.[10] Additionally, an immunofluorescence foci assay (IFA) may detect RSV in a mucus culture or nasal washing.[11]

Treatment

Outpatient treatment and supportive care are common options for infants with mild distress. RSV prophylaxis with a palivizumab (Synagis) injection is indicated in high-risk infants and helps decrease the risk of hospitalization.[6] Palivizumab should be administered every month during RSV season (maximum five doses) to premature infants (i.e., infants born before 29 weeks gestation)

under 1 year of age, as well as premature infants born before 32 weeks gestation who present with chronic lung disease.[3,12] Infants may likewise be considered for palivizumab if they present with hemodynamically significant heart disease or would be immunocompromised during RSV season.[12,13]

Asthma

Overview

Asthma is a respiratory disease that is characterized by widespread narrowing of the airways and is distinguished by an increased responsiveness of the bronchi and trachea to a variety of stimuli. These stimuli trigger diffuse airway inflammation, which results in bronchoconstriction.[14] Severity of asthma may decrease either spontaneously or due to direct treatment.[3]

The pathophysiology of asthma involves acute inflammation and plugging of the airways by thick, viscous mucus. The airways are likewise narrowed by hypertrophy of smooth muscle and remodeled via thickening of the epithelial basement membrane.[3,14] Other pathophysiological features of asthma include mucosal edema and hyperemia.[15]

The most common asthma allergens are encountered indoors and include dust mites, indoor molds, respiratory infections, stress, cold air, pets, cockroaches, and smoke. Asthma may be triggered by exercise, especially in environments that are cold or dry.[14] Certain medications, such as aspirin and other NSAIDs, may also cause asthma.[16] Other contributing factors include airway irritants, such as cigarettes, air pollution, wood smoke, perfumes, aerosol sprays, paints or sealants, and cleaning agents.[17]

Presentation

Asthma is characterized by a pattern of respiratory symptoms that occur when the patient is exposed to triggers of the condition.[18] These symptoms may include coughing, wheezing, chest tightness, and respiratory distress; the patient may also experience difficulty speaking in sentences and may present with diaphoresis and hyperresonance.[19]

More ominous signs of asthma include absent breath sounds, cyanosis, and inability to maintain recumbency. Another ominous sign is pulsus paradoxus, which is indicated by a change in systolic blood pressure amplitude greater than 10 mmHg in between inspiration and expiration.[20]

Workup

When a diagnosis of asthma is suspected, the patient should undergo a pulmonary function test to assess for abnormalities typical of obstructive dysfunction.[14] Hospitalization is recommended if the peak flow is under 60 L/min initially or if there is no improvement in ventilation after aerosol treatment. Laboratory findings, such as slight white

Table 13.1	Asthma Severity Classification			
Classification	Intermittent	Mild Persistent	Moderate Persistent	Severe Persistent
Symptoms	≤ 2 days/week	> 2 days/week	Daily	Throughout the day
Nighttime awakenings	≤ 2/month	3 to 4/month	More than once per week but not nightly	Nightly
Rescue inhaler use	≤ 2 days/week	> 2 days/week but not daily	Daily	Several times per day
Interference with normal activity	None	Minor limitation	Some limitation	Extremely limited
Lung function	FEV1 > 80% predicted and normal between exacerbations	FEV1 > 80% predicted	FEV1 60% to 80% predicted	FEV1 less than 60% predicted

Used with permission from Barkley TW Jr. Pediatric Primary Care Nurse Practitioner Certification Review/Clinical Update Continuing Education Course. West Hollywood, CA: Barkley and Associates; 2015.

blood cell elevation with eosinophilia, are helpful in excluding other diagnoses. A chest x-ray is usually unnecessary but may be used to rule out other conditions.[3,21]

The severity of a patient's asthma can be classified according to table 13.1.[3]

Treatment (see table 13.2)

According to the 2007 National Heart, Lung, and Blood Institute/National Asthma Education and Prevention Program Asthma Guidelines at a Glance, asthma treatment should focus on achieving and maintaining control of asthma symptoms.[22] In the treatment for persistent asthma, inhaled corticosteroids (ICS) commonly see use in all age groups.[22] Combination therapy is recommended when treatment needs to be stepped up; in patients over the age of 12 years, long-acting beta-2 adrenergic agonists are preferred for combination with ICS. Guidelines for asthma management are divided into three distinct age groups with consideration for current impairment and future risk. These age groups are 0–4 years of age, 5–11 years of age, and 12 years of age and older. More frequent monitoring should initially be conducted every 2–4 weeks until control is achieved. If the patient's asthma remains uncontrolled, the NP should move to the next step of treatment and check back with the patient at least every 2 weeks. If there is continued control for 3 months, however, the NP should step down therapy.[3,22]

Pneumonia

Overview

Pneumonia is a respiratory disorder characterized by inflammation of the lower respiratory tract. This condition typically produces when microorganisms gain access through aspiration, inhalation, or hematogenous dissemination. Although the majority of pneumonia cases are viral, the condition may be caused by a variety of other organisms, such as bacteria and fungi.[3,23] Additionally, the presentation of pneumonia typically differs depending on if the condition is acquired in the community or hospital.[24]

The most common bacterial cause of pneumonia includes group B *Streptococcus*, but can also include *Chlamydophila pneumoniae*, *Escherichia coli*, *Haemophilus influenzae*, and *Streptococcus pneumoniae*.[3,25] RSV also causes pneumonia, particularly in infants and children younger than 6 years of age.[26] Immunocompromised or malnourished patients are particularly susceptible to pneumonia caused by fungi or *Pneumocystis jiroveci*.[27]

Presentation

Signs and symptoms of pneumonia in pediatric patients vary based on age group. Fever and cough are common findings of pneumonia in all patients older than 1 month, but viral forms of pneumonia may present with low temperature or no fever at all. Toddlers and preschoolers commonly present with tachypnea and congestion, whereas older children and adolescents may experience constitutional symptoms such as headache and chest pain.[24,28] A physical exam may note lung consolidation, and pulse oximetry will show decreased oxygenation in the event of severe distress.[3]

Workup

If pneumonia is suspected, the NP may order diagnostic tests such as chest x-rays, pulse oximetry, and blood tests.[23] A sputum culture is warranted if the patient presents with a productive cough.[29]

Radiographic characteristics of pneumonia differ depending on the causative organism. For instance, lobar consolidation is indicative of *H. influenzae*, *S. pneumoniae*, and *Klebsiella pneumoniae*. Pneumocystis infections, on the other hand, are

Table 13.2 Assessing Asthma Control and Adjusting Therapy in Children

Components of control		Well controlled		Not well controlled		Very poorly controlled	
		Ages 0–4	Ages 5–11	Ages 0–4	Ages 5–11	Ages 0–4	Ages 5–11
Impairment	Symptoms	2 days/week or less, but not more than once a day		More than 2 days/week or multiple times on 2 days/week or more		Throughout the day	
	Nighttime awakenings	1x/month or less		More than 1x/ month	2x/month or more	More than 1x/ week	2x/week or more
	Interference with normal activity	None		Some limitation		Extremely limited	
	SABA use for symptom control (not EIB prevention)	2 days/week or less		More than 2 days/week		Several times per day	
	Lung function FEV$_1$	N/A	> 80%	N/A	60%–80%	N/A	< 60%
	Lung function FEV$_1$/FVC		> 80%		75%–80%		< 75%
Risk	Exacerbations requiring oral systemic corticosteroids	0–1x/year		2–3x/year	2x/year or more	>3x/year	2x/year or more
	Reduction in lung growth	N/A	Requires long-term followup	N/A	Requires long-term followup	N/A	Requires long-term followup
	Treatment-related adverse effects	Medication side effects can vary in intensity from none to very troublesome and worrisome. The level of intensity does not correlated to specific levels of control but should be considered in the overall assessment of risk.					
Recommended action for treatment		Maintain current step. Regular followup every 1–6 months. Consider step down if well controlled for at least 3 months		Step up 1 step.	Step up at least 1 step.	Consider short course of systemic corticosteroids. Step up 1–2 steps.	

Notes. 1. Before stepping up, review adherence to medication, inhaler technique, and environmental control. If alternative treatment was used, discontinue it and use preferred treatment for that step. 2. Re-evaluate the level of asthma control in 2–6 weeks to achieve control every 1–6 months to maintain control. Children 0–4 years old: If no clear benefit is observed in 4–6 weeks, consider alternative diagnoses or adjusting therapy. Children 5–11 years old: Adjust therapy accordingly. For side effects: consider alternative treatment options. EIB=exercise-induced bronchospasm; FEV$_1$=forced expiratory volume in 1 second; FVC$_1$=forced vital capacity; ICU=intensive care unit; N/A=not applicable. For more information on treatment, see "Stepwise approach for managing asthma for treatment steps" at http://www.nhlbi.nih.gov/files/docs/guidelines/asthsumm.pdf. Source: National Heart, Lung, and Blood Institute, National Institutes of Health. Assessing Asthma Control and Adjusting Therapy in Children. http://www.nhlbi.nih.gov/files/docs/guidelines/asthsumm.pdf. Published 2007. Retrieved April 2015. Reproduced with permission.

characterized by diffuse interstitial, alveolar, apical, or upper lobe infiltrates. Patchy infiltrates are characteristic of *E. coli*, *Staphylococcus aureus*, and *Pseudomonas aeruginosa*. *E. coli* infections may also be indicated by pleural effusion, whereas *P. aeruginosa* infections may also present with cavitation.[3,30]

Treatment

Viral pneumonia is treated by supportive measures such as hydration, antipyretics, humidified oxygen, chest physiotherapy, and bronchodilators, which help improve airway clearance. In viral cases, antibiotics only see use in the event of secondary bacterial infections.[31,32]

For patients with community-acquired pneumonia, pharmacological therapy is determined by the infecting organism. Penicillin is indicated for *S. pneumoniae* infections, whereas *Moraxella catarrhalis* infections are treated by macrolides such as azithromycin.[33,34] Amoxicillin and cephalosporin are indicated for *H. influenzae* infections.[35]

Cystic Fibrosis

Overview

Cystic fibrosis (CF) is the most common autosomal recessive disorder in the Caucasian population.[36] The condition is caused by a chromosome 7 long arm mutation. The mutation causes a defect in epithelial chloride transport, resulting in dehydrated, thick secretions. As a result of mucus buildup, patients may experience digestion problems and life-threatening lung infections.[37] Nearly all exogenic glands are affected by CF, including the respiratory, hepatobiliary, gastroenterology, and reproductive tracts.[3,37] CF is also characterized by progressive obstructive pulmonary disease, recurrent endobronchial infections, and pancreatic insufficiency with intestinal malabsorption. The median survival age of CF is 36.9 years, with males typically living longer than females.[38]

Presentation

Newborns with CF may present with meconium ileus, failure to thrive, or salty-tasting skin.[36,39] CF also presents with recurrent respiratory infections and chronic coughing, among other respiratory findings. Malabsorption causes large, liquid, bulky, and foul stool (i.e., steatorrhea). A nasal exam may reveal rhinorrhea, and gastrointestinal findings may include hepatosplenomegaly or fat-soluble vitamin deficiencies.[3,38] Delayed puberty is more common in CF patients than the general population. Infertility also frequently occurs in CF patients. [37]

Workup

Most cases are discovered during the universal newborn screening and confirmed through a pilocarpine iontophoresis sweat test.[36] Pulmonary function tests reveal an obstructive pattern, and a chest radiograph may detect cystic lesions and atelectasis.[3] Lastly, blood gas and serum electrolyte levels may detect chronic alkalosis.[37]

Treatment

CF patients should be referred to a CF center for care. Although there is no cure for CF, a number of treatment options exist to help reduce symptoms and complications.[40] The main goals of CF treatment are to maintain normal lung function and ensure normal growth through nutritional therapy.[38] Pulmonary treatment is aimed at preventing airway obstruction and also includes prophylaxis against pulmonary infections.[36] Exercise and dietary modifications are also beneficial for CF patients.[39]

References

1. Bickley LS, Szilagyi PG. *Bates' Guide to Physical Examination and History Taking*. 11th ed. Philadelphia, PA: Lippincott, Williams & Wilkins; 2011.

2. Taylor C, Gfeller P, Ring T. Respiratory examination. Learn Pediatrics Web site. http://learnpediatrics.com/files/2011/01/Respiratory-video-script.pdf. Accessed May 19, 2015.

3. Barkley TW Jr. *Pediatric Primary Care Nurse Practitioner Certification Review/Clinical Update Continuing Education Course*. West Hollywood, CA: Barkley and Associates; 2015.

4. Sawicki G, Haver K. Asthma in children younger than 12 years: Initial evaluation and diagnosis. In: Basow DS, ed. *UpToDate*. Waltham, MA: UpToDate; 2015. http://www.uptodate.com/contents/asthma-in-children-younger-than-12-years-initial-evaluation-and-diagnosis. Last updated January 4, 2015. Accessed April 19, 2015.

5. Healthwise, Inc. Obstructive and restrictive lung disease. WebMD Web site. http://www.webmd.com/lung/obstructive-and-restrictive-lung-disease. Reviewed September 4, 2012. Accessed April 19, 2015.

6. Caserta MT. Respiratory syncytial virus (RSV) and human metapneumovirus infections. In: Porter RS, Kaplan JL, eds. The Merck Manual Online. http://www.merckmanuals.com/professional/pediatrics/miscellaneous-viral-infections-in-infants-and-children/respiratory-syncytial-virus-rsv-and-human-metapneumovirus-infections. Last reviewed November 2014. Accessed April 19, 2015.

7. DeNicola LK, Maraqa NF, Custodio HT, & Udeani J. Bronchiolitis. In: Steele RW, ed. Medscape. http://emedicine.medscape.com/article/961963-overview. Updated November 10, 2014. Accessed April 19, 2015.

8. Piedra PA, Stark AR. Bronchiolitis in infants and children: Clinical features and diagnosis. In: Basow DS, ed. *UpToDate*. Waltham, MA: UpToDate; 2015. http://www.uptodate.com/contents/bronchiolitis-in-infants-and-children-clinical-features-and-diagnosis. Last updated January 19, 2015. Accessed April 19, 2015.

9. Tidy C. Bronchiolitis. Patient.co.uk Web site. http://www.patient.co.uk/doctor/bronchiolitis-pro. Last reviewed June 28, 2013. Accessed April 19, 2015.

10. Bronchiolitis. A.D.A.M. Medical Encyclopedia. http://www.nlm.nih.gov/medlineplus/ency/article/000975.htm. Updated August 22, 2013. Accessed April 19, 2015.

11. Pankaj K. Methods for rapid virus identification and quantification. *Mater Methods*. 2013; 3: 207.

12. Committee on Infectious Diseases, Bronchiolitis Guidelines Committee. Updated guidance for palivizumab prophylaxis among infants and young children at increased risk of hospitalization for respiratory syncytial virus infection. *Pediatrics*. 2014; 134(2): 415–420. doi: 10.1542/peds.2014-1665

13. Bollani L, Pozzi M. The prevention of respiratory syncytial virus infection. *Ital J Pediatr*. 2014; 40 (Suppl 2): A35. doi: 10.1186/1824-7288-40-S2-A35

14. Miles MC, Peters SP. Asthma. In: Porter RS, Kaplan JL, eds. The Merck Manual Online. http://www.merckmanuals.com/professional/pulmonary-disorders/asthma-and-related-disorders/asthma. Last reviewed July 2014. Accessed April 19, 2015.

15. Ball DR, McGuire BE. Airway pharmacology. In: Hagberg C, ed. *Benumof and Hagberg's Airway Management*. 3rd ed. Philadelphia, PA: Elsevier Saunders; 2013: 159–183.

16. Asthma. A.D.A.M. Medical Encyclopedia. http://www.ncbi.nlm.nih.gov/pubmedhealth/PMH0062942. Last updated June 11, 2014. Accessed April 19, 2015.

17. United States Department of Health and Human Services, Centers for Disease Control and Prevention. Common asthma triggers. http://www.cdc.gov/asthma/triggers.html. Last reviewed December 14, 2010. Last updated August 20, 2012. Accessed April 19, 2015.

18. Fanta CH. Diagnosis of asthma in adolescents and adults. In: Basow DS, ed. *UpToDate*. Waltham, MA: UpToDate; 2015. http://www.uptodate.com/contents/diagnosis-of-asthma-in-adolescents-and-adults. Last updated March 7, 2014. Accessed April 19, 2015.

19. United States Department of Health and Human Services, National Institutes of Health (NIH), National Heart, Lung, and Blood Institute (NHLBI). What are the signs and symptoms of asthma? http://www.nhlbi.nih.gov/health/health-topics/topics/asthma/signs.html. Updated August 4, 2014. Accessed April 19, 2015.

20. Heuer AJ, Scanlan CL, Wilkins RL. *Wilkins' Clinical Assessment in Respiratory Care*. 7th ed. Maryland Heights, MO: Elsevier Mosby; 2014: 43–45.

21. Morris MJ. Asthma workup. In: Mosenifar Z, ed. Medscape. http://emedicine.medscape.com/article/296301-workup. Updated September 30, 2014. Accessed April 19, 2015.

22. United States Department of Health and Human Services, NIH, NHLBI. Asthma care quick reference: Diagnosing and managing asthma (NIH Publication No. 12-5075). http://www.nhlbi.nih.gov/guidelines/asthma/asthma_qrg.pdf. Revised September 2012. Accessed April 19, 2015.

23. Mayo Clinic Staff. Pneumonia. Mayo Clinic web site. http://www.mayoclinic.com/health/pneumonia/DS00135. Updated March 14, 2015. Accessed April 19, 2015.

24. Pneumonia. A.D.A.M. Medical Encyclopedia. http://www.ncbi.nlm.nih.gov/pubmedhealth/PMH0063028. Updated June 11, 2014. Accessed April 19, 2015.

25. Kamangar N, Harrington A. Bacterial pneumonia. In: Byrd RP Jr, ed. Medscape. http://emedicine.medscape.com/article/300157-overview#showall. Updated October 8, 2014. Accessed April 19, 2015.

26. Understanding RSV. American Lung Association Web site. http://www.lung.org/lung-disease/respiratory-syncytial-virus/understanding-rsv.html. Accessed April 19, 2015.

27. Bennett NJ, Gilroy SA. Overview of pneumocystis jiroveci pneumonia. In: Bronze MS, ed. Medscape. http://emedicine.medscape.com/article/225976-overview. Updated September 2, 2014. Accessed April 19, 2015.

28. Bennett NJ, Domachowske J. Pediatric pneumonia clinical presentation. In: Steele RW, ed. Medscape. http://emedicine.medscape.com/article/967822-clinical. Updated April 28, 2014.

29. Ibrahim M. Sputum culture. In: Staros EB, ed. Medscape. http://emedicine.medscape.com/article/2119232-overview. Updated May 7, 2014. Accessed April 19, 2015.

30. Amanullah S, Posner DH, Farhad M, Lessnau K-D. Typical bacterial pneumonia imaging. In: Garg K, ed. Medscape. http://emedicine.medscape.com/article/360090-overview#showall. Updated May 22, 2013. Accessed April 19, 2015.

31. Lee FE, Treanor J. Viral infections. In: Mason RJ, Broaddus VC, Martin T, et al, eds. *Murray and Nadel's Textbook of Respiratory Medicine*. 5th ed. Philadelphia, PA: Elsevier Saunders; 2010: 661–698.

32. Limper AH. Overview of pneumonia. In: Goldman L, Schafer AI, eds. *Goldman's Cecil Medicine*. 24th ed. Philadelphia, PA: Elsevier Saunders; 2011: 587–595.

33. Falcó V, Sánchez A, Pahissa A, Rello J. Emerging drugs for pneumococcal pneumonia. *Expert Opin Emerg Drugs*. 2011; 16(3): 459–477. doi: 10.1517/14728214.2011.576669

34. Parnham MJ, Erakovic Haber V, Giamarellos-Bourboulis EJ, Perletti G, Verleden GM, Vos R. Azithromycin: Mechanisms of action and their relevance for clinical applications. *Pharmacol Ther*. 2014; 143(2): 225–245. doi: 10.1016/j.pharmthera.2014.03.003

35. Paterson DL, Daveson K. Cefoxitin, cefotetan, and other cephamycins (cefmetazole and flomoxef). In: Grayson ML, Crowe SM, McCarthy JS, eds. *Kucers' The Use of Antibiotics*. 6th ed. Boca Raton, FL: CRC Press; 2010: 301–310.

36. Katkin JP. Cystic fibrosis: Clinical manifestations and diagnosis. In: Basow DS, ed. *UpToDate*. Waltham, MA: UpToDate; 2015. http://www.uptodate.com/contents/cystic-fibrosis-clinical-manifestations-and-diagnosis. Last updated June 25, 2014. Accessed April 19, 2015.

37. Rosenstein BJ. Cystic fibrosis. In: Porter RS, Kaplan JL, eds. The Merck Manual Online. http://www.merckmanuals.com/professional/pediatrics/cystic-fibrosis-cf/cystic-fibrosis. Last reviewed January 2014. Accessed April 19, 2015.

38. Sharma GD. Cystic fibrosis. In: Bye MR, ed. Medscape. http://emedicine.medscape.com/article/1001602-overview#aw2aab6b2b6aa. Updated March 19, 2015. Accessed April 19, 2015.

39. Cystic fibrosis. A.D.A.M. Medical Encyclopedia. http://www.ncbi.nlm.nih.gov/pubmedhealth/PMH0063023. Last updated June 11, 2014. Accessed April 19, 2015.

40. Mayo Clinic Staff. Cystic fibrosis. Mayo Clinic Web site. http://www.mayoclinic.com/health/cystic-fibrosis/DS00287/DSECTION=treatments-and-drugs. Updated June 13, 2012. Accessed April 19, 2015.

Chapter 14

Musculoskeletal Disorders

1. You are conducting an assessment for a 12-year-old whose feet point slightly inward, though he walks normally without a limp. His chief complaint is pain in the "front, bottom part" of his knee, pointing towards the tibial tubercle. He indicates that he began playing soccer year-round 7 months prior without any significant incident or injury. The pain began 3 weeks ago and has been constant since. Which of the following conditions is the patient most likely experiencing?

    a. Genu valgum

    b. Osgood-Schlatter disease

    c. Grade I knee sprain

    d. Legg-Calvé-Perthes disease

2. Which of these clinical tests would be most useful in evaluating the degree of a patient's scoliosis?

    a. Genetic testing

    b. Radiograph

    c. Ultrasound

    d. Joint fluid aspiration

3. A 6-month-old appears to have a shorter left leg, which turns outward slightly further than her right leg. Given this finding, which of the following signs would you least expect to present during the diagnostic assessment?

    a. Galeazzi sign

    b. Barlow sign

    c. Gower's sign

    d. Allis' sign

4. Your patient has significant edema and ecchymoses around the elbow. After ordering a radiograph, you notice a fat pad sign on the x-ray but no visible fracture. What would be the best course of action to take regarding treatment?

    a. Refer the patient to orthopedics

    b. Administer non-steroidal anti-inflammatory drugs

    c. Employ the RICE method

    d. Supinate the arm to correct subluxation

5. Which of the following is the most specific test for muscular dystrophy?

    a. Transaminase level

    b. Prolactin level

    c. Creatine kinase determination

    d. Polymerase chain reaction result

6. A 4-year-old presents with an awkward walk and run, without any pain and with full range of motion. The physical exam reveals that the distance between his ankles exceeds 3 inches. Which of these conditions would be the most likely diagnosis?

a. Genu varum

b. Muscular dystrophy

c. Genu valgum

d. Slipped capital femoral epiphysis

7. A 6-year-old male presents to your office with a limp and complains of pain in his groin. Upon further examination, you notice stiffness in the hip area on the affected side, as well as significant muscle loss in the upper thigh due to limited motion. Which of the following diagnostics would be most helpful in confirming Legg-Calvé-Perthes disease?

a. Radiograph

b. Ultrasound

c. Muscle biopsy

d. Electromyography

8. Which of these diagnostics is not routinely recommended for patients presenting with classic symptoms of slipped capital femoral epiphysis?

a. Radiography

b. Bone scans

c. Endocrine studies

d. Computed tomography

9. A 6-year-old patient arrives at your clinic with a painful limp that seemed to develop out of nowhere. While examining the patient, you discover that the internal rotation of the hip causes spasms. Suspecting toxic synovitis, you order a series of lab panels and imaging studies for confirmation. Which of these procedures would not typically be ordered?

a. Ultrasonography

b. Creatine kinase test

c. Magnetic resonance imaging

d. Erythrocyte sedimentation rate test

10. All of these statements are true of slipped capital femoral epiphysis except:

a. The condition typically occurs in girls prior to menarche.

b. The condition usually occurs without sudden severe force or trauma.

c. There is an increased incidence of the condition amongst obese adolescents.

d. The condition is more common in males and Caucasian adolescents.

RATIONALES

1. b

Pain at the tibial tubercle is commonly a strong indicator for Osgood-Schlatter disease. Though the patient appears to be pigeon-toed, this does not typically indicate that the knees point inward, as seen in genu valgum. A mild knee sprain is possible, but the patient did not indicate any injury; extraneous sports-related activity and pain isolated at the tibial tubercle would commonly make Osgood-Schlatter disease the more likely condition of the two. Although Legg-Calvé-Perthes disease may also indicate limp and knee pain, the patient's hip is not affected, as it commonly would be in cases of this condition.

2. b

Although scoliosis can be diagnosed with Adam's Forward Bend Test, radiographs are often recommended to determine the actual curvature of the spine. Genetic testing can be used to predict the development of scoliosis, but is more often used to diagnose muscular dystrophy. An ultrasound is more often used to diagnose developmental dysplasia of the hip. Lastly, joint fluid aspiration is commonly used to diagnose toxic synovitis.

3. c

Gower's sign, which is usually indicated when the hands are used to walk back towards the legs in order to attain a standing position due to weakness of the proximal muscles, is typically seen in patients with muscular dystrophy and would not likely present in this patient, who shows signs more indicative of developmental dysplasia of the hip (DDH). Signs of DDH would commonly produce positive results for the Galeazzi and Barlow test, though the latter would not typically present after 6 months of age. The Galeazzi sign is indicated by asymmetry in knee height while the infant lies supine with knees and hips flexed. The Barlow sign is indicated when the hip becomes dislocated upon pressure applied posteriorly by the nurse practitioner while the patient lies supine with knees flexed and hip adducted. Allis' sign is another name for the Galeazzi sign and would be present in the diagnostic assessment for a patient with DDH.

4. a

An elbow fracture may present with edema and ecchymosis, and is more often indicated with radiographs that show the presence of the fat pad sign, rather than the presence of any visible fracture; hence, you would refer the patient to orthopedics to be treated for fracture. Administering non-steroidal anti-inflammatory drugs and employing the RICE method are both appropriate steps for managing ankle sprains and other soft tissue injuries. Supinating the injured arm to correct subluxation is recommended for treatment of nursemaid elbow.

5. c

A creatine kinase determination aids in detecting the presence of inflammation or muscle damage stemming from muscular dystrophy (MD). Transaminase levels are used to detect disorders of the liver, whereas prolactin levels are used to measure erectile dysfunction in men and menstrual irregularities in women. A polymerase chain reaction test is used to diagnose viruses such as human papillomavirus and HIV, not genetic conditions such as MD.

6. c

Genu valgum, or knock-knees, typically manifests with abnormally close knees and increased ankle space; common signs and symptoms include no pain, full range of motion, and an awkward gait. The condition typically evolves to normal alignment by 7 years of age; if genu valgum persists past this age or unilaterally, further examination will often be necessary. Genu varum, or bowleg, is characterized by knees that remain apart while the feet and ankles are touching; these patients also typically have a full range of motion, and the condition is usually considered normal until 2 years of age. Muscular dystrophy may present with an awkward gait and posture, but patients may also experience pain and commonly exhibit limited range of motion. Common signs and symptoms of slipped capital femoral epiphysis include pain in the groin, the inability to properly flex the hip, and possible presentation of limb shortening.

7. a

The patient's limp, groin pain, stiffness of the hip, and muscle loss in the upper thigh most likely indicate Legg-Calvé-Perthes disease; radiograph studies would be most useful for both visualizing bone damage caused by this condition and confirming a diagnosis. Ultrasounds are more useful in the diagnosis of developmental dysplasia of the hip, and muscle biopsies and electromyography are often useful in the diagnosis and monitoring of muscular dystrophy.

8. c

Endocrine studies may be ordered in patients presenting with symptoms of slipped capital femoral epiphysis (SCFE) but are typically reserved for if the patient presents with atypical symptoms or has a medical history that would indicate a condition that may present with endocrine disorders. Radiography of the hips is typical in diagnosis of SCFE, with bone scans or magnetic resonance imaging serving to confirm the diagnosis.

9. b

Creatine kinase determination is used to detect inflammation of muscles, not joints, and would serve little use in confirming a diagnosis of toxic synovitis. The presence of inflammation stemming from toxic synovitis is usually detected through a complete blood count, an erythrocyte sedimentation rate test, or a C-reactive protein test. Ultrasonography is used to detect intracapsular effusion, whereas magnetic resonance imaging is used to rule out other potential causes of pain.

10. d

Slipped capital femoral epiphysis (SCFE) is most common in male and African American, not Caucasian, adolescents. Female adolescents are also likely to experience the condition during growth spurts and prior to menarche. SCFE also shows a higher incidence amongst children who are obese or who have sedentary lifestyles and often presents without sudden force or trauma.

DISCUSSION

Osgood-Schlatter Disease

Overview

Osgood-Schlatter disease is a common musculoskeletal condition among pediatric patients experiencing pubertal growth spurts. The disease is characterized by the growth of a painful lump due to inflammation at the tibial tubercle, just below the knee.[1] Incidence is usually seen in children between the ages of 11 and 14 and is especially prevalent in active children who play sports.[2]

Presentation

Patients often present with mild-to-severe swelling of the proximal tibia below one or both kneecaps. Patients may also complain of knee pain that is usually exacerbated by high-impact activities such as running, jumping, and climbing stairs.[3]

Workup

A clinical examination is usually all that is necessary to diagnose Osgood-Schlatter disease. X-rays are primarily ordered to rule out other possible conditions, such as neoplasms, osteomyelitis, and infection. Often, a radiograph will show a prominent, elevated tubercle with anterior soft-tissue swelling. A radiograph that shows ossicles separated from the tibial tuberosity indicates a more severe manifestation.[4,5]

Treatment

Because the disease is a self-limiting condition, pediatric patients should regulate their activity in order to control pain. To manage the condition, children and adolescents should practice the treatments that comprise the acronym R-I-C-E (Rest, Ice, Compress, and Elevate). However, complete activity restriction is not advised. Knee immobilizers may provide some relief, and non-steroidal anti-inflammatory drugs (NSAIDs) are often recommended for pain management.[6]

Toxic Synovitis

Overview

Toxic synovitis (i.e., transient synovitis) is a self-limiting inflammation of the hip that most often has a viral etiology.[7] This condition is most prevalent in children between 2 and 6 years of age but may also occur anywhere from ages 1 to 15. Toxic synovitis is more common in males than females and typically has an insidious onset.[1]

Presentation

Acute hip pain is the most common symptom of toxic synovitis. Pain may either be unilateral or present in both hips. Patients typically present with a painful limp, and additional findings may include spasms caused by internal rotation of the hip. There are usually no obvious signs of infection upon inspection or palpation.[1,8]

Workup

The diagnosis of toxic synovitis is a process of exclusion to rule out septic arthritis and osteomyelitis. Imaging studies may help to confirm toxic synovitis, with radiographs showing an increase in medial joint space and ultrasonography detecting intracapsular effusion. Patients with the condition will also typically show elevated white blood cells (WBC) on a complete blood count (CBC), as well as elevated erythrocyte sedimentation rate (ESR) and C-reactive protein levels.[7,9] Additional tests may be conducted to rule out other causes of pain, including a bone scan, magnetic resonance imaging (MRI), or aspiration of fluid from the hip joint.[7]

Treatment

Analgesics and bed rest should be given as needed. Full unrestricted activity can resume once the limp and pain have resolved. Hospitalization should be considered if the patient presents with a fever, limited range of motion (ROM), or other potential signs of septic arthritis.[7]

Legg-Calvé-Perthes Disease (LCPD)

Overview

Legg-Calvé-Perthes disease (LCPD) is a temporary pediatric condition caused by a lack of blood flow to the femoral head. The area often becomes inflamed and avascular necrosis of bone tissue can occur, which can cause the thigh bone to collapse. The stiffness in the hip joint that causes LCPD varies for each child, but most children with the condition present with a limp.[10] LCPD most commonly occurs in pediatric patients between 4 and 10 years of age who tend to be physically active. The condition also commonly occurs in children who are small for their age, but there is no known reason for this increased incidence.[11]

Presentation

Patients with LCPD usually present with an insidious onset of a limp accompanied by knee pain that may migrate to the groin and lateral hip area. Although the hip pain associated with LCPD is similar to transient synovitis and septic arthritis, LCPD pain is less acute than either condition. Patients with LCPD may be afebrile, which helps to distinguish the disease from osteomyelitis.[1,12]

Workup

Imaging tests, such as x-rays and an MRI, can be used to assess for LCPD. Although a CBC with measurement of ESR may be ordered to assess for inflammation, results may be normal.[12]

Treatment

Patients with LCPD should be referred to an orthopedic specialist. Restoring the patient's ROM while maintaining the femoral head within the acetabulum is the primary goal in treating LCPD. Measures to help alleviate pain include bed rest, limiting the amount of physical activity, and the use of anti-inflammatories. Treatment typically involves the use of orthotic devices. Surgical intervention may be necessary in severe cases. Observation and periodic x-rays are indicated for cases in which full ROM is preserved, the patient is younger than 6 years of age, and if less than half of the femoral head is involved.[1,13] Progress should be monitored through subsequent follow-ups.

Slipped Capital Femoral Epiphysis (SCFE)

Overview

Slipped capital femoral epiphysis (SCFE) is a condition of the adolescent hip characterized by spontaneous dislocation of the femoral head in both a downward and backward position relative to the femoral neck. As a result, the femoral head slips through the epiphyseal plate.[1]

Although etiology is unknown, SCFE may be precipitated by puberty-related hormone changes. The condition is not usually associated with injury but can occur with sudden or severe trauma to the area. The condition typically presents during the adolescent growth spurts or prior to menarche in girls.[1] Incidence is highest in obese adolescents with sedentary lifestyles.[14] The condition is rare, reported in 10.8 cases out of 100,000 adolescent patients. African-American adolescents have a higher incidence rate than adolescents of other races and ethnicities.[1]

Presentation

Patients typically present with pain in the hip that usually has an acute onset. Hip pain may be severe, and the patient may be unable to ambulate or move the hip. Pain may also be reported in the knee, thigh,

or groin because the pain may be referred from the hip via the obturator nerve.[1,14]

Workup

The NP should assess both hips for passive and active ROM during the physical examination. The patient should be in the prone position with knees flexed at 90° for the assessment. In most cases of SCFE, internal rotation of the hip is decreased and often painful. Gentle passive hip flexion may result in external rotation and abduction of the lower extremity.[14]

Diagnostics include radiographs of the pelvis or bilateral hips.[15] Bone scans or an MRI may be used to confirm the diagnosis.[14] Laboratory tests should be ordered for patients who present with atypical presentations of endocrine disorders or other medical conditions, including Down syndrome and short stature.[14]

Treatment

Early diagnosis and treatment is paramount to a good outcome. The NP should refer the patient to an orthopedist, who will typically oversee a surgical course of correction for the condition. The NP should also monitor the patient's other hip for indications of SCFE.[1] NSAIDs may be prescribed to manage pain stemming from SCFE. Although most patients recover well, limb shortening may result from the proximal displacement of the metaphysis in more severe cases.[15]

Genu Varum (Bowleg)

Overview

Genu varum (i.e., bowleg) is a lateral bowing of the tibia that often occurs due to joint laxity. Bowleg is considered to be normal in toddlers younger than 2 years of age. By age 3, bowleg usually resolves and children should be able to stand with their ankles apart and their knees close together. Genu varum should be suspected in children older than age 3 if the knees remain wide apart while the child stands with feet and ankles close together.[1,16]

Presentation

Pediatric patients with bowleg present are unable to stand with their knees touching when the ankles are together. The condition is confirmed if the intercondylar distance is more than 2 inches.[17] Bowing is not typically a cause for concern in children younger than age 3, and if bowing does not increase after the child begins walking and the retains full ROM in the legs.

Workup

Diagnosis of genu varum can be determined by observation alone. Diagnostic tests or labs are often unnecessary. A radiograph may help to confirm an uncertain diagnosis. A genetic assessment may be required if an underlying syndrome is suspected.[1,16]

Treatment

No treatment is necessary for pediatric patients younger than age 2 if the condition appears as a normal variant. If genu varum persists after the age of 2, is unilateral, or becomes progressively worse after the first year, the patient should be referred to an orthopedist.[18]

Genu Valgum (Knock-Knee)

Overview

Genu valgum (i.e., knock-knee) is a condition characterized by a person's knees being abnormally close with the ankle space increased. Knock-knee most commonly presents during preschool age, but the condition typically resolves by age 7.[17]

Presentation

Patients with knock-knee present with knees touching while the legs are straightened. The ankles are spread apart and separated by a distance of more than 3 in. when the knees are together. Patients with knock-knee typically experience no pain and have full ROM. However, some patients may walk or run awkwardly. If the condition persists past 7 years of age, complications such as pain, dislocation, and meniscal tears may produce.[19]

Workup

The patient can be diagnosed through observation alone. Radiographs are only necessary if the patient is older than age 7 or if unilateral involvement is present.[1]

Treatment

In younger patients, knock-knee often requires no treatment.[1] Patients older than age 7 should be referred to orthopedics for potential surgical intervention.[1,19]

Scoliosis

Overview

Scoliosis is a lateral curvature of the spine that most commonly develops during adolescence. The condition is usually idiopathic but tends to run in families; approximately 70% of all cases of scoliosis are familial. Congenital and neuromuscular types of scoliosis are less common. Females are 8 times more likely than males to develop scoliosis.[1,20]

Presentation

Scoliosis patients often present with no distinctive symptoms. Characteristic indications include intense back pain with asymmetry of the shoulders, ribs, hips, and waistline.[21]

Workup

The Adam's Forward Bend Test is the standard physical exam to screen for scoliosis. Radiographs may be ordered for further evaluation.[22]

Treatment

Patients with mild scoliosis should be evaluated every 4 to 6 months for changes in pain. If no pain is present and if spine curvature is less than 25 °, the patient may be observed rather than treated. If the adolescent patient experiences pain or spine curvature that is more than 25 °, the patient should be referred to orthopedics.[1,23,24]

Developmental Dysplasia of the Hip (DDH)

Overview

Developmental dysplasia of the hip (DDH) is abnormal dislocation (i.e., luxation or subluxation) of the hip, which causes the femoral head to become either partially or completely displaced from the acetabulum.[25]

Presentation

Infants with DDH may present with Galeazzi's sign—asymmetrical knee height while the infant is supine and the hips and knees are flexed.[26] A positive Galeazzi test is not specific for DDH, though; other conditions may cause leg length discrepancy.[27] The combination of the Barlow and Ortolani maneuvers has a high specificity for DDH. The Barlow maneuver is performed with light posterior pressure applied to abducted hips, with a palpable dislocation indicating DDH.[27] The Ortolani maneuver is performed by flexing the infant's hips and knees to 90 °, then gently abducting the thighs. If a "clunk" sound is heard when the patient's hip shrinks into the acetabulum while the hip is abducted, DDH is indicated.[28]

Until age 1, DDH is painless. If not detected in infancy, the child may begin to walk with a limp. In older children, DDH may present with decreased hip abduction.[1,26]

Workup

Patients should be examined for DDH within the first few days of life and at every Well Child Check until the child begins to walk normally. Although the Ortolani and Barlow maneuvers are preferred because of the high specificity and absence of radiation, imaging studies may be used to diagnose the condition. Plain radiography relies on metrics such as the Hilgenreiner line to ensure the hips and femurs are properly aligned. Ultrasounds are used to assess for abnormal ranges in the alpha and beta angles.[29]

Treatment

Pediatric patients with DDH should be referred to orthopedics for treatment. Bracing measures, such as a Pavlik harness or abduction brace, may see use in patients younger than 6 months of age. Older pediatric patients typically require closed or open reduction.[29]

Muscular Dystrophy

Overview

Muscular dystrophy (MD) is a chronic progressive genetic disorder that commonly originates in the lower extremities and progresses to the upper extremities and torso. MD is the most commonly inherited neuromuscular disease in pediatric patients and affects 1 out of every 3,500 males.[1] Duchenne MD, which is the most common pediatric form of MD, affects males almost exclusively because it is an x-linked disease.[30] Duchenne MD usually presents between the ages of 3 and 5 and is caused by a lack of dystrophin, a protein that maintains muscle. MD varies in how it affects the muscular system, with some cases affecting the cardiac muscles. The age of onset and rate of progression also vary.[31]

Presentation

Pediatric patients with MD may present with a combination of symptoms, including abnormalities of gait and posture. Patients may also experience developmental clumsiness and have difficulty keeping up with their peers. Gower's maneuver, in which individuals push themselves up to a standing position by using their hands to "walk up" their own body, is a common sign of Duchenne MD.[32]

Calves may appear firm, large, and woody; this appearance indicates that the healthy muscle has been replaced by degenerative tissue. Patients often experience decreased proximal muscle strength[33]; up to 82% of all males age 10 to 14 with Duchenne or Becker MD require the use of a wheelchair.[34]

Workup

A creatine kinase (CK) lab detects inflammation or muscle damage. In males, CK is markedly elevated if MD is a cause of the muscle weakness; for example, CK would fall between 15,000–35,000 IU/L in a patient with MD.[1,35] An electromyography can be used to detect myopathic changes.[32,36] Because MD may cause cardiac issues, an electrocardiogram can be conducted to assess the rate and frequency of heartbeats.[37] Other tests for MD include a muscle biopsy to detect necrotic degenerating muscle fibers, and a DNA test for analysis of genes.[38]

Treatment

There is no cure for MD, but the condition can be managed to control symptoms, delay progression, and maintain strength, and mobility.

Ankle Sprain

Overview

Ankle sprains are the most common sports-related musculoskeletal injury. Ankle sprains are characterized by the stretching or tearing of the ligaments around the ankle. Usually, the lateral ligament complex is affected. Ankle sprain injuries are usually caused by actions or movement resulting in a forced inversion or eversion of the ankle.[1,39]

Presentation

Ankle sprains are graded by the severity of the patient's injury. A grade I ankle sprain occurs when there is stretching with no tearing of the ligaments around the ankle and no joint instability. This grade of ankle sprain is characterized by local tenderness and minimal edema, with the ability to bear weight on the ankle retained. Ecchymoses is typically insignificant or absent. The full ROM may remain, but the patient usually experiences discomfort.[40,41]

A grade II ankle sprain causes partial tearing of the ligaments with some joint instability but a definite endpoint to laxity. The pain after a grade II ankle sprain typically occurs immediately upon injury and is often significant with weight bearing. Edema and ecchymosis are typically localized with this type of sprain, and ROM is often limited.[40,41]

A grade III ankle sprain involves the complete tear of a ligament. Grade III ankle sprains result in severe pain immediately upon injury, with significant edema along the foot and ankle. As a result, the pediatric patient cannot bear weight upon the ankle and has significant loss of ROM.[40,41]

Workup

An ankle sprain can be diagnosed with a physical examination that confirms tenderness and swelling. For pediatric patients 5 years of age and older, Ottawa ankle rules for use of radiography should be followed when diagnosing ankle sprains. An ankle x-ray should be ordered if a patient exhibits pain in the malleolar zone and bone tenderness at (a) the posterior edge or tip of the lateral malleolus or (b) the posterior edge or tip of the medial malleolus. Additionally, an ankle x-ray should be ordered if the patient cannot bear weight immediately after the injury and in the examining room.

A foot x-ray should be ordered if the patient exhibits pain in the midfoot zone and bone tenderness at (a) the base of the fifth metatarsal or (b) the navicular. Additionally, an ankle x-ray should be ordered if the patient cannot bear weight immediately after the injury and in the examining room. If none of these symptoms are present, a physical examination may suffice in diagnosing the condition.[41]

Treatment

All grades of ankle sprains respond well to the R-I-C-E treatment standards. The ankle should be rested, especially during the first couple days. The patient can bear some weight as tolerated for daily activities, but sports should be curtailed. The compression bandage should be applied immediately after the injury to minimize swelling, and ice should be applied on top of the compression dressing as quickly as possible after the injury. Ice should be applied in alternating periods of 30 minutes at a time. The patient should also elevate the ankle for several days after injury in order to reduce pain and swelling and promote recovery. NSAIDs can be used for pain relief. In grade III ankle sprains, surgery may be required to repair the torn ligament.[41,42]

Elbow Fracture

Overview

Patients can experience a fracture in several places on and around the elbow, including the following: above the elbow (supracondylar), at the elbow knob (condylar), at the inside of the elbow tip (epicondylar), at the growth plate (physis), or on the forearm. The fracture may also manifest as a dislocation.[1,43]

Presentation

Even though an elbow fracture may occur in several places, signs and symptoms for most elbow injuries are the same and typically including pain, swelling, and limited ROM.[44]

Workup

Elbow fractures can be diagnosed with follow-up radiographs with an oblique view. If the radiograph cannot provide a clear indication of the fracture, elevation of the anterior and posterior fat pads will suggest the presence of an occult fracture.[45]

Treatment

Pediatric patients with elbow fractures should be referred to orthopedics for proper treatment and assessment for the possibility of neurovascular injury. NSAIDs may be administered to control pain.[45]

Nursemaid Elbow

Overview

Nursemaid elbow is a common injury in children between 1 and 4 years of age that results from swinging or pulling the child's arm, which causes radial head subluxation.[46]

Presentation

Common signs and symptoms of nursemaid elbow include the inability or refusal to use the affected arm and pain with supination. Patients may also hold their affected arm against the body, with the thumb and forearm turned inward.

Workup

Manipulation of the elbow can typically diagnose the condition without ordering any imaging studies. However, ultrasonography can assess for annular ligamentous injury and displacement of the radial head from the capitellum. An MRI may be used to confirm subluxation with a ligament tear.[48] Radiographs are not standard in diagnosis, as imaging results are often normal; however, if significant swelling and bruising are present, or attempts to correct subluxation are unsuccessful, radiographs may be ordered to check for fractures or to rule out other conditions.[1,47,48]

Treatment

If nursemaid elbow has been confirmed, the NP should manipulate the arm in order to return the elbow to its proper condition. This involves supporting the elbow with one hand while placing a thumb laterally over the radial head of the child's elbow, grasping the child's hand, and deliberately supinating and externally rotating the forearm while flexing the elbow. If the subluxation is corrected, the patient should feel immediate relief and be able to use the arm again in a matter of minutes. A splint may be recommended for the next few days in order to ensure comfort, especially if the injury persisted for hours before being corrected.[49] NSAIDs may also be recommended for supportive care.[1]

References

1. Barkley TW Jr. Musculoskeletal issues and disorders. In: Barkley TW Jr, ed. *Pediatric Primary Care Nurse Practitioner Certification Review/Clinical Update Continuing Education Course*. West Hollywood, CA: Barkley and Associates; 2015: 130–137.

2. Mayo Clinic Staff. Osgood-Schlatter disease. Mayo Clinic Web site. http://www.mayoclinic.com/health/osgood-schlatter-disease/DS00392. Updated February 28, 2014. Accessed April 20, 2015.

3. Mayo Clinic Staff. Osgood-Schlatter disease: Symptoms. Mayo Clinic Web site. http://www.mayoclinic.com/health/osgood-schlatter-disease/DS00392/DSECTION=symptoms. Updated February 28, 2014. Accessed April 20, 2015.

4. Weiler R, Ingram M, Wolman R. Osgood-Schlatter disease. *Praxis*. 2011; 100(22): 1369–1370. doi:10.1024/1661-8157/a000715

5. Sullivan JA. Osgood-Schlatter disease workup. In: Young CC, ed. Medscape. http://emedicine.medscape.com/article/1993268-workup#showall. Updated July 15, 2014. Accessed April 24, 2015.

6. Sullivan JA. Osgood-Schlatter disease treatment & management. In: Young CC, ed. Medscape. http://emedicine.medscape.com/article/1993268-treatment. Updated July 15, 2014. Accessed April 20, 2015.

7. Sankar WN, Horn BD, Wells L, Dormans JP. Transient monoarticular synovitis (toxic synovitis). In: Kliegman RM, Stanton BF, St. Geme JW III, Schor NF, Behrman RE, eds. *Nelson Textbook of Pediatrics*. 19th ed. Philadelphia, PA: Elsevier Saunders; 2011: 2360.

8. Whitelaw CC, Schikler KN. Transient synovitis. In: Jung LK, ed. Medscape. http://emedicine.medscape.com/article/1007186-overview#showall. Updated October 9, 2014. Accessed April 20, 2015.

9. Gutierrez K. Transient synovitis. In: Long SS, Pickering LK, Prober CG, eds. *Principles and Practice of Pediatric Infectious Diseases*. 4th ed. London, UK: Elsevier Churchill Livingstone; 2012: 485–486.

10. Legg-Calve-Perthes disease. A.D.A.M. Medical Encyclopedia. http://www.nlm.nih.gov/medlineplus/ency/article/001264.htm. Updated August 22, 2013. Accessed April 20, 2015.

11. Sankar WN, Horn BD, Wells L, Dormans JP. Legg-Calve-Perthes disease. In: Kliegman RM, Stanton BF, St. Geme JW III, Schor NF, Behrman RE, eds. *Nelson Textbook of Pediatrics*. 19th ed. Philadelphia, PA: Elsevier Saunders; 2011: 2361–2362.

12. McQuillen KK. Musculoskeletal disorders. In: Marx JA, Hockberger RS, Walls RM, et al., eds. *Rosen's Emergency Medicine: Concepts and Clinical Practice*. 8th ed. Philadelphia, PA: Elsevier Saunders; 2014: 2250–2270.

13. Kim HKW, Herring JA. Legg-Calvé-Perthes disease. In: Herring JA, ed. *Tachdijan's Pediatric Orthopaedics*. 5th ed. Philadelphia, PA: Elsevier Saunders; 2013: 580–629.

14. Walter KD, Lin DY, Schwartz E. Slipped capital femoral epiphysis. In: Young CC, ed. Medscape. http://emedicine.medscape.com/article/91596-overview#showall. Updated December 17, 2014. Accessed April 20, 2015.

15. Germann CA, Fix ML. Hip and femur injuries. In: Wolfson AB, Cloutier RL, Hendey GW, Ling LJ, Rosen CL, Schaider JJ, eds. *Harwood-Nuss' Clinical Practice of Emergency Medicine*. 6th ed. Philadelphia, PA: Wolters Kluwer Health/Lippincott Williams & Wilkins; 2015: 285–288.

16. Stevens PM. Pediatric genu varum. In: Grogan DP, ed. Medscape. http://emedicine.medscape.com/article/1355974-overview#showall. Updated August 29, 2013. Accessed April 24, 2015.

17. Wells L, Sehgal K. Coronal plane deformities. In: Kliegman RM, Stanton BF, St Geme JW III, Schor NF, Behrman RE, eds. *Nelson Textbook of Pediatrics*. 19th ed. Philadelphia, PA: Elsevier Saunders; 2011: 2348–2349.

18. Canale ST. Osteochondrosis or epiphysitis and other miscellaneous affections. In: Canale ST, Beatty JH, eds. *Campbell's Operative Orthopaedics*. 12th ed. Philadelphia, PA: Elsevier Mosby; 2012: 1133–1201.

19. Stevens PM, Holmstrom MC. Pediatric genu valgum. In: Grogan DP, ed. Medscape. http://emedicine.medscape.com/article/1259772-overview#a0112. Updated April 24, 2014. Accessed April 20, 2015.

20. Hresko MT. Clinical practice: Idiopathic scoliosis in adolescents. *N Engl J Med*. 2013; 368(9): 834–841. doi: 10.1056/NEJMcp1209063

21. Idiopathic scoliosis: Adolescents. Scoliosis Research Society Web site. http://www.srs.org/patient_and_family/scoliosis/idiopathic/adolescents. Accessed April 20, 2015.

22. Mayo Clinic Staff. Scoliosis. Mayo Clinic Web site. http://www.mayoclinic.com/health/scoliosis/DS00194. Updated February 3, 2012. Accessed April 20, 2015.

23. Scherl SA. Adolescent idiopathic scoliosis: Management and prognosis. In: Basow DS, ed. *UpToDate*. Waltham, MA: UpToDate; 2015. http://www.uptodate.com/contents/adolescent-idiopathic-scoliosis-treatment-and-prognosis. Last updated September 2, 2014. Accessed May 22, 2015.

24. Ullrich PF Jr. Scoliosis treatment. Spine-Health Web site. http://www.spine-health.com/conditions/scoliosis/scoliosis-treatment. Updated January 20, 2012. Accessed April 24, 2015.

25. Sankar WN, Horn BD, Wells L, Dormans JP. The hip. In: Kliegman RM, Stanton BF, St. Geme JW III, Schor NF, Behrman RE, eds. *Nelson Textbook of Pediatrics*. 19th ed. Philadelphia, PA: Elsevier Saunders; 2011: 2355–2364.

26. Tamai J, McCarthy JJ. Development dysplasia of the hip. In: Jaffe WL, ed. Medscape. http://emedicine.medscape.com/article/1248135-overview#showall. Updated March 31, 2014. Accessed April 20, 2015.

27. Rosenfeld SB. Developmental dysplasia of the hip: Clinical features and diagnosis. In: Basow DS, ed. *UpToDate*. Waltham, MA: UpToDate; 2015. http://www.uptodate.com/contents/developmental-dysplasia-of-the-hip-clinical-features-and-diagnosis. Last updated April 14, 2015. Accessed May 22, 2015.

28. Sewell MD, Eastwood DM. Screening and treatment in developmental dysplasia of the hip – where do we go from here? *Int Orthop*. 2011; 35(9): 1359–1367. doi: 10.1007/s00264-011-1257-z

29. Blanco JS, Doyle SM, Scher DM, Sink EL, Widmann RF. Developmental pediatric hip dysplasia – an overview. Hospital for Special Surgery Web site. http://www.hss.edu/conditions_developmental-pediatric-hip-dysplasia-overview.asp. Reviewed and updated December 18, 2012. Accessed May 22, 2015.

30. Duchenne muscular dystrophy: Causes/inheritance. Muscular Dystrophy Association Web site. http://www.mda.org/disease/duchenne-muscular-dystrophy/causes-inheritance. Accessed April 24, 2015.

31. U. S. Department of Health and Human Services, National Institutes of Health, National Institute of Neurological Disorders and Stroke, Office of Communications and Public Liaison. NINDS muscular dystrophy information page. http://www.ninds.nih.gov/disorders/md/md.htm. Last updated April 8, 2015. Accessed April 20, 2015.

32. Darras BT. Clinical features and diagnosis of Duchenne and Becker muscular dystrophy. In: Basow DS, ed. UpToDate. Waltham, MA: UpToDate; 2015. http://www.uptodate.com/contents/clinical-features-and-diagnosis-of-duchenne-and-becker-muscular-dystrophy?source=search_result&search=Duchenne+becker&selectedTitle=1~79. Last updated November 18, 2014. Accessed April 20, 2015.

33. Darras BT. Patient information: Overview of muscular dystrophies (beyond the basics). In: Basow DS, ed. UpToDate. Waltham, MA: UpToDate; 2015. http://www.uptodate.com/contents/overview-of-muscular-dystrophies-beyond-the-basics. Last updated October 2, 2013. Accessed April 20, 2015.

34. U.S. Department of Health and Human Services, Centers for Disease Control and Prevention, National Center on Birth Defects and Developmental Disabilities. http://www.cdc.gov/ncbddd/musculardystrophy/data.html. Last updated March 23, 2015. Accessed April 24, 2015.

35. American Association for Clinical Chemistry. CK: The test. Lab Tests Online Web site. http://labtestsonline.org/understanding/analytes/ck/tab/test. Last reviewed February 25, 2013. Last updated February 24, 2015. Accessed April 20, 2015.

36. Mayo Clinic Staff. Electromyography (EMG). Mayo Clinic Web site. http://www.mayoclinic.com/print/emg/MY00107/METHOD=print&DSECTION=all. Updated October 25, 2012. Accessed April 20, 2015.

37. Muscular dystrophy. A.D.A.M. Medical Encyclopedia. http://www.nlm.nih.gov/medlineplus/ency/article/001190.htm. Updated February 24, 2014. Accessed April 20, 2015.

38. Darras BT. Treatment of Duchenne and Becker muscular dystrophy. In: Basow DS, ed. UpToDate. Waltham, MA: UpToDate; 2015. http://www.uptodate.com/contents/treatment-of-duchenne-and-becker-muscular-dystrophy. Last updated October 15, 2014. Accessed April 20, 2015.

39. Mayo Clinic Staff. Sprained ankle. Mayo Clinic Web site. http://www.mayoclinic.com/health/sprained-ankle/DS01014. Updated August 21, 2014. Accessed April 20, 2015.

40. Maughan KL. Ankle sprain. In: Basow DS, ed. UpToDate. Waltham, MA: UpToDate; 2015. http://www.uptodate.com/contents/ankle-sprain. Last updated April 3, 2015. Accessed April 20, 2015.

41. Tiemstra JD. Update on acute ankle sprains. Am Fam Physician. 2012; 85(12): 1170–1176. http://www.aafp.org/afp/2012/0615/p1170.html.

42. Young CC. Ankle sprain. In: Ho SSW, ed. Medscape. http://emedicine.medscape.com/article/1907229-overview#showall. Updated December 16, 2014. Accessed April 20, 2015.

43. Nishijima DK, Goldman M. Elbow fracture. In: Kulkarni R, ed. Medscape. http://emedicine.medscape.com/article/824654-overview#showall. Updated February 26, 2014. Accessed April 20, 2015.

44. Bachman D, Santora S. Orthopedic trauma. In: Fleisher GR, Ludwig S, Bachur RG, Gorelick MH, Shaw KN, Ruddy RM, eds. Textbook of Pediatric Emergency Medicine. 6th ed. Philadelphia, PA: Wolters Kluwer Health/Lippincott Williams & Wilkins; 2010: 1335–1375.

45. Blanco JS, Doyle SM, Green DW, Scher DM, Sink EL, Widmann RF. Elbow fractures in children: An Overview. Hospital for Special Surgery Web site. http://www.hss.edu/conditions_elbow-fractures-children-overview.asp. Reviewed and updated December 12, 2012. Accessed May 22, 2015.

46. Wolfram W, Boss DN. Nursemaid elbow: Overview. In: Bachur RG, ed. Medscape. http://emedicine.medscape.com/article/803026-overview#a0104. Updated February 7, 2014. Accessed April 20, 2015.

47. Mayo Clinic Staff. Dislocated elbow. Mayo Clinic Web site. http://www.mayoclinic.com/health/dislocated-elbow/DS01165. Updated April 3, 2015. Accessed April 20, 2015.

48. Wolfram W, Boss DN. Nursemaid elbow workup. In: Bachur RG, ed. Medscape. http://emedicine.medscape.com/article/803026-workup. Updated February 7, 2014. Accessed April 24, 2015.

49. Sigman LJ. Procedures. In: Tschudy MM, Arcara KM, eds. The Harriet Lane Handbook. 19th ed. Philadelphia, PA: Elsevier Mosby; 2011: 57–88.

Chapter 15
Neurologic Disorders

1. In what area of the brain do childhood tumors predominately occur?

    a. Infratentorial region

    b. Supratentorial region

    c. Tentorium cerebelli

    d. Occipital lobes

2. Which cranial nerve controls hearing and equilibrium?

    a. CN II

    b. CN IV

    c. CN VI

    d. CN VIII

3. The practitioner knows that which of the following prophylactic drugs is not used in pediatric migraine management?

    a. Doxepin

    b. Bisoprolol

    c. Ibuprofen

    d. Amitriptyline

4. Which of the following characteristics is not typically associated with febrile seizures?

    a. Fever with rectal temperature of 102 °F or above

    b. Generally manifests in early infancy by 3 months of age

    c. There is usually a family history of febrile seizures

    d. There is typically a loss of consciousness with this type of seizure

5. Tension and psychogenic headaches are commonly associated with what mechanism of headache pain?

    a. Vascular dilation

    b. Traction

    c. Muscular contraction

    d. Inflammation

6. Jamie, a 4-year-old male, presents to the clinic in a sleepy, afebrile state. His mother mentions that, after his afternoon nap, he started screaming in their brightly-lit den and began vomiting. When she tried to talk to him, he spoke nonsense. When you talk to Jamie, he rouses, exhibits normal speech, and says he feels fine. What is the most likely source of Jamie's symptoms?

    a. Viral meningitis

    b. Brain tumor

    c. Neurofibromatosis

    d. Confusional migraine

7. A patient has been referred to your practice by an optometrist, who found Lisch nodules in the patient's irises. Which finding would best help to confirm the suspected diagnosis?

    a. Photophobia

    b. Failure to thrive

    c. Axillary freckling

    d. Aphasia

8. Which of the following best defines a simple partial seizure?

    a. Staring for 25 seconds prior to onset of minor autonomic symptoms

    b. Minor motor symptoms with no loss of consciousness

    c. Staring for 10 seconds with brief onset and termination

    d. Partial loss of consciousness with increased muscle tone

9. Which of these signs would indicate meningitis in a patient?

    a. Pain upon external rotation of the knee

    b. Pain upon extension of the leg when the hip is flexed 90°

    c. Sciatic pain when both legs are elevated off the exam table

    d. Pain with internal rotation of the flexed right thigh

10. In a patient with tic disorders, all of the following presentations would typically be recognized as a simple tic except:

    a. Blinking for 30 seconds without interruption

    b. Extensive clearing of the throat

    c. Jerking the head back and forth

    d. Repeating a word another person said

RATIONALES

1. a

Seventy to 80% of childhood brain tumors occur in the infratentorial region of the brain. Despite ongoing research, the etiology of these tumors is unknown. The supratentorial region, tentorium cerebelli, and occipital lobes may develop tumors; however, these regions are not predominating areas of occurrence of brain tumors in children.

2. d

CN VIII is known as the acoustic nerve, which controls hearing and equilibrium. CN II, on the other hand, controls vision. CN IV controls downward and inward eye movement, whereas CN VI controls lateral eye movement.

3. a

Doxepin is a tricyclic antidepressant used to treat depression and anxiety disorders, but is not suitable for migraine prophylaxis and is not approved for pediatric patients. Although tricyclic antidepressants are generally not used in migraine management, amitriptyline may see use when the migraines are accompanied by chronic pain, insomnia, or depression. Bisoprolol and other beta-blockers are thought to interfere with arterial dilation, and thus are commonly considered a drug of choice for preventing chronic migraine. Lastly, ibuprofen belongs to the class of NSAIDs widely used in migraine treatment.

4. b

Febrile seizures do not generally manifest before 6 months of age; such an early manifestation should call for a referral to a pediatric neurologist. Febrile seizures generally develop between 6 months of age and 5 years of age, with peak incidence in the toddler years. A patient with a familial history of febrile seizures often stands a higher risk of developing the condition. Febrile seizures often present when rectal temperature exceeds 102 °F and generally cause a loss of consciousness.

5. c

Tension and psychogenic headaches are closely associated with muscular contraction. Vascular dilation, on the other hand, is a mechanism of pain associated with migraine headaches. Traction is associated with space-occupying lesions, such as hematomas and increased intracranial pressure. Lastly, inflammation is associated with infections of parts of the body, such as the meninges.

6. d

Confusional migraines may present with confusion, aphasia, vomiting, photophobia, and agitation; once these symptoms pass, the patient may fall into a deep sleep, only to wake up feeling well. Since confusional migraine is commonly a diagnosis of exclusion, it warrants a work-up to rule out organic causes. Brain tumors may also produce aphasia, vomiting, and photophobia, and sleepiness; in children, however, tumors typically also present with headache that is at its worst in the morning. Viral meningitis produces vomiting and photophobia as well, but also typically exhibits fever. Neurofibromatosis is characterized by seizures and multiple café au lait spots.

7. c

Lisch nodules in the irises and axillary freckling are part of the diagnostic criteria for neurofibromatosis type 1; inguinal freckling would also indicate the condition. Photophobia would more likely indicate bacterial meningitis or migraines, aphasia more commonly produces as a result of migraines or brain tumor, and failure to thrive more often arises from disease or dysfunction of multiple bodily systems.

8. b

A simple partial seizure presents with no loss of consciousness and minor motor, autonomic, or sensory symptoms. A complex partial seizure will present with the same symptoms, but is accompanied by an episode of staring longer than 20 seconds that presents before, during, or after the symptoms. An absence, or petit mal, seizure is characterized by a brief staring episode of 10–20 seconds with brief onset and termination. Partial or complete loss of consciousness accompanying increased muscle tone indicates a tonic seizure.

9. b

Kernig's sign, a hallmark indicator of meningitis, presents as pain when the leg is elevated 90° from the hip and extended. Pain upon external rotation of the knee is Lachman's test, an indicator of damage to the anterior or posterior cruciate ligament of the knee. The positive straight leg raise test, meant to diagnose lower back pain, presents as radiating or sciatic pain when both legs are elevated off the exam table. Pain with internal rotation of the flexed right thigh is the Obturator sign, an indicator of appendicitis.

10. d

Repetition of another person's words, or echolalia, is typically recognized as a complex tic, not a simple tic. In tic disorders, simple tics are those which involve a single muscle group or a simple sound. Such simple tics may include sustained blinking, jerking the head back and forth, or throat clearing.

DISCUSSION

Headache

Overview

Headaches consist of pain in any part of the head, which is caused by activation of specific pain-sensitive structures.[1] Headaches may present for a multitude of reasons and can be difficult to evaluate. Although headaches commonly occur, serious causes are rare.[2] Proper evaluation of the history of the patient's headache and its associated symptoms is essential to making an accurate diagnosis.

Presentation

There are four primary mechanisms of headache pain: vascular pain, muscle contraction, traction, and inflammation.[2] Vascular dilation, which occurs in migraine headaches, consists of cranial artery distension caused by dilation or swelling of the blood vessels.[3] Causes of vascular dilation include fever, vasodilator drugs, metabolic disturbance, and systemic infections.[4] Muscular contraction, which occurs in tension headaches, involves tension of the head and neck muscles.[5] Traction pain may be caused by increased intracranial pressure and space-occupying lesions such as brain tumors, mass lesions, abscesses, and hematomas.[4] Lastly, headaches related to inflammation are often caused by infections in the meninges, sinuses, and teeth.[6]

For assessment of headache symptoms, the nurse practitioner (NP) may use the OLD CART system. This mnemonic reminds NPs to evaluate headache based on onset, location of pain, duration of headache, distinctive characteristics, aggravating factors, remedial and alleviating factors, and effective methods of treatment.[4]

Headache Considerations

Overview

Headache considerations in febrile patients include meningitis, which may be bacterial, viral, tuberculous, or aseptic. Brain abscess or other intracranial infections, encephalitis, and hypoglycemia should also be considered in febrile patients, as well as dehydration and sinusitis. Headache patients may also present with associated infections such as strep throat, influenza, mononucleosis, or rubeola.[4]

Headache considerations for afebrile patients include subarachnoid and intraparenchymal hemorrhages, postictal headaches, cerebral ischemia, severe hypertension, acute dental disease, and acute glaucoma. Space-occupying conditions such as brain tumors and hydrocephalies may also be suspected.[4]

Meningitis

Overview

Meningitis is an inflammation of the meninges, which envelop the brain and spinal cord. Although meningitis may occur in patients of any age, infants are at a higher risk for developing the condition.[7]

Most cases of meningitis in the United States are caused by viruses.[8] Enteroviruses are the most common source of viral meningitis; these infections usually occur in the summer and early autumn but may develop in sporadic cases throughout the year.[9] Bacterial meningitis, on the other hand, makes up only a small percentage of meningitis cases; when it does occur, it is extremely serious and is considered a medical emergency.[10] The most common bacterial causes of meningitis in children are *Streptococcus pneumoniae* and *Neisseria meningitidis*, the latter of which can cause death within hours.[11] Other causative agents of bacterial meningitis include group B *Streptococcus*, *Haemophilus influenzae*, and *Escherichia coli*, among others.[7]

Presentation

Meningitis is often indicated by temperatures higher than 101.8 °F (38.8 °C).[4,12] The classic triad of meningitis symptoms consists of fever, headache, and nuchal rigidity; however, many meningitis patients do not present with this triad of symptoms.[13] For example, most signs and symptoms of meningitis in pediatric patients are behavioral responses such as tantrums and sleep disturbance.[4,12] Newborns and young infants may present with other signs and symptoms such as irritability, lethargy, poor feeding, and a bulging fontanel.[14] Older infants and children may also present with headaches and irritability. Other typical signs and symptoms of meningitis include nausea and vomiting, photophobia, confusion, hyperesthesia, cranial nerve palsy, and ataxia.[4,15] Back pain may also occur in cases of meningitis caused by *Staphylococcus aureus* and other bacteria.[11]

Furthermore, nuchal rigidity can be demonstrated by both Kernig's and Brudzinski's signs.[16] A positive Kernig's sign consists of pain on extension of the leg when the hip is flexed at 90 °. A positive Brudzinski's sign is indicated by involuntary flexion of the legs when the neck is flexed.[17,18]

Workup

When meningitis is suspected, patients should undergo a cerebrospinal fluid (CSF) analysis via lumbar puncture.[19] A confirmatory finding will appear cloudy and show white blood cells, increased protein, and decreased glucose.[4]

Treatment

Antibiotics are the mainstay of treatment for bacterial meningitis,[11] and the choice of antibiotic typically depends on the type of bacteria that causes the patient's condition. Ceftriaxone and cefotaxime often see use against gram-negative organisms, whereas vancomycin may see use if *S. pneumoniae* is believed to be the causative pathogen.[19] Most cases of viral meningitis resolve on their own, and patients can be treated with bed rest, fluids, and over-the-counter medications.[8]

Brain Tumors

Overview

Brain tumors form as masses of abnormal cells, which may be either benign or malignant.[20] Although the cause of brain tumors is unknown, these masses are a leading cause of cancer-related deaths, as well as the most common type of solid cancer in children younger than 15 years of age.[21] Infratentorial brainstem tumors comprise the majority of tumors in children.[22]

Presentation

Frequently, headaches are the worst symptom in brain tumor patients. Headaches commonly appear in older children with brain tumors; upon manifestation, these headaches usually increase in frequency, are typically followed by vomiting, and are worse in the morning. Seizures are also a common symptom of brain tumors in both adult and pediatric patients.[20] Certain signs and symptoms depend on the location of the tumor; for example, ataxia is often associated with brain tumors located in the cerebellum.[21] Moreover, the patient may present with other abnormal neurologic or ocular findings, such as hemiparesis, cranial nerve palsies, somnolence, and papilledema. Additional abnormal neurologic findings include a positive Babinski sign, behavioral changes, loss of fine motor control, and diabetes insipidus. Finally, certain signs and symptoms are found specifically in infants and may include the following: increased head circumference, irritability, head tilt, failure to thrive, the loss of developmental milestones, and a tense, bulging fontanel.[4]

Workup

In most cases of brain tumors, magnetic resonance imaging (MRI) is the only diagnostic test needed.[23] Brain tumors may also be diagnosed with other imaging tests such as a computerized axial tomography (CAT) scan and computed tomography (CT) scan. A lumbar puncture (LP) may be used, but this test should only be performed after a neurological examination, and the NP should approach an LP with caution due to technical considerations.[24]

Treatment

Treatment of brain tumors is determined by the location and grade of the tumor.[21] Tumors are graded numerically from 1 to 4 according to their microscopic appearance and abnormality. Grade 1 tumors appear close to normal, whereas higher grade tumors appear abnormal and spread more rapidly.[25] Surgical removal of the tumor is often possible, and radiation therapy and chemotherapy are procedures that may be used if removal is not possible.[26]

Migraine Headaches (Vascular Headaches)

Overview

Migraine headaches are vascular headaches that are caused by dilation and excessive pulsation of branches of the external carotid artery. Females are more often affected by migraine headaches than males, and often there is a family history of migraines.[27] A variety of "triggers" associated with migraines include emotional or physical stress, lack or excess sleep, missed meals, and nitrate-containing foods. Alcoholic beverages, menstruation, and use of oral contraceptives may trigger migraines in adolescents.[28]

Visual and sensory symptoms of migraine headaches are known collectively as an aura, and onset usually occurs before the patient experiences head pain.[29] The presence or absence of an aura helps distinguish between classic and common migraines, as an aura typically appears in classic migraines, not common migraines. Furthermore, common migraines are the most frequent type of migraine in childhood, whereas classic migraines occur less frequently in children.[28]

Presentation

Migraines present with a dull or throbbing headache that may occur on one or both sides of the patient's head, accompanied by focal neurologic disturbances such as field defects and luminous visual hallucinations.[27] A number of other prominent signs and symptoms occur along with the headache, including nausea and vomiting, photophobia, and phonophobia.[1] The patient may also present with aphasia, numbness, tingling, clumsiness, and weakness.[4]

Confusional migraines are a type of migraine that commonly occur in younger children, and typically consist of a period of confusion and disorientation that is followed by vomiting and deep sleep, after which the patient awakens feeling well. Pediatric patients may or may not report a headache.[4] Another childhood periodic syndrome is abdominal migraines, which present with episodic abdominal pain, not head pain, as well as nausea and vomiting.[30]

Workup

Migraine headaches are commonly diagnosed by a physical examination, which helps detect characteristic signs and symptoms.[1] Additional studies are indicated by the patient's history and physical exam findings, and may also help to rule out other diagnoses.[29] Blood chemistries, basic metabolic panel, complete blood count (CBC), and an erythrocyte sedimentation rate test should be considered to rule out infection. A Venereal Disease Research Laboratory test may be used to rule out syphilis, and a CT scan of the head may rule out tumors.[4]

Treatment

When managing migraine headaches, avoidance of trigger factors is very important, and the NP should advise the patient to keep a headache diary.[27] A balanced diet, aerobic exercise, and regular sleep are recommended to improve general health, and relaxation and stress management can also help to reduce headaches.[27,28,29] Moreover, the patient should eliminate monosodium glutamate (MSG) and nitrates, or nitrites, from his or her diet. It is also recommended that the patient either reduce or eliminate his or her caffeine intake.[4]

Prophylactic therapy should be considered if attacks occur more than 3 or 4 times per month or if migraines interfere with the patient's daily functioning.[29] Non-steroidal anti-inflammatory drugs (NSAIDs) may be given in chronic low doses daily. Other prophylactic agents include propanolol, amitriptyline, and topiramate.[31] Imipramine, an antidepressant with tumor-fighting properties, is given in doses of 10–150 mg daily, whereas verapamil, a calcium channel blocker that exhibits antiproliferative action, is prescribed in doses of 15–30 mg/kg by mouth twice a day.[4]

The NP may manage an acute migraine attack by prescribing antiemetics as well as having the patient rest in a dark, quiet room.[4] Additionally, a simple analgesic such as ibuprofen taken immediately may provide some relief.[32] The NP should prescribe ibuprofen in doses of 7.5–10 mg/kg in younger children; doses may be increased up to 800 mg in older teens.[4]

Triptans are recommended when over-the-counter analgesics are not effective.[33] These triptans may include almotriptan, which is approved for children 12 years and older and is administered in doses of 6.25 mg. Rizatriptan is given in 5 mg doses, and sumatriptan and zolmitriptan are both given nasally in 5 mg doses. Sumatriptan tablets are less expensive, but they may not work as well due to slower absorption. All triptans noted above have been found to have the greatest effect in adolescents, whereas triptans recommended for ages 6–11 years include rizatriptan (Maxalt) 5 mg and sumatriptan (Imitrex) nasal 5 mg. The patient may take triptans at the first sign of a headache, and then repeat in 2 hours if needed; however, triptans should be avoided in children who are at risk for heart disease.[4]

Seizure Disorder

Overview

Seizure disorders consist of transient disturbances of cerebral function due to an abnormal paroxysmal neuronal discharge in the brain. There are several types of seizures, each with different presentations, diagnostic findings, and treatments. The term epilepsy denotes any disorder characterized by recurrent seizures; however, many individuals who have a seizure never experience a second one.[34] Moreover, fevers can lower the seizure threshold and, thus, make it easier for patients to develop seizures.[35]

Seizures may be caused by congenital abnormalities. Perinatal injuries may result in seizures presenting in infancy and early childhood. Among adolescents, trauma is a major cause of seizures. Metabolic disorders have also been linked to seizures, including hypocalcaemia, hypoglycemia, pyridoxine deficiency, renal failure, and acidosis. Furthermore, seizures can be caused by infectious diseases such as bacterial meningitis, herpes encephalitis, and neurosyphilis. Lastly, seizures are common in patients with brain tumors.[36]

Presentation

Seizures may be either partial or generalized. Partial seizures are concentrated in a limited area of the brain and do not typically affect the patient's awareness or memory. However, there may be a variety of other motor, autonomic, and sensory symptoms, such as abnormal perceptions, hallucinations, or uncontrollable muscle contraction.[37] Complex partial seizures, on the other hand, commonly impair the patient's awareness and memory during, before, and after the seizure.[37]

There are a variety of types of generalized seizures, which are typically bilateral and involve both hemispheres. Distinguishing between different types of seizures can be difficult, though eyewitness accounts and recorded evidence of the seizure can aid in diagnosis.[38]

Absence, or petit mal, seizures almost always begin in childhood and consist of brief "staring" episodes that usually last only a few seconds.[39]

Tonic seizures, on the other hand, cause a sudden increase in muscle tone, producing a number of characteristic postures that may make it difficult for the patient to breathe.[40] During the onset of tonic seizures, consciousness is usually partially or completely lost; postictal alteration of consciousness is usually brief and may last several minutes.[4]

Tonic-clonic (i.e., grand mal) seizures often present with a sudden loss of consciousness and arrested respirations during the tonic phase; subsequently, the patient enters the clonic phase, which involves increased muscle tone followed by rhythmic jerks.[40] Moreover, urinary or fecal incontinence may occur in the clonic phase. The postictal state can last minutes to hours, and is characterized by deep sleep for up to an hour, headaches, disorientation, muscle discomfort, and nausea.[4]

Lastly, atonic seizures cause sudden loss of muscle tone and may result in the patient falling to the ground or dropping his or her head.[41]

Workup

When investigating the underlying cause of the patient's seizures, an electroencephalogram (EEG) is an essential component of the patient's evaluation.[42] Additional tests may help rule out suspected causes that may be indicated by the patient's age and history, such as a CT scan, an MRI scan, and an LP.[14,43] A CBC, glucose test, renal and liver function test, and serologic test for syphilis should also be performed to assess the patient's overall health and to detect underlying conditions that may be causing the patient's seizures, such as anemia and diabetes mellitus.[4,43]

Treatment

The initial management of seizures is supportive, as most seizures are self-limiting. The NP should maintain an open airway, protect the patient from injuries, and administer oxygen if the patient is cyanotic. It is important, however, not to force artificial airways or objects between the patient's teeth, as this may result in chips, cracks, or other dental injuries.[4] Parenteral anticonvulsants, including benzodiazepines such as lorazepam, are used to stop convulsive seizures.[44] The NP should consider a referral to neurology or the emergency room if the patient's seizures continue despite therapeutic monitoring through anticonvulsant levels, if there is a regression of cognitive function or developmental skills, or if the patient's side effect profile is unacceptable.[4]

Febrile Seizures

Overview

Febrile seizures occur during the course of, and as a result of, fevers. Although febrile seizures occur in only a small percentage of children, these seizures are the most common type of seizure in pediatric patients.[45] After the onset of a fever, most febrile seizures develop within 24 hours; conversely, if a seizure occurs more than 24 hours after onset of fever, it is likely due to an infection.[4,46] Some pediatric patients have a family history that puts them at risk for febrile seizures.[47] Other risk factors for febrile seizures include tobacco use by mothers during pregnancy, prematurity, neonatal hospitalization for more than 28 days, and frequent infections in the first year of age.[4]

Presentation

The majority of febrile seizures are either clonic or tonic-clonic, and episodes typically last less than 5 minutes.[4,46] The NP should perform a physical exam to rule out meningitis and other infectious causes of seizures such as chickenpox, tonsillitis, herpes simplex virus, and the flu.[48]

Workup

Although diagnostic testing is usually unnecessary for patients with febrile seizures, an LP is indicated in cases where meningitis is suspected.[49] EEGs, chemistries, and serologies are not indicated, as febrile seizure patients typically do not need a full seizure workup.[47]

Treatment

Febrile seizures should be treated if they continue for more than 5 minutes.[49] During treatment, the NP should protect the patient's airway and place him or her in a side-lying position. Cooling measures and acetaminophen are recommended to treat febrile seizures as well. Seizure prophylaxis in collaboration with a neurologist is indicated based on considerations such as a family history of seizures, a prior abnormal neurological exam, previous seizures, and more than one seizure in 24 hours. Furthermore, prophylaxis is also warranted if the patient experiences recurring seizures.[4]

Neurofibromatosis (von Recklinghausen Disease)

Overview

Neurofibromatosis (NF) is a neurocutaneous syndrome characterized by numerous café-au-lait spots (CLS) on the skin, as well as nerve tumors on the skin and in the body. The condition is usually diagnosed in childhood or early adulthood, and may either be inherited or caused by a mutation in the patient's genes.[50,51] NF does not affect the patient's intelligence, and the severity of the condition is highly variable.[4] There are two common types of NF: Type 1 NF, also known as von Recklinghausen disease, is the more prevalent of the two and presents with neurologic and cutaneous manifestations; type 2 NF, on the other hand, only accounts for a small percentage of NF cases and primarily manifests itself as acoustic neuromas.[52]

Presentation

NF commonly presents with multiple CLS, which are usually the earliest clinical findings in patients with the condition.[53] To confirm a diagnosis of NF, the patient's presentation must include at least two of the following criteria: six or more CLS that are either larger than 5 mm in diameter in prepubertal children or larger than 15 mm in postpubertal children; two or more cutaneous neurofibromas; axillary or inguinal freckling; two or more iris Lisch nodules; distinctive osseous lesions; and an autosomal dominant NF1 gene mutation present in a first-degree relative.[54]

Workup

NF is usually diagnosed based on the patient's physical examination and medical history.[55] If neurologic signs and symptoms are present,

the patient should undergo an MRI, which is the preferred imaging study for diagnosis. A CT scan may also be used for imaging screening of NF. Both imaging studies may be used to detect the presence of optic gliomas or acoustic neuromas.[4,52,53]

Treatment

Treatment of NF depends on the type of tumor and complications that appear in the patient's presentation.[56] Surgery may be used to remove the patient's tumors, and nerve resection can be accomplished by most surgeons.[53] Radiation or chemotherapy may also be needed if the tumors are cancerous.[51] Furthermore, NF patients should be referred to a neurologist, and genetic counseling may be recommended.[52]

Tic Disorders

Overview

Tic disorders consist of brief, abrupt, non-purposeful movements or utterances. Movements usually involve the face, neck, or shoulders, and may sometimes involve muscles of the limbs or other parts of the body. The onset of tic disorders usually occurs during school age; etiology is unknown, although tic disorders may be genetically inherited.[22,57] Frequently, tic disorders are unrecognized as a movement disorder in children. Many cases of tic disorders either resolve by themselves or become less severe by the time patients reach adulthood.[58]

The most common tic disorder is Tourette syndrome, which onsets before adulthood and is characterized by motor and vocal tics lasting more than 1 year.[59,60] Tic disorders are often caused by other psychobehavioral problems such as attention deficit hyperactivity disorder (ADHD).[61] Moreover, tic disorders may be associated with medications such as methylphenidate, pemoline, and amphetamines.[4]

Presentation

Patients with tic disorders present with movements that can be classified as simple or complex tics. Simple motor tics may include movements such as blinking or grimacing, among other behaviors.[58] Complex motor tics, on the other hand, last longer and may appear intentional because they involve recognizable words and gestures.[60] These tics may include copropraxia (i.e., obscene gestures), coprographia (i.e., obscene writing), coprolalia (i.e., obscene speech), palilalia (i.e., repeating one's own words), and echolalia (i.e., repeating another's words). In addition to recognizable words, other vocal tics may consist of nonsense words or phrases, as well as oropharyngeal, nasopharyngeal, or laryngeal sounds, consonants, or syllables.[4]

Workup

A diagnosis of tic disorders is based on clinical features. Typically, no further workup is necessary after the NP finds indications of Tourette syndrome or other tic disorders but may be required if the patient's history indicates the tic disorder is an abnormal presentation.[59]

Treatment

Pharmacotherapy is recommended for treatment of tic disorders if the patient's tics are interfering with daily living.[62] Clonidine, an antihypertensive that serves to treat ADHD, may be effective in controlling tics. Antipsychotics may likewise help to manage tics. It is important to treat comorbidities as well.[60] Furthermore, treatment is administered in collaboration with neurology.

References

1. Silberstein SD. Migraine. In: Porter RS, Kaplan JL, eds. The Merck Manual Online. http://www.merckmanuals.com/professional/neurologic_disorders/headache/migraine.html?qt=migrainealt=sh. Last reviewed April 2014. Accessed April 20, 2015.

2. Headaches. Mayo Clinic web site. http://www.mayo.edu/research/departments-divisions/department-neurology/programs/headaches. Accessed April 20, 2015.

3. Vascular headache. MedicineNet web site. http://www.medicinenet.com/script/main/art.asp?articlekey=5962. Last reviewed August 28, 2013. Accessed April 20, 2015.

4. Barkley TW Jr. *Pediatric Primary Care Nurse Practitioner Certification Review/Clinical Update Continuing Education Course.* West Hollywood, CA: Barkley and Associates; 2015.

5. Tension headache. A.D.A.M. Medical Encyclopedia. http://www.nlm.nih.gov/medlineplus/ency/article/000797.htm. Updated October 29, 2013. Accessed April 20, 2015.

6. United States Department of Health and Human Services, National Institutes of Health (NIH), National Institute of Neurological Disorders and Stroke (NINDS), Office of Communications and Public Liaison. NINDS headache information page. http://www.ninds.nih.gov/disorders/headache/headache.htm. Last updated February 23, 2015. Accessed April 20, 2015.

7. United States Department of Health and Human Services, Centers for Disease Control and Prevention. Bacterial meningitis. http://www.cdc.gov/meningitis/bacterial.html. Last updated April 1, 2014. Accessed April 20, 2015.

8. Mayo Clinic Staff. Meningitis. Mayo Clinic web site. http://www.mayoclinic.org/diseases-conditions/meningitis/basics/definition/con-20019713. Updated March 19, 2013. Accessed April 20, 2015.

9. Greenlee JE. Viral meningitis. In: Porter RS, Kaplan JL, eds. The Merck Manual Online. http://www.merckmanuals.com/professional/neurologic_disorders/meningitis/viral_meningitis.html. Last reviewed February 2013. Accessed April 20, 2015.

10. Hasbun R. Meningitis. In: Bronze MS, ed. Medscape. http://emedicine.medscape.com/article/232915-overview#showallHeadache. Updated January 28, 2015. Accessed April 20, 2015.

11. Greenlee JE. Acute bacterial meningitis. In: Porter RS, Kaplan JL, eds. The Merck Manual Online. http://www.merckmanuals.com/home/brain_spinal_cord_and_nerve_disorders/meningitis/acute_bacterial_meningitis.html. Updated February 2013. Accessed April 20, 2015.

12. Garralda E, Als L. What are the behavioural, emotional and cognitive impacts of meningitis and septicaemia on children? Meningitis Research Foundation web site. http://www.meningitis.org/impact-in-children. Accessed April 20, 2015.

13. Fraimow HS, Reboli AC. Specific infections with critical care implications. In: Parrillo JE, Dellinger RP, eds. *Critical Care Medicine: Principles of Diagnosis and Management in the Adult.* 4th ed. Philadelphia, PA: Elsevier Saunders; 2013: 936–964.

14. Mayo Clinic Staff. Epilepsy. Mayo Clinic web site. http://www.mayoclinic.org/diseases-conditions/epilepsy/basics/tests-diagnosis/con-20033721. Updated November 22, 2014. Accessed April 20, 2015.

15. Green NA. Meningitis. http://kidshealth.org/parent/infections/lung/meningitis.html#. Reviewed April 2013. Accessed April 20, 2015.

16. Tunkel AR. Clinical features and diagnosis of acute bacterial meningitis in adults. In: Basow DS, ed. *UpToDate.* Waltham, MA: UpToDate; 2015. http://www.uptodate.com/contents/clinical-features-and-diagnosis-of-acute-bacterial-meningitis-in-adults. Last updated April 28, 2014. Accessed April 20, 2015.

17. Kernig's sign of meningitis. A.D.A.M. Medical Encyclopedia. http://www.nlm.nih.gov/medlineplus/ency/imagepages/19077.htm. Updated October 6, 2012. Accessed April 20, 2015.

18. Brudzinski's sign of meningitis. A.D.A.M. Medical Encyclopedia. http://www.nlm.nih.gov/medlineplus/ency/imagepages/19069.htm. Updated October 6, 2012. Accessed April 20, 2015.

19. Meningitis. A.D.A.M. Medical Encyclopedia. http://www.nlm.nih.gov/medlineplus/ency/article/000680.htm. Updated October 6, 2012. Accessed April 20, 2015.

20. Brain tumor – primary – adults. A.D.A.M. Medical Encyclopedia. http://www.nlm.nih.gov/medlineplus/ency/article/007222.htm. Updated October 30, 2013. Accessed April 20, 2015.

21. What is neuroblastoma? American Cancer Society web site. http://www.cancer.org/cancer/neuroblastoma/detailedguide/neuroblastoma-what-is-neuroblastoma. Last revised March 10, 2015. Accessed April 20, 2015.

22. Rull G, Tidy C. Brain tumors in children. Patient.co.uk web site. http://www.patient.co.uk/doctor/brain-tumours-in-children. Last updated June 22, 2011. Accessed April 21, 2015.

23. Wong ET, Wu JK. Clinical presentation and diagnosis of brain tumors. In: Basow DS, ed. *UpToDate*. Waltham, MA: UpToDate; 2015. http://www.uptodate.com/contents/clinical-presentation-and-diagnosis-of-brain-tumors. Last updated September 26, 2014. Accessed April 21, 2015.

24. Shlamovitz GZ, Shah NR. Lumbar puncture. In: Lutsep HL, ed. Medscape. \http://emedicine.medscape.com/article/80773-overview#showall. Updated December 2, 2014. Accessed April 21, 2015.

25. U.S. Department of Health and Human Services, NIH, National Cancer Institute. Tumor grade. http://www.cancer.gov/cancertopics/factsheet/detection/tumor-grade-fact-sheet. Reviewed May 3, 2013. Accessed April 21, 2015.

26. Childhood brain tumors. A.D.A.M. Medical Encyclopedia. http://www.nlm.nih.gov/medlineplus/childhood-braintumors.html. Accessed April 21, 2015.

27. Mayo Clinic Staff. Migraine. Mayo Clinic web site. http://www.mayoclinic.org/diseases-conditions/migraine-headache/basics/definition/CON-20026358. Updated June 4, 2013. Accessed April 21, 2015.

28. Cleveland Clinic Staff. Migraines in children. Cleveland Clinic web site. http://my.clevelandclinic.org/disorders/pediatric_headache/ns_migraines.aspx. Accessed April 21, 2015.

29. Chawla J. Migraine headache. In: Lutsep HL, ed. Medscape. http://emedicine.medscape.com/article/1142556-overview. Updated September 15, 2014. Accessed April 21, 2015.

30. Draper R, Tidy C. Migraine in children. Patient.co.uk web site. http://www.patient.co.uk/doctor/Migraine-in-Children.htm. Last updated October 22, 2014. Accessed April 21, 2015.

31. Shahein R, Beiruti K. Preventive agents for migraine: Focus on the antiepileptic drugs. *J Cent Nerv Syst Dis*. 2012; 4: 37–49. doi:10.4137/JCNSD.S9049

32. Healthwise, Inc. Drugs for migraine and headache pain. WebMD web site. http://www.webmd.com/migraines-headaches/pain-relief-headaches. Reviewed April 18, 2015. Accessed April 21, 2015.

33. Kenny T, Tidy C. Triptans. Patient.co.uk web site. http://www.patient.co.uk/health/triptans. Last updated July 31, 2014. Accessed April 21, 2015.

34. Adamolekun B. Seizure disorders. In: Porter RS, Kaplan JL, eds. The Merck Manual Online. http://www.merckmanuals.com/professional/neurologic_disorders/seizure_disorders/seizure_disorders.html?qt=-seizures&alt=sh. Last reviewed May 2013. Accessed April 21, 2015.

35. Donner EJ. What causes seizures? About Kids' Health web site. http://www.aboutkidshealth.ca/en/resource-centres/epilepsy/aboutepilepsy/anoverviewofepilepsy/pages/what-causes-seizures.aspx. Published February 4, 2010. Accessed April 21, 2015.

36. Seizures. American Brain Tumor Association web site. http://www.abta.org/brain-tumor-information/symptoms/seizures.html. Accessed April 21, 2015.

37. Partial (focal) seizure. A.D.A.M. Medical Encyclopedia. http://www.nlm.nih.gov/medlineplus/ency/article/000697.htm. Updated February 20, 2014. Accessed April 21, 2015.

38. Borton C, Tidy C. Managing epilepsy in primary care. Patient.co.uk web site. http://www.patient.co.uk/doctor/Managing-Epilepsy-in-Primary-Care.htm. Last updated March 14, 2012. Accessed April 21, 2015.

39. Absence seizure. A.D.A.M. Medical Encyclopedia. http://www.nlm.nih.gov/medlineplus/ency/article/000696.htm. Updated February 20, 2014. Accessed April 21, 2015.

40. Tonic and clonic seizures. Johns Hopkins Medicine web site. http://www.hopkinsmedicine.org/neurology_neurosurgery/specialty_areas/epilepsy/seizures/types/tonic-and-clonic-seizures.html. Accessed April 21, 2015.

41. Healthwise, Inc. Epilepsy: Atonic seizures – Topic overview. WebMD web site. http://www.webmd.com/epilepsy/atonic-seizures. Last updated March 12, 2014. Accessed April 21, 2015.

42. Sheth RD. EEG in common epilepsy syndromes. In: Benbadis SR, ed. Medscape. http://emedicine.medscape.com/article/1138154-overview#showall. Updated October 8, 2014. Accessed April 21, 2015.

43. Healthwise, Inc. Epilepsy health center – Diagnosis & tests. WebMD web site. http://www.webmd.com/epilepsy/guide/epilespy-diagnosis-tests. Accessed April 21, 2015.

44. Healthwise, Inc. Epilepsy – Medications. WebMD web site. http://www.webmd.com/epilepsy/tc/epilepsy-medications. Reviewed March 12, 2014. Accessed April 21, 2015.

45. Tejani NR. Febrile seizures. In: Bechtel KA, ed. Medscape. http://emedicine.medscape.com/article/801500-overview. Updated September 12, 2014. Accessed April 21, 2015.

46. McBride MC. Febrile seizures. In: Porter RS, Kaplan JL, eds. The Merck Manual Online. http://www.merckmanuals.com/professional/pediatrics/neurologic_disorders_in_children/febrile_seizures.html. Last reviewed August 2013. Accessed April 21, 2015.

47. Febrile seizures. A.D.A.M. Medical Encyclopedia. http://www.nlm.nih.gov/medlineplus/ency/article/000980.htm. Updated February 26, 2014. Accessed April 21, 2015.

48. National Health Service (UK). Febrile seizures – Causes. http://www.nhs.uk/Conditions/Febrile-convulsions/Pages/Causes.aspx. Last reviewed June 10, 2014. Accessed April 21, 2015.

49. Fishman MA. Patient information: Febrile seizures (Beyond the Basics). In: Basow DS, ed. UpToDate. Waltham, MA: UpToDate; 2015. http://www.uptodate.com/contents/febrile-seizures-beyond-the-basics. Last updated August 30, 2013. Accessed April 21, 2015.

50. Mayo Clinic Staff. Neurofibromatosis. Mayo Clinic web site. http://www.mayoclinic.org/diseases-conditions/neurofibromatosis/basics/definition/con-20027728. Updated January 3, 2013. Accessed April 21, 2015.

51. United States Department of Health and Human Services, NIH, NINDS, Office of Communications and Public Liaison. NINDS neurofibromatosis information page. http://www.ninds.nih.gov/disorders/neurofibromatosis/neurofibromatosis.htm. Last updated February 23, 2015. Accessed April 21, 2015.

52. McBride MC. Neurofibromatosis. In: Porter RS, Kaplan JL, eds. The Merck Manual Online. http://www.merckmanuals.com/professional/pediatrics/neurocutaneous_syndromes/neurofibromatosis.html?qt=neurofibromatosis&alt=sh. Last reviewed September 2013. Accessed April 21, 2015.

53. Hsieh DT, Rohena LO. Neurofibromatosis type 1. In: Kao A, ed. Medscape. http://emedicine.medscape.com/article/1177266-overview. Updated December 16, 2014. Accessed April 21, 2015.

54. Peltonen S, Pöyhönen M. Clinical diagnosis and atypical forms of NF1. In: Upadhyaya M, Cooper DN, eds. *Neurofibromatosis Type 1: Molecular and Cellular Biology*. Berlin: Springer; 2013: 17–30.

55. Mayo Clinic Staff. Meningitis. Mayo Clinic web site. http://www.mayoclinic.org/diseases-conditions/meningitis/basics/definition/con-20019713. Updated March 19, 2013. Accessed April 22, 2015.

56. Korf BR. Neurofibromatosis type 1 (NF1): Management and prognosis. In: Basow DS, ed. *UpToDate*. Waltham, MA: UpToDate; 2015. http://www.uptodate.com/contents/neurofibromatosis-type-1-nf1-management-and-prognosis. Last updated March 25, 2015. Accessed April 22, 2015.

57. United States Department of Health and Human Services, Centers for Disease Control and Prevention. Tourette syndrome (TS). http://www.cdc.gov/ncbddd/tourette/facts.html. Last updated August 8, 2014. Last reviewed March 9, 2015. Accessed April 22, 2015.

58. Jankovic J. Tourette syndrome. In: Basow DS, ed. *UpToDate*. Waltham, MA: UpToDate; 2015. http://www.uptodate.com/contents/tourette-syndrome. Last updated April 9, 2015. Accessed April 22, 2015.

59. Robertson WC Jr. Tourette syndrome and other tic disorders. In: Kao A, ed. Medscape. http://emedicine.medscape.com/article/1182258-overview. Updated April 30, 2014. Accessed April 22, 2015.

60. McBride MC. Tic disorders and Tourette syndrome in children and adolescents. In: Porter RS, Kaplan JL, eds. The Merck Manual Online. http://www.merckmanuals.com/professional/pediatrics/neurologic_disorders_in_children/tic_disorders_and_tourette_syndrome_in_children_and_adolescents.html?qt=tic%20disorders&alt=sh. Last reviewed August 2013. Accessed April 22, 2015.

61. Myers EF, Zinner SH. Attention deficit hyperactivity disorder and co-occurring tics. *Contemp Pediatr.* 2013; 30(4): 24. http://contemporarypediatrics.modernmedicine.com/contemporary-pediatrics/news/modernmedicine/welcome-modernmedicine/attention-deficit-hyperactivity-d?page=full

62. Roessner V, Schoenefeld K, Buse J, Bender S, Ehrlich S, Münchau A. Pharmacological treatment of tic disorders and Tourette syndrome. *Neuropharmacology*, 2013; 68: 143–149. doi:10.1016/j.neuropharm.2012.05.043

Chapter 16

Hematologic and Oncologic Disorders

QUESTIONS

1. A 6-year-old female who is new to this country presents with a racing heart, rapid breathing, and pale-colored skin. During the physical examination, you notice splenomegaly and a very bony facial structure. Based on the patient's findings, which of the following would be most likely to present?

    a. MCV: 82 fl; MCHC: 32%; reticulocyte count: 2%

    b. MCV: 72 fl; MCHC: 30%; reticulocyte count: 3%

    c. MCV: 70 fl; MCHC: 34%; reticulocyte count: 1%

    d. MCV: 88 fl; MCHC: 36%; reticulocyte count: 1%

2. Joey, an 11-month-old infant, is brought in by his mother because he's been sleeping more than usual. A physical examination indicates pallor, palpitations, and tachycardia. In discussing recent events with the mother, she says that she has been alternating between breast milk and formula for Joey; when pressed for time and lacking formula, she gives him whole milk instead. After he responded well to the taste, she replaced breast milk with whole cow's milk. Joey most likely has which of these dietary insufficiencies?

    a. Insufficient iron

    b. Insufficient folic acid

    c. Insufficient fiber

    d. Insufficient vitamin D

3. Which of the following is <u>least</u> likely to result in lead poisoning?

    a. A red wagon from the 1970s

    b. Mexican soft drinks

    c. Inner-city playgrounds near major highways

    d. Indian herbal remedies

4. A febrile 5-year-old patient with sickle cell anemia has continued bedwetting. You order a urinalysis. Which of the following findings would you expect?

    a. Proteinuria

    b. Red blood cells

    c. Leukocyte esterase

    d. Specific gravity of 1.008

5. Which form of leukemia accounts for about 20% of all childhood leukemias and occurs primarily in infants and adolescents?

    a. Chronic myelogenous leukemia

    b. Chronic lymphocytic leukemia

    c. Acute myelogenous leukemia

    d. Acute lymphocytic leukemia

6. A toddler who presents with iron-deficiency anemia is also at increased risk for lead poisoning due to pica. After moving to a house built in 1965, the mother brings the child in for venous blood level testing. While going over the results, you explain that chelation therapy is not recommended because the toddler's venous blood level concentrations do not reach which threshold?

   a. Level 35 µg/dl

   b. Level 45 µg/dl

   c. Level 65 µg/dl

   d. Level 75 µg/dl

7. A mother brings her adopted 6-year-old to see you after he bruised his elbow bumping it on the kitchen counter. She became concerned the day after the injury because he said his elbow was tingling. After finding a normal complete blood count, you order a coagulation panel because you are most concerned about which disorder?

   a. Hemophilia

   b. Platelet disorder

   c. Anemia

   d. Leukemia

8. An otherwise healthy 4-year-old presents with bruises that the parents cannot explain. The parents first noticed the bruises a few days ago. The complete blood count results show the platelet count is low, hemoglobin is 12 g/dl, hematocrit is 36%, and her white blood cell count is 7,000/mm³. Which of the following is the most likely diagnosis?

   a. Suspected child abuse

   b. Iron deficiency anemia

   c. Immune thrombocytopenic purpura

   d. Leukemia

9. A toddler recently diagnosed as anemic is found to have a reticulocyte count of 0.3%. All of the following may explain these findings except:

   a. Iron deficiency anemia

   b. Hemolytic anemia

   c. Folic acid deficiency

   d. Bone marrow failure

10. A 5-year-old is brought to your clinic by his mother because she is concerned about the multiple bruises on his extremities and back. The boy's mother also states that he looks pale. During your physical examination, you detect scattered, enlarged lymph nodes. Which of the following actions are you most likely to do?

    a. Order a peripheral smear

    b. Refer the patient to a hematologist-oncologist

    c. Do a bone marrow aspiration and biopsy

    d. Consult a child protective agency

RATIONALES

1. b

Values of MCV=72 fl, MCHC=30%, and reticulocyte count=3%, respectively, are suggestive of thalassemia, which may present with tachypnea, tachycardia, pale skin, splenomegaly, and frontal bossing. Thalassemia is a microcytic, hypochromic anemia with a high reticulocyte count. Patients with MCVs of 82 fl and 88 fl fall within the normocytic range. The normal range for mean corpuscular hemoglobin concentration (MCHC) is 32%–36%, so patients with an MCHC of either 32% or 36% would be normochromic, not hypochromic. A reticulocyte count of 1%–2% is considered normal, not elevated.

2. a

Iron deficiency anemia often presents with palpitations, lethargy, and tachycardia. In infants, this condition may be caused by an intake of whole milk before the age of 9 months, which may produce a microhemorrhage in the gut. Folic acid deficiency would be more likely if the child was on a goat's milk diet. Fiber deficiency is more likely to lead to constipation, not tachycardia or lethargy. Vitamin D deficiency is very rare in infancy, but may present with muscle twitching, muscle weakness, and softening or thinning of the skull.

3. b

Although certain Mexican foods and candies have been flagged for high lead content, Mexican soda is not likely to cause lead poisoning. Other common sources of lead poisoning include contaminated soil, especially when near freeways; toys that may contain lead paint, such as toys from the 1970s or earlier; and ethnic folk remedies, such as Indian Ayurvedic preparations.

4. d

The urinalysis for a child with sickle cell anemia is usually hypoconcentrated, as indicated by a urine specific gravity of 1.008. Presence of white blood cells, leukocyte esterase, or red blood cells would not be expected in a urinalysis of a child with sickle cell anemia. Proteinuria may be found in adult patients with sickle cell anemia because of sickle cell nephropathy, but pediatric sickle cell disease patients typically have normal renal function.

5. c

Acute myelogenous leukemia is a form of leukemia that accounts for about 20% of all leukemias and occurs primarily in infants and adolescents. Acute lymphocytic leukemia accounts for about 75% of pediatric leukemia cases, rather than 20%, and peak incidence occurs in children younger than 5 years of age. Chronic myelogenous leukemia and chronic lymphocytic leukemia rarely occur in children.

6. a

Chelation therapy is recommended for venous blood level concentrations that meet or exceed 45 mcg/dl. At levels below 45 mcg/dl, removing lead sources from the child's environment is considered to be more effective than chelation therapy. At levels above 70 mcg/dl, hospitalization for chelation, hydration, and close observation is recommended.

7. a

Easy bruising and joint tingling, a symptom of joint bleeding, may be indicative of a coagulation disorder, such as hemophilia. Platelet disorders, anemia, and leukemia would not likely present with joint tingling. Immunoglobulin assays are often performed in pediatric patients when platelet disorders are suspected. A complete blood count (CBC) would not be normal in individuals with anemia or leukemia. A CBC would show low red blood cells in individuals with anemia, which may also indicate leukemia.

8. c

The most likely diagnosis is immune thrombocytopenic purpura since the platelet count alone is shown to be abnormal. The child is not anemic because the hemoglobin and hematocrit are normal. Leukemia is also possible but less likely because only one blood component is abnormal. Although unexplained bruising may indicate child abuse, the abnormal platelet count makes immune thrombocytopenia purpura more likely than child abuse.

9. b

In hemolytic anemia, the destruction of red blood cells causes the bone marrow to produce an elevated reticulocyte count. A reticulocyte count of 0.3% is below the normal range of 1%–2%. A low reticulocyte count may indicate iron deficiency anemia, folic acid deficiency, or bone marrow failure.

10. a

A peripheral smear should be ordered to detect malignant cells. If malignant cells are detected, the next step would be a referral to a hematologist-oncologist who would likely perform a bone marrow aspiration and biopsy. Although abuse must be considered, especially with bruises on the back, enlarged lymph nodes would not be expected in suspected cases of child abuse.

DISCUSSION

Anemias

Overview

Anemias are a group of disorders characterized by a pathological process in which either the hemoglobin (Hgb) concentration in red blood cells (RBCs) or RBC mass is abnormally low.[1]

Anemias encompass various disorders that affect the patient's RBC count, quality of Hgb, or volume of packed RBCs. These disorders are classified according to both RBC size, which is determined by mean corpuscular volume (MCV), and Hgb content, which is determined by mean corpuscular hemoglobin concentration (MCHC).[1] Anemias are considered normocytic if the patient has an MCV of 80–100 fl; MCV values under 80 fl are classified as microcytic, whereas values over 100 fl are classified as macrocytic. Likewise, an anemia that presents with an MCHC of 32%–36% is considered normochromic, whereas an MCHC under 32% is considered hypochromic. An anemia that presents with MCHC greater than 36% is considered hyperchromic; many texts do not recognize this classification, however, on the grounds that it is impossible for an RBC to be "too red."[2]

Microcytic, hypochromic anemias, such as iron deficiency anemia, thalassemia, and lead poisoning, are more prevalent among pediatric patients. Macrocytic, normochromic anemias, such as vitamin B12 deficiency and pernicious anemia, are more prevalent among adults. Normocytic, normochromic anemias include anemia of chronic disease, acute blood loss, and early iron deficiency anemia.[2]

Iron Deficiency Anemia

Overview

Iron deficiency anemia is a microcytic, hypochromic anemia characterized by a defect in Hgb synthesis that reduces the capacity of the blood to deliver oxygen to body cells and tissues.[3] Iron deficiency anemia is caused by an overall deficiency of iron due to decreased iron intake or blood loss.[2]

Iron deficiency anemia develops in three stages: iron depletion, iron-deficient erythropoiesis, and iron deficiency anemia. Complications associated with iron deficiency include impaired cognitive and psychomotor function, as well as decreased leukocyte and lymphocyte function.[3]

Iron deficiency in children and infants is frequently attributed to nutritional factors. The risk of developing iron deficiency increases in toddlers and infants who rely on whole milk diets. Whole milk does not supply enough iron to meet dietary intake needs and can cause gastrointestinal bleeding in very young infants.[2]

A common cause of iron deficiency among adolescents is increased iron requirements related to rapid growth during the pubertal development stages. In males, iron intake requirements peak during puberty because of expanding blood volume.[4] Adolescent females who have experienced menarche require higher dietary intake of iron to compensate for menstrual blood loss.[2,4,5]

Presentation

Signs and symptoms of iron deficiency anemia depend on severity. Most pediatric patients with mild to moderate cases appear asymptomatic.[3] However, patients appearing asymptomatic may exhibit pica, pagophagia, or signs of impaired cognitive, psychomotor, or mental development.[3]

Severe cases of iron deficiency anemia may include presentations of lethargy, irritability, pallor, and poor feeding. Cardiovascular symptoms may include tachypnea and tachycardia. Shortness of breath and heart palpitations may also indicate cardiomegaly.[3] Other presenting signs include weakness, headache, irritability, brittle hair, and pale, dry skin and mucous membranes.[2,4]

Workup

The most common, cost-efficient method to screen for iron deficiency is to measure Hgb and hematocrit (Hct) levels for anemia. A presumptive diagnosis can be determined with findings of low Hgb and Hct.[1]

When screening for iron deficiency anemia, it is important to consider that Hgb and Hct levels vary among adolescents according to age and gender. The threshold for defining anemia is two standard deviations below the mean for the age- and sex-specific reference population.[1]

Following a presumptive diagnosis, the patient should be administered iron therapy and then evaluated for a response. Iron therapy is usually administered in the form of oral ferrous sulfate and is primarily recommended for confirming a diagnosis of iron deficiency in infants up to 24 months of age.[3] A presumptive diagnosis is supported if Hgb levels improve after administration of iron therapy. Patients who do not respond to iron therapy after a month should be screened to rule out other conditions, such as sickle cell trait, parasitic infections, or other types of anemia.[3] For older patients and infants who do not respond to ferrous sulfate iron therapy, additional assessment tests include a complete blood count (CBC), a reticulocyte count, and a peripheral blood smear.[3]

Confirmatory diagnostic findings include low serum ferritin and low Hgb and Hct levels.[1,6] Additional diagnostic findings include low serum iron, low MCV, low MCHC, low RBCs, increased total iron binding capacity (TIBC), and increased red cell distribution width (RDW).[2]

Treatment

Treatment should focus on raising Hgb levels and replacing iron stores. Dietary modifications should be made to increase vitamin C and iron intake.[6] Treatment should include oral iron therapy until iron levels have reached the age-adjusted normal range and iron storage pools have been replaced.[2,6]

Depending on severity and the patient's age, the recommended dose for pediatric patients is 3–6 mg/kg of elemental iron once or twice daily until Hgb normalizes.[6] This dosage should be taken between meals and preferably with juice rich in vitamin C to improve iron absorption. Once a reticulocyte response is seen, which may take up to 72 hours in severe cases, treatment should be reduced to 2–3 mg/kg/day of oral iron therapy for several months until iron stores are replaced.[2,6]

Prevention of iron deficiency anemia is recommended for infants and toddlers. Infants should undergo a risk assessment for iron deficiency at 4, 18, and 24 months of age, and a universal laboratory screening between 9 and 12 months of age. Parents should ensure infants are breastfed exclusively for the first 4–6 months, and toddlers are fed iron-fortified foods and foods rich in vitamin C.[6]

Screening recommendations vary for adolescents. Menstruating females should be screened annually during adolescence, and males should be screened at least once during the peak growth period.[4]

Thalassemia

Overview

Thalassemia is a group of hereditary disorders characterized by a partial or complete deficiency of α- or β-globin chain synthesis. This deficiency impairs production of globin chains and causes a reduction in the amount of Hgb deposited into each RBC.[7] This reduction of Hgb leads to a microcytic, hypochromic anemia with presentations that vary according to the classification of thalassemia.

Thalassemia is the second most common cause of microcytic anemias.[2] Classification of thalassemia is determined by which globin chain is affected, resulting in either α thalassemia or β thalassemia, and is further sub-classified according to the severity of impairment to globin chain synthesis.[7,8] Incidence of thalassemia is highest among Mediterranean, Middle Eastern, Indian, and Southeast Asian populations, as well as groups from the tropic and subtropic regions of Africa.[8]

Presentation

Presenting signs of thalassemia depend on the classification of the disease and the patient's age. Thalassemia is usually suspected in patients presenting with a hypochromic, microcytic anemia who do not respond to oral iron therapy.[7] Most pediatric patients with mild cases are asymptomatic but may feel tired from mild anemia. In addition to symptoms of mild anemia, mild to moderate cases may present with slowed growth, delayed puberty, brittle bones, or an enlarged spleen.[7,9]

In severe thalassemia cases, symptoms usually occur within the first 2 years of life. Patients typically have severe anemia but may also present with dark urine, pallor, lethargy, and slowed growth.[1,9] Bone marrow expansion may lead to bone abnormalities, such as frontal bossing.[9] Patients may also present with abdominal swelling and an enlarged heart with hyperdynamic precordium.[2,7] Patients who are not receiving blood transfusion therapy may develop debilitating symptoms, such as neuropathy and paralysis.[7] In older children and adolescents, presentations may include growth retardation, delayed puberty, mild to moderately severe jaundice, and iron overload from multiple blood transfusions. Signs of iron overload include bleeding tendencies, frequent infections, and organ dysfunction.[2,7]

Workup

A CBC count and peripheral blood smear examination are usually performed in suspected cases. Initial laboratory findings include a low MCV and low MCHC.[7] Lab findings that help to differentiate thalassemia from other microcytic, hypochromic anemias include normal to increased levels of ferritin and serum iron, normal TIBC, decreased Hgb, and decreased α- or β-globin chains.[9]

Classifying the type of thalassemia involves a bone marrow examination or Hgb electrophoresis.[7] Additional tests may involve β-globin gene mapping or evaluating ferritin and total bilirubin levels.[2]

Treatment

Patients should be referred to a hematologist for treatment.[2] Mild cases generally do not require treatment. In moderate and severe cases, treatment usually involves chronic blood transfusions, but chronic transfusions can cause severe iron overload and result in severe organ failure.[10] Iron overload can also damage the hypothalamic pituitary axis, which can adversely affect pubertal growth and sexual development. To counter the effects of iron overload, chelation therapy is recommended. Patients should also receive annual endocrine evaluations, bone mass evaluation, and nutritional counseling.[8]

For pediatric patients in the first decade of life, normal growth and development can be achieved by maintaining near-normal pretransfusion Hgb levels of 9–10 grams/dl.[8] Dietary recommendations include a high intake of folic acid, small doses of vitamin C and vitamin E, and avoidance of iron.[7] In very rare cases, a splenectomy may be required, particularly if the patient's spleen becomes hyperactive. However, this procedure can lead to excessive destruction of RBCs and an increased need for frequent blood transfusions. Because the spleen is a store for nontoxic iron, early removal of the spleen may be harmful, and caution should be taken to avoid further complications. As such, this procedure is usually delayed until the patient is at least 4 or 5 years of age.[7]

Sickle Cell Anemia

Overview

Sickle cell diseases are blood disorders caused by an autosomal recessive condition in which the Hgb S gene develops instead of Hgb A.[11] Sickle cell anemia, the most common form of sickle cell disease, is a hereditary anemia that typically manifests in early childhood. The mutated Hgb causes RBCs to be crescent- or sickle-shaped. These sickle-shaped RBCs block blood flow in the blood vessels, resulting in a chronic, hemolytic anemia. In sickle cell anemia, abnormal sickle cells have a significantly shorter life span than normal RBCs, and the bone marrow is often unable to make new RBCs to adequately replace those that have died.[12]

Pain, progressive organ damage, and increased risk of infection are associated with sickle cell disease, as well as cerebrovascular disease and cognitive impairment.[12,13] Young children are at increased risk of bacterial infection, splenic sequestration, and stroke. Indications of end-organ damage may manifest in adolescents and adults.[9]

Patients who are sickle cell trait carriers are clinically asymptomatic.[11,14] Carriers have some resistance to malaria, which can be a benefit in regions where malaria is common.[11]

The incidence of sickle cell disease is highest among populations of African or African-American ancestry.[13] The sickle cell gene is carried in 8% of African Americans.[2]

Presentation

Signs and symptoms of sickle cell anemia vary depending on age but typically manifest within the first year of life as levels of fetal Hgb (Hgb F), which inhibit deoxy-Hb S polymerization in the red blood cells, begin to fall.[11]

All patients present with hemolytic anemia, but signs and symptoms vary and may include fatigue, anemia, cholelithiasis, and possible development of vasculopathy.[13] Vaso-occlusive crisis, characterized by sudden, excruciating pain occurring in the back, chest, abdomen, and long bones, is the most common clinical presentation among patients with sickle cell disease.[11] Patients also may present with a low-grade fever, infection, or blood loss. Other manifestations include jaundice, retinopathy, delayed puberty, hepatosplenomegaly, an enlarged heart with hyperdynamic precordium, and systolic murmur.[2] In rare cases, end-organ damage may occur. Signs of end-organ damage include pulmonary hypertension, renal disease, stroke, leg ulcers, and chronic pain syndromes.[15]

Carriers of the sickle cell trait usually present with no clinical symptoms. Patients may, however, experience painful acute symptoms under conditions leading to hypoxia and may present with isosthenuria and hematuria.[2,11,14]

Workup

A diagnosis of sickle cell disease is determined through an Hgb analysis, which typically detects the disease in newborns during mandatory screening programs.[13] An analysis is usually performed through a hemoglobin electrophoresis; findings that show the presence of Hgb SS can confirm sickle cell anemia, whereas findings that show the presence of Hgb S and Hgb A can confirm sickle cell trait.[11,13]

Laboratory findings include decreased Hgb (5–9 grams/dl), decreased Hct (17%–29%), and an elevated total leukocyte count (12,000–20,000 cells/mm³) with a predominance of neutrophils.[11] Additional lab findings may include indirectly elevated bilirubin and platelets above 400,000/μl. The reticulocyte count is usually elevated between 10% and 25% but may vary depending on the extent of baseline hemolysis. Further diagnostic findings include a peripheral blood smear that demonstrates target cells, characteristic sickle-shaped erythrocytes, and cells that appear elongated.[2] RBCs containing nuclear remnants, known as Howell-Jolly bodies, indicate asplenic conditions in the patient.[11] Urinalysis is usually hypoconcentrated.

Antenatal testing for sickle cell disease can be conducted for parents who are at risk of having a baby with the disease. An antenatal diagnosis can be made in the first trimester through chorionic villus biopsy or in the second trimester through amniocentesis.[13]

Treatment

Patients diagnosed with sickle cell anemia should be referred to a pediatric hematologist for treatment and management, with a focus on preventing associated complications.[2]

Both acute and chronic complications must be treated when dealing with sickle cell anemia. Management of acute complications may include fluids for dehydration, analgesics for pain, and oxygen for hypoxemia.[2,12] Blood transfusions may also be used to manage acute and chronic complications by correcting anemia, decreasing the percentage of Hgb S, suppressing Hgb S synthesis, and reducing hemolysis.[13] Hydroxyurea at 35 mg/kg/day is recommended for patients experiencing frequent painful episodes, severe symptomatic anemia, and severe chronic pain that is unmanageable through other medications.[2] Hydroxyurea, which stimulates Hgb F, is recommended for patients with a history of acute chest syndrome, stroke or high risk of stroke, and other severe vaso-occlusive events.[11]

Antibiotics are recommended for cases of infection and are given prophylactically until at least 5 years of age.[11] Immunization with Pneumovax is recommended at 2 and 5 years of age.[2,16] Vaccines to immunize against *Haemophilus influenzae*, *Neisseria meningitidis*, hepatitis B, and influenza are also recommended.[17]

Hemophilia A (X-Linked Recessive)

Overview

Hemophilia A is an X-linked recessive disorder caused by a deficiency of functional factor VIII (FVIII), which is a trace plasma glycoprotein that is vital to normal blood coagulation. This condition results in bleeding in the joints and muscles, with severe forms occurring in about 48% of all cases.[2,18]

Hemophilia A occurs in about 1 out of every 7,000 males.[2] Males inherit a hemophilic gene from the mother and a male chromosome from the father.[19] The frequency of carrier females is about 1 in 3,500. Among those female carriers, each pregnancy carries a 25% risk of having an affected son, a 25% risk of having a carrier daughter, and a 50% chance of having a healthy, non-carrier child.[2]

Presentation

Patients with hemophilia A are generally phenotypically normal at birth but may display easy bruising patterns or inadequate clotting following a traumatic injury.[2] Characteristic signs and symptoms include spontaneous and provoked bleeding of the mucocutaneous, joint, muscle, gastrointestinal, and central nervous systems. If left untreated or undertreated, bleeds can lead to major morbidity and even mortality.[20] Pediatric patients experiencing musculoskeletal hemorrhaging may complain of tingling or cracking sensations in the joints and refuse to use the affected joint. Additionally, patients may complain of warmth, pain, or stiffness in the joints. Gastrointestinal signs include hematemesis, melena, and abdominal pain. Genitourinary symptoms include hematuria, renal colic, and post-circumcision bleeding.[21]

In severe cases, spontaneous hemorrhaging may occur after a traumatic injury. General signs of hemorrhage include weakness, orthostasis, tachycardia, and tachypnea.[21]

Workup

Diagnosis of hemophilia A includes a CBC, coagulation studies, and an assay of FVIII.[21] Mild cases can be determined with FVIII measuring greater than 0.05 IU/ml. Moderate cases are supported by FVIII levels measuring between 0.05 and 0.01 IU/ml. A severe case of hemophilia A is determined with a finding of FVIII measuring less than 0.01 IU/ml.[18,21] CBC findings may indicate normal to low levels of Hgb and Hct, as well as normal platelet count. Coagulation studies include normal bleeding and prothrombin times.[21]

Treatment

Patients with hemophilia A should be referred to a comprehensive hemophilia care center for treatment. Treatment should involve management of hemostasis and bleeding episodes, replacement of FVIII, and rehabilitation of patients with hemophilia synovitis.[21] For severe cases, the current standard of care for pediatric patients is primary prophylaxis to prevent joint destruction.[18]

Lead Poisoning

Overview

Lead poisoning is a preventable chronic disease of toxic levels of lead in the body resulting from prolonged exposure. Lead exposure is dangerous to the developing brain in children because lead is easily absorbed in the nervous system and gastrointestinal tract.[22] Consequently, children younger than 6 years of age, especially young children between 12 and 36 months of age, are highly susceptible to the toxic effects of lead.[23] Lead poisoning can affect nearly every system in the body, including the peripheral and central nervous systems, and can impair several areas of cognitive, behavioral, and physical development. In severe cases, brain damage, coma, and even death may occur.[22,24]

Lead can be ingested or inhaled through toxins in the environment. Lead can be found in contaminated soil, gasoline emissions, food, and drinking water. The prevalence of lead poisoning is highest in poor, inner-city areas where housing built prior to 1978 still contains lead-based paint. Additional sources of lead include overseas products, such as toys or other household items, and herbal folk remedies or spices of Asian, Mexican-American, or Indian origin.[2,25]

Presentation

Signs and symptoms of lead poisoning depend upon the degree of exposure and the age of the patient. Presentations are usually vague or nonspecific in mild cases, and even in some severe cases.[23] Regardless, symptoms of lead poisoning usually involve the gastrointestinal, neuromuscular, and neurological systems.[26]

Classic presentations of lead poisoning found in pediatric patients include irritability, loss of appetite, weight loss, and sluggishness.[23] Gastrointestinal symptoms include abdominal pain, constipation, vomiting, and anorexia. Additional signs include muscle weakness, pallor, peripheral palsies, papilledema, and iron deficiency anemia. Cognitive defects may also present, such as inattentiveness, impulsiveness, distractibility, and learning problems. Encephalopathy may also result, and may be accompanied by lethargy, headaches, convulsions, and coma.[2,23,26,27]

Lead lines, also known as Burtonian lines, are a characteristic sign that rarely manifest but most often are a result of severe and prolonged lead exposure. A Burtonian line is a bluish-black line along the gingival border resulting from circulating lead reacting with sulfur ions released by oral bacteria.[2,23,28]

Diagnosis is normally made through a lead screening program. Patients suspected of having lead poisoning should undergo a complete physical examination and a patient history. The physical exam should focus on the neurologic portion of the examination, as well as psychological and language development, to assess possible neurologic consequences of lead toxicity.[23]

The history portion should assess the patient's nutritional, environmental, medical, and developmental history. When assessing nutritional history, particular attention should be given to the patient's iron and calcium intake. An environmental history should focus on potential sources of lead exposure. Such sources could be the patient's residence, surrounding soil, outside play areas, and any indoor or outdoor dust and dirt. Medical and developmental history should determine if there is a family history of lead poisoning or a patient history of pica. The patient's developmental milestones should also be evaluated. An assessment should also include an evaluation of behaviors, occupations, and hobbies of immediate family members, as well as exposure to imported products.[2,23]

Workup

To confirm a diagnosis of lead poisoning, the patient's blood lead levels (BLL) should be evaluated through venous sampling and compared to family members or other children who live near or with the patient.[27] Venous blood level concentrations are evaluated to categorize the degree of lead poisoning according to the following indications[2]:

Class I   Less than or equal to 10 µg/dl
Class IIA   10–14 µg/dl
Class IIB   15–19 µg/dl
Class III   20–44 µg/dl
Class IV   45–69 µg/dl
Class V   Higher than 70 µg/dl

Treatment

Therapy mainly depends on BLL, but treatment should primarily focus on managing the toxicity level and preventing further exposure to lead.[27] General treatment options include decontamination, chelation, and supportive therapy.[26] Patients should also be closely observed for hemoglobinopathies, impaired renal function, and vitamin D deficiencies.[2]

Patients with class IIA lead poisoning and higher should be referred to a hematologist. Patients with class IV lead poisoning should be recommended for chelation therapy, which involves injections of chemicals that bind to lead and draw it out of the tissues so that it can be excreted.[29] The injections must be administered over several weeks and can prevent death, but do not prevent brain damage.[22] Patients with class V lead poisoning should be hospitalized for chelation and hydration.

Leukemias

Overview

Leukemia is a cancer that encompasses a group of malignant hematological diseases characterized by abnormal, poorly differentiated lymphocytes (i.e., blast cells) replacing normal bone marrow elements. These blast cells may either fail to develop into mature cells or fail to mature correctly. Leukemia can be either acute or chronic. Acute leukemias spread quickly as many undeveloped malignant blast cells replace normal cells in the blood and marrow. Chronic leukemias develop slowly and with more mature-looking cells.[30]

Acute lymphocytic leukemia (ALL) and acute myelogenous leukemia (AML) are the two most prevalent forms of leukemia among pediatric patients. ALL, also known as acute lymphoblastic leukemia, is the most common type of leukemia diagnosed in pediatric patients, accounting for approximately 75% of all pediatric cancer cases. ALL is more prevalent among Caucasians and occurs predominantly in males.[2] The peak age of incidence of ALL is between 2 and 5 years of age.[2,31]

The etiology for ALL is unknown, although a variety of genetic and environmental factors have been related to incidence.[31] ALL originates in the lymphoid cells in the bone marrow, where lymphoblasts proliferate, thus affecting production

of normal blood cells. These lymphoblasts also proliferate in the liver, spleen, and lymph nodes, and can infiltrate the testes, tonsils, adenoids, and orbital tissues.[31,32]

AML—also known as acute myelocytic, myeloid, or myoblastic leukemia—replaces normal bone marrow cells with abnormal, primitive hematopoietic cells. AML can be classified into eight different subtypes, depending on which type of bone marrow cells—myoblasts, monoblasts, erythroblasts, and megakaryoblasts—are being affected. The long-term survival rate of AML is 60% among pediatric patients.[33]

Etiology of AML has been associated with several risk factors that include genetic disorders, physical and chemical exposures, radiation exposure, and prior chemotherapy.[33]

Presentation

Generally, leukemia patients do not exhibit any symptoms in the early stages. Some of the general signs and symptoms of leukemia are flu or cold symptoms, minor fever or history of frequent infections, fatigue and pallor associated with anemia, and bone and joint pain. Signs associated with thrombocytopenia and neutropenia are also general signs of leukemia.[2,31,32]

With ALL, clinical presentations are most often acute but can evolve insidiously over the course of several months. Fever, fatigue, lethargy, and bone and joint pain are the most common symptoms of ALL, as well as a bleeding diathesis related to thrombocytopenia. Additional findings of ALL include lymphadenopathy, anemia, neutropenia, and either leucopenia or leukocytosis.[31,32]

Signs and symptoms of AML depend on the type of AML the patient has. Cytopenia, anemia, hemorrhage, and fever are attributed to a deficiency of normally functioning cells. In leukemia patients whose AML is characterized by proliferation and infiltration of the abnormal leukemic cell mass and infiltrative disease, typical findings include extramedullary infiltration, mediastinal mass, abdominal masses, and gingival hyperplasia or central nervous system (CNS) infiltration.[33]

Workup

Patients suspected of having leukemia should undergo a CBC with differential WBC, platelet counts, and reticulocyte counts. Further diagnostic tests include a peripheral blood smear, which may indicate malignant cells, and a bone marrow aspiration, which may show the poorly differentiated blast cells that have been replacing healthy bone marrow tissue. Anemia is a common finding of leukemia, and thrombocytopenia is present in up to 85% of all cases.[2]

The most common diagnostic findings of ALL include anemia, thrombocytopenia, neutropenia, and either leucopenia or leukocytosis. Additional

HEMATOLOGIC AND ONCOLOGIC DISORDERS   521

findings may include hyperleukocytosis, which is found in approximately 15% of all pediatric patients, and elevated levels of serum uric acid and lactate dehydrogenase (LDH).[31] ALL can be distinguished from other malignant lymphoid disorders by the immunophenotype of the cells, which is similar to B- or T-precursor cells.[32]

The hallmark sign of AML is the reduction or absence of normal hematopoietic elements; a bone marrow examination can establish a diagnosis. Typical diagnostic findings of AML include a normocytic anemia, a low reticulocyte count, and decreased Hgb. Findings also include elevated or decreased WBC count and elevated levels of serum acid, serum muramidase, and LDH. A peripheral blood smear may indicate primitive granulocyte or monocyte precursors.

Immunophenotyping, such as cytogenic testing and human leukocyte antigen (HLA) typing, is used to further characterize leukemic cells for different cell lineages and stages of development. Cytogenic tests confirm the diagnosis, and HLA typing identifies HLA-matched family donors if a bone marrow transplant is required. Imaging studies are not required to diagnose AML but are useful for managing possible complications, such as sinusitis. Lastly, a lumbar puncture and cerebral spinal fluid examination may be required for diagnostic and therapeutic purposes.[33]

Treatment

Pediatric patients should be referred to an oncologist.[2] Chemotherapy and blood transfusions are the primary treatments for leukemia patients; however, some patients may undergo additional procedures that include radiation therapy and stem cell transplantation. For all leukemia patients, treatment intensity should be adjusted according to prognostic factors associated with the risk of recurrence.

Treatment of ALL varies according to the patient's presenting features, leukemia features, and response to early therapy. Treatment should focus on eliminating residual leukemia, preventing or eradicating CNS leukemia, and ensuring continuation of remission. Therapy should be adapted according to the level of risk for relapse, degree of supportive care, and optimization of chemotherapy drugs.[31]

Treatment is generally broken down into separate phases: the remission-induction phase, intensification and consolidation phase, and continuation therapy targeted at eliminating disease.[32]

In most treatment centers, ALL treatment involves short-term intensive chemotherapy with a combination of high-dose antineoplastic agents and corticosteroids.[31] Antineoplastic agents include methotrexate (Trexall) and cytarabine. Corticosteroids include dexamethasone (Baycadron, Maxidex, Ozurdex) and prednisone.[32] Antimicrobials

and antifungals are used in conjunction with chemotherapy to prevent infection and to provide further supportive therapy. Antimetabolite therapy should be considered for patients with a low risk of relapse. High-risk patients and patients showing either induction failure or persistent minimal residual disease after the first 2 weeks of induction therapy should be considered for more aggressive therapy and for allogeneic hematopoietic stem-cell transplantation.[31] CNS or testicular leukemia requires aggressive treatment, as these systems are poorly penetrated by chemotherapeutic agents. Although radiation therapy may be warranted to treat these sites in adults, the procedure is not recommended for pediatric patients; rather, an aggressive, directed course of conventional chemotherapy is the best first option for treatment in children.[31] Additional supportive care for patients may include blood transfusions, or antibiotics to manage complications associated with ALL therapy.[32]

The goals of AML therapy are to quickly destroy leukemic cells and prevent the emergence of a resistance clone. Therefore, patients with AML are normally transferred to pediatric cancer centers and hospitalized for extended periods of time, with intensive chemotherapy as an essential component of treatment. Hospitalization is also beneficial because it allows the patient to receive supportive care, particularly during extended periods of pancytopenia, until the bone marrow achieves hematologic remission and is again producing normal hematopoietic cells. Blood transfusions are critical to correcting anemia, thrombocytopenia, and other coagulopathies.[33]

Radiation may be recommended in AML cases where chloromas and other masses are pressing on a vital structure. Chemotherapeutic agents, such as purine antimetabolite (e.g., cytarabine) and daunomycin (Cerubidine), are used to destroy myeloblasts. Other drugs included in AML therapy in conjunction with chemotherapeutic agents include antiemetics, such as ondansetron (Zofran), to prevent nausea and vomiting; prophylactic broad-spectrum antimicrobials, such as sulfamethoxazole and trimethoprim (Bactrim), to prevent infection; and prophylactic antifungals, such as fluconazole (Diflucan), to treat and decrease host colonization of candidiasis. The role of surgery is limited; however, some patients may be referred for allogeneic or autologous bone marrow transplant therapy following chemotherapy and radiation treatment.[33]

References

1. Sandoval C. Approach to the child with anemia. In: Basow DS, ed. *UpToDate.* Waltham, MA: UpToDate; 2015. http://www.uptodate.com/contents/approach-to-the-child-with-anemia?source=search_result&search=thalassemia&selectedTitle=28~150#H9. Last updated September 25, 2013. Accessed April 22, 2015.

2. Barkley TW Jr. Hematological issues and disorders. In: Barkley TW Jr, ed. *Pediatric Primary Care Nurse Practitioner Certification Review/Clinical Update Continuing Education Course.* West Hollywood, CA: Barkley & Associates; 2015: 148–155.

3. Mahoney DH Jr. Iron deficiency in infants and young children: Screening, prevention, clinical manifestations, and diagnosis. In: Basow DS, ed. *UpToDate.* Waltham, MA: UpToDate; 2015. http://www.uptodate.com/contents/iron-deficiency-in-infants-and-young-children-screening-prevention-clinical-manifestations-and-diagnosis?detectedLanguage=en&source=search_result&search=iron+deficiency+anemia&selectedTitle=1~150&provider=noProvider#H1. Last updated February 2, 2015. Accessed April 22, 2015.

4. Abrams SA. Iron requirements and iron deficiency in adolescents. In: Basow DS, ed. *UpToDate.* Waltham, MA: UpToDate; 2015. http://www.uptodate.com/contents/iron-requirements-and-iron-deficiency-in-adolescents?detectedLanguage=en&source=search_result&search=iron+deficiency+anemia&selectedTitle=3~150&provider=noProvider#H1. Last updated December 8, 2014. Accessed April 22, 2015.

5. United States Department of Health and Human Services, National Institutes of Health (NIH), Office of Dietary Supplements. Iron. http://ods.od.nih.gov/factsheets/Iron-HealthProfessional. Reviewed February 19, 2015. Accessed April 22, 2015.

6. Mahoney DH Jr. Iron deficiency in infants and young children: Treatment. In: Basow DS, ed. *UpToDate.* Waltham, MA: UpToDate; 2015. http://www.uptodate.com/contents/iron-deficiency-in-infants-and-young-children-treatment?source=search_result&search=iron+deficiency+anemia&selected Title=2~150. Last updated February 2, 2015. Accessed April 22, 2015.

7. Yaish HM. Pediatric thalassemia. In: Coppes MJ, ed. Medscape. http://emedicine.medscape.com/article/958850#showall. Updated April 24, 2013. Accessed April 22, 2015.

8. Rachmilewitz EA, Giardina PJ. How I treat thalassemia. *Blood.* 2011; 118(13): 3479–3488. doi:10.1182/blood-2010-08-300335

9. Benz EJ Jr. Clinical manifestation and diagnosis of the thalassemias. In: Basow DS, ed. *UpToDate.* Waltham, MA: UpToDate; 2015. http://www.uptodate.com/contents/clinical-manifestations-and-diagnosis-of-the-thalassemias?source=search_result&search=thalassemia&selectedTitle=1~150. Last updated December 17, 2014. Accessed April 22, 2015.

10. Disease & treatment. Thalassemia Foundation of Canada Web site. http://www.thalassemia.ca/disease-treatment. Accessed April 22, 2015.

11. Maakaron JE. Sickle cell anemia. In: Besa EC, ed. Medscape. http://emedicine.medscape.com/article/205926-overview#showall. Updated September 15, 2014. Accessed April 22, 2015.

12. United States Department of Health and Human Services, NIH, National Heart, Lung, and Blood Institute (NHLBI). What is sickle cell anemia? http://www.nhlbi.nih.gov/health/health-topics/topics/sca. Updated September 28, 2012. Accessed April 22, 2015.

13. Rees DC, Williams TN, Gladwin MT. Sickle-cell disease. *The Lancet.* 2010; 376(9757): 2018–2031. doi:10.1016/S0140-6736(10)61029-X

14. United States Department of Health and Human Services, NIH, NHLBI. What causes sickle cell anemia? http://www.nhlbi.nih.gov/health/health-topics/topics/sca/causes. Updated September 28, 2012. Accessed April 22, 2015.

15. United States Department of Health and Human Services, NIH, NHLBI. What are the signs and symptoms of sickle cell anemia? http://www.nhlbi.nih.gov/health/health-topics/topics/sca/signs. Updated September 28, 2012. Accessed April 22, 2015.

16. Quinn CT, Rogers ZR, McCavit TL, Buchanan GR. Improved survival of children and adolescents with sickle cell disease. *Blood.* 2010; 115(17): 3447–3452. doi:10.1182/blood-2009-07-233700

17. Booth C, Inusa B, Obaro SK. Infection in sickle cell disease: A review. *Int J Infect Dis.* 2010; 14(1): e2–e12. doi:10.1016/j.ijid.2009.03.010

18. Gouw SC, van der Bom JG, Ljung R, et al. Factor VIII products and inhibitor development in severe hemophilia A. *N Engl J Med.* 2013; 368(3): 231–239. doi:10.1056/NEJMoa1208024

19. United States Department of Health and Human Services, Centers for Disease Control and Prevention. Hemophilia. http://www.cdc.gov/ncbddd/hemophilia/facts.html. Last updated August 26, 2014. Accessed April 22, 2015.

20. Wong TE, Majumdar S, Adams E, et al. Overweight and obesity in hemophilia: A systematic review of the literature. *Am J Prev Med.* 2011; 41(6S4): S369–S375. doi:10.1016/j.amepre.2011.09.008

21. Zaiden RA. Hemophilia A. In: Dronen SC, ed. Medscape. http://emedicine.medscape.com/article/779322-overview#showall. Updated November 7, 2014. Accessed April 22, 2015.

22. Lead. American Cancer Society Web site. http://www.cancer.org/cancer/cancercauses/othercarcinogens/athome/lead. Last reviewed May 27, 2014. Accessed April 22, 2015.

23. Hurwitz RL, Lee DA. Childhood lead poisoning: Clinical manifestations and diagnosis. In: Basow DS, ed. *UpToDate.* Waltham, MA: UpToDate; 2015. http://www.uptodate.com/contents/childhood-lead-poisoning-clinical-manifestations-and-diagnosis?detectedLanguage=en&source=search _result&search=lead+poisoning&selectedTitle=2~102&provider=noProvider. Last updated July 15, 2014. Accessed April 22, 2015.

24. Tiwari S, Tiwari HL, Tripathi IP. Lead effects on health. *Int Res J Environment Sci*. 2013; 2(8): 83–87. http://www.isca.in/IJENS/Archive/v2/i8/14.ISCA-IRJE-vS-2013-149.pdf

25. Minnesota Department of Health. Lead poisoning in children: Early detection, intervention and prevention. http://www.health.state.mn.us/divs/fh/mch/webcourse/lead. Accessed April 22, 2015.

26. Badawy MK. Pediatric lead toxicity clinical presentation. In: Conners GP, ed. Medscape. http://emedicine.medscape.com/article/1009587-clinical#showall. Updated June 26, 2013. Accessed April 22, 2015.

27. Hurwitz RL, Lee DA. Childhood lead poisoning: Management. In: Basow DS, ed. *UpToDate*. Waltham, MA: UpToDate; 2015. http://www.uptodate.com/contents/childhood-lead-poisoning-management. Last updated November 17, 2014. Accessed April 22, 2015.

28. Babu MS, Murthy KV, Sasidharan S. Burton's line. *Am J Med*. 2012; 125(10): 963–964. doi: 10.1016/j.amjmed.2012.04.004

29. United States Department of Health and Human Services, Centers for Disease Control and Prevention. Blood lead levels in children. http://www.cdc.gov/nceh/lead/acclpp/lead_levels_in_children_fact_sheet.pdf. Accessed April 22, 2015.

30. Leukemia. Cedars-Sinai Web site. http://www.cedars-sinai.edu/Patients/Health-Conditions/Leukemia.aspx?gclid=CP3rwPHxo7sCFYF7QgodAmEA0A. Accessed April 22, 2015.

31. United States Department of Health and Human Services, NIH, National Cancer Institute. Childhood acute lymphoblastic leukemia treatment (PDQ). http://www.cancer.gov/cancertopics/pdq/treatment/childALL/HealthProfessional/page1/AllPages. Updated April 8, 2015. Accessed April 22, 2015.

32. Kanwar VS. Pediatric acute lymphoblastic leukemia. In: Arceci RJ, ed. Medscape. http://emedicine.medscape.com/article/990113-overview#showall. Updated December 5, 2014. Accessed April 22, 2015.

33. Weinblatt ME. Pediatric acute myelocytic leukemia. In: Arceci RJ, ed. Medscape. http://emedicine.medscape.com/article/987228-overview#showall. Updated April 25, 2014. Accessed April 22, 2015.

Chapter 17

Endocrine Disorders

1. A 17-year-old female who is obese undergoes a diabetes screening every 2 years. Which set of risk factors related to the patient's heritage and medical history would best justify this screening?

    a. Pacific Islander with polycystic ovarian disease

    b. Caucasian with hypertension

    c. Hispanic with dysmenorrhea

    d. Native American with hypotension

2. A 5-year-old male presents with weakness, muscle fatigue, and arthralgias. A physical examination reveals dry skin, diminished heart sounds, and diminished deep tendon reflexes. Suspecting hypothyroidism, you order a series of lab studies. Which of the following findings would confirm a diagnosis of hypothyroidism?

    a. Low liver enzymes

    b. Low serum cholesterol

    c. Elevated serum T3

    d. Increased thyroid-stimulating hormone

3. You are providing nutritional education to the parents of a 12-year-old male who has been newly diagnosed with type 1 diabetes mellitus. All of the following statements regarding proper nutrition would be appropriate except:

    a. Consume no less than 2,000 calories per day.

    b. Carbohydrates should make up the majority of the diet.

    c. Protein should account for roughly 20% of caloric intake.

    d. The diet should be high in fiber.

4. During routine screening, a 22-month-old patient shows signs of short stature. The medical history, which reveals poor weight gain and recurrent gastrointestinal symptoms that include vomiting and chronic diarrhea, lead you to suspect celiac disease. Which of the following findings would enable you to establish this diagnosis and determine the etiology of the patient's short stature?

    a. Human leukocyte antibodies

    b. Endomysial antibodies

    c. Serum antinuclear antibodies

    d. Growth hormone antibodies

5. Margaret, an 11-year-old female diagnosed with type 1 diabetes mellitus, is experiencing hypoglycemia at 3 a.m. and elevated blood sugar at 7 a.m. What is the proper treatment for her?

    a. Reduce or eliminate the dose of insulin before bed

    b. Increase the dose of metformin before bed

    c. Add or increase the dose of insulin before bed

    d. Advise a snack before bed

6. Metformin is not recommended as a first line therapy for type 2 diabetes mellitus patients presenting with which of the following?

    a. Children less than 10 years of age

    b. Hypoglycemia

    c. Polydipsia

    d. Renal failure

7. You are treating Cynthia, age 9, who has recently been diagnosed with hyperthyroidism. What two drugs should you recognize as typical first-line treatment?

   a. Methimazole and levothyroxine

   b. Propranolol and methimazole

   c. Levothyroxine and propranolol

   d. Insulin and propylthiouracil

8. Which of these laboratory values would most likely be decreased in a patient with hyperthyroidism?

   a. Free thyroxine index

   b. Serum antinuclear antibodies

   c. Thyroid-stimulating hormone

   d. Triiodothyronine

9. Which of the following best describes the state of the pancreatic islet cells at symptom presentation in pediatric patients with type 1 diabetes mellitus?

   a. Pancreatic islet cells have shrunken in numbers but grown in size.

   b. Most pancreatic islet cells have been destroyed.

   c. The number of pancreatic islet cells is near normal levels but shrinking rapidly.

   d. Pancreatic cells produce insulin at a lower rate but their number doesn't change.

10. You are treating an overweight 7-year-old Hispanic female diagnosed with hypertension. She has a family history of type 2 diabetes mellitus (DM). Which of the following is true regarding risk factors and screening for type 2 DM for this patient?

   a. The patient should not be screened until age 10 or onset of puberty.

   b. The patient should be screened as soon as possible due to her hypertension.

   c. The patient should have been screened before the age of 7.

   d. The patient should be screened as soon as possible due to risk factors related to her ethnicity.

RATIONALES

1. a

For individuals with obesity and at least two risk factors, screening for diabetes mellitus (DM) should typically be conducted every 2 years, beginning around the onset of puberty. One risk factor is being Asian/Pacific Islander, African American, Native American, or Hispanic. Signs of insulin resistance, evidenced by polycystic ovarian disease, acanthosis nigricans, hypertension, or dyslipidemia, are also risk factors. Caucasians are not generally at an increased risk of developing DM. Hypotension and dysmenorrhea are also not considered to be risk factors for DM.

2. d

The thyroid-stimulating hormone (TSH) test is the standard diagnostic procedure for hypothyroidism, which is characterized by high TSH levels. An individual with hypothyroidism may present with high serum cholesterol, rather than low serum cholesterol. The T3 is generally elevated in thyrotoxicosis, not hypothyroidism. Patients with hypothyroidism may present with elevated liver enzymes rather than low liver enzymes.

3. a

The caloric intake of a child with type 1 diabetes mellitus (DM) is commonly determined by the child's weight and growth patterns. A 2,000 calorie diet may be appropriate for one child, but not for another. Carbohydrates are the main energy source and should make up the majority of daily calories. Protein, which delays the absorption of carbohydrates, should account for about 20% of daily calories. Individuals with type 1 DM should generally consume about 25 grams of fiber per 1,000 calories, which equates to a high-fiber diet. High-fiber diets may help to control blood sugar levels and A1C.

4. b

Serologic testing for endomysial antibodies is commonly used to diagnose celiac disease, which is a condition that often causes short stature and presents with gastrointestinal symptoms. Human leukocyte antibodies are more relevant in cases of diabetes mellitus, and serum antinuclear bodies are a diagnostic of hyperthyroid conditions such as Addison's disease. Growth hormone deficiency may be seen in patients with short stature but is not indicative of celiac disease.

5. a

Reducing or eliminating insulin before bed is a common method of treating the Somogyi effect, which occurs when nocturnal hypoglycemia stimulates a surge of counter regulatory hormones that raise blood sugar. To treat the dawn phenomenon, which occurs when blood sugar levels peak at around 7 a.m. because of progressively elevated glucose levels during the night, bedtime insulin should be increased or added to the patient's regimen. Metformin does not stimulate insulin action and would not be appropriate to treat the Somogyi effect.

6. d

Patients with hepatic or renal failure should not be prescribed metformin, which is commonly used to control high blood glucose and reduce gluconeogenesis in patients with type 2 diabetes mellitus (DM). Metformin is known to upset the gastrointestinal tract and exacerbate lactic acidosis. Metformin does not generally produce or exacerbate hypoglycemia in DM patients. Polydipsia may present as a symptom in type 1 or type 2 DM patients, but is not a contraindication for metformin.

7. b

Propranolol and thiourea drugs, such as methimazole (Tapazole), are commonly used in managing hyperthyroidism. Propranolol blocks the beta adrenergic activity of hyperthyroid disease, such as palpitations and anxiety. Thiourea drugs, such as methimazole, and propylthiouracil block the synthesis of the thyroid hormones. Levothyroxine, on the other hand, is often used when treating hypothyroidism, while insulin is typically used in the management of diabetes mellitus.

8. c

Levels of thyroid-stimulating hormone are typically decreased in patients with hyperthyroidism. Conversely, hyperthyroidism patients will likely present with elevated levels of triiodothyronine, free thyroxine index, and serum antinuclear antibodies.

9. b

By the time of symptom presentation of type 1 diabetes mellitus (DM), most of the pancreatic islet cells are destroyed due to production of islet cell autoantibodies. The reduction in number of islet cells would have typically occurred before type 1 DM symptoms present, when the number of cells may still approximate normal levels. The pancreatic cells do not regenerate.

10. a

Screening for type 2 diabetes mellitus (DM) does not need to be conducted until age 10 or the onset of puberty unless the child is overweight and has at least two risk factors for type 2 DM. The patient in the scenario displays three risk factors for type 2 DM (i.e., hypertension, Hispanic ethnicity, and family history of type 2 DM) and is also overweight. Therefore, she should be screened for type 2 DM at either the age of 10 or the onset of puberty, whichever comes first.

DISCUSSION

Diabetes Mellitus

Overview

Diabetes mellitus (DM) is defined as inappropriate hyperglycemia and disordered metabolism arising from either a reduction in the biologic effectiveness of insulin or an absolute deficiency of its secretion.[1] Classifications for DM fall into type 1 and type 2.[2] Type 1 DM produces ketosis if left untreated, whereas type 2 DM usually does not.[1]

Type 1 Diabetes Mellitus

Overview

Type 1 DM was previously known as insulin-dependent, or juvenile, diabetes. The presence of certain human leukocyte antigens (HLAs), such as HLA-DR3 and HLA-DR4, is strongly associated with the development of type 1 DM. By the time of symptom onset, most of the pancreatic islet cells are destroyed, and islet cell antibodies are detected through the autoimmune process. Type 1 DM is believed to be the result of an infectious disease, toxic environmental insult, or autoimmune destruction of pancreatic B cells.[3]

Presentation

Polyuria, polydipsia, and polyphagia are classic symptoms of type 1 DM.[3] Other presentations typically include nocturnal enuresis, weight loss with increased hunger, fatigue, weakness, parasthesia, dehydration, and dysfunction of peripheral sensory nerves. The patient's consciousness levels may change, ranging from mild cases of irritability to a comatose state. Muscle wasting and loss of subcutaneous fat are suggestive of an insidious onset. In advanced stages, an ophthalmic exam may detect the presence of cotton wool spots or microaneurysms; diminished deep tendon reflexes (DTRs) and evidence of peripheral vascular insufficiency may also present.[3]

Workup

A serum fasting blood sugar test producing results greater than or equal to 126 mg/dL on two separate occasions is a diagnostic of type 1 DM; results ranging from 100 to 125 mg/dL indicate impaired glucose tolerance, or prediabetes.[4] Glucosuria and ketonuria, as well as the presence of plasma ketones, are other typical laboratory findings of type 1 DM. Serum blood urea nitrogen, creatinine, and hemoglobin A1C levels may all be elevated. The presence of polyuria, polydipsia, and weight loss, along with a random blood sugar level greater than or equal to 200 mg/dL, indicate the diagnosis should be confirmed with fasting tests.

Baseline studies must first be established before initiating treatment. A family history should be taken, and a full physical evaluation should include a neurologic exam, a foot exam, and an assessment of peripheral pulses. The age of disease onset should be noted, as well as the presence of cardiac risk factors such as obesity. An electrocardiogram, as well as cholesterol and triglyceride fasting tests, should also be ordered to screen for potential cardiovascular complications. Ketone and antibody levels should be assessed. Whether or not administration of insulin is required is often determined on the basis of blood glucose levels.[5]

Treatment

Dietary competency, preferably with the aid of a dietitian, is of paramount importance in the management of type 1 DM. Caloric intakes must be noted. Maintaining proper caloric intake is necessary in order to achieve, and retain, ideal body weight.[1] Carbohydrates should account for 50%–60% of all calories; fats should account for 25%–30% of all calories; protein should account for 10%–20% of all calories; and 25 grams of fiber should be consumed for every 1,000 calories. Self-testing for blood glucose will help the patient to better tailor the regimen to his or her needs, minimizing the risk of complications resulting from DM.[6] The patient and family should both be trained in the process of self-tests.

Initiation of insulin is a necessity for patients who present with ketones in the blood or urine, as this signals the potential development of diabetic ketoacidosis. The benchmark for starting a course of insulin is 0.5 units/kg/day, with two-thirds of the dose administered in the morning and the other one-third given in the evening.[5]

Somogyi Effect and the Dawn Phenomenon

There are two conditions that produce early morning hyperglycemia; however, these conditions have separate etiologies and different management strategies. One is the Somogyi effect, which results when increased insulin levels in the evening produce a decrease in blood sugar. This nocturnal hypoglycemic state then triggers a rush of counterregulatory hormones that raise blood sugar. The patient will typically be hypoglycemic at 3 a.m., and will rebound around 7 a.m. with a corresponding rise in blood sugar. The treatment is aimed at reducing or eliminating the bedtime dose of insulin.

The other condition is the Dawn phenomenon, which occurs when tissue becomes desensitized to insulin over the course of the night. Blood sugar subsequently increases throughout the night, and typically peaks at 7 a.m. The tissue desensitization is most likely due to a nocturnal rise and spike in growth hormone levels. Proper treatment calls for adding an insulin regimen at bedtime or increasing the dose in an already present regimen.[1]

Type 2 Diabetes Mellitus

Overview

Type 2 DM was previously referred to as non-insulin-dependent DM. It is not linked to the HLA system, and no islet cell antibodies are identified. Although it is more common in adults, the presence of obesity increases the risk of type 2 DM in children.[6] A family history of type 2 DM is also considered a major risk factor.

Presentation

In early disease, physical findings typically do not present; insidious onset of hyperglycemia may also be asymptomatic with type 2 DM. The first symptom of type 2 DM in women is typically recurrent vaginitis. As in type 1 DM, peripheral neuropathies and blurred vision may present, but these findings are more common in type 2. Chronic skin infections typically present with type 2 DM, as do generalized pruritus and acanthosis nigricans. Polydipsia, polyphagia, and polyuria may be present,[7] but these are less common in type 2 than type 1. In women, symptoms of type 2 DM may warrant screening for polycystic ovarian disease, as the condition leads to increased insulin resistance.[8]

Workup

The workup for type 2 DM is the same as type 1; however, the presence of ketones in blood and urine is not expected. Screening for type 2 DM must be considered if the patient is obese and presents with two of the following risk factors: family history of type 2 DM; Hispanic, Native American, African American, or Asian/Pacific Islander ethnicity; or signs associated with insulin resistance, such as acanthosis nigricans, hypertension, dyslipidemia, or polycystic ovarian disease. Screening should be initiated at age 10 or at the onset of puberty,[9] whichever occurs first, and should be repeated every 2 years.

Treatment

Baseline data, as outlined for type 1 DM, should first be obtained; establishing weight management should follow. Metformin (Glucophage), 500 mg three times a day or 850 mg twice a day, may be used for the management of type 2 DM.[1] The drug does not trigger insulin action, but instead works to reduce gluconeogenesis. Metformin may cause significant gastrointestinal upset and minor hypoglycemia, though the gastrointestinal upset is typically transient. Metformin should not be given to patients with hepatic or renal failure, or patients prone to hypoxia. Administration of metformin should cease 48 hours before surgeries or tests that use contrast dye.[10]

In cases of severe hyperglycemia or ketoacidosis, insulin therapy should be employed in addition to the metformin regimen. In moderate to severe cases of ketoacidosis, fluids should be administered in order to remedy dehydration.

Hyperthyroidism

Overview

Hyperthyroidism, sometimes referred to as thyrotoxicosis, covers a group of clinical disorders characterized by increased circulating levels of free thyroxine (T4) or triiodothyronine (T3). Graves' disease, which is the most common manifestation of overt hyperthyroidism in children, is associated with diffuse enlargement and hyperactivity of the thyroid gland, as well as the presence of antibodies acting against different portions of the gland.[11]

Hyperthyroidism is more common in females by an 8:1 ratio. The onset is typically from 12 to 14 years of age. Common causes of hyperthyroidism include toxic adenoma, thyroid-stimulating hormone (TSH)-secreting pituitary tumor, subacute thyroiditis, and high-dosage amiodarone therapy.

Presentation

Patients with hyperthyroidism may complain of nervousness, restlessness, muscle cramps, chest pains, and migraines in the basilar region. Patients may also present with fine hair and heart palpitations, and female adolescent patients may exhibit menstrual irregularities. Heat intolerance may result, leading to increased sweating and warm, moist skin. Weight changes may also manifest, commonly producing as weight loss.[12] Physical findings typically include atrial fibrillation, tachycardia, and thyroid goiter, often without bruit. Graves' ophthalmopathy and hyperactive DTRs may also be present.

Workup

Mandatory newborn screenings often detect congenital hyperthyroidism in young patients. The TSH test is the most sensitive diagnostic for hyperthyroidism; TSH levels will typically be decreased in patients with a positive diagnosis. Elevated T3 and T4 levels are also diagnostics of hyperthyroidism.[13] Moreover, serum antinuclear antibodies (ANAs) are usually elevated without evidence of lupus.

Treatment

The first step in treating hyperthyroidism is to refer the patient to pediatric endocrinology. Pharmacologic treatment includes propranolol for symptomatic relief; dosing should begin at 10 mg, and may be titrated to 80 mg four times daily. For patients with mild cases of hyperthyroidism, or with small goiters or fear of isotopes, thiourea drugs (e.g., propylthiouracil, methimazole) may be utilized. Other treatments may include radioactive iodine 131-I or thyroid surgery. Before thyroid surgery can be performed, however, the patient must achieve a euthyroid state through medication.[14] Additionally, patients should receive 2–3 drops of Lugol's solution once a day for 10 days to diminish the vascularity of the gland.

Hypothyroidism

Overview

Hypothyroidism is a condition resulting in a lack of circulating thyroid hormone. The condition may occur due to disease that directly affects the thyroid gland, or due to a deficiency of pituitary TSH or hypothalamic thyrotropin-releasing hormone (TRH). Most often, hypothyroidism occurs due to autoimmune thyroiditis; however, other causes typically include deficient pituitary, iodine deficiency, and destruction of the gland by external radiation, surgery, or trauma.[1]

Hypothyroidism may be congenital or juvenile acquired. Congenital hypothyroidism may affect the fetus in the first trimester, and can lead to absence or underdevelopment of the thyroid gland, inherent dysfunction in transportation or assimilation of iodine, or development of hypothalamic or pituitary disorder.[15] Congenital hypothyroidism occurs in 1:4,000 live births.[1] Patients with juvenile acquired hypothyroidism may develop Hashimoto's thyroiditis, pituitary deficiency of TSH, hypothalamic deficiency of TRH, iodide deficiency, or damage to the gland.

Presentation

Signs and symptoms of hypothyroidism in neonates and infants are not obvious in the first month of life. However, signs that may appear after the first month include lethargy and poor feeding. Prolonged bilirubin elevation, growth deceleration, large fontanels, bradycardia, and hypotonia are other common findings in neonates and infants with hypothyroidism.

Older children with hypothyroidism may feel weak and achy, and can present with muscle fatigue, arthralgia, cramps, and lethargy. Constipation and weight gain are also common findings. Hypothyroidism may cause delayed bone age resulting in poor bone growth; dry skin, thinning hair, and brittle nails may also present. Various forms of swelling often occur; macroglossia and edema in the hands and face are typically found. Other manifestations of hypothyroidism in older children may include ascites, slowed DTRs, diminished heart sounds, and poor motor.[16]

Workup

Hypothyroidism screening for newborns is mandatory. Elevated TSH and serum cholesterol levels are indicative of hypothyroidism, as is an increase in liver enzymes. T4 and free T4 levels will typically be decreased in patients with hypothyroidism.[17] Lab findings indicating hyponatremia, hypoglycemia, and anemia are also typically present in cases of hypothyroidism.

Treatment

Treatment for hypothyroidism requires referral to a pediatric endocrinologist. Hormone replacement therapy with Synthroid[17]—as opposed to generic levothyroxine—is preferred for keeping thyroid levels consistent.

Short Stature

Overview

Short stature is defined as height measuring less than two standard deviations below the mean, or a distinct deviation from a previously established growth curve.[18] Short stature is also defined as a failure to achieve more than 4 cm of growth per year. Approximately 5% of the population is afflicted with short stature.

Proportional short stature may be caused by intrauterine growth retardation, maternal or fetal infection, chromosomal abnormalities, or a failure to thrive. Various endocrine conditions—including hypopituitarism, growth hormone deficiency, diabetes, and hypothyroidism—may also result in proportional short stature.[19] Disproportionate short stature commonly manifests as a result of dwarfism or rickets.

Presentation

Normal variants of the condition include a familial genetic variant and constitutional delay. The familial genetic variant is characterized by a normal linear growth rate with a short target height. Constitutional delay is marked by a consistency with bone age and height age; a slow growth rate is often seen for the first 2–3 years of life, followed by a low-normal growth rate. A family history of short stature and a delayed onset of puberty are often present in patients with constitutional delay.[1]

Workup

The presentation of short stature should warrant an assessment for chronic disease, neglect, and endocrine deficiencies. Proportion of short stature should first be determined, followed by investigation of underlying causes.

Tests for the condition include a complete blood count,[20] liver function tests, an electrolyte panel, a urinalysis, a thyroid function test, and an erythrocyte sedimentation rate. Bone age should be determined; a skeletal survey may be utilized if disproportionate features are present. Antiendomysial and antigliadin antibody tests should be performed to rule out celiac disease, and a sweat test is performed to rule out cystic fibrosis in cases of recurrent bronchitis. A stool test for ova and parasites may be ordered to determine an infectious cause. Growth hormone levels may also be checked.[20]

Treatment

Treatment for short stature depends on etiology; a referral to a sub-specialist may be warranted in some cases. Family support, however, is healthy for management of all cases.[19]

References

1. Barkley TW Jr. Endocrine issues and disorders. In: Barkley TW Jr, ed. *Pediatric Primary Care Nurse Practitioner Certification Review/Clinical Update Continuing Education Course*. West Hollywood, CA: Barkley & Associates; 2015: 156–164.

2. Diabetes. A.D.A.M. Medical Encyclopedia. http://www.nlm.nih.gov/medlineplus/ency/article/001214.htm. Updated August 5, 2014. Accessed April 23, 2015.

3. Levitsky LL, Misra M. Epidemiology, presentation, and diagnosis of type 1 diabetes mellitus in children and adolescents. In: Basow DS, ed. *UpToDate*. Waltham, MA: UpToDate; 2015. http://www.uptodate.com/contents/epidemiology-presentation-and-diagnosis-of-type-1-diabetes-mellitus-in-children-and-adolescents. Last updated June 10, 2014. Accessed April 23, 2015.

4. American Diabetes Association. Standards of medical care in diabetes. *Diabetes Care*. 2011; 34(Suppl 1); S11–S61. doi: 10.2337/dc11-S011

5. Laffel LMB, Wood JRS. Diabetes mellitus in children and adolescents. In: Bope ET, Kellerman RD, eds. *Conn's Current Therapy 2012*. Philadelphia, PA: Elsevier Saunders; 2012: 1063–1070.

6. Mayo Clinic Staff. Type 2 diabetes. Mayo Clinic web site. http://www.mayoclinic.com/health/type-2-diabetes/DS00585. Updated July 24, 2014. Accessed April 23, 2015.

7. Diabetes symptoms. American Diabetes Association web site. http://www.diabetes.org/diabetes-basics/symptoms/?loc=DropDownDB-symptoms&print=t. Last reviewed August 1, 2013. Last edited September 12, 2014. Accessed April 23, 2015.

8. Barber TM, Franks S. The link between polycystic ovary syndrome and both type 1 and type 2 diabetes mellitus. *Womens Health*. 2012; 8(2): 147–154. doi: 10.2217/whe.11.94

9. United States Department of Health and Human Services, National Institutes of Health, National Institute of Diabetes and Digestive and Kidney Diseases. Diagnosis of diabetes and prediabetes. http://diabetes.niddk.nih.gov/dm/pubs/diagnosis/#3 . Published June 2014. Last updated September 10, 2014. Accessed April 23, 2015.

10. McCulloch DK. Patient information: Diabetes mellitus type 2: Treatment (Beyond the Basics). In: Basow DS, ed. *UpToDate*. Waltham, MA: UpToDate; 2015. http://www.uptodate.com/contents/diabetes-mellitus-type-2-treatment-beyond-the-basics. Last updated March 14, 2014. Accessed April 23, 2015.

11. LaFranchi S. Clinical manifestations and diagnosis of hyperthyroidism in children and adolescents. In: Basow DS, ed. *UpToDate*. Waltham, MA: UpToDate; 2015. http://www.uptodate.com/contents/clinical-manifestations-and-diagnosis-of-hyperthyroidism-in-children-and-adolescents. Last updated April 1, 2015. Accessed April 23, 2015.

12. Sinha S. Pediatric hyperthyroidism clinical presentation. In: Kemp S, ed. Medscape. http://emedicine.medscape.com/article/921707-clinical#showall. Updated June 3, 2013. Accessed April 23, 2015.

13. Sinha S. Pediatric hyperthyroidism workup. In: Kemp S, ed. Medscape. http://emedicine.medscape.com/article/921707-workup#showall. Updated June 3, 2013. Accessed April 23, 2015.

14. Lee SL, Ananthakrishnan S. Hyperthyroidism treatment & management: Thyroidectomy. In: Khardori R, ed. Medscape. http://emedicine.medscape.com/article/121865-treatment#showall. Updated September 4, 2014. Accessed April 23, 2015.

15. Mayo Clinic Staff. Hypothyroidism (underactive thyroid) - causes. Mayo Clinic web site. http://www.mayoclinic.org/diseases-conditions/hypothyroidism/basics/causes/con-20021179. Updated December 1, 2012. Accessed April 23, 2015.

16. Mayo Clinic Staff. Hypothyroidism (underactive thyroid): Symptoms. http://www.mayoclinic.com/health/hypothyroidism/DS00353/DSECTION=symptoms. Updated December 1, 2012. Accessed April 23, 2015.

17. Gaitonde DY, Rowley KD, Sweeney LB. Hypothyroidism: An update. *Am Fam Physician*. 2012; 86(3): 244–251. http://www.aafp.org/afp/2012/0801/p244.html

18. Rogol AD. Diagnostic approach to children and adolescents with short stature. In: Basow DS, ed. *UpToDate*. Waltham, MA: UpToDate; 2015. http://www.uptodate.com/contents/diagnostic-approach-to-children-and-adolescents-with-short-stature. Last updated September 11, 2014. Accessed April 23, 2015.

19. Short stature. A.D.A.M. Medical Encyclopedia. http://www.nlm.nih.gov/medlineplus/ency/article/003271.htm. Updated August 22, 2013. Accessed April 23, 2015.

20. Sinha S. Short stature workup. In: Kemp S, ed. Medscape. http://emedicine.medscape.com/article/924411-workup#showall . Updated August 1, 2014. Accessed April 23, 2015.

Chapter 18

Genitourinary Disorders

QUESTIONS

1. In male infants, cryptorchidism occurs in 20%–30% of which specific population?

   a. Infants 6 months of age

   b. Brothers of males who experienced cryptorchidism

   c. Premature infants

   d. Sons of males who experienced cryptorchidism

2. What is the preferred over-the-counter analgesic for the treatment of dysmenorrhea?

   a. Aspirin

   b. Acetaminophen

   c. Ibuprofen

   d. Indomethacin

3. In which of the following age groups is primary dysmenorrhea most commonly seen?

   a. Early adolescence in individuals with precocious puberty

   b. Women over the age of 30

   c. Late adolescence

   d. Pre-menopausal women

4. A 1-month-old male is brought to the clinic for a regular check-up. He exhibits irritability and a fever of 100.2 °F, and shows signs of dehydration and documented weight loss. A urinalysis is positive for leukocytes and nitrites. Given the most likely diagnosis, what is the first step that should be taken in treating his underlying condition?

   a. Home course of oral cephalosporins

   b. Surgical intervention

   c. Oral desmopressin

   d. Hospitalization

5. Which of the following medications is least likely to be recommended for the treatment of enuresis?

   a. Desmopressin

   b. Oxybutynin

   c. Flavoxate

   d. Nitrofurantoin

6. Michael, a 5-year-old patient, is experiencing involuntary urination during waking hours. His parents point out that Michael historically exhibited bladder control until 2 weeks ago. As he does not demonstrate any signs of psychological distress, you suspect Michael's condition may be neurogenic in origin. How would you best classify Michael's enuresis?

   a. Primary enuresis

   b. Nocturnal enuresis

   c. Functional enuresis

   d. Diurnal enuresis

7. Which of the following conditions is <u>least</u> likely to present as asymptomatic in males?

    a. Gonorrhea

    b. Cryptorchidism

    c. Chlamydia

    d. Testicular torsion

8. Why must circumcision <u>not</u> be performed on patients with hypospadias?

    a. It makes the patient susceptible to infection.

    b. There is no foreskin to remove.

    c. The foreskin is used in repair.

    d. Complications often cause death.

9. Concerned parents bring their 2-month-old son with hypospadias to the clinic. They say they wish to learn more about the likelihood of other genitourinary conditions that may occur alongside hypospadias. The nurse practitioner should explain that all of the following disorders may potentially present in conjunction with hypospadias <u>except</u>:

    a. Undescended testicles

    b. Urinary tract infection

    c. Inguinal hernia

    d. Hydrocele

10. You determine that a 12-year-old male presents with testicular torsion. What is your treatment priority?

    a. Recommend cilostazol to improve blood flow

    b. Write release from physical education for the next 5 days

    c. Advise to make appointment with urology

    d. Refer to the emergency department for immediate surgical evaluation

RATIONALES

1. c

Cryptorchidism occurs in about 20%–30% of all premature male newborns. About 3% of all male infants are born with the condition, but by 1 year of age, the rate drops to 1%. Heritability in first-degree male relatives is estimated to be 7%, with about 2% of fathers of patients with cryptorchidism experiencing the condition themselves.

2. c

Ibuprofen is the preferred over-the-counter analgesic for the treatment of dysmenorrhea due to its fast onset, ability to rapidly achieve peak serum concentrations, and low cost as a generic drug. Ibuprofen tablets have been shown to reduce elevated levels of prostaglandin activity during the menstrual cycle. Aspirin is generally less effective in treating dysmenorrhea than other NSAIDs. Acetaminophen may only be useful as an adjunct treatment for mild menstrual pain, whereas indomethacin is often avoided due to the high incidence of adverse effects.

3. c

Primary dysmenorrhea is most commonly seen in late adolescence and early adulthood. Young adolescents with precocious puberty do not yet fall into this category, and women in older populations typically experience decreasing incidence of dysmenorrhea with age.

4. d

The patient's irritability, fever, dehydration, weight loss, and a urinalysis positive for leukocytes and nitrites all indicate a urinary tract infection (UTI); children under the age of 2 months who present with a UTI should be considered for hospitalization and treatment with parenteral antibiotics. A course of oral cephalosporins is recommended by national guidelines as the preferred oral course of treatment in older populations. Surgical intervention is recommended for hypospadias and testicular torsion, and oral desmopressin is a common course of treatment for enuresis.

5. d

Nitrofurantoin is an antibiotic commonly recommended for treatment of urinary tract infections, not enuresis. Desmopressin is often the treatment of choice for enuresis, with oxybutynin and flavoxate typically recommended for children who also experience daytime symptoms. Other methods of management, such as an enuresis alarm, positive reinforcement, and bladder control training, are often recommended before using medication.

6. d

Involuntary urination during waking hours is known as diurnal enuresis. In a child who has previously had control, evaluation for the presence of a urinary tract infection or constipation as a contributing factor may be indicated, as treatment may ameliorate symptoms. Primary enuresis, on the contrary, is only applicable to children who have never established bladder control. Nocturnal enuresis refers to incontinence during sleep, whereas functional enuresis refers to enuresis that has no neurogenic or anatomic cause.

7. d

Testicular torsion is not likely to present as asymptomatic, and is often heralded by sudden, severe pain in one testicle. Gonorrhea, cryptorchidism, and chlamydia are all often asymptomatic in males.

8. c

Circumcision should not be performed on patients born with hypospadias because the foreskin may be needed in correcting the condition. Hypospadias repair is usually performed when the child is between 6 and 24 months old. Susceptibility to infection and complications that can cause death are not common reasons to avoid circumcising patients with hypospadias. Lastly, patients born with hypospadias are typically born with foreskin; however, the foreskin may be incompletely formed in some cases.

9. b

A urinary tract infection is not known to accompany hypospadias, although patients who have undergone hypospadias corrective surgery are at an increased risk for urinary tract infections, especially if hair-bearing skin was used in the operation. Undescended testicles, inguinal hernia, and hydrocele are genitourinary anomalies that may potentially occur alongside hypospadias.

10. d

In patients with testicular torsion, acute pain occurs as a result of an interruption of vascular flow; this interruption warrants a referral for immediate urological surgery to restore normal blood flow. Although cilostazol dilates arteries and improves blood flow and oxygen, this medication is typically used for peripheral vascular disease and improving blood flow to the legs. Testicular torsion is not a self-resolving condition; thus, a temporary withdrawal from physical activity will not properly treat it. Recommending an appointment to be made with urology may take days, and the testicular tissue would most likely be dead from a lack of blood flow.

DISCUSSION

Enuresis

Overview

Enuresis is a disorder of involuntary urination that presents at an age when voluntary control is typically present. Enuresis is classified as diurnal if it occurs during waking hours, or nocturnal if it occurs at night. The disorder is further divided into primary and secondary forms: Primary enuresis is the involuntary passage of urine in children who have never established control; secondary enuresis occurs when children begin wetting after being dry for at least 6 months.[1]

Although the rate of enuresis amongst the general population is difficult to determine, the condition is common in children younger than 5 years of age.[2] Physical, psychological, and emotional problems rarely cause enuresis; rather, the great majority of cases of enuresis are functional.[3,4,5] Functional enuresis involves involuntary voiding of urine without a neurogenic or anatomic cause.

Presentation

The evaluation of the patient should be aimed at isolating the source of the patient's bed wetting through the process of exclusion. A thorough history is a key component of the evaluation, which should include a review of present illnesses and therapy, the patient's history of voiding patterns, and symptoms that may suggest a neurogenic or anatomic etiology.[5,6]

Workup

The patient's history and a physical examination may help rule out physical causes of enuresis (e.g., spinal defects or obstructive sleep apnea).[7] The most important test is urinalysis, which can screen for various indications. Abnormal urinalysis findings may show the presence of white blood cells (WBCs), which may indicate cystitis as the underlying disorder. Findings of red blood cells (RBCs) may indicate urinary obstruction, and the presence of glucose may indicate diabetes mellitus.[4]

Treatment

Parent education is the most important aspect of enuresis treatment.[6] Preliminary management is aimed at behavior modification and helped by positive reinforcement measures.[4,5] Once behavioral training techniques are implemented, an enuresis alarm helps to optimize treatment of bedwetting.[3] Bladder control training also aids in treatment by conditioning the patient's bladder to hold more urine.[8]

When pharmacological treatment is necessary, the preferred medication is desmopressin, which may be administered orally or by nasal spray.[4] Tricyclic medications, such as imipramine, may help to decrease bladder contractility and increase outlet resistance, aiding in urine storage.[4] Anticholinergics with antispasmodic activity are also useful in treating patients with diurnal enuresis due to voiding dysfunction.[6,7] This category of medications includes oxybutynin, which is administered to patients 6 years of age and older in order to manage detrusor muscle hyperactivity, which commonly stems from neurological disorders such as spina bifida.[9] Oxybutynin is typically administered orally in 5 mg doses twice per day, but may be administered up to three times per day if required.[5]

Alternative methods of treatment used in place of medications include hypnosis and self-hypnosis; some practitioners believe that hypnosis methods are more effective than medications despite the lack of data to definitively assess the effectiveness of such alternative treatments.[3,5] Additional treatment or therapy may be required if secondary conditions such as urinary tract infections (UTIs) are detected.

Urinary Tract Infection

Overview

UTIs are common during childhood and may involve both the kidneys and the bladder, which can possibly lead to other complications.[10,11] Children with vesicoureteral reflux (VUR), which may result in renal scarring, hypertension, and kidney failure, are also at an increased risk of developing a UTI.[12]

UTIs are most frequently caused by infections due to bacteria residing in the bowels. The most common bacterium is *Escherichia coli*, although other types include *Staphylococcus aureus*. In the first year of life, bacterial UTIs are more common in uncircumcised males.[13] In the general population, however, UTIs occur more frequently in females.[14,15] Predisposing factors include urinary stasis and congenital or acquired obstructive lesions, as well as non-obstructive causes such as neurogenic bladder, constipation, poor hygiene, and sexual intercourse.[5] Sexual abuse and neglect should also be considered as potential causes of UTIs.[16]

Presentation

Infants with UTIs may be asymptomatic. Presenting symptoms that may appear in infants include failure to thrive, irritability, dehydration, and weight loss.[5,13] Older children may present with poor weight gain.[17] Other presenting indications in children and adolescents include dysuria, frequency, urgency, nocturia, suprapubic and lower abdominal discomfort, hematuria, and fever.[5,11] As UTIs may produce sepsis in younger patients, patients presenting with fever and chills should be assessed for the disease.

Workup

Diagnosis of a UTI is determined by collecting and analyzing a sample of the patient's urine for indications of pyuria or bacteriuria.[13] The method of urine collection depends on the child's age.[18] For children who can void voluntarily, a clean-catch specimen often sees use in cases with mild symptoms and follow-up examinations.[5,13] For infants and toddlers still wearing diapers, a plastic collection bag may be used.[18] A straight catheter is indicated for culture and sensitivity in those who cannot void voluntarily. Urinalysis findings indicative of a UTI include leukocytes, nitrites, WBCs, RBCs, and increased pH, among others.[19]

A urine culture may be indicated to determine the type of bacterium causing the UTI and can also aid in determining the most appropriate method of treatment.[15] Although not required, additional diagnostic methods may include blood studies, evaluation of renal function, and imaging studies.[13]

Treatment

Patients with UTIs who do not present with findings indicative of sepsis may be treated initially with oral antibiotics such as amoxicillin, ciprofloxacin, and nitrofurantoin.[13,15] The nurse practitioner (NP) should follow up with the patient in 2 days and change the patient's antibiotics if no improvement is seen; subsequently, the NP should follow up in 1–2 weeks, then every 1–3 months for 1 year.[5] Children younger than 2 months of age who present with a UTI should undergo hospitalization and a course of treatment with parenteral antibiotics. Parenteral antibiotics are also recommended for children with a presentation indicative of sepsis or those who are unable to retain oral intake.[11]

A voiding cystourethrography (VCUG) is indicated if ultrasound findings are reflective of recurrent UTIs, as well as bladder or renal abnormalities. A VCUG and antimicrobial prophylaxis are not indicated after first febrile UTI; furthermore, antimicrobial prophylaxis is not indicated for prevention of UTI recurrences.[20]

Frequent bladder emptying and proper wiping is also important in the treatment of UTIs.[21] Fluid intake should be encouraged; studies have shown that cranberry juice may help prevent symptomatic recurrence of UTIs in children and may prevent bacteria from adhering to uroepithelial cells.[5,22]

Hypospadias

Overview

Hypospadias is a relatively common congenital abnormality in males where the urethral opening forms on the underside, or ventral surface, of the penis rather than at the tip.[23] The cause of hypospadias is unknown, but the condition is often inherited. Current hypotheses hold hypospadias to be a deformity rather than a malformation; regardless, the condition is considered to be one of the most common congenital abnormalities in infants and live births. Hypospadias usually begins developing when the male fetus is in the ninth week of gestation as the external genitalia begin to differentiate between sexes.[24] The condition is also linked to an increased likelihood of other genitourinary (GU) abnormalities, such as undescended testicles, inguinal hernia, and hydrocele.[5]

Presentation

The characteristic findings of hypospadias include presentation of a dorsally hooded foreskin, downward aim of the patient's urinary stream, and ventral bowing of the penis (i.e., chordee).[25]

Workup

Diagnosis is made by clinical findings; evaluation of the patient should include a history, examining the patient's genitalia, and identifying other congenital anomalies.[24] Imaging tests are only required if the patient presents with anomalies in other organ systems, such as the renal system.[26]

Treatment

Patients with hypospadias should be referred to a urologist at birth. Surgery should be performed between 6 and 12 months of age, and involves straightening and correcting the opening by using tissue grafts from the foreskin.[5,23] Because the foreskin is used in repair, circumcision should not be done prior to surgery.[26]

Cryptorchidism (Undescended Testes)

Overview

Cryptorchidism is the failure of one or both testes to descend from the abdomen into the scrotal sac in utero. Since testes normally descend during the last trimester, the majority of cases of cryptorchidism are diagnosed at birth.[5,27] Although cryptorchidism occurs rarely in newborn males, it is the most common congenital abnormality of the genitourinary tract and is found in up to 30% of all premature male newborns.[5,28,29]

Presentation

The main sign of cryptorchidism is inability to palpate a testicle where it is expected; this sign is often described as an empty scrotum.[30,31] Cryptorchidism typically presents with no additional signs or symptoms.[32]

Workup

Cryptorchidism does not typically require laboratories or diagnostics to confirm a diagnosis if the patient presents with unilateral undescended testes.[5] For patients with bilateral undescended testes, however, consultation with an endocrinologist or a geneticist is recommended for diagnosis. An ultrasound and karyotyping for chromosomal abnormalities, such as prune belly syndrome, may also be ordered.[5,28]

Treatment

In most cases of cryptorchidism, the testes descend into the scrotum by 1 year of age.[31] If the testes are undescended at 1 year of age, the NP should refer the patient to a urologist. If the testes are palpable and undescended, surgical repair may be necessary. Surgical repair is recommended by 3–6 months of age in order to improve fertility potential and reduce risk of testicular cancer later in life.[27] Post-surgery, the surgeon should monitor the patient via a physical exam, ultrasound, or assessing hormone levels. Parents should monitor testicular development by regularly checking testicular positioning. Later in life, especially as the patient reaches puberty, the patient should be taught how to perform a testicular self-examination to ensure early detection of tumors.[30]

Testicular Torsion

Overview

Testicular torsion is the twisting and strangulation of the spermatic cord, which interrupts the vascular flow and produces acute pain. When the condition presents, it necessitates emergency surgical intervention with the goal of preventing necrotic testicles and infertility. Testicular torsion occurs primarily in neonates and adolescents, and is most often observed in patients between 10 and 20 years of age.[5,33]

Presentation

The most common signs of testicular torsion include sudden, severe pain in one testicle; redness and swelling within one side of the scrotum; and one testicle that rests higher than the other.[34] Additional signs and symptoms include lightheadedness, nausea and vomiting, a testicular lump, and presence of blood in the semen.[35] Testicular torsion does not present with a fever, irritative voiding symptoms, or systemic symptoms.[5]

Workup

Testicular torsion can often be treated on the basis of a clinical diagnosis alone and does not usually require laboratories or diagnostics to confirm.[36] In uncertain cases, an ultrasonography with Doppler color flow is the imaging test of choice. Radionuclide scans and magnetic resonance imaging may also be useful.[37]

Treatment

Patients with testicular torsion usually require immediate surgical intervention.[34] The success rate of surgical treatment of testicular torsion is approximately 95% if it is performed within 6 hours of onset but declines to 20% after 24 hours.[38]

Dysmenorrhea

Overview

Dysmenorrhea is pain and cramping associated with menstruation. Dysmenorrhea can be either primary or secondary, depending on its presentation and underlying cause. Primary dysmenorrhea has an absence of any pelvic pathology and is currently considered to be hormonal and endocrine-related in nature. Primary dysmenorrhea commonly starts to manifest 6–12 months after menarche, with symptoms gradually presenting more often until patients are in their mid-20s.[5] Secondary dysmenorrhea is commonly caused by organic underlying conditions such as pelvic inflammatory disease (PID), pregnancy, and endometriosis.[5,39] Secondary dysmenorrhea usually presents in adulthood, except in cases that are caused by congenital malformations such as bicornuate uterus.[40]

Presentation

Dysmenorrhea typically presents with dull, throbbing, or cramping pain in the lower abdomen that may radiate to the back and is typically strongest during the first few days of bleeding.[5,40,41] Additional signs and symptoms of dysmenorrhea include nausea, fatigue, headaches, and diarrhea.[42]

Workup

Primary dysmenorrhea is diagnosed clinically. Laboratory tests are useful in determining the underlying cause of secondary dysmenorrhea.[5] Imaging studies may include a pelvic ultrasound to determine the presence of comorbid conditions such as uterine fibroids, adenomyosis, and endometriosis.[43]

Treatment

Pharmacotherapy is the most effective method of relieving dysmenorrhea.[39] Non-steroidal anti-inflammatory drugs (NSAIDs) are recommended for moderate to severe dysmenorrhea and are very effective in reducing pain associated with the condition.[5,43] Patients may also be given oral contraceptives or other forms of hormonal birth control as needed to reduce the severity of menstrual cramps, prevent ovulation, and diminish the uterine contractions and menstrual bleeding that contribute to discomfort associated with dysmenorrhea.[41,43] Less severe cases of dysmenorrhea may necessitate over-the-counter analgesics as a support measure, preferably ibuprofen. Ibuprofen is given in doses of 400 mg every 4–6 hours, starting with the onset of the menstrual cycle and continuing for 24–72 hours.[5]

Additional support measures include heat application, psychological support, and referral as needed. Dysmenorrhea patients should be educated about menstruation and proper diet, as diets high in vitamin E and fish oil may decrease symptoms of dysmenorrhea.[39] It is also important for patients to get adequate exercise and sleep.[40]

Chlamydia

Overview

Chlamydia is a parasitic sexually transmitted infection (STI) that is caused by the bacteria *Chlamydia trachomatis* and may result in severe reproductive tract complications in both males and females. Chlamydiae are intracellular obligates that closely resemble gram-negative bacteria and cause diseases such as STIs and pneumonias.[5,44] Furthermore, chlamydia is the most common bacterial STI in the United States and is also the leading cause of urethritis and cervicitis in adolescents.[5,45]

Presentation

Although signs and symptoms may vary among males and females, both sexes are often asymptomatic.[46] Symptoms that may appear in female chlamydia patients include abnormal vaginal discharge after intercourse, dysuria, dyspareunia, intermenstrual spotting, postcoital bleeding, and lower abdominal or pelvic pain.[5,45] Males may present with dysuria and a thick, cloudy penile discharge. Testicular pain and swelling may also present, but these findings are less common.[47]

Workup

Although a diagnosis of chlamydia can sometimes be made solely on the basis of a clinical evaluation, testing is recommended for patients at risk for STIs because many chlamydia patients are asymptomatic.[44] Urine checks are recommended for adolescent patients. A culture is the most definitive diagnostic of chlamydia but results may take 3–9 days. An enzyme immunoassay, on the other hand, yields results in 30–120 minutes and can be performed at a low cost.[5]

Treatment

Antibiotics are the usual treatment for chlamydia.[45] *C. trachomatis* is particularly susceptible to tetracyclines and macrolides, the first-line agents of which are azithromycin (Zithromax) and doxycycline, respectively.[49] Azithromycin is given to chlamydia patients in a single dose of 1 gram orally, whereas doxycycline is given in doses of 100 mg orally twice a day for 7 days.[49] Additionally, it is recommended by the Centers for Disease Control and Prevention (CDC) that all confirmed cases of *C. trachomatis* infection be reported to the health department.[49]

Gonorrhea

Overview

Gonorrhea is a bacterial STI caused by *Neisseria gonorrhoeae*, which may be spread by sexual contact or by transmission during childbirth.[50] *N. gonorrhoeae* is a gram-negative diplococcus that may take root in the genitourinary tract, oropharynx, conjunctiva, or anorectum. Gonorrhea is the second most common communicable disease in the United States and is a major cause of cervicitis in women and urethritis in men.[51] Moreover, gonorrhea is also the leading cause of infertility among females.[52]

Presentation

Gonorrhea is often asymptomatic, especially in females.[5] Both males and females, however, may present with dysuria and urinary frequency, among other signs and symptoms. Additional signs and symptoms in men include testicular pain and penile discharge, which may be white, yellow, or green in color.[53] Female gonorrhea patients, on the other hand, may present with mucopurulent vaginal discharge, labial pain and swelling, lower abdominal pain, or dysmenorrhea.[54] Fever, chills, nausea, and vomiting may also appear in female patients with gonorrhea who develop PID, although these findings are less common.[50]

Workup

A diagnosis of gonorrhea may be confirmed when gonococci are detected by a Gram stain or culture.[55] Urine checks should be performed in adolescent patients, with these urine samples often serving as the base for cultures. A Gram stain is a rapid and inexpensive test and may show gram-negative diplococci and WBCs in the patient's discharge.[5,50] Cervical cultures for *N. gonorrhoeae* are processed using Thayer-Martin or Transgrow media and are particularly useful in isolating the bacteria from any site.[5,51]

Treatment

For antibiotic treatment of gonorrhea, uncomplicated cases should be treated with ceftriaxone in combination with azithromycin or doxycycline.[54] Patients should also be co-treated for chlamydia, as about half of all female gonorrhea patients experience a concomitant chlamydial infection. Ceftriaxone, distributed under the brand name Rocephin, is given intramuscularly in a 250 mg single dose. This dose should be given in combination with either azithromycin (Zithromax) 1 gram orally in a single dose or doxycycline 100 mg by mouth twice a day for 7 days, in order to cover concomitant chlamydial infection.[50] Additionally, all gonorrhea patients should be contacted and tested by the health department.[53]

Syphilis

Overview

Syphilis is an STI that is caused by the spirochete bacteria *Treponema pallidum* and involves multiple organ systems. Syphilis infections usually result from sexual contact, although *T. pallidum* may be transmitted by skin contact or through the placental barrier.[55]

Presentation

There are four clinical stages of syphilis. In the primary stage, the first sign of syphilis is a chancre that appears at the site of transmission.[56] The secondary stage presents with flu-like symptoms as well as a generalized maculopapular rash that appears on various parts of the body, especially the palms and soles.[57] Latent syphilis is seropositive, but asymptomatic.

The latent stage may persist indefinitely or be followed by late-stage syphilis (i.e., tertiary syphilis).[55] Approximately one-third of all untreated cases of the disease develop into tertiary syphilis, which often presents with leukoplakia and cardiac insufficiencies such as aortitis, aneurysms, and aortic regurgitation.[5] At the tertiary stage, the condition may damage parts of the body, such as the bones and liver, and may produce central nervous system disorders such as meningitis, hemiparesis, and hemiplegia, among others.[5,56]

Workup

Syphilis is most commonly diagnosed by serologic testing, the two primary methods of which are treponema-specific tests and non-treponemal reaginic tests.[58,59] Non-treponemal antibody tests such as the Venereal Disease Research Laboratory test or the rapid plasma reagin test are given first. A diagnosis is then confirmed with treponemal tests such as a fluorescent treponemal antibody absorption test or a microhemagglutination assay for antibody to *T. pallidum*.[5]

In addition to serologic testing, spirochetes can be directly identified through darkfield microscopy, which will show treponemes in almost all chancres that appear in primary syphilis.[58] Primary syphilis can also be diagnosed by a typical lesion or newly positive syphilis screen. Furthermore, a syphilis screen will typically be strongly reactive in cases of secondary syphilis, whereas the screen will show serologic evidence of untreated syphilis in the latent and tertiary stages.[5]

Treatment

Penicillin is the preferred treatment in all stages of syphilis.[60] Most syphilis infections are treated by benzathine penicillin G, which is given in a single dose of 2.4 million units intramuscularly.[55] For patients who are allergic to penicillin, the NP may prescribe alternatives such as doxycycline or tetracycline.[49] Patients with tertiary syphilis will likely also require surgical care for treatment of complications such as aortitis. In addition to antibiotic treatment, the NP should report all cases of syphilis to the health department.

Bacterial Vaginosis

Overview

Bacterial vaginosis is a vaginal infection in which "harmful" species of bacteria produce an alteration in the normal functioning of vaginal flora. In this alteration, lactobacilli decrease and anaerobic pathogens overgrow.[62] Bacterial vaginosis is not considered an STI; however, it manifests more often in women who are sexually active, and the development of this condition is associated with sexual activity.[5,63] Although the cause of bacterial vaginosis is unknown, it is the most common type of infectious vaginitis, as well as the most common cause of vaginal discharge in women of childbearing age.[6,62]

Presentation

A large percentage of patients with bacterial vaginosis are asymptomatic.[64] Symptomatic patients often present with an increased milky discharge that is thin and grayish white.[65] A malodorous, "fishy" discharge is also usually present and is most evident after sexual intercourse, when the discharge is more alkaline.[62] Other physical findings may include pain during urination as well as pruritus around the vagina.[66] On a physical exam, the patient's cervix, uterus, and adnexa will usually appear normal.[5,63]

Workup

Bacterial vaginosis is diagnosed upon detection of clue cells—epithelial cells covered with bacteria that appear with poorly defined borders and small dots or specks.[63] Clue cells are detected by microscopic examination of a saline wet mount, which also detects decreasing or absent lactobacilli as well as few or absent white blood cells.[5,62] A positive amine "whiff" test detects a fishy odor when potassium hydroxide is added to the slide.[67]

Treatment

Antibiotics are the mainstay of bacterial vaginosis treatment.[63] Medications that may be used in treatment include metronidazole; common preparations include 500 mg oral doses administered twice a day for 7 days, or a 0.75% gel administered in 5 gram doses inserted intravaginally once a day for 5 days. Clindamycin cream (2%) may be given in 5 gram doses intravaginally at bedtime for 7 days.[49]

Herpes

Overview

Herpes is a recurrent, viral STI that is associated with painful lesions and caused by two types of herpes simplex virus (HSV), known as types 1 and 2. HSV type 1 is found on the lips, face, and mucosa, whereas HSV type 2 is found on the genitalia.[68] Transmission of herpes occurs by direct contact with the virus across broken skin or intact mucosa.[69]

Presentation

Presentation of herpes varies depending on the clinical designation of the patient's condition. The three clinical designations of herpes are primary, non-primary first episode, and recurrent.[70] Initial signs and symptoms of herpes include fever, malaise, and dysuria, as well as painful and pruritic ulcers lasting for approximately 12 days. Non-primary first episodes follow the same pattern of symptoms, but tend to present with fewer lesions and less systemic symptoms. Recurrent herpes also presents with ulcers, but these ulcers are less painful and pruritic than those of primary herpes and usually last for only 5 days.[5]

Workup

A diagnosis of herpes can often be made clinically based on the appearance of characteristic lesions.[71] The most definitive laboratory test to confirm an HSV infection is a tissue culture, which isolates the virus.[72] Additionally, HSV may be detected by a Papanicolaou or Tzanck stain.[5]

Treatment

There is no curative treatment for herpes, and the patient's symptoms may disappear without treatment in 1–2 weeks.[73] Patients may be given drying and antipruritic agents for symptomatic treatment. Medication options include acyclovir (Zovirax), given orally at 400 mg three times a day for 7–10 days or 200 mg orally five times a day for 7–10 days. Valacyclovir, 1 gram orally twice a day for 7–10 days, may also be used. Treatment may be extended if healing is incomplete after the recommended length of therapy.[49]

Acquired Immune Deficiency Syndrome (AIDS)

Overview

AIDS is the final stage of HIV infection. This stage occurs the patient's immune system becomes damaged, leaving the patient vulnerable to opportunistic infections.[74] AIDS is typically transmitted prenatally by perinatal transmission from mother to child by shared blood circulation; postnatally, breastfeeding is the primary vertical route in infants and neonates.[5,75]

Presentation

Neonates with AIDS present with a low birth weight. Such patients also typically demonstrate a falling ratio of head circumference to height and weight. Additional signs and symptoms of AIDS in pediatric patients may include recurrent infections, diminishing activity, developmental delays, hepatosplenomegaly, and generalized lymphadenopathy.[5]

Workup

HIV polymerase chain reaction testing is used to test for the genetic material of the virus and is particularly recommended for children born to HIV-positive mothers.[76] Older children are screened with the ELISA test, which is the most common type of HIV test and has greater than 99.9% sensitivity.[5,77] If the HIV patient shows progress towards AIDS, the western blot test confirms this diagnosis.[76]

The patient's CD4 lymphocyte percentage of white blood cells should be assessed to confirm a diagnosis of AIDS. The risk of progression to AIDS is high if the patient's CD4 lymphocyte count is below 20%, whereas a normal absolute CD4 lymphocyte count is greater than 800 cells/μL.[5] Ideally, the patient's viral load should be less than 5,000 copies, which may be described as "zero" or "undetectable."[78]

Treatment

The patient should be referred to an HIV infectious disease specialist for care. Although there is no available cure for AIDS, a number of treatments can help improve the patient's quality of life and diminish signs and symptoms.[75] To help prevent pneumocystic pneumonia, Bactrim may be given to treat *Pneumocystis jiroveci*. The patient should also be monitored for cytomegalovirus. Antiretroviral therapy includes combination treatment; although decisions on when to start antiretroviral therapy typically vary based on age and presentation of symptoms, various studies indicate that treatment should ideally be started by the time the patient has a CD4 of 350 cells/μL.[5,79] Because drug resistance may develop rapidly, the patient should be taught to take medications exactly as prescribed and at the same time every day.[80]

References

1. Knott L, Tidy C. Nocturnal enuresis in children. Patient. co.uk web site. http://www.patient.co.uk/doctor/nocturnal-enuresis-in-children. Last updated March 26, 2014. Accessed April 23, 2015.

2. Tu ND, Baskin LS. Nocturnal enuresis in children: Management. In: Basow DS, ed. *UpToDate*. Waltham, MA: UpToDate; 2015. http://www.uptodate.com/contents/nocturnal-enuresis-in-children-management. Last updated August 13, 2014. Accessed April 23, 2015.

3. Drutz JE, Tu ND. Patient information: Bedwetting in children (Beyond the Basics). In: Basow DS, ed. *UpToDate*. Waltham, MA: UpToDate; 2015. http://www.uptodate.com/contents/bedwetting-in-children-beyond-the-basics. Last updated January 9, 2013. Accessed April 23, 2015.

4. Robson WML. Enuresis. In: Cendron M, ed. Medscape. http://emedicine.medscape.com/article/1014762-overview. Updated February 19, 2014. Accessed April 23, 2015.

5. Barkley TW Jr. *Pediatric Primary Care Nurse Practitioner Certification Review/Clinical Update Continuing Education Course*. West Hollywood, CA: Barkley and Associates; 2015.

6. Figueroa TE. Incontinence in children. In: Porter RS, Kaplan JL, eds. The Merck Manual Online. http://www.merckmanuals.com/professional/pediatrics/incontinence_in_children/urinary_incontinence_in_children.html?qt=enuresis&alt=sh. Last reviewed October 2014. Accessed April 23, 2015.

7. Bedwetting. A.D.A.M. Medical Encyclopedia. http://www.nlm.nih.gov/medlineplus/ency/patientinstructions/000703.htm. Updated March 19, 2014. Accessed April 23, 2015.

8. Urinary incontinence (Enuresis). Lucile Packard Children's Hospital at Stanford web site. http://www.lpch.org/DiseaseHealthInfo/HealthLibrary/growth/enuresis.html. Accessed April 23, 2015.

9. Oxybutynin. A.D.A.M. Medical Encyclopedia. http://www.nlm.nih.gov/medlineplus/druginfo/meds/a682141.html. Last revised May 15, 2014. Accessed April 23, 2015.

10. Shaikh N, Hoberman A. Urinary tract infections in children: Epidemiology and risk factors. In: Basow DS, ed. *UpToDate*. Waltham, MA: UpToDate; 2015. http://www.uptodate.com/contents/urinary-tract-infections-in-children-epidemiology-and-risk-factors. Last updated December 8, 2014. Accessed April 23, 2015.

11. Weinberg GA. Urinary tract infection in children (UTI). In: Porter RS, Kaplan JL, eds. The Merck Manual Online. http://www.merckmanuals.com/professional/pediatrics/ miscellaneous_infections_in_infants_and_children/urinary_tract_infection_in_children_uti.html?qt=urinary%20tract%20infection&alt=sh. Last reviewed March 2010. Accessed April 23, 2015.

12. United States Department of Health and Human Services, National Institutes of Health (NIH), National Institute of Diabetes and Digestive and Kidney Diseases (NIDDK), National Kidney and Urologic Diseases Information Clearinghouse (NKUDIC). Vesicoureteral reflux. http://kidney.niddk.nih.gov/kudiseases/pubs/vesicoureteralreflux. Published September 2011. Last updated June 29, 2012. Accessed April 23, 2015.

13. Fisher DJ. Pediatric urinary tract infection. In: Steele RW, ed. Medscape. http://emedicine.medscape.com/article/969643-overview#aw2aab6b2b. Updated August 18, 2014. Accessed April 23, 2015.

14. Mersch J. Urinary tract infections (UTIs) in children. In: Stöppler MC, ed. MedicineNet. http://www.medicinenet.com/urinary_tract_infections_in_children/article.htm. Reviewed February 5, 2015. Accessed April 23, 2015.

15. Mayo Clinic Staff. Urinary tract infection (UTI). Mayo Clinic web site. http://www.mayoclinic.org/diseases-conditions/urinary-tract-infection/basics/definition/con-20037892. Updated August 29, 2012. Accessed April 23, 2015.

16. Pediatric urinary tract infections. American Urological Association web site. http://www.auanet.org/education/pediatric-urinary-tract-infections.cfm. Accessed April 23, 2015.

17. Shaikh N, Hoberman A. Urinary tract infections in infants and children older than one month: Clinical features and diagnosis. In: Basow DS, ed. *UpToDate*. Waltham, MA: UpToDate; 2015. http://www.uptodate.com/contents/urinary-tract-infections-in-infants-and-children-older-than-one-month-clinical-features-and-diagnosis. Last updated March 17, 2015. Accessed April 23, 2015.

18. United States Department of Health and Human Services, NIH, NIDDK, NKUDIC. Urinary tract infections in children. http://kidney.niddk.nih.gov/kudiseases/pubs/utichildren. Published November 2011. Last updated November 16, 2011. Accessed April 23, 2015.

19. Bates BN. Interpretation of urinalysis and urine culture for UTI treatment. *US Pharm*. 2013; 38(11): 65–68. http://www.uspharmacist.com/content/c/44877/?t=men%27s_health,urology

20. Voiding cystourethrogram. A.D.A.M. Medical Encyclopedia. http://www.nlm.nih.gov/medlineplus/ency/article/003784.htm. Updated October 9, 2012. Accessed April 23, 2015.

21. Minnesota Department of Public Health and Human Services. Best practice guidelines: Urinary tract infections. https://dphhs.mt.gov/Portals/85/dsd/documents/DDP/MedicalDirector/UrinaryTractInfections.pdf. Published 2010. Accessed April 23, 2015.

22. Jepson R, Williams GJ, Craig JC. Cranberries for preventing urinary tract infections. *Cochrane Database Syst Rev*. 2012; 10: CD001321. doi: 10.1002/14651858.CD001321.pub5

23. Hypospadias. A.D.A.M. Medical Encyclopedia. http://www.nlm.nih.gov/medlineplus/ency/article/001286.htm. Updated October 9, 2012. Accessed April 23, 2015.

24. Baskin LS. Hypospadias. In: Basow DS, ed. *UpToDate*. Waltham, MA: UpToDate; 2015. http://www.uptodate.com/contents/hypospadias. Last updated April 20, 2015. Accessed April 23, 2015.

25. Mayo Clinic Staff. Hypospadias. Mayo Clinic web site. http://www.mayoclinic.org/diseases-conditions/hypospadias/basics/definition/con-20031354. Updated October 1, 2013. Accessed April 23, 2015.

26. Gatti JM, Kirsch AJ, Snyder HM III. Hypospadias. In: Cendron M, ed. Medscape. http://emedicine.medscape.com/article/1015227-workup. Updated May 2, 2013. Accessed April 23, 2015.

27. Rabinowitz R, Cubillos J. Congenital renal and genitourinary anomalies. In: Porter RS, Kaplan JL, eds. The Merck Manual Online. http://www.merckmanuals.com/professional/pediatrics/ congenital_renal_and_genitourinary_anomalies/penile_and_urethral_anomalies.html?qt=hypospadias&alt=sh. Last reviewed May 2013. Accessed April 23, 2015.

28. Sumfest JM, Kolon TF, Rukstalis DB. Cryptorchidism. In: Kim ED, ed. Medscape. http://emedicine.medscape.com/article/438378-overview#a0199. Updated November 19, 2014. Accessed April 23, 2015.

29. Kolon TF, Herndon CD, Baker LA, et al. Evaluation and treatment of cryptorchidism: AUA guideline. *J Urol*. 2014; 192(2): 337–345. doi: 10.1016/j.juro.2014.05.005.

30. Mayo Clinic Staff. Undescended testicle (cryptorchidism). Mayo Clinic web site. http://www.mayoclinic.com/health/undescended-testicle/DS00845/DSECTION=symptoms. Updated April 11, 2013. Accessed April 23, 2015.

31. Undescended testicle. A.D.A.M. Medical Encyclopedia. http://www.nlm.nih.gov/medlineplus/ency/article/000973.htm. Updated October 2, 2013. Accessed April 23, 2015.

32. Undescended testicle – topic overview. WebMD web site. http://www.webmd.com/parenting/baby/tc/undescended-testicle-topic-overview. Last updated December 28, 2012. Accessed April 23, 2015.

33. Ogunyemi OI, Weiker M, Abel EJ. Testicular torsion. In: Kim ED, ed. Medscape. http://emedicine.medscape.com/article/2036003-overview#a0101. Updated November 17, 2014. Accessed April 23, 2015.

34. Testicular torsion repair. A.D.A.M. Medical Encyclopedia. http://www.nlm.nih.gov/medlineplus/ency/article/002994.htm. Updated October 2, 2013. Accessed April 23, 2015.

35. Testicular torsion. A.D.A.M. Medical Encyclopedia. http://www.nlm.nih.gov/medlineplus/ency/article/000517.htm. Updated October 2, 2013. Accessed April 23, 2015.

36. Shenot PJ. Penile and scrotal disorders. In: Porter RS, Kaplan JL, eds. The Merck Manual Online. http://www.merckmanuals.com/professional/genitourinary_disorders/penile_and_scrotal_disorders/testicular_torsion.html?qt=testicular%20torsion&alt=sh. Last reviewed December 2012. Accessed April 23, 2015.

37. Hittelman AB. Neonatal testicular torsion. In: Basow DS, ed. *UpToDate*. Waltham, MA: UpToDate; 2015. http://www.uptodate.com/contents/neonatal-testicular-torsion. Last updated January 14, 2014. Accessed April 23, 2015.

38. Mayo Clinic Staff. Testicular torsion. Mayo Clinic web site. http://www.mayoclinic.com/health/testicular-torsion/DS01039. Updated March 12, 2015. Accessed April 23, 2015.

39. Calis KA, Popat V, Dang DK, Kalantaridou SN, Erogul M. Dysmenorrhea. In: Rivlin ME, ed. Medscape. http://emedicine.medscape.com/article/253812-overview. Updated December 1, 2014. Accessed April 23, 2015.

40. Pinkerton JV. Dysmenorrhea. In: Porter RS, Kaplan JL, eds. The Merck Manual Online. http://www.merckmanuals.com/professional/gynecology_and_obstetrics/menstrual_abnormalities/dysmenorrhea.html?qt=dysmenorrhea&alt=sh. Last reviewed August 2012. Accessed April 23, 2015.

41. Mayo Clinic Staff. Menstrual cramps. Mayo Clinic web site. http://www.mayoclinic.com/health/menstrual-cramps/DS00506/DSECTION=symptoms. Updated May 8, 2014. Accessed April 23, 2015.

42. Painful periods (dysmenorrhea) – Symptoms. NHS Choices web site. http://www.nhs.uk/Conditions/Periods-painful/Pages/Symptoms.aspx. Last reviewed November 5, 2014. Accessed April 23, 2015.

43. Smith RP, Kaunitz AM. Patient information: Painful menstrual periods (dysmenorrhea) (Beyond the basics). In: Basow DS, ed. *UpToDate*. Waltham, MA: UpToDate; 2015. http://www.uptodate.com/contents/painful-menstrual-periods-dysmenorrhea-beyond-the-basics. Last updated April 13, 2015. Accessed April 23, 2015.

44. Hammerschlag MR. Chlamydia. In: Porter RS, Kaplan JL, eds. The Merck Manual Online. http://www.merckmanuals.com/professional/infectious_diseases/chlamydia_and_mycoplasmas/chlamydia.html?qt=chlamydia&alt=sh. Last reviewed February 2014. Accessed April 23, 2015.

45. Chlamydia. A.D.A.M. Medical Encyclopedia. http://www.nlm.nih.gov/medlineplus/ency/article/001345.htm. Updated June 11, 2014. Accessed April 23, 2015.

46. Marrazzo J. Clinical manifestations and diagnosis of chlamydia trachomatis infections. In: Basow DS, ed. *UpToDate*. Waltham, MA: UpToDate; 2015. http://www.uptodate.com/contents/clinical-manifestations-and-diagnosis-of-chlamydia-trachomatis-infections. Last updated March 13, 2015. Accessed April 23, 2015.

47. United States Department of Health and Human Services, Centers for Disease Control and Prevention. Chlamydia – CDC fact sheet. http://www.cdc.gov/std/chlamydia/STDFact-chlamydia-detailed.htm. Last reviewed November 29, 2012. Last updated December 16, 2014. Accessed April 23, 2015.

48. Marrazzo J. Treatment of Chlamydia trachomatis infection. In: Basow DS, ed. *UpToDate*. Waltham, MA: UpToDate; 2015. http://www.uptodate.com/contents/treatment-of-chlamydia-trachomatis-infection. Last updated December 23, 2014. Accessed April 23, 2015.

49. Workowski KA, Bolan GA. Sexually transmitted diseases treatment guidelines, 2015. *MMWR Morb Mortal Wkly Rep*. 2015; 64(3): 1–137. http://www.cdc.gov/std/tg2015/tg-2015-print.pdf

50. Wong B. Gonorrhea. In: Chandrasekar PH, ed. Medscape. http://emedicine.medscape.com/article/218059-overview. Updated April 16, 2014. Accessed April 23, 2015.

51. Leone PA. Epidemiology, pathogenesis, and clinical manifestations of Neisseria gonorrhoeae infection. In: Basow DS, ed. *UpToDate*. Waltham, MA: UpToDate; 2015. http://www.uptodate.com/contents/epidemiology-and-pathogenesis-of-neisseria-gonorrhoeae-infection. Last updated June 26, 2014. Accessed April 23, 2015.

52. Crosta P. What is gonorrhea? What causes gonorrhea? Medical News Today web site. http://www.medicalnewstoday.com/articles/155653.php. Last updated September 26, 2014. Accessed April 23, 2015.

53. Gonorrhea. A.D.A.M. Medical Encyclopedia. http://www.nlm.nih.gov/medlineplus/ency/article/007267.htm. Updated April 25, 2013. Accessed April 23, 2015.

54. Mayo Clinic Staff. Gonorrhea. Mayo Clinic web site. http://www.mayoclinic.com/health/gonorrhea/DS00180/DSECTION=symptoms. Updated January 2, 2014. Accessed April 23, 2015.

55. McCutchan JA. Overview of sexually transmitted diseases. In: Porter RS, Kaplan JL, eds. The Merck Manual Online. http://www.merckmanuals.com/professional/infectious_diseases/sexually_transmitted_diseases_std/overview_of_sexually_transmitted_diseases.html. Last reviewed September 2013. Accessed April 23, 2015.

56. Mayo Clinic Staff. Syphilis. Mayo Clinic web site. http://www.mayoclinic.org/diseases-conditions/syphilis/basics/definition/con-20021862. Updated January 2, 2014. Accessed April 23, 2015.

57. United States Department of Health and Human Services, Centers for Disease Control and Prevention. Syphilis – CDC fact sheet. http://www.cdc.gov/std/syphilis/stdfact-syphilis.htm. Last reviewed January 29, 2014. Last updated July 8, 2014. Accessed April 23, 2015.

58. Hicks CB. Diagnostic testing for syphilis. In: Basow DS, ed. *UpToDate*. Waltham, MA: UpToDate; 2015. http://www.uptodate.com/contents/diagnostic-testing-for-syphilis. Last updated October 16, 2014. Accessed April 23, 2015.

59. Waseem M, Aslam M. Pediatric syphilis. In: Steele RW, ed. Medscape. http://emedicine.medscape.com/article/969023-workup#showall. Updated April 1, 2013. Accessed April 23, 2015.

60. Mayo Clinic Staff. Syphilis. Mayo Clinic web site. http://www.mayoclinic.com/health/syphilis/DS00374/DSECTION=treatments-and-drugs. Updated January 2, 2014. Accessed April 23, 2015.

61. Healthwise Staff. Antibiotics for syphilis. WebMD web site. http://www.webmd.com/sexual-conditions/antibiotics-for-syphilis. Last updated October 8, 2013. Accessed April 23, 2015.

62. Soper DE. Bacterial vaginosis. In: Porter RS, Kaplan JL, eds. The Merck Manual Online. http://www.merckmanuals.com/professional/gynecology-and-obstetrics/vaginitis-cervicitis-and-pelvic-inflammatory-disease-pid/bacterial-vaginosis?qt=bacterialvaginosis&alt=sh. Last reviewed January 2015. Accessed April 23, 2015.

63. Girerd PH. Bacterial vaginosis. In: Rivlin ME, ed. Medscape. http://emedicine.medscape.com/article/254342-overview#aw2aab6b2b2aa. Updated March 27, 2014. Accessed April 23, 2015.

64. Sobel JD. Bacterial vaginosis. In: Basow DS, ed. *UpToDate*. Waltham, MA: UpToDate; 2015. http://www.uptodate.com/contents/bacterial-vaginosis. Last updated March 18, 2015. Accessed April 23, 2015.

65. Mayo Clinic Staff. Bacterial vaginosis. Mayo Clinic web site. http://www.mayoclinic.com/health/bacterial-vaginosis/DS01193/DSECTION=symptoms. Updated April 20, 2013. Accessed April 23, 2015.

66. United States Department of Health and Human Services, NIH, National Institute of Allergy and Infectious Diseases. Bacterial vaginosis. http://www.niaid.nih.gov/topics/bacterialvaginosis/Pages/default.aspx. Last updated January 31, 2013. Accessed April 23, 2015.

67. Healthwise Staff. Tests for bacterial vaginosis. WebMD web site. http://www.webmd.com/sexual-conditions/tests-for-bacterial-vaginosis. Last updated March 12, 2014. Accessed April 23, 2015.

68. Herpes simplex: Herpes types 1 and 2. WebMD web site. http://www.webmd.com/genital-herpes/pain-management-herpes. Last updated September 30, 2014. Accessed April 23, 2015.

69. Straface G, Selmin A, Zanardo V, De Santis M, Ercoli A, Scambia G. Herpes simplex virus infection in pregnancy. *Infect Dis Obstet Gynecol.* 2012; 2012: 385697. doi: 10.1155/2012/385697

70. Albrecht MA. Epidemiology, clinical manifestations, and diagnosis of genital herpes simplex virus infection. In: Basow DS, ed. *UpToDate*. Waltham, MA: UpToDate; 2015. http://www.uptodate.com/contents/epidemiology-clinical-manifestations-and-diagnosis-of-genital-herpes-simplex-virus-infection. Last updated July 2, 2014. Accessed April 23, 2015.

71. Kaye KM. Herpes simplex viruses (HSV) infections. In: Porter RS, Kaplan JL, eds. The Merck Manual Online. http://www.merckmanuals.com/professional/infectious_diseases/herpesviruses/herpes_simplex_virus_hsv_infections.html?qt=herpes&alt=sh. Last updated April 2013. Accessed April 23, 2015.

72. Salvaggio MR, Lutwick LI, Seenivasan M, Kumar S. Herpes simplex. In: Bronze MS, ed. Medscape. http://emedicine.medscape.com/article/218580-overview. Updated November 14, 2014. Accessed April 23, 2015.

73. Oral herpes (cold sore). A.D.A.M. Medical Encyclopedia. http://www.ncbi.nlm.nih.gov/pubmedhealth/PMH0001631. Accessed April 23, 2015.

74. United States Department of Health and Human Services. HIV/AIDS 101: What is HIV/AIDS? AIDS.gov web site. https://aids.gov/hiv-aids-basics/hiv-aids-101/what-is-hiv-aids. Last revised April 29, 2014. Accessed April 23, 2015.

75. HIV/AIDS. A.D.A.M. Medical Encyclopedia. http://www.ncbi.nlm.nih.gov/pubmedhealth/PMH0001620. Accessed April 23, 2015.

76. United States Department of Health and Human Services. HIV testing: Get the basics. AIDS.gov web site. http://aids.gov/hiv-aids-basics/prevention/hiv-testing/hiv-test-types. Last revised March 27, 2015. Accessed April 23, 2015.

77. Lancaster JB. HIV testing resources. TeensHealth web site. http://kidshealth.org/teen/sexual_health/stds/hiv_tests.html#. Reviewed November 2013. Accessed April 23, 2015.

78. HIV viral load testing. WebMD web site. http://www.webmd.com/hiv-aids/hiv-viral-load-what-you-need-to-know?page=2. Reviewed April 17, 2014. Accessed April 23, 2015.

79. United States Department of Health and Human Services. Guidelines for the use of antiretroviral agents in pediatric HIV infection. http://aidsinfo.nih.gov/guidelines/html/2/pediatric-arv-guidelines/70/when-to-initiate-therapy-in-antiretroviral-naive-children. Last updated April 27, 2015. Accessed April 28, 2015.

80. AIDS treatment. University of California San Francisco Medical Center web site. http://www.ucsfhealth.org/conditions/aids/treatment.html. Accessed April 23, 2015.

Index